Nutritional Deficiencies: Causes, Effects and Management

Nutritional Deficiencies: Causes, Effects and Management

Edited by Lisa Jordan

SYRAWOOD
PUBLISHING HOUSE
New York

Published by Syrawood Publishing House,
750 Third Avenue, 9th Floor,
New York, NY 10017, USA
www.syrawoodpublishinghouse.com

Nutritional Deficiencies: Causes, Effects and Management
Edited by Lisa Jordan

International Standard Book Number: 978-1-68286-434-0 (Hardback)

Cataloging-in-publication Data

Nutritional deficiencies : causes, effects and management / edited by Lisa Jordan.
p. cm.
Includes bibliographical references and index.
ISBN 978-1-68286-434-0
1. Deficiency diseases. 2. Nutrition disorders. 3. Nutritionally induced diseases. 4. Vitamin D deficiency.
5. Nutrition disorders in children. I. Jordan, Lisa.
RC623.5 .N88 2017
616.39--dc23

Printed in China.

TABLE OF CONTENTS

PREFACE

Nutritional deficiency can be defined as the consumption of a diet consisting of nutrients less than the required amount. This book on nutritional deficiencies covers a wide range of topics including malnutrition aid and ideal supplements and nutritional substitutes. The topics included in this book on nutritional deficiencies are of utmost significance and bound to provide insights to readers. It unfolds the innovative aspects revolving around the causes of nutritional deficiencies along with their effects and management techniques which will be crucial for the progress of this discipline. Students and academicians in the field of nutrition and diet will find this book to be extremely useful.

This book is a result of research of several months to collate the most relevant data in the field.

When I was approached with the idea of this book and the proposal to edit it, I was overwhelmed. It gave me an opportunity to reach out to all those who share a common interest with me in this field. I had 3 main parameters for editing this text:

1. Accuracy - The data and information provided in this book should be up-to-date and valuable to the readers.
2. Structure - The data must be presented in a structured format for easy understanding and better grasping of the readers.
3. Universal Approach - This book not only targets students but also experts and innovators in the field, thus my aim was to present topics which are of use to all.

Thus, it took me a couple of months to finish the editing of this book.

I would like to make a special mention of my publisher who considered me worthy of this opportunity and also supported me throughout the editing process. I would also like to thank the editing team at the back-end who extended their help whenever required.

Editor

1

Continuous Quality Improvement in Daily Clinical Practice: A Proof of Concept Study

Jonathan A. Lorch[1], Victor E. Pollak[2,3]*

1 Department of Medicine, Weill Cornell Medical College and The Rogosin Institute, New York, New York, United States of America, 2 Department of Medicine, University of Colorado Health Sciences Center, Aurora, Colorado, United States of America, 3 MIQS, Inc., Boulder, Colorado, United States of America

Abstract

Continuous Quality Improvement (CQI) is an iterative process of: planning to improve a product or process, plan implementation, analyzing and comparing results against those expected, and corrective action on differences between actual and expected results. It is little used in clinical medicine. Anemia, a complex problem in End Stage Renal Disease patients, served to test the ability of an unique electronic medical record (EMR) optimized for daily care to empower CQI in practice. We used data collected during daily care, stored in the EMR, and organized to display temporal relationships between clinical, laboratory, and therapeutic events. Our aims were optimal hemoglobin with minimum epoetin, and maintaining stable hemoglobin and epoetin. The study was done on 250 patients treated by maintenance hemodialysis (HD), receiving epoetin prior to February 1, 2010 and followed to July 31, 2011. Repleting iron, ensuring iron sufficiency, slow epoetin reduction, and decision support tools enabling data display over long periods in patient-centered reports were key elements. Epoetin dose, adjusted 6–8 weekly, was based on current clinical conditions and past responses. Hemoglobin increased by months 1–2; epoetin decreased from month 4. By months 16–18, epoetin had decreased 42% to 9,720 units/week while hemoglobin increased 8% to 123.6 g/L. Hemoglobin and epoetin were stable from month 7 onward. New epoetin orders decreased 83%. Transferrin saturation increased after the study start. Individual patient hemoglobin variation decreased by 23%, range by 27%. Mortality, 11.78 per 100 patient years, was 42% less than United States dialysis patient mortality. Allowable epoetin charges decreased by $15.33 per treatment and were $22.88 less than current Medicare allowance. The study validates the hypothesis that an EMR optimized for daily patient care can empower CQI in clinical medicine and serve to monitor medical care quality and cost.

Editor: Mercedes Susan Mandell, University of Colorado, United States of America

Funding: VEP received salary support from MIQS, Inc. The funders had no role in study design, data collection and analysis, decision to publish, or preparation of the manuscript.

Competing Interests: VEP is Founder, Member of the Board of Directors, owner of stock, and fulltime employee of MIQS, Inc. JAL is owner of stock of MIQS, Inc. This does not alter the authors' adherence to all the PLOS ONE policies on sharing data and materials.

* E-mail: vpollak@miqs.com

Introduction

The statistical approach to continuous quality improvement (CQI) was invented by Shewhart over 50 years ago [1], and applied in industrial manufacturing and service industries by W. Edwards Deming [2]. He demonstrated repeatedly its capacity to improve quality and reduce costs of manufacturing and services. CQI is an iterative and continuing process of improvement that involves: (1) planning to improve a product or process, (2) implementation of the plan, (3) analyzing results and comparing results against those expected, and (4) taking corrective action on significant differences between actual and expected results. Critical to effective CQI implementation are, among others: deciding to adopt the CQI philosophy, constancy of purpose toward improvement of service, leadership to help people do a better job, training to achieve that end, and an education and self-improvement program [2]. At its heart, CQI concerns itself with taming variability. In industry the focus is on processes that affect quality of the final product, whereas in clinical medicine it is on the varied responses to therapeutic interventions determined at least in part by the biology of individual patients, their co-morbidities, and details of their illnesses.

Care of chronic diseases that now predominate in medical practice accounts for >75% of US medical care costs [3]. In chronic disease, Fries wrote over 35 years ago "a major failure of the traditional chart is its inability to indicate adequately complex temporal relationships between clinical, laboratory, and therapeutic events" [4]. One of us (VEP) postulated that "successful management and treatment of patients and the important individual manifestations of a chronic disease require complex feedback systems that relate therapeutic interventions to clinical and laboratory information relevant to multi-organ systems over prolonged periods" [5]. Although testing this postulate seems to us to depend at least in part on collecting and viewing relevant data sequentially over time, this process is far from routine. We found little literature on CQI in clinical medicine, and sparse reports on the effect of electronic medical records (EMRs) on quality improvement in any chronic disease [6].

The patient-centered, comprehensive, coded, analyzable EMR used herein, first developed 30 years ago, was designed specifically to enable CQI in medical practice [5,7]. Discrete practice details for diseases affecting multiple organ systems were transformed into coded data, enabling rearrangement of data elements at the point-of-care to facilitate clinical practice and observations over many years.

End Stage Renal Disease (ESRD) is complex, costly, and affects >600,000 patients in the United States [8]. Because ESRD is highly regulated with mandated criteria to start dialysis treatment and frequent State and Federal oversight, ESRD has unique advantages as a model for a proof of concept study. Treatments, devices, drugs used, and dialysis procedures are largely standardized, but outcomes vary greatly between dialysis facilities [9] even though standardized treatment protocols are used widely.

In protocol-driven health care delivery some individuals will not benefit from the parameters of the protocol; without individual scrutiny of care choices patients could actually be harmed. Increasing epoetin alfa (EPO) given to HD patients has led to administration of very large amounts, now acknowledged to adversely affect survival at least in patients with moderate anemia (Hb 100–130 g/L) [10,11].

For the present study we examine the effects of treatment of anemia, a chronic condition in HD patients with ESRD. Underlying causes include deficiency of iron stores and the erythrocyte stimulating hormone erythropoetin. EPO has played a major role in anemia treatment for >20 years [12]. Adequate iron stores are needed for optimal EPO response [13]. Iron deficiency is common in patients treated by HD [14] and those with decreased renal function not on dialysis [15]. Yet many studies of EPO use in chronic renal failure were done on patients iron deficient when EPO was administered [16–18]. When EPO is administered to patients deficient or marginally sufficient in iron, demands for iron for hemoglobin (Hb) production are likely to deplete iron available for other essential metabolic processes.

We have reported favorable effects of treatment with IV iron but not with oral iron [14]. Later, retrospective analysis of clinical practice from 1998 to 2007 clearly demonstrated the importance of iron in long-term survival of HD patients, and that survival was better with relatively low EPO doses [19]. The practice at that time was to administer EPO using a standardized protocol in doses aimed to maintain patient Hb within the 100–120 g/L range; to decrease or withhold EPO solely on when the latest patient Hb was >125 or >130 g/L; and to resume and even increase EPO administration when Hb had not responded or when the latest Hb decreased to <90 or <100 g/L [20].

Analysis showed that this approach was associated with wide Hb swings and frequent prolonged periods with low Hb levels. We therefore developed a prospective patient-centered CQI approach, and report on its design and testing under the leadership of one of the authors (JAL). We made use of patient-specific data collected during daily care and stored in the EMR. Our objectives were: to achieve optimal Hb with minimum required EPO, and maintain stable Hb and EPO dose.

Methods

The Participants

The study was done on all 264 patients treated by maintenance in-center HD in one of three dialysis unit managed by The Rogosin Institute (New York, NY) and affiliated with New York Presbyterian Hospital and Weill Medical College of Cornell University. Before February 2010, intravenous (IV) iron and EPO had been prescribed using a protocol consistent with the Kidney Disease Outcomes Quality Initiative (KDOQI) guidelines [20], and influenced by Centers for Medicare and Medicaid Services (CMS) mandates. The 250 patients, who had been receiving EPO in October 2009 to February 2010, are the subjects of this analysis. They were followed until July 31, 2011.

The EMR

The EMR (MIQS Inc, Boulder, CO) employs a relational database (SAP Sybase Adaptive Server Enterprise, SAP AG, Walldorf, Germany), running on a server computer (Oracle, Redwood Shores CA). Its architecture is shown diagrammatically in Figure 1. It is accessed using a custom toolset (4D, Inc., San Jose, CA) from client personal computers in dialysis units and other practice sites [21]. All clinical, administrative, and financial data are immediately accessible at all times on patients ever entered into the database. Subject to security considerations, lifetime patient data relevant to pertinent caregiver needs are accessed whenever and wherever needed.

Coded data elements include diagnoses, procedures, symptoms, signs, medications, allergies, and hospitalizations. HD treatment screens record all details at the time of treatment. HD orders and medications to be given during HD automatically populate treatment screen fields.

Accuracy and completeness of data on EPO and IV iron administered during HD treatments are facilitated and ensured by full software integration of billing and clinical information. Accuracy and completeness of data on hospital admissions are also facilitated and ensured by software integration of billing and clinical information.

To provide clinically useful point-of-care reports MIQS-designed embedded query tools are incorporated. They provide classes of reports (including single patient tabular, multi-patient tabular, and aggregate reports) to organize data quickly in any way desired over any time span, to make knowledge available about individual patients, and groups. User created reports can be updated and organized at the point-of-care, and are designed to facilitate clinical decisions based on timely, complete, relevant,

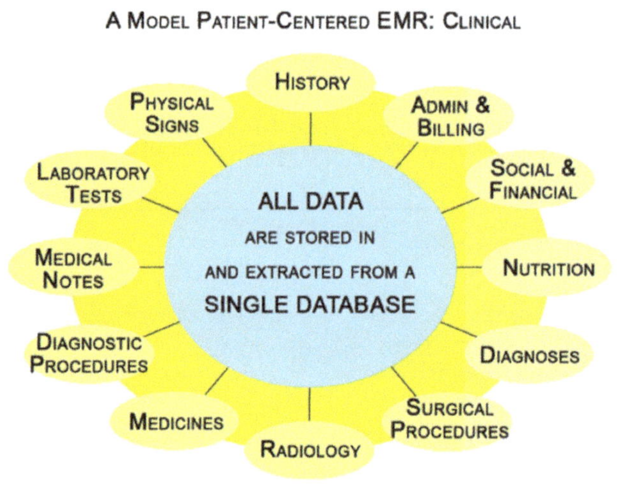

Figure 1. A model of a patient-centered EMR that, with a single database, accommodates multiple clinical functions and domains of information. As shown these include symptoms, physical signs, laboratory tests, medicines, diagnoses, diagnostic and surgical procedures, radiology, medical notes, nutrition, and social work. The single database also accommodates and includes the needs of: caregivers and other staff; data entry and reporting of physicians, nurses, dietitians, social workers, pharmacists, administrators, and clerical, billing, and accounting staff; multiple locations including main and remote dialysis units, peritoneal dialysis unit, home HD, chronic kidney disease, renal and other transplant, physician office, hospital outpatient; non-clinical functions such as insurance, fee tables, charges, physician billing, dialysis unit billing, electronic remittance and explanation of benefits.

patient-specific, time-oriented data. Individual patient reports include contemporaneous medications and laboratory tests, comprehensive lifetime lists of diagnoses, surgical procedures, diagnostic procedures, allergies, adverse drug reactions, immunizations, and hospitalizations.

The Framework for the CQI Study

Based on our previous study [19] we developed a framework for hematinic medication administration in individual patients treated by HD. It was not a protocol to be applied uniformly to a heterogeneous patient population. Rather, the elements of the framework represented goals that had been shown to result in optimum patient survival using a minimum amount of EPO. To achieve the desired goals required knowledge of each patient, familiarity with factors causing apparent EPO resistance, and visual access in a single report to the domains of data that might effect application of the framework in individual patients.

The goals within the framework included: Iron replete patients were to receive IV iron 200 mg monthly as a single dose. Patients not iron sufficient (TSAT <25% and/or serum ferritin <300 µg/L) were to receive iron 200 mg during 5 consecutive HD treatments, thereafter 200 mg monthly. EPO and iron dose changes were to be evaluated monthly. EPO changes were to be made only 6–8 weekly as normal erythrocyte lifespan is ≈120 days [22], and because we had observed that large Hb variations accompanied frequent EPO changes.

Other details were:

- Patients with Hb<120 g/L and/or EPO>27,000 units/week were examined and data reviewed to determine possible cause(s) for EPO resistance. If considered resistant EPO dose was held unchanged until resistance judged by clinical examination, increased serum albumin and decreased C reactive protein, was considered unlikely.
- In patients unresponsive to EPO, the dose was reduced stepwise to the last level at which a response to EPO occurred.
- Before EPO was increased, a previously responsive patient with stable Hb<115 g/L was evaluated for inflammatory states and other possible reasons for unresponsiveness.
- If Hb was <110 g/L, EPO dose changes were made to try to attain a new goal of 120 g/L.
- If not iron sufficient, IV iron was given to achieve iron sufficiency, leaving EPO dose unchanged. EPO dose was changed only after iron sufficiency was established and maintenance iron initiated.
- If Hb was >125 g/L on 3 consecutive occasions EPO was reduced by 20%, but never to 0 (zero).
- EPO dose was not to be raised to >27,000 units/week without close consideration.
- When iron sufficient, EPO naive patients received EPO 90 units/Kg/week initially. The dose was not adjusted for 6–8 weeks, and the starting dose was not changed before there was evidence of iron sufficiency. Once a response was achieved (Hb 115–125 g/L), EPO was reduced by 20%. With assurance of iron repletion and sufficiency, EPO dose was then modified as in EPO established patients.

Implementation

Implementation required a new approach to prescribing hematinic drugs and managing the process. The prevailing practice had been that the medical director or attending physicians signed EPO orders previously written by designated nurses. Guiding the protocol used for EPO prescription was the then current CMS policy that penalized reimbursement when the Hb was >130 g/L. The prevailing widely used practice was that EPO dose could be increased, decreased, or discontinued every two weeks based only on the most currently available Hb. In addition, individual physicians might also write anemia medication orders. We found by retrospective data analysis that this practice had had an adverse effect on patient Hb (Figure 2).

To enable the new CQI study framework EPO administration was brought under the anemia management team, a core group of caregivers charged with reviewing all patients with a clear understanding of the clinical condition and past response to EPO doses of each patient. Prior to the start, the results of the retrospective analysis and the rationale underlying the new framework were communicated to and discussed with the team by one of the authors (JAL). Orders were to be written only by the anemia management team. Orders by individual physicians were stopped. Senior management endorsed the process to ensure that it was carried out.

Patient-centered EPO administration required first-hand knowledge of each patient and data that might affect the response. Therapeutic decisions were made systematically at one-month intervals by caregivers knowledgeable about each patient's course. These included physicians, nurses and nurse practitioners. Also participating were the unit administrator, nurse manager and physician responsible for implementation of the CQI framework.

To review individual patients, data from HD treatments, medications administered, and laboratory domains were aggregated monthly for the prior 18-months using the aggregate class of reports. Projection on a 140 cm television screen wall mounted in a conference room enabled all team members to see the data simultaneously and participate in decision making. Adjustments to IV iron and EPO were made as needed, consistent with the CQI framework. For acute problems, data aggregated weekly were displayed over a shorter time span. For chronic and perplexing problems, data were aggregated quarterly over several years.

Controls

The other two other dialysis units administered by The Rogosin Institute served as contemporaneous controls. Both used the EMR in daily practice, were aware of the approach undertaken by the study unit, and of the desirability of reducing EPO administered in view of the upcoming changes in HD treatment reimbursement. An EPO dosing strategy was not imposed, but was left to each unit. Physicians and clinical staff had no training in the processes of CQI.

Data Analysis

For analysis, the aggregate report was used to abstract data monthly for the historical period 12 months before and the CQI period 18 months after start of the study. Data captured included the number of HD treatments, mean post dialysis weight, Hb, TSAT, serum ferritin, serum albumin, C reactive protein and number of injections, total given, and mean dose of EPO and iron. Mean EPO/week, EPO/Kg/week, IV iron/month, and iron/Kg/month were calculated (Figure 3). Other reports abstracted new and discontinued EPO and IV iron orders. All Hb, TSAT, EPO and iron administration values were exported to JMP software (SAS Institute Inc., Cary, NC) to calculate monthly patient means and percentiles.

Using the Lab - Multiple Patients report, Hb values were abstracted for the two historical 6-month periods before and three 6-month periods after the study start. Data were exported to SAS JMP. Means, standard deviations (SD), coefficients of variation

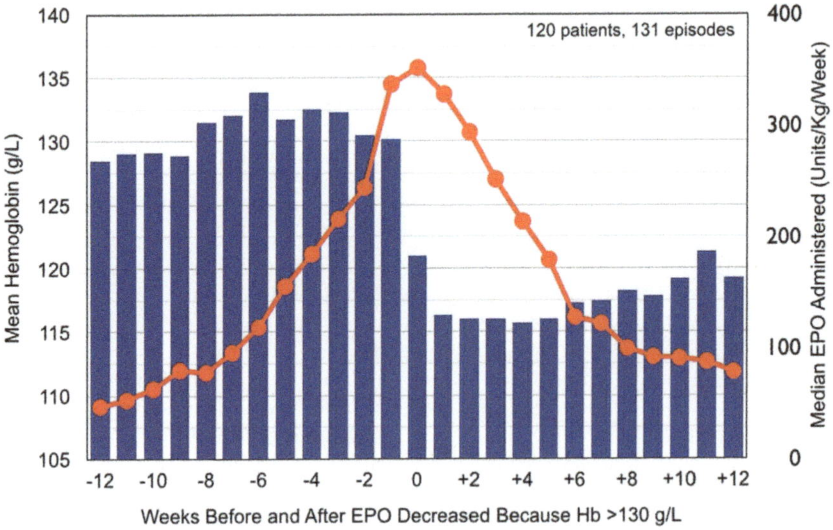

Figure 2. Summary of findings for 12 weeks before and after EPO administration was decreased because Hb was >130 g/L in 120 patients (131 episodes) in the study dialysis unit during the protocol period in calendar year 2009. EPO reduction (blue bars) was followed by pronounced and prolonged reduction of Hb (red dots) to <115 g/L. Similar observations were made in 2 other dialysis units that deployed the EMR.

year-month	2009-11	2009-12	2010-1	2010-2	2010-3	2010-4	2010-5	2010-6	2010-7	2010-8
HD Treatments & Lab Tests										
HD Treatments	13	13	13	12	14	13	12	13	13	13
HD Duration (min)	206	212	209	207	209	207	212	212	209	209
Blood processed (L)	65.9	73.8	77.6	70.9	67.7	70.7	68.5	65.1	66.7	66.3
Weight (kg) Post-HD	56.0	57.7	57.5	59.0	57.8	59.2	58.4	59.2	59.8	59.9
Serum creatinine (umol/L)	787	707	734	787	1,078	712	999	866	999	782
Kt/V	1.95	1.48	1.44	1.48	1.04	2.69	1.44	1.44	3.17	1.40
Serum albumin (g/L)	36	33	37	42	43	40	43	41	42	43
C Reactive Protein (mg/L)				11.3	2.5	2.0	5.4	35.1	1.6	10.4
Hemoglobin (g/L)	**88**	**100**	**115**	**118**	**140**	**132**	**132**	**150**	**135**	**147**
RBC (10^12/L)	2.86	3.38	3.71	3.72	4.65	4.38	4.26	5.19	4.71	4.77
Hematocrit (%)	28.7	32.6	37.6	37.3	44.6	41.8	41.2	47.5	43.8	47.1
MCV (fl)	91.0	89.0	92.0	90.0	90.0	97.4	93.0	96.1	93.0	99.4
MCH (pg)	28.4	26.1	27.7	28.8	28.1	30.8	29.7	30.5	30.4	31.7
MCHC (g/L)	312	294	300	320	314	317	318	318	326	320
TSAT (%)	33	20	35	12	18	33	20	55	44	39
Serum ferritin (ug/L)			280			455			672	
Platelet count (10^9/L)	442	292	251	170	194	149	221	165	181	202
Medications Given during HD										
EPO units (count)	12	13	13	12	13	13	12	13	13	10
EPO units (total)	48,400	93,500	100,100	92,400	100,100	91,300	79,200	66,000	39,600	22,000
EPO units (mean)	4,033	7,192	7,700	7,700	7,700	7,023	6,600	5,077	3,046	2,200
EPO units/Week (mean)	**10,275**	**19,850**	**21,252**	**21,252**	**19,734**	**19,383**	**18,216**	**14,013**	**8,407**	**4,671**
EPO units (mean) /Kg/Week	184	344	370	360	342	327	312	237	141	78
Venofer mg iron (count)	0	5	0	5	6	1	6	1	1	1
Venofer mg iron (total)		1,000		1,000	1,200	200	1,200	200	200	200
Venofer mg iron (mean)		200		200	200	200	200	200	200	200
Total iron counts	0	5	0	5	6	1	6	1	1	1
Total iron given (mg)	0	1,000	0	1,000	1,200	200	1,200	200	200	200
Iron given mg (mean/injection)		200		200	200	200	200	200	200	200
Total iron (mean/HD)	0	77	0	83	86	15	100	15	15	15
Total iron given (mg/month)	**0**	**939**	**0**	**1,018**	**1,047**	**188**	**1,221**	**188**	**188**	**188**
Total iron given (mg/Kg/month)	0.0	16.3	0.0	17.3	18.1	3.2	20.9	3.2	3.1	3.1

Figure 3. Aggregate report used for CQI in a 44 year old female patient treated by dialysis for 23 years. Although the report was run monthly for the latest 18-months, for clarity only a 10-month time span is shown. This report automatically calculated data for monthly intervals during 2009. Displayed are HD treatments, data relevant to the erythron and iron status, and the EPO and IV iron administered. In November 2009 to January 2010, despite EPO administration of 355–445 units/Kg/week, hemoglobin was low and falling; the low TSAT and relatively low MCH pointed to iron insufficiency. She received 3.4 g of iron intravenously between February and May 2010. An increase in Hb, TSAT, MCH, and serum albumin was evident in May, and continued.

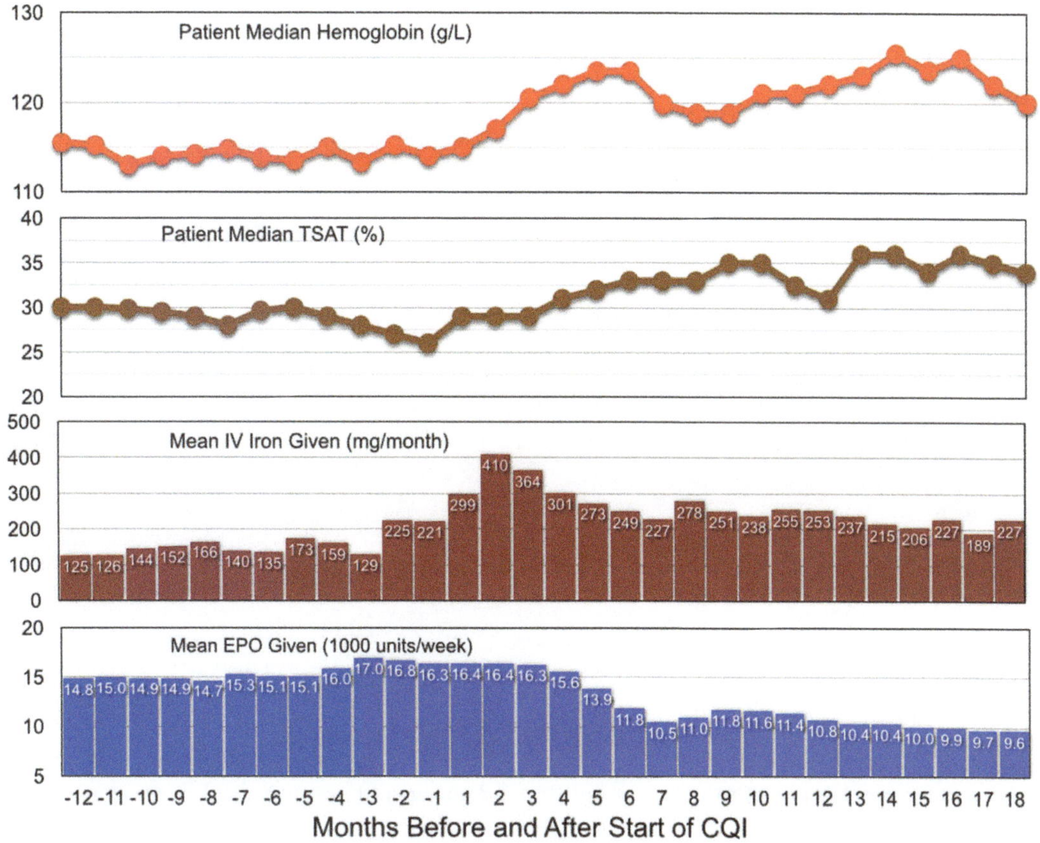

Figure 4. For all study patients, patient median Hb, median TSAT, mean IV iron and mean EPO administered in the protocol period 12 months before study start and the 18-month CQI period.

and ranges were calculated as measures of variability, for Hb values of each patient during each 6-month period. Means, medians, SD, ranges, and coefficients of variation were then calculated for all patients.

Mortality per 100 patient years was calculated as is done by USRDS [8], by dividing the number of deaths by the total time in years that the patients were treated by HD, and multiplying by 100.

Medicare Part B allowable charges for EPO and IV iron were calculated using Centers for Medicare and Medicaid Services (CMS) published data (accessed 06/18/2010) and from the amount of each drug given during any month divided by the number of HD treatments during that month. Included were treatments both for patients studied longitudinally and for all others treated in that month.

Study Approval

The Institutional Review Board did not require informed consent as (1) the study of quality improvement was considered to be a part of routine clinical care of the patients, and (2) the data were analyzed anonymously. The study was approved by the Institutional Review Board of Weill Medical College of Cornell University.

Results

Mean patient age was 59±16.2 years; 55% were male, 34% White, 46% Black, 20% of other ethnic groups. Primary renal disease was: glomerulonephritis in 35%, hypertension in 30%, diabetic nephropathy in 21%. From February 1, 2010 to July 31, 2011, 17 patients received a kidney transplant, 9 were transferred to peritoneal and nocturnal home HD, 22 to another dialysis unit, and one was lost to follow up.

In the 12-month historical period prior to study start, patient monthly median Hb varied between 113.0 and 115.5 g/L, TSAT between 26% and 30%, with the lowest values immediately before study start (Figure 4). IV iron given varied between 124 mg and 159 mg per month, with larger amounts in the last two months before study start. EPO administration varied between 14,800 and 17,000 units per week.

IV iron administered increased in month 1, peaked at 410 mg/month in month 2, and decreased to ≈250 mg/month by month 6. In months 13–18, an average of 215 mg was given monthly. Hb increased in month 1, and was consistently higher thereafter. In months 13–18 patient monthly median Hb was 120 to 125 g/L. EPO administered decreased slightly in month 4, and further in months 5 and 6. In months 16–18 mean EPO dose was 9,720 units/week.

To provide more details of changes over time, percentiles of TSAT, serum ferritin, Hb, and EPO administered are displayed monthly. Median serum ferritin, measured 3-monthly, increased from 552 µg/L before study start to 1148 µg/L in months 13–18 (Figure 5a). TSAT levels increased steadily from CQI months 1 to 9 for all percentiles (Figure 5b). In months 13–18, the 10th and 25th percentiles were 23.7% and 29,1% respectively, indicating that iron insufficiency was then uncommon. Hb levels increased steadily from CQI month 1 onward (Figure 5c). In months 13–18, levels were 142.7 g/L for the 90th percentile, 132.5 g/L for the

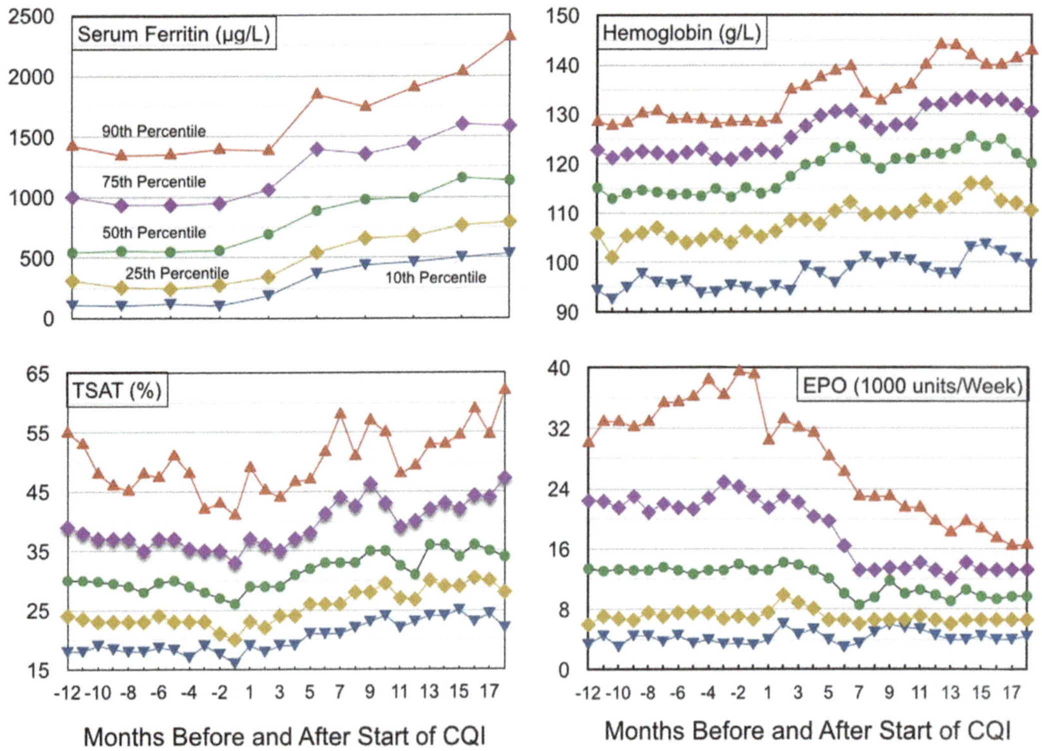

Figure 5. Percentiles of patients by (a) serum ferritin, (b) TSAT, (c) hemoglobin, and (d) administered EPO for 12 months before and 18 months after study start.

75th, 122.7 g/L for the 50th, 113.3 g/L for the 25th, and 101.2 g/L for the 10th percentile. EPO administration levels decreased steadily from CQI months 3 to 6, indicating that administered EPO decreased whether initially very high or more modest (Figure 5d). The most striking decreases occurred in the 90th and 75th percentiles. The 50th percentile changed negligibly in months 1–4, and decreased to an average of 9,786 units/week (134 units/Kg/week) in months 13–18.

There were 2.10 new and 2.08 discontinued IV iron orders per patient year in the historical period (Figure 6). New IV iron orders doubled in the first 6 CQI months and then decreased to 1.44 per year in months 13–18, when discontinued orders were 0.86 per patient year. New EPO orders, 6.77 per patient year in the

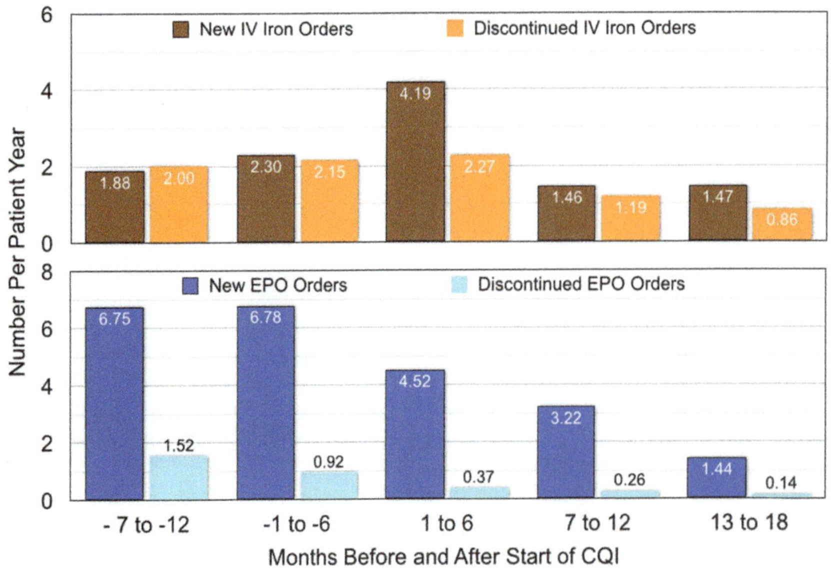

Figure 6. New orders and discontinued orders for IV iron and for EPO for two 6-month periods before and three 6-month periods after the start of the CQI process.

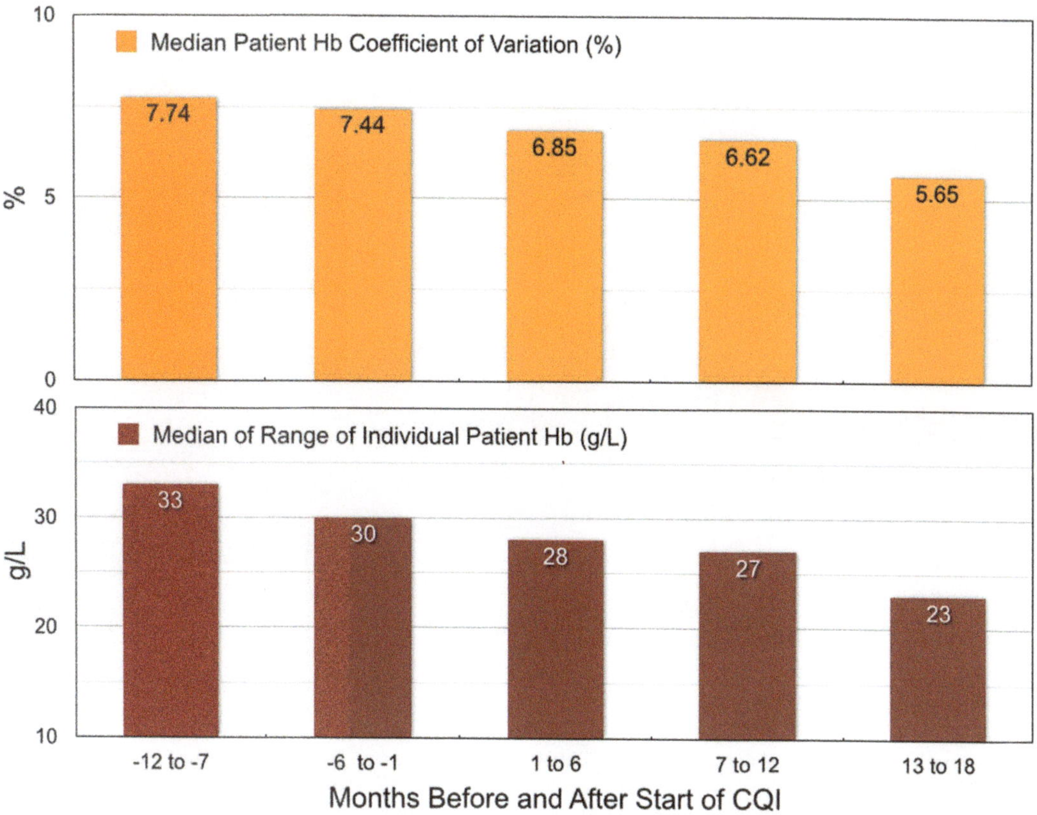

Figure 7. Patient median Hb coefficients of variation and median Hb ranges for two 6-month periods before and three 6-month periods after the start of the CQI process.

historical period, decreased 83% in CQI months 13–18 to 1.12. EPO discontinuation orders, 1.20 per patient year in the historical period, decreased 84% in CQI months 13–18 to 0.19.

With 3 caregivers reviewing the data, 12 caregiver hours were needed at study start for the review of 250 patients; another 3 hours were needed for one caregiver to enter new and changed orders. With experience and increased stability of Hb and TSAT, and of EPO and IV iron orders, fewer caregiver hours were needed: in CQI months 13–18, 6 caregiver hours for the monthly review, and 1.5 caregiver hours to enter new and changed orders. Thus anemia management which consumed 15 caregiver hours per month at study start required only 7.5 caregiver hours per month at the end of the CQI study.

The individual patient coefficient of variation and range of Hb values in individual patients were analyzed in five 6-month periods (Figure 7). The coefficient of variation and range decreased after the study start and were least in CQI months 13–18. Coefficients of variation for all Hb measurements for each individual patient, 7.53% (IQR 5.68, 10.63) in the historical period, decreased by 23% to 5.82% (IQR 4.13, 9.04) in CQI months 13–18. The variation of Hb measurements decreased by 27% from 31.5 g/L to 23 g/L.

Table 1. Selected data on patients in the study unit who died and who were alive at the end of the study.

	Died (n = 35)	Alive (n = 215)	p
Age at study start (years)	70.6±14.4	58.6±14.7	<0.001
Admissions per patient year	4.65	1.27	<0.001
Hb (g/L)	112.5 (100.5, 120.5)	121.0 (114.0, 126.0)	<0.001
TSAT (%)	29.5 (23.5, 35.1)	33.0 (29.0, 37.4)	<0.01
Serum ferritin (µg/L)	1080 (607, 1305)	922 (568, 1328)	NS
Serum albumin (g/L)	37.0 (33.0, 38.5)	40.5 (38.0, 42.0)	<0.001
C-reactive protein (mg/L)	12.3 (6.1, 36.0)	6.33 (2.65, 13.10)	<0.005
EPO given (1000 units/week)	13.53 (7.59, 18.98)	10.25 (6.58, 15.75)	<0.05

Laboratory test results and EPO administered are median values and interquartile range (IQR).

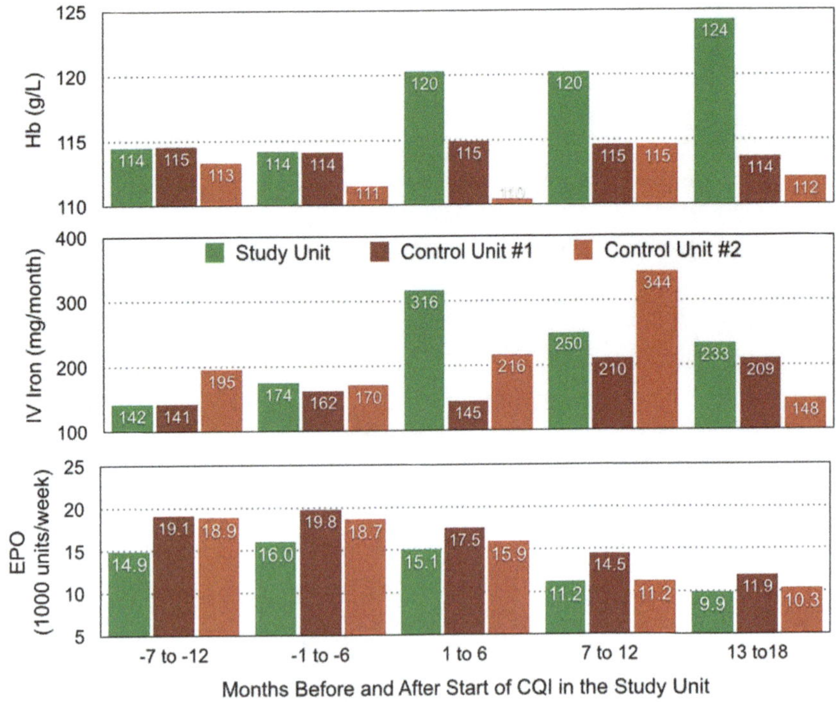

Figure 8. Patient median Hb and mean IV iron and EPO administered in the CQI study and two control units. Data are summarized for two 6-month periods before and three 6-month periods after start of the CQI process in the CQI study unit.

Using data from all patients treated in the unit from 2004 to 2011 with 10 or more Hb values per year, we analyzed by calendar year the per patient range of Hb levels. This historical perspective showed that from 2004–2009 the range was ≤20 g/L in only 4% of patients, and ≤30 g/L in 15%. In 2011, by contrast, the proportion meeting these low ranges had increased to 9% and 33% respectively.

In the 12 months before CQI start patients were followed for a total of 219.77 years and there were 331 hospital admissions (1.51 per year). During the 18-month CQI period the patients were followed for a total of 297.06 years, and there were 422 admissions to hospital (1.42 per year).

Thirty-five patients died during the CQI study. The mortality rate, 11.78 per 100 patient years, was 42% less than the 2009 United States rate for all dialysis patients of 19.95 per 100 years

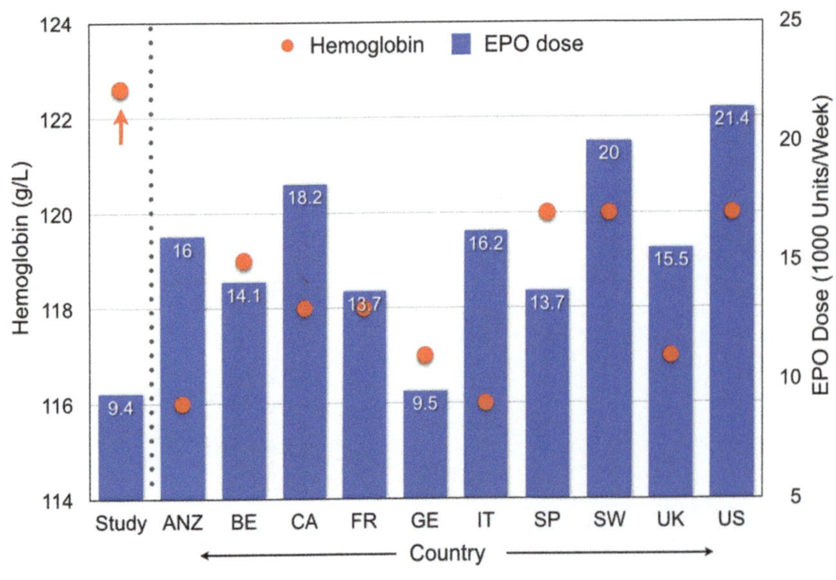

Figure 9. EPO dose and Hb in 2005–2008 in ten countries [26] and in the study unit (Study) in February–July, 2011. (Abbreviations: ANZ = Australia and New Zealand; BE = Belgium; CA = Canada; Fr = France; GE = Germany; IT = Italy; SP = Spain; SW = Sweden; UK = United Kingdom; US = United States).

Table 2. Selected data on patients in the study and two control units in months 13–18 after start of CQI in the study unit.

	Study Unit	Control Unit #1	Control Unit #2
Hemoglobin			
Patient median Hb (g/L)	123.6	114	112
Change from 6 months before CQI start in study unit	+8.8%	0%	+1%
Median patient coefficient of variation (%)	5.65%	6.51%	7.55%
EPO			
EPO administered (units/week)	9,867	11,874	10,264
Change from 6 months before CQI start in study unit	−35.5%	−37.7%	−45.5%
EPO new orders per patient year	1.44	7.91	6.44
IV iron			
IV iron administered (mg/month)	233	209	148
IV iron new orders per patient year	1.47	7.04	7.30

[8] and did not differ significantly from that before study start. Compared with those who survived the 35 patients who died were 12 years older, had lower serum albumin, lower TSAT, higher C-reactive protein, and a more frequent rate of hospital admission (Table 1). Slightly more EPO was administered in those who died.

In control units #1 and# 2 there were 202 and 175 patients, average age 63.1 and 64.0 years, who received EPO in the 4 months before February 2010. During 216 and 170 years of follow up, deaths were respectively 14.2 and 18.8 per 100 patient years. Little attention was paid to iron administration and EPO was reduced without a defined plan; in unit #2 EPO was reduced in the first 6 months before IV iron administration was increased (Figure 8). TSAT increased to 30.7% and 36.0% by months 13–18 in the two units, serum ferritin to 854 and 1,170 µg/L, but Hb was unchanged (Figure 9). EPO was reduced to a comparable level in all 3 units. New orders for EPO per patient year in months 13–18 were 5.4 and 4.5 times more frequent in the control units than in the study unit; new orders for IV iron were 4.8 and 5.0 times more frequent (Table 2). The median coefficient of variation of Hb was 15% and 34% higher in the control than in the study units.

The allowable charges for the hematinic medications administered to all patients in the study unit were summarized in five 6-month periods. The allowable charges for EPO administered, $48.99 per HD treatment in the 12-month historical period before CQI start, decreased to $33.69 per treatment in the 13–18 months after CQI start. That of IV iron increased from $4.50 to $7.19.

For comparison, the Medicare 2012 per treatment "bundle" allowance was $56.82 for erythrocyte stimulating agents (EPO and darbepoetin alfa) per HD treatment and $6.54 for IV iron. Thus the allowable charges of $40.88 for CQI study patient use of these two hematinic drugs in months 13–18 was $22.88 (34.8%) less than the Medicare "bundle" allowance.

Discussion

Standardized protocols are used widely in the United States, where recent EPO use has decreased 40%, with a 6.7% decrease in Hb from 120 to 112 g/L [23]. In the present study the control units used the same EMR as the CQI study unit, but continued a protocol-based approach to anemia treatment. Over 18 study months, EPO administration decreased 41% with little change in Hb. In the CQI study unit, by contrast, EPO administration decreased 42%, but Hb increased by 8.8%; there was also less Hb variation than in the controls (Table 2). EPO administered weekly in the CQI study unit was also much less than that in 9 countries in a recent study of a randomly selected group of 300 patients from each of 10 countries [24]. Yet, Hb in the CQI unit was 2.6 to 6.6 g/L higher than in each of these 10 countries.

There have been concerns about adverse effects of Hb>120 g/L in renal failure [16–18]. Re-analysis, however, showed the lowest mortality was associated with the highest achieved Hb [25,26]. In other studies, patient mortality was highest with Hb≤ 110 g/L, lowest with Hb>120 g/L [27–31]. In the CQI study

Table 3. Percentage of patients with various TSAT levels in the last 3 months of three studies over 14 years from 1997 to 2011.

IV iron administration	Years of Study	CQI	TSAT (%)			
			≤15	≤20	≤25	≤30
Previous Studies						
Iron insufficient at study start, prospective [12]	1996–1997	Yes	1	9	30	48
Clinical practice, retrospective [17]	1998–2007	No	5	16	29	51
Present Study						
CQI Study Unit	2009–2011	Yes	1	5	11	26
Control Unit #1	2009–2011	No	5	17	40	62
Control Unit #2	2009–2011	No	5	11	27	45

unit, patient median Hb was 121.0 g/L in survivors, 112.5 g/L in those who died. Hospital admissions were 3.66 times more frequent in those who died. Arranged in ranks (≤100; 100.1–110; 110.1–120; >120 g/L) Hb distribution differed in the two groups ($\chi^2_{[3]} = 19.6$, $p<0.0003$). These data are consistent with an association of mortality with age and morbidity rather than with high Hb.

We investigated the importance of iron and effect of Hb on survival in a 9.5-year retrospective study of 1774 patients [19]. Multifactorial analysis demonstrated the favorable effect of Hb> 120 g/L. As compared with the 442 patients with Hb>120 g/L, the hazard ratios for death for Hb 110–120, 100–110, and < 100 g/L were respectively 1.67, 2.69, and 2.83. In the last 3 months of the present study, TSAT was ≤20% in 5%, ≤25% in 11% of patients in the CQI study unit, (Table 3), while in control units #1 and #2 respectively the proportions were higher: ≤20% in 17% and 11% of patients, ≤25% in 40% and 27%.

This suggested that the conventional method of IV iron administration in intermittent courses, without systematic feedback, was associated with suboptimal results; patients were probably cycling between iron deficiency and repletion, without being continuously iron sufficient. In the CQI study group only 6% of patients had TSAT ≤20% in the last 3 months, suggesting that continuous long-term modulation of interrelationships between IV iron, EPO dose and Hb was probably enabled by the CQI process.

In contrast to the current widely used approach that strongly encourages application of population-based guidelines or protocols to individual patient care, CQI enables clinicians to assess variables such as severity of symptoms, illness, comorbidity, and other clinical nuances [32] with clinically pertinent reports immediately available at the point-of-care. Skilled clinicians can thereby generate patient and practice specific knowledge on a day-to-day basis for each patient as an individual, and practice medicine based on scientific judgment conditioned by the totality of available up-to-date evidence of the state of the patient [33].

The application to patient care of protocols without critical oversight of details of individual patients neither promotes nor enables consideration by caregivers of details of the patient illness; it may result in treating patients without regard specifically to factors such as age, race, gender, and co-morbid conditions that may impair or enhance treatment responses. This is particularly so with protocols based on ensuring that certain predetermined numbers are met. By contrast, the CQI process promotes and enables attention to many details of care of patients as individuals, and as individual members of a patient population. It enables caregivers to inquire of the reasons why therapeutic objectives were not met, promotes correction of underlying problems or complications, and does so repeatedly and particularly.

We have shown that a disciplined, classic CQI process wedded to an appropriately designed EMR can lead to better outcome and reduce cost. Neither alone suffices. To facilitate decisions repeatedly over long time spans access serially to relevant time-oriented information including laboratory tests and medications is essential; these data must be organized to display feedback over time between treatments and their effects. Without an EMR that so displays data in spreadsheet (or graphic) metaphor the task is personnel intensive and overwhelming. Needed for introduction and implementation of CQI is clinical and administrative leadership and education and encouragement of physicians, nurses, and other caregivers.

The present study has limitations. It was applied to a single clinical problem, and needs testing with others. It was tested in a dialysis unit treating patients with chronic renal failure, and requires testing in other populations and practice environments. It should also be tested with other EMRs that display feedback over time between treatments and their effects.

Conclusions

Medical therapies are often based on randomized studies where patient variability is intentionally filtered out, or protocols assembled from relevant literature; these are rarely tested in diverse populations. Physicians are also bereft of tools and techniques to apply randomized study results or protocols to each particular individual patient. CQI is an iterative process to understand and contain the effects of variability that, in clinical medicine, stems from the biologic uniqueness of individual patients and their co-morbid conditions.

A recent Institute of Medicine report concluded: "Although unprecedented levels of information are available, patients and clinicians often lack access to guidance that is relevant, timely, and useful for the circumstances at hand. Overcoming this challenge will require applying computing capabilities and analytic approaches to develop real-time insights from routine patient care, disseminating knowledge using new technological tools, and addressing the regulatory challenges that can inhibit progress" [34].

The CQI process is sustainable, practical and appropriate for most complex, expensive therapies now used in chronic disease patient care. We suggest that it provides a model to address both the issues raised by the recent Institute of Medicine report, and an approach to design of methodologies to optimize physician decision making for individual patient care in heterogeneous patient populations.

Acknowledgments

The authors wish to thank John P. Flynn whose work in software design over the past 20 years enabled this study.

Author Contributions

Conceived and designed the experiments: JAL VEP. Performed the experiments: JAL. Analyzed the data: VEP. Wrote the paper: VEP.

References

1. Shewhart W (1986) Statistical Method from the Viewpoint of Quality Control. Mineola, NY: Dover.
2. Deming WE (1982) Out of the Crisis. Cambridge, England: Cambridge University Press.
3. Heffler S, Smith S, Keehan S, Borger C, Clemens MK, et al. (2005) U.S. health spending projections for 2004–2014. Health Aff (Millwood) Suppl Web Exclusives: W5-74-W5-85.
4. Fries JF (1972) Time-oriented patient records and a computer data bank. JAMA 222: 1536–1542.
5. Pollak VE, Buncher CR, Donovan ER (1977) On-line computerized data handling system for treating patients with renal disease. Arch. Int. Med 137: 446–456.
6. Buntin MB, Burke MF, Hoaglin MC, Blumenthal D (2011) The benefits of health information technology: a review of the recent literature shows predominantly positive results. Health Aff (Millwood) 30: 464–471.
7. Pollak VE (1985) The computer in medicine: its application to medical practice, quality control, and cost containment. JAMA 253: 62–68.
8. U.S. Renal Data System, USRDS (2011) Annual Data Report: Atlas of Chronic Kidney Disease and End-Stage Renal Disease in the United States, National Institutes of Health, National Institute of Diabetes and Digestive and Kidney Diseases, Bethesda, MD, 2011. U.S. Renal Data System, USRDS 2011.
9. Goodkin DA, Bragg-Gresham JL, Koenig KG, Wolfe RA, Akiba T, et al (2003) Association of comorbid conditions and mortality in hemodialysis patients in

Europe, Japan, and the United States: the Dialysis Outcomes and Practice Patterns Study (DOPPS). J Am Soc Nephrol 14: 3270–3277.
10. Weinhandl ED, Gilbertson DT, Collins AJ (2011) Association of Mean Weekly Epoetin Alfa Dose with Mortality Risk in a Retrospective Cohort Study of Medicare Hemodialysis Patients. Am J Nephrol 34: 298–308.
11. Servilla KS, Singh AK, Hunt WC, Harford AM, Miskulin D, et al. (2009) Anemia Management and Association of Race with Mortality and Hospitalization in a Large Not-for-profit Dialysis Organization." Am J Kidney Dis 54: 498–510.
12. Eschbach JW, Egrie JC, Downing MR, Browne JK, Adamson JW (1987) Correction of the anemia of end-stage renal disease with recombinant human erythropoietin. Results of a combined phase I and II clinical trial. N Engl J Med 316: 73–78.
13. Eschbach JW (1991) Erythropoietin 1991—an overview. Am J Kidney Dis 18: 3–9.
14. Pollak VE, Lorch JA, Means RTJ (2001) Unanticipated favorable effects of correcting iron deficiency in chronic hemodialysis patients. J Investig Med 49: 173–183.
15. Hsu CY, McCulloch CE, Curhan GC (2002) Iron status and hemoglobin level in chronic renal insufficiency. J Am Soc Nephrol 13: 2783–2786.
16. Besarab A, Bolton WK, Browne JK, Egrie JC, Nissenson AR, et al (1998) The effects of normal as compared with low hematocrit values in patients with cardiac disease who are receiving hemodialysis and epoetin. N Engl J Med 339: 584–590.
17. Drueke TB, Locatelli F, Clyne N, Eckardt KU, Macdougall IC, et al (2006) Normalization of Hemoglobin Level in Patients with Chronic Kidney Disease and Anemia. N Engl J Med 355: 2071–2084.
18. Singh AK, Szczech L, Tang KL, Barnhart H, Sapp S, et al (2006) Correction of Anemia with Epoetin Alfa in Chronic Kidney Disease. N Engl J Med 355: 2085–2098.
19. Pollak VE, Lorch JA, Shukla R, Satwah S (2009) The importance of iron in long-term survival of maintenance hemodialysis patients treated with epoetin-alpha and intravenous iron: analysis of 9.5 years of prospectively collected data. BMC Nephrol 10: 6.
20. (2006) KDOQI Clinical Practice Guidelines and Clinical Practice Recommendations for Anemia in Chronic Kidney Disease. Am J Kidney Dis 47: S11–145.
21. Pollak VE, Lorch JA (2007) Effect of electronic patient record use on mortality in End Stage Renal Disease, a model chronic disease: retrospective analysis of 9 years of prospectively collected data. BMC Med Inform Decis Mak 7: 38.
22. Eschbach JW, Funk D, Adamson J, Kuhn I, Scribner BH, et al. (1967) Erythropoiesis in patients with renal failure undergoing chronic dialysis. N Engl J Med 276: 653–658.
23. Fuller DS, Pisoni RL, Bieber BA, Robinson BM (2013) The DOPPS Practice Monitor for US Dialysis Care: Trends Through December 2011. Am J Kidney Dis 61: 342–346.
24. McFarlane PA, Pisoni RL, Eichleay MA, Wald R, Port FK, et al. (2010) International trends in erythropoietin use and hemoglobin levels in hemodialysis patients. Kidney Int 78: 215–223.
25. Besarab A, Frinak S, Yee J (2009) What is so bad about a hemoglobin level of 12 to 13 g/dL for chronic kidney disease patients anyway? Adv Chronic Kidney Dis 16: 131–142.
26. Agarwal R (2010) Individualizing decision-making—resurrecting the doctor-patient relationship in the anemia debate. Clin J Am Soc Nephrol 5: 1340–1346.
27. Ofsthun N, Labrecque J, Lacson E, Keen M, Lazarus JM (2003) The effects of higher hemoglobin levels on mortality and hospitalization in hemodialysis patients. Kidney Int 63: 1908–1914.
28. Hampl H, Hennig L, Rosenberger C, Amirkhalily M, Gogol L, et al (2005) Effects of Optimized Heart Failure Therapy and Anemia Correction with Epoetin Beta on Left Ventricular Mass in Hemodialysis Patients. Am J Nephrol 25: 211–220.
29. Regidor DL, Kopple JD, Kovesdy CP, Kilpatrick RD, McAllister CJ, et al (2006) Associations between Changes in Hemoglobin and Administered Erythropoiesis-Stimulating Agent and Survival in Hemodialysis Patients. J Am Soc Nephrol 17: 1181–1191.
30. Portoles J, Lopez-Gomez JM, Aljama P (2007) A prospective multicentre study of the role of anaemia as a risk factor in haemodialysis patients: the MAR Study. Nephrol Dial Transplant 22: 500–507.
31. Fort J, Cuevas X, García F, Pérez-García R, Lladós F, et al (2010) Mortality in incident haemodialysis patients: time-dependent haemoglobin levels and erythropoiesis-stimulating agent dose are independent predictive factors in the ANSWER study. Nephrol Dial Transplant 25: 2702–2710.
32. Feinstein AR, Horwitz RI (1997) Problems in the "evidence" of "evidence-based medicine". Am J Med 103: 529–535.
33. Rawlins M (2009) De testimonio: on the evidence for decisions about the use of therapeutic interventions. Lancet 372: 2152–2161.
34. National Research Council (2012) Best Care at Lower Cost: The Path to Continuously Learning Health Care in America. Washington, DC: The National Academies Press.

2

Suboptimal Vitamin D Status in a Population-Based Study of Asian Children: Prevalence and Relation to Allergic Diseases and Atopy

Tsung-Chieh Yao[1,2]*, Yu-Ling Tu[1,2,3], Su-Wei Chang[4], Hui-Ju Tsai[5,6,7], Po-Wen Gu[8], Hsian-Chen Ning[8], Man-Chin Hua[2,9], Sui-Ling Liao[2,9], Ming-Han Tsai[2,9], Chih-Yung Chiu[2,9], Shen-Hao Lai[2,10], Kuo-Wei Yeh[1,2], Jing-Long Huang[1,2]* and for the PATCH study group¶

1 Division of Allergy, Asthma, and Rheumatology, Department of Pediatrics, Chang Gung Memorial Hospital and Chang Gung University College of Medicine, Taoyuan, Taiwan, **2** Community Medicine Research Center, Chang Gung Memorial Hospital at Keelung, Keelung, Taiwan, **3** Graduate Institute of Clinical Medical Sciences, Chang Gung University College of Medicine, Taoyuan, Taiwan, **4** Clinical Informatics and Medical Statistics Research Center, Chang Gung University College of Medicine, Taoyuan, Taiwan, **5** Division of Biostatistics and Bioinformatics, Institutes of Population Health Sciences, National Health Research Institutes, Miaoli, Taiwan, **6** Department of Pediatrics, Feinberg School of Medicine, Northwestern University, Chicago, Illinois, United States of America, **7** Department of Genome Medicine, Kaohsiung University, Kaohsiung, Taiwan, **8** Department of Laboratory Medicine, Chang Gung Memorial Hospital, Taoyuan, Taiwan, **9** Department of Pediatrics, Chang Gung Memorial Hospital at Keelung, Keelung, Taiwan, **10** Division of Pediatric Pulmonology, Department of Pediatrics, Chang Gung Memorial Hospital, Taoyuan, Taiwan

Abstract

Background: New evidence shows high prevalence of vitamin D deficiency in many countries and some studies suggest a possible link between vitamin D status and allergic diseases. The objectives of this study were to determine the prevalence of suboptimal vitamin D status in a population sample of Asian children and to investigate the relationship of vitamin D status with allergic diseases and atopy.

Methods: Children aged 5–18 years (N = 1315) in the Prediction of Allergies in Taiwanese CHildren (PATCH) study were evaluated using questionnaires, anthropometric measurements, and serum levels of 25-hydroxyvitamin D [25(OH)D] and total and specific immunoglobulin E (IgE).

Results: The mean concentration of serum 25(OH)D was 20.4 ng/mL (SD: 7.1 ng/mL). Vitamin D deficiency (defined as serum 25(OH)D<20 ng/mL) was present in 670 subjects (51.0%), while vitamin D insufficiency (defined as serum 25(OH)D<30 ng/mL) was observed in 1187 subjects (90.3%). Older age ($P<0.001$), female gender ($P<0.001$), higher body mass index ($P = 0.001$), winter and spring seasons (compared to summer; P both<0.001), and passive smoking ($P = 0.011$) were independently associated with low serum 25(OH)D levels. After adjusting for potential confounders, serum 25(OH)D status had no association with asthma, rhinitis, eczema, atopy, or total serum IgE (all $P>0.05$).

Conclusions: Low serum 25(OH)D levels are remarkably common in this population sample of Asian children, suggesting that millions of children living in Taiwan may have suboptimal levels of vitamin D, which should be a matter of public health concern. Our results provides epidemiological evidence against the association of vitamin D status with various allergic diseases and atopy in Asian children.

Editor: Jung Eun Lee, Sookmyung Women's University, Republic of Korea

Funding: This work was funded by the National Science Council of Taiwan (grants NSC 101-2314-B-182A-044, NSC 102-2314-B-182A-048, and NSC 101-2314-B-400-009-MY2) and by Chang Gung Memorial Hospital (grants CMRPG260291~260293, CMRPG2B0071~2B0073, and CMRPG4B0031~4B0033). The funders only provided financial support for conducting this study. The funders had no role in study design, data collection and analysis, decision to publish, or preparation of the manuscript.

Competing Interests: The authors have declared that no competing interests exist.

* E-mail: yao@adm.cgmh.org.tw (TCY); long@adm.cgmh.org.tw (JLH)

¶ Membership of the PATCH (Prediction of Allergies in Taiwanese CHildren) study group is provided in the Acknowledgments.

Introduction

The understanding of vitamin D in human physiology has expanded tremendously in the last years. Historically, vitamin D is well known for its role in calcium absorption and maintenance of healthy bones, and its deficiency results in rickets in children and osteomalacia in adults. Recently, a number of studies have identified previously unanticipated roles of vitamin D in the immune system, cardiovascular system, and cancer prevention [1]. There are growing data in several countries that vitamin D deficiency is a prevalent and unrecognized health problem. It has been estimated that 1 billion people worldwide may have vitamin D deficiency or insufficiency [1]. In the NHANES III, approximately 25% to 57% of American adults and adolescents are vitamin D deficient [2]. In addition, studies in Australia, India,

Lebanon, Saudi Arabia, Turkey, and the United Arab Emirates, have reported that 30 to 50% of adults and children have vitamin D deficiency [3,4,5,6]. However, vitamin D status in Asian children is largely underreported.

Allergic diseases are the most common chronic diseases among children. In a global survey [7], Taiwan has the highest prevalence of allergic rhinoconjunctivitis among 6–7-year-old children in the world and the prevalence has increased by 166% during a 7-year period, attracting considerable attention to the burden of childhood allergies in this country. Our recent epidemiological study [8] has revealed that 48% of children in Keelung, Taiwan are currently symptomatic for at least 1 of 3 allergic diseases (asthma, rhinitis, and eczema).

Over the past few years, some studies have reported the relationship of vitamin D with asthma [9,10,11], allergic rhinitis [12], atopic dermatitis [13], and immunoglobulin E (IgE) sensitization [11,14,15]. Most published studies on these topics were conducted in Western populations and not population-based. The objectives of this study were to determine the prevalence of suboptimal vitamin D status in a large and well-characterized population-based cohort study of Asian children in Taiwan and to investigate the relationship of vitamin D status with allergic diseases and atopy (also called allergic sensitization).

Methods

Study subjects

The Prediction of Allergies in Taiwanese CHildren (PATCH) study is a population-based prospective cohort study that was launched in 2007 in Keelung (25°N latitude), Taiwan, to investigate the epidemiology and predictive factors of asthma and allergies in children. Detailed descriptions of subject recruitment and data collection have been reported previously [8,16,17,18,19]. The subject flow diagram of the current study is presented in **Figure 1**. Briefly, study subjects were enrolled from a school-based sample of 5351 children (2616 boys, 48.9%; age, 10.4±2.9 years) in an International Study of Asthma and Allergies in Childhood (ISAAC) epidemiologic survey. Thereafter, a random sample of 1,900 subjects were invited to undergo a thorough examination and 1717 agreed to participate, representing an overall participation rate of 90.4%. Parents of all study subjects answered a questionnaire regarding demographic data, general health information, and questions related to clinical symptoms and diagnosis of allergic diseases. Serum levels of 25-hydroxyvitamin D [25(OH)D)] and allergen-specific IgE were measured in 1315 subjects whose parents agreed to blood sampling. There was no significant difference in terms of age, sex, and prevalence of allergic diseases between these 1315 subjects who provided blood samples and the original 5351 cohort members, indicating a sampling cohort representative of the general population. All subjects were born to parents who were Asian descent. The Institutional Review Board of Chang Gung Medical Foundation approved the study. The parents of all subjects provided written informed consent on behalf of their children.

Serum 25(OH)D

Blood samples were centrifuged promptly and serum samples was stored frozen in aliquots until analysis. The stored samples were then sent to the laboratory for measurement of serum 25(OH)D at the same time. Serum 25(OH)D levels were measured by a new automated electrochemiluminescense-based assay, Elecsys Vitamin D total assay (Roche Diagnostics, Mannheim, Germany), in the central laboratory at the Chang Gung Memorial Hospital (Taoyuan, Taiwan), which is accredited by the College of American Pathologists (CAP) since 2003 with an accuracy-based 25(OH)D survey offered by the CAP being conducted semiannually. This new assay employs a competitive test principle using recombinant vitamin D binding protein allowing measurement of both 25(OH)D_2 and 25(OH)D_3, instead of using a monoclonal antibody against 25(OH)D_3 in the former Elecsys Vitamin D3 assay that showed underperformance [20]. The assay is standardized against liquid-chromatography tandem mass spectrometry (LC-MS/MS) with traceability to the National Institute of Standards and Technology (NIST) standard reference material 972 [20]. In-house precision testing showed intra-assay coefficients of variation (CVs) of 3.7% and 3.4% at 15 and 32 ng/mL, respectively, and inter-assay CVs of 7.9% and 5.4% at 17 and 33 ng/mL, respectively.

Total and allergen-specific serum immunoglobulin E

The serum level of total IgE was determined by ImmunoCAP (Phadia, Uppsala, Sweden). Specific IgE was determined by a commercial assay for IgE (ImmunoCAP Phadiatop Infant; Phadia) against the most common inhalant and food allergens (i.e. house dust mite, cat, dog, birch, timothy, ragweed, wall pellitory, egg white, cow's milk, peanut and shrimp) [21].

Definitions of allergic diseases and atopy

Information of current and past allergic symptoms and diagnosis of allergic diseases was collected using a modified ISAAC questionnaire [22]. Asthma was defined as ever having asthma and either the occurrence of wheeze in the last 12 months or current use of asthma medications. Rhinitis and eczema were defined as ever having the two diseases, respectively, and either the presence of symptoms in the last 12 months or current use of medication for the two diseases, respectively. Atopy was defined as a positive Phadiatop Infant test result (≧0.35 PAU/L).

Potential confounders

The following were considered potential confounding factors because of their known or plausible associations with serum 25(OH)D and outcomes: age, gender, body mass index (BMI), season of sampling, recent upper respiratory infection (URI) symptoms in the past 2 weeks, active smoking, passive smoking, and premature birth. Age and BMI were considered as continuous variables while season of sampling was categorized as spring (March to May), summer (June to August), autumn (September to November), and winter (December to February).

Statistical analysis

All data analyses were performed using the SPSS statistical package version 15.0 for Windows (SPSS, Chicago, IL, USA). A P-value<0.05 was considered statistically significant. We categorized serum 25(OH)D levels as ≧30 ng/mL, between 20 and 30 ng/mL, and <20 ng/mL. Univariate analysis was performed using Student's t-test or ANOVA for comparing continuous variables, as appropriate, and chi-square test for comparing categorical variables. Variables with a P-value<0.1 in univariate analyses were included in the multivariate regression model for exploring factors associated with serum 25(OH)D. Multivariate logistic or linear regression, as appropriate, was used to examine the relationship between serum 25(OH)D status and allergic phenotypes, both unadjusted and adjusted for factors independently associated with serum 25(OH)D. We also examined serum 25(OH)D as either a dichotomous variable or a continuous

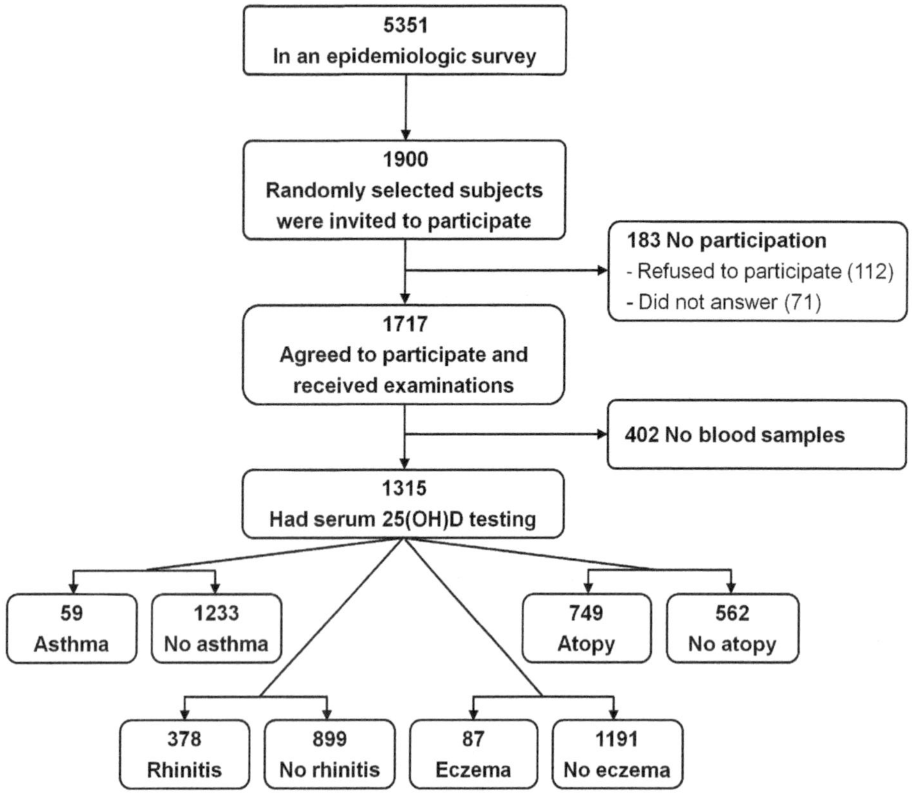

Figure 1. Schematic presentation of the recruitment process of the study subjects.

variable in the analysis. Subjects with missing data on variables of interest (<3.5%) were excluded from analysis.

Results

Subject characteristics

The characteristics of the 1,315 subjects (645 boys; age: 10.3±2.7 years [range 5–18]) are listed in **Table 1**. The mean BMI in the study population was 18.7 kg/m^2 (SD: 3.6). Blood samples were drawn more frequently in the spring (44.6%) and winter (33.3%), and relatively less frequently in the summer (15.7%) and autumn (6.5%). Approximately four of every ten subjects (40.6%) had recent URI symptoms in the past 2 weeks. The prevalence of active smoking was extremely low (0.7%), whereas the prevalence of passive smoking was fairly high (54.1%). A small proportion of the subjects (6.3%) were born prematurely. The prevalence of asthma, rhinitis, eczema, and atopy in the study population was 4.6%, 29.6%, 6.8%, and 57.1%, respectively.

Serum 25(OH)D levels

The mean concentration of serum 25(OH)D in the 1315 subjects was 20.4 ng/mL (SD: 7.1 ng/mL), with a range of 3.0 to 41.8 ng/mL. **Figure 2** showed the distribution of serum 25(OH)D levels in this population. Surprisingly, vitamin D deficiency (defined as serum 25(OH)D<20 ng/mL) was present in 670 of 1315 subjects (51.0%), while vitamin D insufficiency (defined as serum 25(OH)D<30 ng/mL) was observed in 1187 of 1315 subjects (90.3%) (**Figure 2**).

Univariate and multivariate analyses of factors associated with serum 25(OH)D

Univariate analysis revealed that age (P<0.001), gender (P< 0.001), BMI (P<0.001), season (P<0.001), and passive smoking (P = 0.005) were associated with serum 25(OH)D status (**Table 1**). Serum 25(OH)D levels significantly decreased with age (r = −0.273, P<0.001; **Figure 3a**). BMI significantly and negatively correlated to serum 25(OH)D (r = −0.179, P<0.001; **Figure 3b**). Girls had significantly lower serum 25(OH)D than boys (mean ± SD, 19.2±6.9 vs. 21.6±7.2 ng/mL, P<0.001; **Figure 3c**). Subjects sampled in the winter (19.7±7.4 ng/mL) or spring (19.1±6.8 ng/mL) had lower serum 25(OH)D levels than did subjects sampled in the summer (24.4±6.3 ng/mL) (both P< 0.001; **Figure 3c**). Subjects exposed to passive smoke at home had lower serum 25(OH)D levels than those did not (19.9±7.0 vs. 21.1±7.3 ng/mL, P = 0.003; **Figure 3c**).

Multivariate linear regression analysis of serum 25(OH)D levels was performed using variables that had a P-value<0.1 in univariate analyses. Older age (P<0.001), female gender (P< 0.001), higher BMI (P = 0.001), winter and spring seasons (compared to summer; P both<0.001), and passive smoking (P = 0.011) were independently associated with low serum 25(OH)D levels (**Table 2**). Multivariate ordinal logistic regression analysis of serum 25(OH)D showed similar results, supporting the association of the aforementioned variables with serum 25(OH)D status (**Table 3**). In addition, similar results were found when we examined serum 25(OH)D as a dichotomous variable in the analysis (data not shown).

Table 1. Characteristics of 1315 subjects according to serum 25(OH)D levels.

Characteristic	All (N=1315)	Serum 25(OH)D level <20 ng/mL (n=670)	20–29.9 ng/mL (n=517)	≧30 ng/mL (n=128)	*P*
Age, years (mean ± SD)	10.3±2.7	10.9±2.6	9.7±2.5	9.5±2.8	**<0.001**
Gender (n [%])					
Male	645 (49.0)	274 (42.5)	294 (45.6)	77 (11.9)	**<0.001**
Female	670 (51.0)	396 (59.1)	223 (33.3)	51 (7.6)	
BMI, kg/m^2 (mean ± SD)	18.7±3.6	19.1±3.8	18.4±3.4	17.6±2.9	**<0.001**
Season (n [%])					
Spring (Mar to May)	586 (44.6)	340 (58.0)	207 (35.3)	39 (6.7)	**<0.001**
Summer (Jun to Aug)	206 (15.7)	53 (25.7)	118 (57.3)	35 (17.0)	
Autumn (Sep to Nov)	85 (6.5)	28 (32.9)	48 (56.5)	9 (10.6)	
Winter (Dec to Feb)	438 (33.3)	249 (56.8)	144 (32.9)	45 (10.3)	
Recent URI (n [%])					
Yes	517 (40.6)	271 (52.4)	196 (37.9)	50 (9.7)	0.572
No	755 (59.4)	373 (49.4)	304 (40.3)	78 (10.3)	
Active smoking (n [%])					
Yes	9 (0.7)	5 (55.6)	2 (22.2)	2 (22.2)	0.339
No	1306 (99.3)	665 (50.9)	515 (39.4)	126 (9.6)	
Passive smoking (n [%])					
Yes	692 (54.1)	368 (53.2)	271 (39.2)	53 (7.7)	**0.005**
No	586 (45.9)	278 (47.4)	233 (39.8)	75 (12.8)	
Premature birth (n [%])					
Yes	80 (6.3)	35 (43.8)	39 (48.8)	6 (7.5)	0.214
No	1190 (93.7)	605 (50.8)	464 (39.0)	121 (10.2)	

25(OH)D, 25-hydroxyvitamin D; BMI, body mass index; URI, upper respiratory infection.

Relationship of serum 25(OH)D with allergic phenotypes

Univariate analysis demonstrated that serum 25(OH)D status was not significantly associated with asthma ($P=0.723$), rhinitis ($P=0.367$), eczema ($P=0.111$), atopy ($P=0.171$), or total IgE levels ($P=0.516$).

Multivariate regression analysis was also undertaken to further explore the relationship of serum 25(OH)D status with allergic diseases and atopy, taking factors associated with serum 25(OH)D into consideration. After adjusting for age, gender, BMI, season of sampling, and passive smoking, serum 25(OH)D status had no association with asthma, rhinitis, eczema, atopy (**Table 4**), or total

(a) Histogram

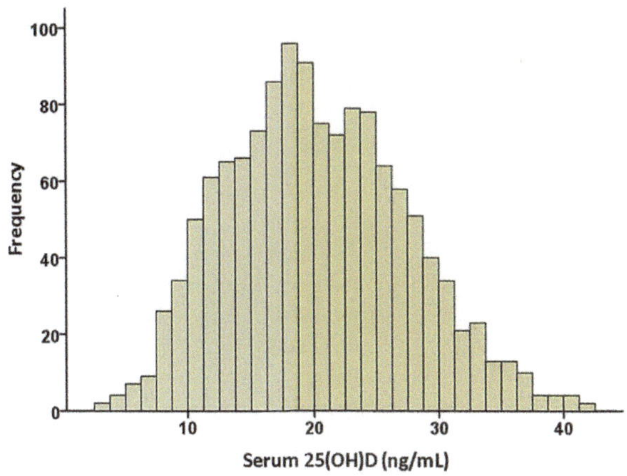

(b) Distribution

25(OH)D	n (%)
<10 ng/mL	82 (6.24%)
10 to 19.9 ng/mL	588 (44.71%)
20 to 29.9 ng/mL	517 (39.32%)
≧30 ng/mL	128 (9.73%)

Figure 2. Serum 25(OH)D levels: (a) histogram, (b) distribution.

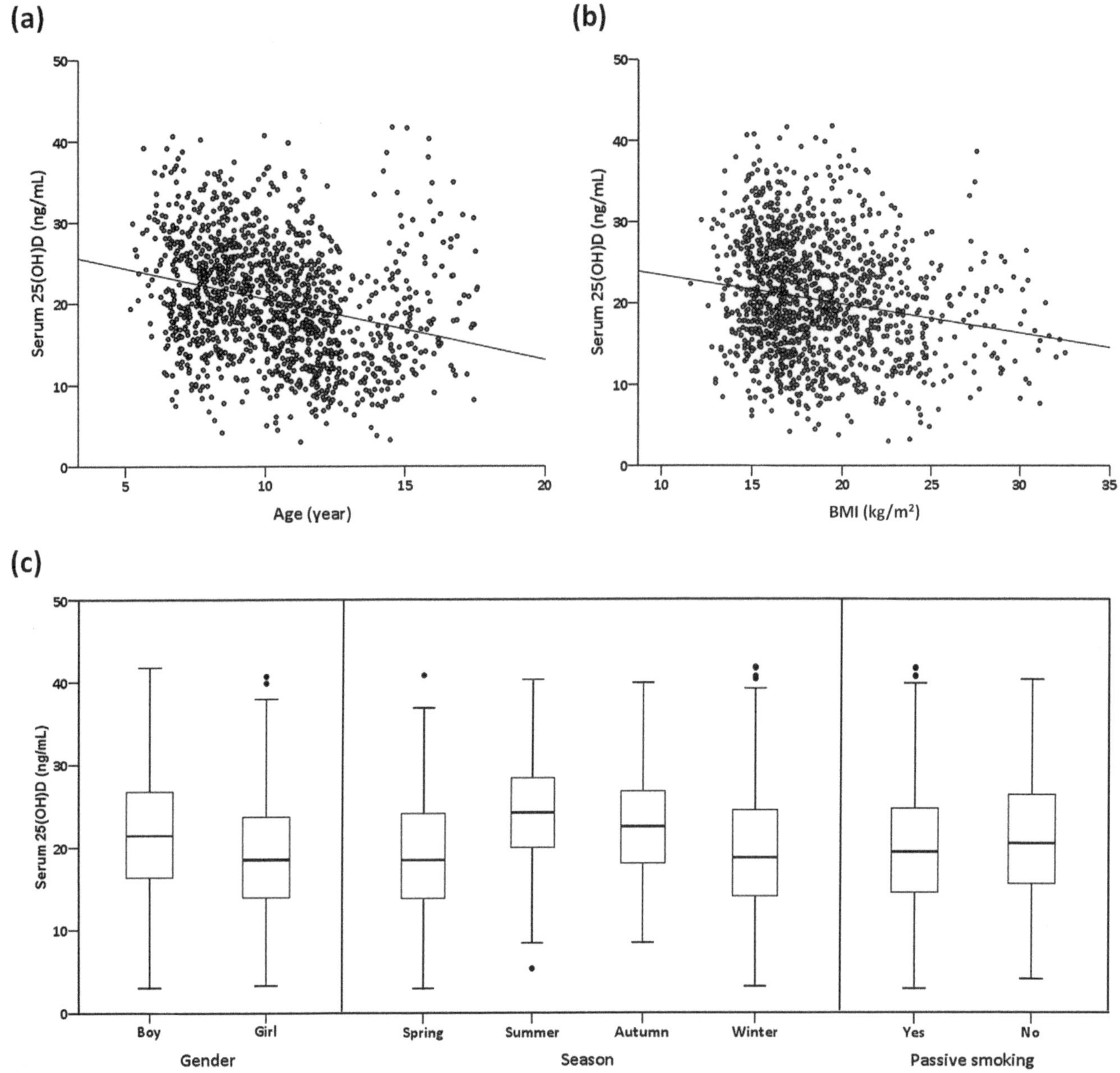

Figure 3. Serum 25(OH)D levels by (a) age ($r = -0.273$, $P < 0.001$), (b) body mass index ($r = -0.179$, $P < 0.001$), and (c) gender ($P < 0.001$), season of sampling ($P < 0.001$), and passive smoking ($P = 0.003$).

IgE levels (**Table 5**). The adjusted odds ratios for asthma seemed to increase across categories of serum 25(OH)D (1.00 [reference] for $\geqq$30 ng/mL, 1.48 [95% CI: 0.50–4.39] for 20–29.9 ng/mL, and 1.74 [95% CI: 058–5.17] for <20 ng/mL), though not statistically significant ($P = 0.481$ and 0.322 for 20–29.9 ng/mL and <20 ng/mL, respectively) (**Table 4**).

To further explore the association of serum 25(OH)D with allergic diseases or atopy, we also examined serum 25(OH)D as a dichotomous variable ($\geqq$30 versus the <30 ng/mL category; likewise, $\geqq$20 versus the <20 ng/mL category) or a continuous variable in the analysis. Univariate or multivariate analysis with the serum 25(OH)D levels as a dichotomous variable or a continuous variable also did not reveal any statistically significant association of serum 25(OH)D with allergic diseases or atopy (data not shown). We also performed the above analyses stratified by gender, which did not yield any statistically significant results (data not shown).

Discussion

New evidence shows high prevalence of vitamin D deficiency in several countries [1] and some studies suggest a possible link between vitamin D status and atopy-related phenotypes [9,10,11,12,13,14,15]. To our knowledge, this is the first large population-based study providing an in-depth examination of the prevalence of vitamin D deficiency and its relation to allergic phenotypes in Asian children. Main findings in the present study highlight a previously under-recognized public health issue that a substantial proportion of Asian children have suboptimal levels of vitamin D, especially those who are older in age, are female, have

Table 2. Multivariate linear regression analyses for serum 25(OH)D levels.

Variable	Coefficient (95% CI)	*P*
Age (years)	−0.025 (−0.033~−0.017)	**<0.001**
Male (vs female)	0.120 (0.080~0.160)	**<0.001**
BMI (kg/m^2)	−0.010 (−0.016~−0.004)	**0.001**
Season (vs summer)		
Spring	−0.214 (−0.273~−0.154)	**<0.001**
Summer	Reference	-
Autumn	−0.046 (−0.138~0.046)	0.322
Winter	−0.183 (−0.245~−0.120)	**<0.001**
Passive smoking (vs no exposure)	−0.051 (−0.091~−0.012)	**0.011**

25(OH)D, 25-hydroxyvitamin D; BMI, body mass index.

a higher BMI, are evaluated in winter or spring season, and are exposed to passive smoke. Another important finding is that our data does not support associations of vitamin D status with allergic diseases and atopy in this population.

In recent years, growing attention has been paid to the vitamin D status of Western populations, but there is a paucity of data in the Asia, particularly in children, on the prevalence and predictors of vitamin D deficiency. Determination of vitamin D status in children is generally more difficult in a large number of children than that in adults because sampling issues are more challenging. This cohort is perhaps one of the largest study to date that measures serum 25(OH)D in a population of 1315 Asian children over a wide range in the community. At present, the best indicator of vitamin D status is the serum 25(OH)D [1]. While there is no universally accepted consensus yet on serum 25(OH)D thresholds to define optimal vitamin D status, vitamin D deficiency is defined by most experts as <20 ng/mL, and insufficiency as <30 ng/mL [1,23], with threshold values based on optimal bone health [24]. When these cut-offs are applied to children aged 5 to 18 years in the current study, more than half (51%) of the children have vitamin D deficiency and 9 of every 10 children have insufficient vitamin D levels. Potential explanations for the remarkably high prevalence of low vitamin D status observed in this population include, but are not limited to, skin pigmentation, the substantial number of rainy days (i.e., an average of 15.9 days with at least 0.1 mm rain per month during the study period), the widespread use of sunscreens on children, and perhaps also dietary factors. This study identifies a previously under-recognized public health issue of vitamin D deficiency in Asian children and therefore calls for careful consideration of vitamin D supplementation particularly in at-risk children to further optimize health.

Given that exposure to sunlight, specifically UVB, is believed to provide most of the vitamin D requirements of the human population [25], the seasonal variation of vitamin D levels in the current study is expected. The inverse association of vitamin D status with age during childhood and adolescence in this population is of interest, which is in accordance with previous studies [26,27,28,29,30]. A plausible explanation is that older children and adolescents may have less exposure to sunlight due to fewer incentives and opportunities for outdoor activities. Indeed, it has been shown previously that a consistent decline in physical activity is found over the school age years, with males decreasing about 2.7% per year and females decreasing about 7.4% per year [31]. Consistent with previous studies [5,27,28,29,30,32,33,34,35],

Table 3. Multivariate ordinal logistic regression analyses for categories of serum 25(OH)D levels*.

Variable	OR (95% CI)	*P*
Age (years)	0.89 (0.85~0.94)	**<0.001**
Male (vs female)	1.97 (1.58~2.47)	**<0.001**
BMI (kg/m^2)	0.96 (0.93~0.99)	**0.027**
Season (vs summer)		
Spring	0.36 (0.26~0.50)	**<0.001**
Summer	1.00 (Reference)	-
Autumn	0.79 (0.49~1.30)	0.354
Winter	0.42 (0.30~0.59)	**<0.001**
Passive smoking (vs no exposure)	0.76 (0.61~0.95)	**0.016**

25(OH)D, 25-hydroxyvitamin D; OR, odds ratio; BMI, body mass index.
*Serum 25(OH)D levels were categorized into 3 ordinal categories of vitamin D status: <20, 20–29.9, and ≧30 ng/mL. The reference group for each variable is given in parentheses. The interpretation of the ORs from the ordinal logistic models is similar to the interpretation of the ORs in the binary logistic regression. For example, the OR for "male subjects (compared with female subjects)" is 1.97, which means that for male subjects, the odds of being in the ≧30 versus the <30 ng/mL category are 1.97 times the odds for female subjects, assuming that all other variables in the model are held constant. Likewise, the odds are the same for the comparison of the ≧20 versus the <20 ng/mL category (on the basis of confirmed proportional odds assumption).

Table 4. Association of serum 25(OH)D status with allergic diseases and atopy.

		Unadjusted		Adjusted**	
	Subjects n/N (%)*	OR (95% CI)	P	OR (95% CI)	P
Asthma					
≧30 ng/mL	4/127 (3.1)	1.00 (Reference)	-	1.00 (Reference)	-
20–29.9 ng/mL	24/509 (4.7)	1.52 (0.52~4.47)	0.445	1.48 (0.50~4.39)	0.481
<20 ng/mL	31/656 (4.7)	1.53 (0.53~4.40)	0.435	1.74 (0.58~5.17)	0.322
Rhinitis					
≧30 ng/mL	41/122 (33.6)	1.00 (Reference)	-	1.00 (Reference)	-
20–29.9 ng/mL	156/508 (30.7)	0.88 (0.58~1.33)	0.535	0.93 (0.60~1.43)	0.736
<20 ng/mL	181/647 (28.0)	0.77 (0.51~1.16)	0.209	0.93 (0.60~1.44)	0.737
Eczema					
≧30 ng/mL	9/126 (7.1)	1.00 (Reference)	-	1.00 (Reference)	-
20–29.9 ng/mL	43/504 (8.5)	1.21 (0.58~2.56)	0.613	1.28 (0.60~2.74)	0.522
<20 ng/mL	35/648 (5.4)	0.74 (0.35~1.59)	0.441	0.92 (0.42~2.04)	0.836
Atopy					
≧30 ng/mL	75/128 (58.6)	1.00 (Reference)	-	1.00 (Reference)	-
20–29.9 ng/mL	309/515 (60.0)	1.06 (0.72~1.57)	0.772	1.07 (0.72~1.60)	0.734
<20 ng/mL	365/668 (54.6)	0.85 (0.58~1.25)	0.410	0.92 (0.62~1.38)	0.689

25(OH)D, 25-hydroxyvitamin D; OR, odds ratio; CI, confidence interval.
*N is the sample size of each category of serum 25(OH)D and n is the number of cases in each category.
**Adjusted for age, gender, body mass index, season of sampling, and passive smoking.

gender and BMI each has an independent effect on serum vitamin D levels in the current study. It has been demonstrated that the prevalence of physical inactivity is higher in girls than boys and is higher in obese children than their normal-weight peers [31]. It is therefore possible that gender and BMI may act as surrogate indicators for sunlight exposure through their association with physical activity. In addition to less sunlight exposure due to sedentary lifestyle, the observed inverse association between BMI and vitamin D levels could be explained by other possibilities, including poor diet and sequestration of vitamin D in fat tissues [36]. The associations in our study between low vitamin D status and exposure to passive smoke, after adjusting for confounders, have not, to our knowledge, been previously reported, and the mechanisms remain unclear and warrant further study.

In the current study, allergic phenotypes including asthma, rhinitis, eczema, atopy, and total IgE levels are not associated with serum 25(OH)D, in contrast with previous studies that demonstrate relationships between various allergic phenotypes and vitamin D status [9,10,11,12,13,14,15]. Two case-control studies provide epidemiological support for the association between vitamin D deficiency and asthma [9,10]. A longitudinal cohort study [11] reveals that serum vitamin D levels at age 6 years are not associated with concurrent asthma at that age but are significant predictors of subsequent asthma at age 14 years. The cross-sectional analysis in the current study shows no significant association between serum 25(OH)D and concurrent asthma, although the role of serum 25(OH)D levels as predictors of subsequent asthma remains to be defined in the longitudinal follow-up of the cohort subjects which is currently underway. Although there is also emerging evidence from recent studies suggesting the association of vitamin D status with allergic rhinitis [12], atopic dermatitis [13], and IgE sensitization [11,14,15], the findings from the current study do not support the previous research. Taken together, the current study provides epidemiological evidence against a strong link between vitamin D status and various allergic phenotypes.

This study has several notable strengths. The representative sampling of children across a broad age range in the community,

Table 5. Association of serum 25(OH)D status with total immunoglobulin E levels.

		Unadjusted		Adjusted*	
25(OH)D (ng/mL)	Subjects	Coefficient (95% CI)	P	Coefficient (95% CI)	P
≧30 ng/mL	128	Reference	-	Reference	-
20–29.9 ng/mL	515	0.159 (−0.153~0.471)	0.319	0.161 (−0.155~0.476)	0.317
<20 ng/mL	668	0.076 (−0.229~0.381)	0.624	0.116 (−0.198~0.431)	0.468

25(OH)D, 25-hydroxyvitamin D; CI, confidence interval.
Total immunoglobulin E levels were logarithmically transformed for analysis.
*Adjusted for age, gender, body mass index, season of sampling, and passive smoking.

large sample size with robust data collection, incorporation of objective markers of atopy, and thorough analysis, all add strengths to the results of this study. This study has some limitations, including its cross-sectional design and lack of data on dietary and supplemental vitamin D intake and physical activity. Some might argue that the small proportion of children with sufficient serum 25(OH)D levels (≧30 ng/mL) might have limited our ability to discern associations. In our opinion, however, the argument is very unlikely since the repeat analyses by treating serum 25(OH)D levels as either a dichotomous variable or a continuous variable do not significantly alter the results. Although it is possible that this relatively large study has not been adequately powered to detect associations of modest effect, the effect size observed in this study is hardly likely to be clinically significant even statistical significance would have been attained with a larger sample size. It will be interesting to investigate in future follow-ups of this longitudinal cohort if serum 25(OH)D levels predict the subsequent development of allergic phenotypes.

In conclusion, low serum 25(OH) D levels are remarkably common in this population-based sample of Asian children aged 5 to 18 years, suggesting that millions of children living in Taiwan may have suboptimal levels of vitamin D, which should be a matter of concern for public health authorities and professionals and also for families with children. This population-based study provides evidence against the association of vitamin D status with allergic diseases and atopy in Asian children. The relationship between vitamin D status and allergic diseases thus merits further study.

Acknowledgments

Members of the PATCH study group are: Jing-Long Huang (Study Coordinator), Tsung-Chieh Yao, Wen-I Lee, Liang-Shiou Ou, Li-Chen Chen, Kuo-Wei Yeh, Yu-Ling Tu, Man-Chin Hua, Ming-Han Tsai, Sui-Ling Liao, and Shen-Hao Lai (Principal Investigators). The authors thank the study subjects, their parents, their teachers and the school nurses, as well as the schools involved, for their active participation in the study. The authors also thank the Department of Education, Keelung City Government, Keelung City, Taiwan for administrative support for the study.

Author Contributions

Conceived and designed the experiments: TY. Performed the experiments: TY PG HN. Analyzed the data: TY SC HT YT. Contributed reagents/materials/analysis tools: MH S-L Liao MT CC S-H Lai KY JH. Wrote the paper: TY YT SC HT. Assisted in participant recruitment/cohort maintenance/data collection: MH S-L Liao MT CC S-H Lai KY JH.

References

1. Holick MF (2007) Vitamin D deficiency. N Engl J Med 357: 266–281.
2. Looker AC, Dawson-Hughes B, Calvo MS, Gunter EW, Sahyoun NR (2002) Serum 25-hydroxyvitamin D status of adolescents and adults in two seasonal subpopulations from NHANES III. Bone 30: 771–777.
3. McGrath JJ, Kimlin MG, Saha S, Eyles DW, Parisi AV (2001) Vitamin D insufficiency in south-east Queensland. Med J Aust 174: 150–151.
4. Marwaha RK, Tandon N, Reddy DR, Aggarwal R, Singh R, et al. (2005) Vitamin D and bone mineral density status of healthy schoolchildren in northern India. Am J Clin Nutr 82: 477–482.
5. El-Hajj Fuleihan G, Nabulsi M, Choucair M, Salamoun M, Hajj Shahine C, et al. (2001) Hypovitaminosis D in healthy schoolchildren. Pediatrics 107: E53.
6. Sedrani SH (1984) Low 25-hydroxyvitamin D and normal serum calcium concentrations in Saudi Arabia: Riyadh region. Ann Nutr Metab 28: 181–185.
7. Asher MI, Montefort S, Bjorksten B, Lai CK, Strachan DP, et al. (2006) Worldwide time trends in the prevalence of symptoms of asthma, allergic rhinoconjunctivitis, and eczema in childhood: ISAAC Phases One and Three repeat multicountry cross-sectional surveys. Lancet 368: 733–743.
8. Yao TC, Ou LS, Yeh KW, Lee WI, Chen LC, et al. (2011) Associations of Age, Gender, and BMI with Prevalence of Allergic Diseases in Children: PATCH Study. J Asthma 48: 503–510.
9. Freishtat RJ, Iqbal SF, Pillai DK, Klein CJ, Ryan LM, et al. (2010) High prevalence of vitamin D deficiency among inner-city African American youth with asthma in Washington, DC. J Pediatr 156: 948–952.
10. Bener A, Ehlayel MS, Tulic MK, Hamid Q (2012) Vitamin D deficiency as a strong predictor of asthma in children. Int Arch Allergy Immunol 157: 168–175.
11. Hollams EM, Hart PH, Holt BJ, Serralha M, Parsons F, et al. (2011) Vitamin D and atopy and asthma phenotypes in children: a longitudinal cohort study. Eur Respir J 38: 1320–1327.
12. Wjst M, Hypponen E (2007) Vitamin D serum levels and allergic rhinitis. Allergy 62: 1085–1086.
13. El Taieb MA, Fayed HM, Aly SS, Ibrahim AK (2013) Assessment of Serum 25-Hydroxyvitamin D Levels in Children with Atopic Dermatitis: Correlation With SCORAD Index. Dermatitis 24: 296–301.
14. Sharief S, Jariwala S, Kumar J, Muntner P, Melamed ML (2011) Vitamin D levels and food and environmental allergies in the United States: results from the National Health and Nutrition Examination Survey 2005–2006. J Allergy Clin Immunol 127: 1195–1202.
15. Hypponen E, Berry DJ, Wjst M, Power C (2009) Serum 25-hydroxyvitamin D and IgE - a significant but nonlinear relationship. Allergy 64: 613–620.
16. Yao TC, Ou LS, Lee WI, Yeh KW, Chen LC, et al. (2011) Exhaled nitric oxide discriminates children with and without allergic sensitization in a population-based study. Clin Exp Allergy 41: 556–564.
17. Yao TC, Lee WI, Ou LS, Chen LC, Yeh KW, et al. (2012) Reference values of exhaled nitric oxide in healthy Asian children aged 5 to 18 years. Eur Respir J 39: 378–384.
18. Tu YL, Chang SW, Tsai HJ, Chen LC, Lee WI, et al. (2013) Total Serum IgE in a Population-Based Study of Asian Children in Taiwan: Reference Value and Significance in the Diagnosis of Allergy. PLoS One 8: e80996.
19. Yao TC, Tsai HJ, Tu YL, Chang SW, Hua MC, et al. (2014) Multiplexed immunoglobulin E sensitization in relation to exhaled nitric oxide in a population sample of children. Allergy 69: 678–682.
20. Emmen JM, Wielders JP, Boer AK, van den Ouweland JM, Vader HL (2012) The new Roche Vitamin D Total assay: fit for its purpose? Clin Chem Lab Med 50: 1969–1972.
21. Ballardini N, Nilsson C, Nilsson M, Lilja G (2006) ImmunoCAP Phadiatop Infant—a new blood test for detecting IgE sensitisation in children at 2 years of age. Allergy 61: 337–343.
22. Asher MI, Keil U, Anderson HR, Beasley R, Crane J, et al. (1995) International Study of Asthma and Allergies in Childhood (ISAAC): rationale and methods. Eur Respir J 8: 483–491.
23. Ross AC, Manson JE, Abrams SA, Aloia JF, Brannon PM, et al. (2011) The 2011 report on dietary reference intakes for calcium and vitamin D from the Institute of Medicine: what clinicians need to know. J Clin Endocrinol Metab 96: 53–58.
24. Henry HL, Bouillon R, Norman AW, Gallagher JC, Lips P, et al. (2010) 14th Vitamin D Workshop consensus on vitamin D nutritional guidelines. J Steroid Biochem Mol Biol 121: 4–6.
25. Ovesen L, Andersen R, Jakobsen J (2003) Geographical differences in vitamin D status, with particular reference to European countries. Proc Nutr Soc 62: 813–821.
26. Mansbach JM, Ginde AA, Camargo CA, Jr. (2009) Serum 25-hydroxyvitamin D levels among US children aged 1 to 11 years: do children need more vitamin D? Pediatrics 124: 1404–1410.
27. Weng FL, Shults J, Leonard MB, Stallings VA, Zemel BS (2007) Risk factors for low serum 25-hydroxyvitamin D concentrations in otherwise healthy children and adolescents. Am J Clin Nutr 86: 150–158.
28. Carpenter TO, Herreros F, Zhang JH, Ellis BK, Simpson C, et al. (2012) Demographic, dietary, and biochemical determinants of vitamin D status in inner-city children. Am J Clin Nutr 95: 137–146.
29. Absoud M, Cummins C, Lim MJ, Wassmer E, Shaw N (2011) Prevalence and predictors of vitamin D insufficiency in children: a Great Britain population based study. PLoS One 6: e22179.
30. Tolppanen AM, Fraser A, Fraser WD, Lawlor DA (2012) Risk factors for variation in 25-hydroxyvitamin D(3) and D(2) concentrations and vitamin D deficiency in children. J Clin Endocrinol Metab 97: 1202–1210.
31. Sallis JF (1993) Epidemiology of physical activity and fitness in children and adolescents. Crit Rev Food Sci Nutr 33: 403–408.
32. Rockell JE, Green TJ, Skeaff CM, Whiting SJ, Taylor RW, et al. (2005) Season and ethnicity are determinants of serum 25-hydroxyvitamin D concentrations in New Zealand children aged 5–14 y. J Nutr 135: 2602–2608.
33. Gordon CM, DePeter KC, Feldman HA, Grace E, Emans SJ (2004) Prevalence of vitamin D deficiency among healthy adolescents. Arch Pediatr Adolesc Med 158: 531–537.
34. Valtuena J, Gonzalez-Gross M, Huybrechts I, Breidenassel C, Ferrari M, et al. (2013) Factors associated with vitamin D deficiency in european adolescents: the HELENA study. J Nutr Sci Vitaminol (Tokyo) 59: 161–171.

35. Gonzalez-Gross M, Valtuena J, Breidenassel C, Moreno LA, Ferrari M, et al. (2012) Vitamin D status among adolescents in Europe: the Healthy Lifestyle in Europe by Nutrition in Adolescence study. Br J Nutr 107: 755–764.

36. Wortsman J, Matsuoka LY, Chen TC, Lu Z, Holick MF (2000) Decreased bioavailability of vitamin D in obesity. Am J Clin Nutr 72: 690–693.

3

Ergocalciferol and Microcirculatory Function in Chronic Kidney Disease and Concomitant Vitamin D Deficiency: An Exploratory, Double Blind, Randomised Controlled Trial

Gavin Dreyer[1,3], Arthur T. Tucker[4], Steven M. Harwood[3], Rupert M. Pearse[2], Martin J. Raftery[1], Muhammad M. Yaqoob[1,3]*

1 Department of Renal Medicine, Barts Health NHS Trust, London, United Kingdom, **2** Department of Critical Care Medicine, Barts Health NHS Trust, London, United Kingdom, **3** Department of Translational Medicine and Therapeutics, Queen Mary University of London, London, United Kingdom, **4** Ernest Cooke Microvascular Unit, Barts Health NHS Trust, London, United Kingdom

Abstract

Background and Objectives: Vitamin D deficiency and endothelial dysfunction are non-traditional risk factors for cardiovascular events in chronic kidney disease. Previous studies in chronic kidney disease have failed to demonstrate a beneficial effect of vitamin D on arterial stiffness, left ventricular mass and inflammation but none have assessed the effect of vitamin D on microcirculatory endothelial function.

Study Design: We conducted a randomised controlled trial of 38 patients with non diabetic chronic kidney disease stage 3–4 and concomitant vitamin D deficiency (<16 ng/dl) who received oral ergocalciferol (50,000 IU weekly for one month followed by 50,000 IU monthly) or placebo over 6 months. The primary outcome was change in microcirculatory function measured by laser Doppler flowmetry after iontophoresis of acetylcholine. Secondary endpoints were tissue advanced glycation end products, sublingual functional capillary density and flow index as well as macrovascular parameters. Parallel *in vitro* experiments were conducted to determine the effect of ergocalciferol on cultured human endothelial cells.

Results: Twenty patients received ergocalciferol and 18 patients received placebo. After 6 months, there was a significant improvement in the ergocalciferol group in both endothelium dependent microcirculatory vasodilatation after iontophoresis of acetylcholine ($p = 0.03$) and a reduction in tissue advanced glycation end products ($p = 0.03$). There were no changes in sublingual microcirculatory parameters. Pulse pressure ($p = 0.01$) but not aortic pulse wave velocity was reduced. There were no significant changes in bone mineral parameters, blood pressure or left ventricular mass index suggesting that ergocalciferol improved endothelial function independently of these parameters. In parallel experiments, expression of endothelial nitric oxide synthase and activity were increased in human endothelial cells in a dose dependent manner.

Conclusions: Ergocalciferol improved microcirculatory endothelial function in patients with chronic kidney disease and concomitant vitamin D deficiency. This process may be mediated through enhanced expression and activity of endothelial nitric oxide synthase.

Trial Registration: Clinical trials.gov NCT00882401

Editor: Giuseppe Danilo, University of Milan, Italy

Funding: This study was funded by grants from the British Renal Society (www.britishrenal.org) (Grant number BRS 09/010) and the Barts and the London charitable Trust (Barts and the London charitable Trust). The funders had no role in study design, data collection and analysis, decision to publish, or preparation of the manuscript.

Competing Interests: The authors have declared that no competing interests exist.

* Email: m.m.yaqoob@qmul.ac.uk

Introduction

Patients with chronic kidney disease (CKD) are far more likely to die of cardiovascular disease (CVD) than progress to end stage kidney disease (ESKD) [1]. Traditional risk factors including age, hypertension, smoking and diabetes mellitus do not entirely account for the excess of CVD mortality in patients with CKD. Vitamin D deficiency, a non-traditional CVD risk factor in patients with all stages of kidney disease [2,3,4], is highly prevalent in patients with CKD [5,6] and is associated with elevated cardiovascular (CV) morbidity and mortality [7,8,9].

Vitamin D deficiency in patients with CKD has been shown to correlate with impairment in endothelial function [10,11]. In pre-clinical [12] and clinical studies [13], endothelial dysfunction has been identified as a non-traditional risk factor for CVD in CKD with improvements in endothelial function reflecting improved global vascular health and a reduced risk of CVD [14].

Observational studies [15,16,17,18,19,20] have provided support for the protective role of vitamin D therapy in reducing the risk of CVD in patients with CKD and ESKD. However, these studies were heterogeneous in design, therapeutic intervention and patient populations (CKD vs ESKD) and have not elucidated the mechanism by which vitamin D reduces CV risk in this patient group. Several *in vitro*, pre-clinical and clinical studies have demonstrated that endothelial and therefore microcirculatory function can be ameliorated after treatment with both activated and nutritional forms of vitamin D [21,22,23,24,25]. However, none of these studies have included patients with CKD. Two previous studies in patients with non-dialysis and CKD and ESKD evaluating the effect of nutritional vitamin D compounds on endothelial biomarkers and conduit artery function have provided conflicting results [26,27].

The microcirculation, defined as blood vessels <150 μm in diameter [28] located within tissue parenchyma, is intricately linked to endothelial function and predicts the function of the microcirculatory beds in renal and cardiac tissue [29,30,31,32,33]. A review of cardiovascular assessment in patients with CKD [34] has highlighted the need for further assessments of microcirculatory dysfunction in patients with CKD as a method for predicting adverse CV outcomes. To date, there have been no prospective, randomized controlled studies investigating the effect of vitamin D on microcirculatory endothelial function or CV endpoints in patients with CKD [35].

We therefore conducted an exploratory, double blind, randomised, controlled trial to determine if therapy with ergocalciferol compared to placebo improves microcirculatory endothelial function in patients with CKD and concomitant vitamin D deficiency. We also conducted parallel *in vitro* experiments to elucidate the mechanistic pathway of ergocalciferol in cultured human endothelial cells.

Methods

Study design

The protocol for this trial and supporting CONSORT checklist are available as supporting information; see Checklist S1 and Protocol S1. This was a single centre, double blind, exploratory randomised controlled trial comparing oral ergocalciferol to placebo in patients with CKD stage 3–4 (estimated glomerular filtration rate (eGFR) 60–15 ml/min/1.73 m^2) and concomitant vitamin D deficiency (defined as a serum 25 hydroxy vitamin D (25 (OH) D) level of <16 ng/ml). The study was conducted at the Royal London Hospital, UK, between 1/5/2009 and 1/9/2010. All patients provided written informed consent and ethical approval was obtained from the East London Research Ethics Committee. The trial was registered at clinicaltrials.gov (Clinical trials number- NCT00882401, http://clinicaltrials.gov/ct2/show/NCT00882401) and conducted in accordance with the Declaration of Helsinki.

Inclusion/exclusion criteria

The principle inclusion criteria were an eGFR between 15 and 60 ml/min/1.73 m^2 with evidence of 2 consecutive measures of eGFR <60 ml/min/1.73 m^2 by the 4 variable MDRD equation [36] at least 3 months apart, serum 25 (OH) D levels <16 ng/ml, age >18 and <80 years, no evidence of diabetes mellitus (fasting blood sugar <128 mg/dl, not taking any diabetic medication), not receiving nor having had renal replacement therapy in the preceding three months

The principle exclusion criteria were current vitamin D therapy of any type, serum calcium above 10.4 mg/dl (based on the upper limit of the laboratory reference range [37]), pregnant or lactating women, presence of conditions which predispose to hypercalcaemia, renal calculi and presence of a disease other than CKD associated with microcirculatory dysfunction.

Intervention and randomization

Patients were randomised to either ergocalciferol (Sanofi Aventis, New Jersey, USA) or a matching placebo. The dose of ergocalciferol was 50,000 IU weekly for one month followed by 50,000 IU monthly for 5 months resulting in a total dose of 450,000 IU over 6 months. This was in line with existing K/DOQI guidelines for the replacement of vitamin D in patients with CKD at the time the study was designed [37]. The dose of ergocalciferol was standardized for all patients to ensure equal dosing of ergocalciferol over the duration of the study to avoid the potentially confounding effect of varying doses of ergocalciferol based on initial serum concentrations of 25 (OH) D. The control arm received a matching placebo given at the same dose schedule as ergocalciferol. All patients received dietary advice appropriate to their stage of CKD from specialist renal dietitians which included advice on dietary intake of calcium, phosphate, sodium, potassium and protein. Patients were reviewed monthly for 6 months. A 2 week washout period for any vitamin D containing drugs or over the counter supplements was included before randomization, however no subjects required vitamin D washout. The randomization schedule was developed by an independent accountant. Sequentially numbered, sealed envelopes were used to achieve allocation concealment. Envelopes were stored and sequentially dispensed to study patients by the hospital clinical trial pharmacy who were blinded to the intervention and allocation as were the remainder of the study team.

Study endpoints

The primary outcome measure was microcirculatory endothelial function assessed by laser Doppler flowmetry (LDF) over forearm skin after iontophoresis of acetylcholine (ACh). Secondary outcome measures were microvascular parameters including skin autofluorescence (AF) and side stream dark field imaging (SDF) of the sub lingual microcirculation as well as macrovascular parameters including blood pressure, pulse pressure, aortic pulse wave velocity (aPWV), left ventricular mass index (LVMI) and bone mineral parameters (see File S1 for details of all techniques).

Clinical assessments

All patients were reviewed at the Royal London Hospital kidney unit. Patients were instructed to wear loose clothing, avoid caffeine and nicotine for 12 hours prior to assessments and rested for 15 minutes in a temperature and humidity controlled room before microcirculatory assessments.

Iontophoresis and laser Doppler flowmetry

Iontophoresis involves the delivery of charged particles to the local microcirculation, through the skin, using electrically repulsive forces. Laser Doppler flowmetry is a non-invasive technique which uses the Doppler principle to measure flux of erythrocytes in sub dermal capillaries. Increasing red cell flux after iontophoresis reflects microcirculatory vasodilatation as a consequence of improved endothelial function. The combination of these techniques is a validated method for studying endothelial function in the microcirculation in various pathologies including CKD. [38,39,40] A 1% solution of both ACh and sodium nitroprusside (SNP) were iontophoresed on the volar aspect of the non-dominant forearm using a low current protocol to reduce galvanic effect [41] with a maximum achieved dose of 75 μA after 7.5 minutes. To eliminate baseline variability, relative percentage change from baseline flux after the maximum iontophoretic dose is the primary outcome measure (see Figure S1 and Table S1 in File S1) [38].

Skin autofluorescence

Tissue advanced glycation end (AGE) product levels are an independent risk predictor of microcirculatory complications and are predictors of CVD in renal failure [42]. The technique utilises the AGE reader (Diagnoptics, Netherlands) which provides a non-invasive measure of AGE in the skin. AGE products correlate with measures of skin AF provided by the output from the AGE reader device [42].

Side stream dark field imaging of the sublingual microcirculation

This is a non-invasive, real time, imaging tool to assess intra-vital capillary blood flow. An analysis of the moving cells in the recorded video images permits the quantitative measurement of red blood cell flow in the capillaries. SDF images were scored and interpreted according to standard guidelines [43].

Macrocirculatory parameters

Aortic pulse wave velocity (Vicorder device, Skidmore Medical, UK) was measured to determine if changes in microcirculatory function occurred independently of changes in large conduit vessels. LVMI was measured by cardiac magnetic resonance imaging (cMRI) to determine if the hypothesized improved microcirculatory function resulted in reduced peripheral resistance leading to reduced cardiac workload and subsequent reductions in LVMI.

Biochemical analysis

All biochemical tests were performed in our hospital laboratory by a Roche modular unit analyser (F. Hoffmann-La Roche Ltd, Switzerland). Serum vitamin D levels were assessed by UPLC-MS/MS, which is a quantitative ultra-performance liquid chromatography tandem mass spectrometry assay. Parathyroid hormone (PTH) levels were assessed by the Roche E170 intact PTH assay (Roche Diagnostics, Mannheim)

Experimental work

Human aortic endothelial cells (HAEC, Promocell, UK) were cultured and incubated for 24 h using either low (12 ng/dl) or high (120 ng/dl) concentrations of ergocalciferol. Real time polymerase chain reaction (RT-PCR) was used to evaluate the effect of ergocalciferol on the expression of endothelial nitric oxide synthase (eNOS). Nitrite levels in cell supernatant, to evaluate the downstream effect of changes in eNOS expression in cells, were measured by a chemiluminescent technique [44] (see File S1 and figures S1-5 for full description of all techniques).

Statistical analysis

At the time of designing the study, there was insufficient available evidence of the effect of ergocalciferol therapy on microcirculatory parameters to undertake a standard power calculation. Our hypothesis was that ergocalciferol would significantly improve the function of the endothelium in patients with CKD and concomitant vitamin D deficiency. Given the profoundly low levels of 25 (OH) D in this patient group, the expected rise in serum 25 (OH) D levels with ergocalciferol and predicted lack of change of 25 (OH) D levels in the placebo group, we estimated that 30% of patients in the placebo group and 80% of the patients in the ergocalciferol group would have an improvement in peripheral LDF measured by relative change from baseline flux after 6 months of therapy. At 80% power and with a significance level of 0.05, this required 19 patients per arm. An intention to treat analysis was performed.

Clinical trial subjects

The two groups were compared for similarity at baseline and after 6 months of therapy using the Student's t test for normally distributed variables, Mann Whitney tests for non-parametric data and Chi squared tests or Fisher's exact test for proportions. Differences in 25 (OH) D levels and change from baseline flux measured by LDF after iontophoresis were analysed using a two way repeated measures ANOVA test followed by Bonferroni post tests for comparisons at pre determined time points (1, 3 and 6 months). We confirmed our findings using a mixed effects model. Forearm laser Doppler flowmetry is expressed as the percentage increase in flux from baseline after iontophoresis of ACh [38]. Four patients in the ergocalciferol group and 1 in the placebo group completed an initial 3 months on therapy before the end of the predetermined study period and this data was included in the analysis. The analysis of data at 6 months includes data from all remaining patients who completed the full follow up period. SDF imaging of the sublingual microcirculation was expressed as functional capillary density (mm^{-1}) and microvascular flow index as described previously [43]. LVMI, SDF imaging, skin AF and bone mineral parameters were analysed using t tests and Mann Whitney tests based on the distribution of the data. A p value of < 0.05 was considered statistically significant. Analysis was conducted on Stata version 10 (www.stata.com) and GraphPad Prism software version 5 (see File S1 and figures S2–S5 for sub-group analysis).

Cell experiments

RT-PCR data were analyzed with ABI 7900HT Prism sequence detector software (SDS Version 2.3, Applied Biosystems) to determine differential gene expression for eNOS compared to β actin. Differences in nitrite levels were assessed using the Student t-test. Ethanol is included since this was used to dilute the ergocalciferol. Statistical analysis was performed using GraphPad Prism software (version 5).

Results

Patient screening, enrolment and randomization are shown in figure 1. The treatment and placebo groups were similar with respect to demographic, clinical (table 1) and laboratory parameters (table 2). Two patients were lost to follow up in the ergocalciferol arm and 1 in the placebo arm. All patients self reported complete compliance and this was confirmed by manual inspection of study medication bottles at each visit. No patients were taking nitrate containing medications that may have acted as vasodilators through the donation of nitric oxide. After 6 months of treatment with ergocalciferol, 25 hydroxy vitamin D (25 (OH) D) levels increased significantly in the treatment group ($p<0.0001$) (figure 2) but there were no significant changes in other biochemical parameters (table 3).

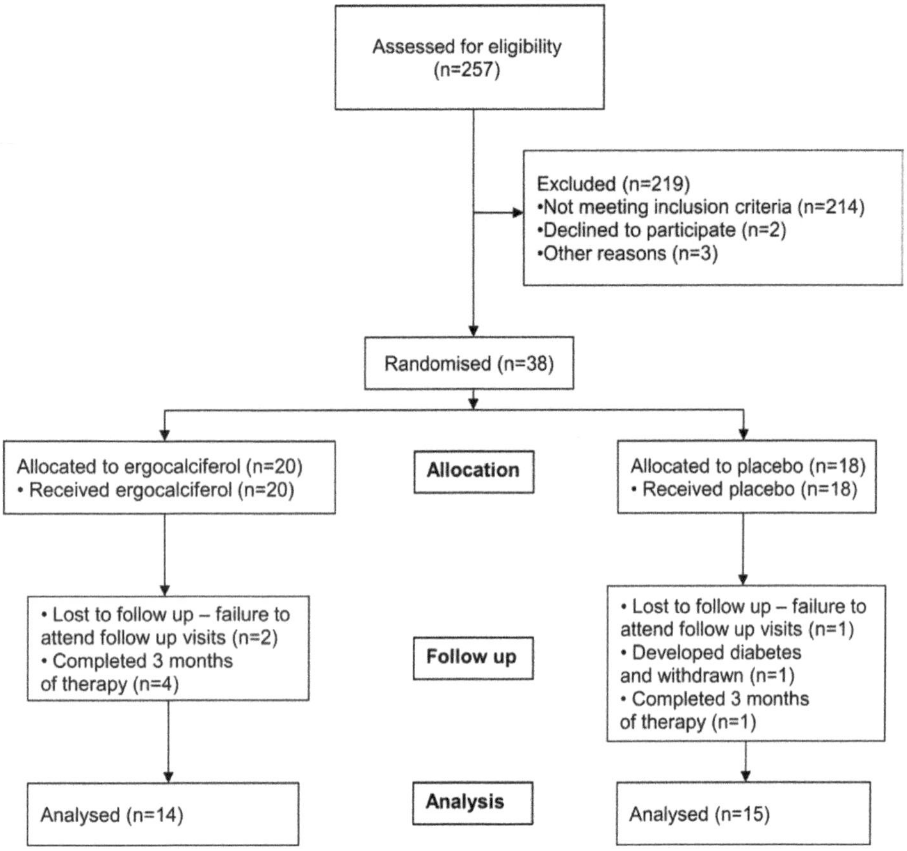

Figure 1. Recruitment schedule for study patients.

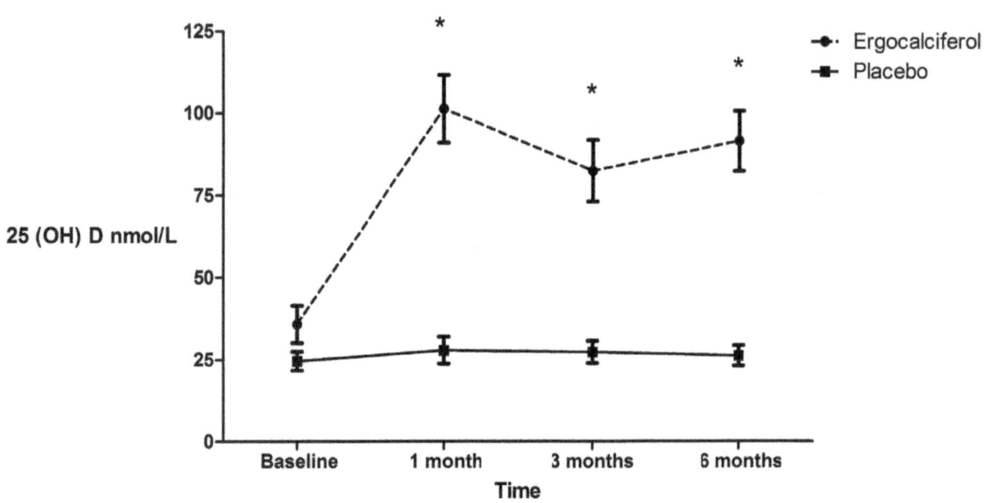

Number at risk

	Baseline	1 month	3 months	6 months
Ergocalciferol	20	19	18	14
Placebo	18	18	16	15

Figure 2. 25 (OH) D levels in patients treated with ergocalciferol and placebo. Bonferroni post tests following two way repeated measures ANOVA at 1,3 and 6 months $p<0.0001$. (* = statistically significant).

Table 1. Baseline demographic and clinical data for patients.

	Ergocalciferol (n = 20)	Placebo (n = 18)	p value
Age years	45.8 (10.0)	48.8 (12.2)	0.39
Sex (% male)	14 (60.9%)	14 (73.7%)	0.22
Body mass index	30.4 (7.1)	29.2 (3.4)	0.51
Ethnicity			0.57
Caucasian	5 (21.8%)	6 (31.6%)	
Non-Caucasian	15 (78.2%)	12 (68.4%)	
Cause of CKD			0.74
Hypertension	5 (25%)	7 (38.9%)	
Glomerulonephritis	8 (40%)	5 (27.8%)	
ADPKD	2 (10%)	1 (5.6%)	
Other~	5 (25%)	5 (27.7%)	
Smoking status			0.59
Current smoker	1 (5%)	2 (11.1%)	
Never/Ex-smoker	19 (95%)	16 (88.9%)	
Presence of endovascular stent devices	0 (0%)	1 (5.6%)	0.47
ACE-I/ARB	16 (80%)	12 (66.7%)	0.33
β Blocker	7 (35%)	6 (33.3%)	0.57
Statin use	9 (45%)	7 (38.9%)	0.84
Anti platelet therapy	2 (10%)	3 (16.7%)	0.48
Folic acid	1 (5.0%)	1 (5.6%)	1.00
Nitrate containing medications#	0 (0%)	0 (0%)	1.00
Medications containing Vitamin D	0 (0%)	0 (0%)	1.00
BP in past history	15 (65.2%)	11 (57.9%)	0.63
Systolic BP (mmHg)	114 (10)	119 (10)	0.11
Diastolic BP (mmHg)	70 (8)	71 (7)	0.57
MAP (mmHg)	84 (8)	87 (8)	0.29
Pulse pressure (mmHg)	45 (7)	48 (6)	0.08
aPWV (m/s)	8.5 (1.1)	8.5 (1.5)	0.66
LVMI (g/m2)	96.1 (36.3)	87.5 (174)	0.55
Skin AF (AU)	2.8 (0.9)	3.1 (0.9)	0.26
FCD (mm-1)	5.2 (0.5)	5.0 (0.5)	0.78
MFI (AU)	2.5 (0.1)	2.4 (0.1)	0.54

Figures in brackets are standard deviation of the mean or % of total in treatment group. ADPKD – autosomal dominant polycystic kidney disease. BP = blood pressure, ACE-I angiotensin converting enzyme inhibitor, ARB – angiotensin receptor blocker, MAP = mean arterial pressure, aPWV = aortic pulse wave velocity, LVMI – left ventricular mass index, AF – auto fluorescence, FCD – functional capillary density, MFI – microvascular flow index. AU – arbitrary units

#- any form of glyceryl trinitrate, isosorbide mononitrate, isosorbide dinitrate or other esters of nitric acid

~- Additional causes of CKD in ergocalciferol group: tubulo-interstitial nephritis (n = 1), reflux nephropathy (n = 2), unknown (n = 2). Placebo group: reflux nephropathy (n = 2), ischaemic nephropathy presumed due to reno-vascular disease (n = 1), unknown (n = 2).

The effect of ergocalciferol on microcirculatory parameters

Treatment with ergocalciferol compared to placebo was associated with a significant increase in change from baseline flux measured by LDF after iontophoresis of ACh (repeated measures 2 way ANOVA $p = 0.03$) with a significant difference between treatment groups observed at 6 months (Bonferroni post test $p = 0.012$) (figure 3). There were no significant differences in change from baseline flux after the iontophoresis of SNP between treatment groups at 6 months (repeated measures 2 way ANOVA $p = 0.18$) (figure 4). The use of a mixed effects model did not change the significance of these findings (change from baseline after iontophoresis at 6 months follow up: ACh $p = 0.03$, SNP $p = 0.36$).

Skin AF was significantly lower in patients treated with ergocalciferol after 6 months, reflecting reduced levels of tissue oxidative stress ($p = 0.03$). At the end of the follow up period, there were no differences in parameters of functional capillary density (FCD) or microvascular flow index (MFI) assessed by SDF imaging of the sublingual microcirculation (table 4).

The effect of ergocalciferol on macrocirculatory parameters

Pulse pressure was significantly lower in patients treated with ergocalciferol after 6 months ($p = 0.01$) but systolic, diastolic and

Table 2. Baseline laboratory data for CKD patients randomised to either ergocalciferol or placebo.

	Ergocalciferol (n = 20)	Placebo (n = 18)	p value
Creatinine (mg/dl)	2.3 (0.8)	2.0 (1.0)	0.60
eGFR (ml/min/1.73 m^2)	33.0 (13.5)	38.7 (15)	0.39
Stage of CKD			0.33
Stage 3	9 (45%)	13 (72.2%)	
Stage 4	11 (55%)	5 (27.8%)	
Hb (g/dl)	12.8 (1.8)	12.6 (1.4)	0.63
Calcium (mg/dl)	8.8 (0.8)	8.8 (0.8)	0.74
Phosphate (mg/dl)	3.8 (0.6)	3.5 (0.6)	0.16
Calcium phosphate product (mg^2/dl^2)	33.0 (4.2)	31.2 (5.1)	0.25
PTH (pg/L)	102.8 (76.4)	118.9 (103.8)	0.60
CRP (mg/L)	7.6 (17.2)	5.9 (9.8)	0.71
Urine P:CR	190.8 (276.4)	102.7 (147.0)	0.32
Total cholesterol (mg/dl)	201 (53)	185 (39)	0.36
High density lipoprotein cholesterol (mg/dl)	57.5 (24.0)	46.7 (15.9)	0.20

Figures in brackets are standard deviation of the mean. eGFR = estimated glomerular filtration rate, 25 (OH) D = 25 hydroxy vitamin D, Hb = haemaglobin, PTH = parathyroid hormone, CRP = C reactive protein, P:CR = protein:creatinine ratio.

mean arterial pressures were similar between treatment groups. There were no differences between the study groups in aPWV or LVMI after 6 months of therapy (table 4).

Safety data

There were no serious adverse events reported. Three patients in each group experienced episodes of gout that resolved with analgesia. The highest 25 (OH) D level recorded was 68.5 ng/ml. There were no recorded episodes of hypercalcaemia (defined as a serum calcium >10.4 mg/dl).

The effect of ergocalciferol on eNOS expression and nitrite levels in cultured human aortic endothelial cells

RT-PCR analysis for the fold-increase of eNOS compared to β-actin as a control gene demonstrated a dose dependent increase in expression with a 2.4-fold increase in eNOS expression after 24 h of incubation with high concentration ergocalciferol (120 ng/dl) compared to a 1.6 fold increase with low dose ergocalciferol (12 ng/dl) ($p = 0.002$). Only high concentration ergocalciferol resulted in a statistically significant increase in fold expression of eNOS compared to the control experiment ($p < 0.001$) (figure 5). There was no significant difference in nitrite levels between control and low dose ergocalciferol treated cells at 24 h. However, high dose ergocalciferol treatment produced a significant rise in nitrite compared to both low dose ($p = 0.007$) and vehicle control ($p = 0.003$) (figure 6).

Discussion

In this study, ergocalciferol therapy over 6 months in patients with CKD and concomitant vitamin D deficiency was associated with improved endothelium dependent microcirculatory function and a reduction in measures of tissue oxidative stress. The increase

Table 3. Laboratory results in both groups after 6 months of therapy.

	Ergocalciferol (n = 14)	Placebo (n = 15)	p value
Creatinine (mg/dl)	2.4 (0.9)	2.3 (1.1)	0.80
eGFR (ml/min/1.73 m^2)	31.4 (10.6)	35.0 (14.5)	0.44
Hb (g/dl)	12.6 (2.1)	12.4 (1.3)	0.73
Calcium (mg/dl)	9.1 (0.7)	8.9 (0.6)	0.43
Phosphate (mg/dl)	3.7 (0.74)	3.7 (1.2)	0.98
Calcium phosphate product (mg^2/dl^2)	33.6 (8.2)	32.6 (3.5)	0.66
PTH (pg/L)	97.2 (74.5)	135.8 (96.2)	0.26
CRP (mg/L)	7.5 (15.0)	9.7 (19.8)	0.76
Urine P:CR	154.0 (210.3)	117.5 (126.3)	0.62
Total cholesterol (mg/dl)	193 (38)	174 (35)	0.21
High density lipoprotein cholesterol (mg/dl)	54.2 (25.2)	50.8 (15.3)	0.67

Figures in brackets are standard deviation of the mean. eGFR = estimated glomerular filtration rate, 25 (OH) D = 25 hydroxy vitamin D, Hb = haemaglobin, PTH = parathyroid hormone, CRP = C reactive protein, P:CR = protein:creatinine ratio.

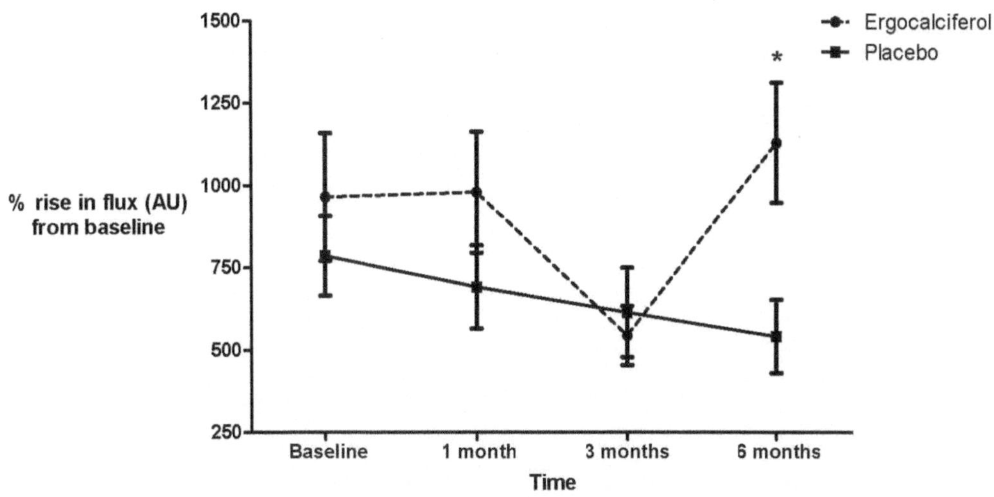

Number at risk

	Baseline	1 month	3 months	6 months
Ergocalciferol	20	19	18	14
Placebo	18	18	16	15

Figure 3. Percentage rise from baseline flux in arbitrary units (AU) after iontophoresis of ACh. Absolute values of percentage change in flux (AU): baseline - ergocalciferol 964.8, placebo 785.9 (p = NS). 1 month - ergocalciferol 979.5, placebo 690.9 (p = NS). 3 months – ergocalciferol 543.7, placebo 613.5 (p = NS). 6 months – ergocalciferol 1130.0, placebo 540.6 (p = 0.012). p values are Bonferroni post test following two way repeated measures ANOVA. (* = statistically significant).

in relative change of flux from baseline after iontophoresis with ACh but not SNP in subjects treated with ergocalciferol indicates improved microcirculatory function occurred through an endothelium dependent mechanism. Reduction in measures of skin AF in the ergocalciferol group correlates with reduced oxidative stress in these patients which will contribute to improved endothelial function and a reduced risk of future CV events [42]. This is in line with previous experimental work that demonstrated the protective effect of calcitriol in human endothelial cells cultured with AGE products [21].

In our study, bone mineral parameters, kidney function, C reactive protein, blood pressure and aPWV were similar at 6

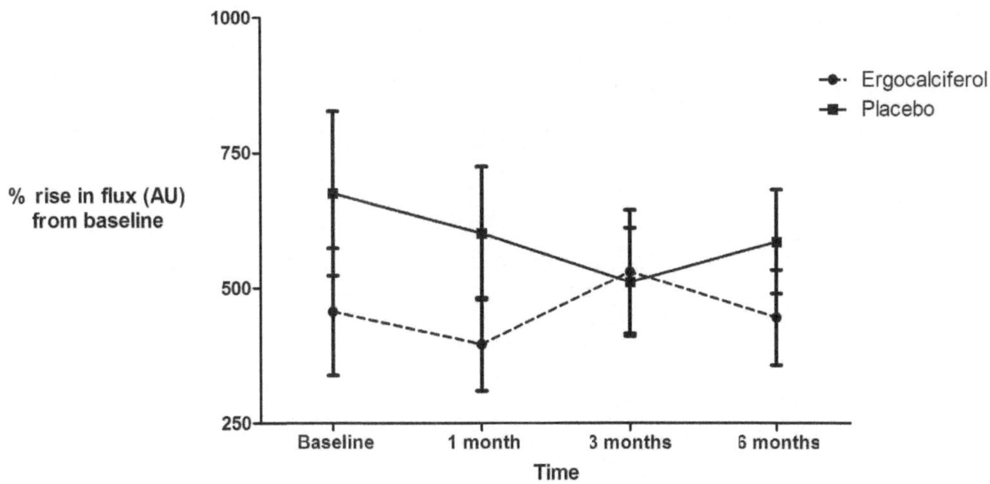

Number at risk

	Baseline	1 month	3 months	6 months
Ergocalciferol	20	19	18	14
Placebo	18	18	16	15

Figure 4. Percentage rise from baseline flux in arbitrary units (AU) after iontophoresis of SNP. Absolute values of percentage change in flux (AU): baseline - ergocalciferol 455.8, placebo 670.1 (p = NS). 1 month - ergocalciferol 395.5, placebo 601.3 (p = NS). 3 months – ergocalciferol 530.2, placebo 511.2 (p = NS). 6 months – ergocalciferol 445.7, placebo 585.9 (p = NS). p values are Bonferroni post test following two way repeated measures ANOVA.

Table 4. Measures of macrovascular parameters in both groups after 6 months of therapy.

	Ergocalciferol (n = 14)	Placebo (n = 15)	p value
Systolic BP (mmHg)	118 (10)	123 (15)	0.26
Diastolic BP (mmHg)	74 (6)	70 (9)	0.15
MAP (mmHg)	89 (7)	88 (10)	0.77
Pulse pressure (mmHg)	44 (8)	53 (12)	0.01
aPWV (m/s)	8.4 (1.3)	8.5 (1.2)	0.78
LVMI (g/m^2)	94.7 (28.4)	110 (54.3)	0.44
Skin AF (AU)	2.8 (0.6)	3.5 (0.9)	0.03
FCD (mm^{-1})	5.3 (0.7)	5.4 (0.8)	0.90
MFI (AU)	2.4 (0.2)	2.4 (0.2)	0.81

Figures in brackets are standard deviation of the mean. BP = blood pressure, MAP = mean arterial pressure, aPWV = aortic pulse wave velocity, LVMI - left ventricular mass index, AF - auto fluorescence, FCD - functional capillary density, MFI - microvascular flow index. AU - arbitrary units.

month follow up suggesting that functional changes to the microcirculation occurred independently of these parameters, adding strength to the argument that ergocalciferol may have a specific mechanism of action within the microcirculation. In contrast to other studies [45,46], proteinuria was unaffected in the ergocalciferol group although the differences in vitamin D compounds, dose schedule, study duration and populations between those studies and ours may explain this difference. aPWV did not decrease in line with the reduction in pulse pressure and this finding may reflect the short duration of the study. Studies with a longer follow up duration are more likely to demonstrate a fall in pulse wave velocity which may occur after a reduction in pulse pressure

After 6 months of therapy with ergocalciferol, there was no increase in the functional capillary density or flow within the microcirculation. This implies that the observed improvements in endothelium dependent microcirculatory function did not involve the recruitment of extra functionally relevant capillaries or changes in blood flow but rather that the endothelium dependent function of the existing microcirculatory network was improved by the direct effect of ergocalciferol.

This hypothesis is supported by the results of parallel *in vitro* experiments in which ergocalciferol, in a dose dependent manner, upregulated eNOS expression measured by RT-PCR. Nitric oxide generation compared to vehicle was numerically but not statistically significantly increased with low dose ergocalciferol but was significantly increased with high dose ergocalciferol. This suggests that higher doses of ergocalciferol are required to increase the functional effect of ergocalciferol on the endothelium and therefore that there may be a threshold 25 (OH) D concentration

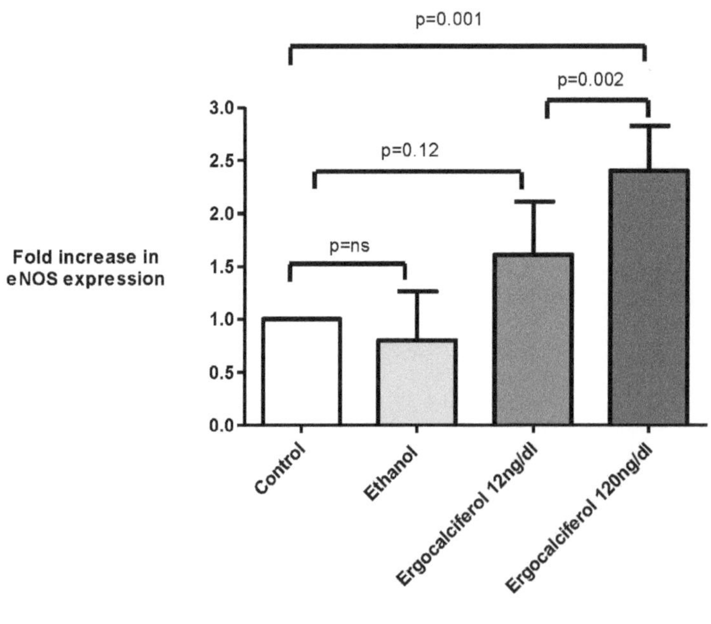

eNOS – endothelial nitric oxide synthase

Figure 5. Fold increase in eNOS expression by RT-PCR in cultured HAEC.

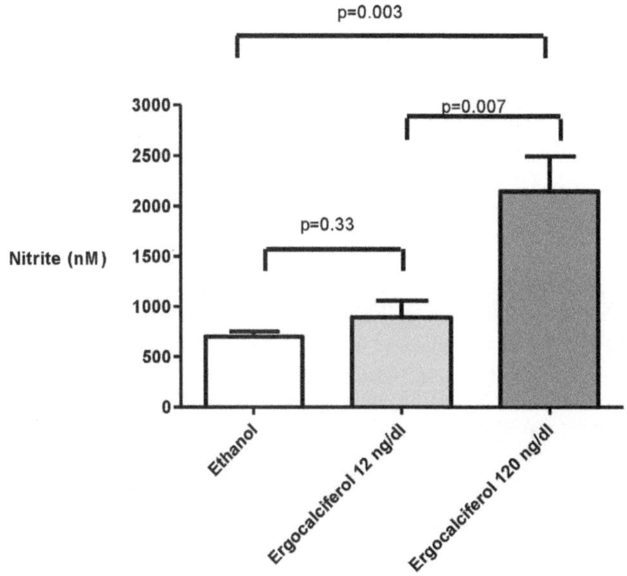

Figure 6. Nitrite levels in supernatants of HAEC. Cultured in low dose (12 ng/dl) and high dose (120 ng/dl) ergocalciferol after 24 h incubation.

above which the maximum effects of ergocalciferol on the microcirculation are achieved.

The present study is the first of its kind to explore the effect of vitamin D on microcirculatory function in patients with CKD and concomitant vitamin D deficiency. The exclusion of patients with diabetes mellitus allowed us to evaluate the effect of ergocalciferol on the microcirculation in CKD without the potentially confounding effect of diabetes on endothelial function.

Prospective studies of the effect of vitamin D therapy in patients with CKD have so far failed to show a beneficial effect of vitamin D on endpoints including LVMI, aPWV, blood pressure and inflammatory biomarkers. [27,47] The effect of nutritional vitamin D compounds on endothelial biomarkers and conduit artery endothelial function in kidney disease has been evaluated in two studies which have produced conflicting results. Marckmann *et al.* [27] compared the effect of 8 weeks of 40,000 IU of weekly cholecalciferol compared to a placebo in patients with both CKD and ESKD treated with haemodialysis. Patients in the control and intervention group were similar at baseline including cause of kidney disease, dialysis status and serum 25 (OH) D, 1,25 $(OH)_2$ D_3 and bone mineral parameters (PTH, Ca, PO_4) levels. There was a significant increase in 25 (OH) D levels in the treatment compared to control group (154.7 nmol/L vs 23.5 nmol/L) and a significant increase in 1,25 $(OH)_2$ D_3 levels although the increase in 1,25 $(OH)_2$ D_3 levels was higher in non-dialysis compared to dialysis requiring CKD (median increase in the CKD group 49 pmol/L ($p<0.01$) compared to 14 pmol/L in the dialysis group ($p>0.05$)). After 8 weeks of treatment, PTH fell significantly in non-dialysis CKD patients but not in dialysis requiring CKD patients. Despite the significant increase in vitamin D levels in the cholecalciferol group, there was no reduction in markers of endothelial dysfunction including D-dimer, von Willebrand factor, fibrinogen and interleukin (IL) 8 or C reactive protein. Additionally, blood pressure, aPWV and aortic augmentation index did not change between the two groups. Specifically, there were no significant differential effects on these parameters when comparing cholecalciferol treated and untreated patients in the dialysis and non-dialysis groups.

Assimon *et al.* [26] have evaluated the effect of ergocalciferol ($n = 20$ on ergocalciferol for a mean of 39.2 weeks and $n = 20$ not receiving ergocalciferol) on markers of vascular endothelial adhesion in a case control study of 40 patients undergoing maintenance haemodialysis. There were no significant differences in baseline parameters including dialysis vintage and both groups were receiving an equivalent dose of doxercalciferol. Serum 25 (OH) D levels were higher in the ergocalciferol group (90.8 nmol/L compared to 60.2 nmol/L, $p = 0.03$). In the ergocalciferol group, there was reduction in levels of vascular adhesion molecules sVCAM-1, sICAM-1, P-selectin and in all patients there was a significant negative correlation between serum 25 (OH) D levels and P-selectin and E-selectin. There was no difference in inflammatory biomarkers including IL-6 and TNF-α. However, the functional response of the endothelium was not evaluated and the case control design of this study means that the causal relationship between endothelial adhesion molecules and ergocalciferol cannot be established.

Despite the prompt and sustained rise in 25 (OH) D levels in our patients, significant differences in key microcirculatory end points were only observed after 6 months of therapy with ergocalciferol even though 25 (OH) D levels were similar at 1,3 and 6 months. Previous clinical studies using high dose ergocalciferol or cholecalciferol in healthy and diabetic patients without significant kidney disease demonstrated improved microcirculatory function between 8–12 weeks [24,25,48]. The delay in attainment of significantly improved microvascular function in the current study and lack of improvement over 8 weeks in Marckmann *et al.* study [27] may be a consequence of the uraemic milieu reducing the response of the microcirculation both to the upregulation of eNOS [49] and its downstream effects [50] in increasing availability of vasodilator moieties.

The findings from our study suggest that treatment with high dose ergocalciferol over an extended period of time is required before there is an improvement in microcirculatory endothelial function. This concept will have important implications for determining both the optimum duration of therapy of ergocalciferol and the optimum serum 25 (OH) D level to ensure a maximally beneficial effect on the microcirculation.

The strengths of our study are its double blind randomised placebo control design, replacement of vitamin D in line with international guidelines [37] that was standardised for all patients and commensurate with baseline serum concentrations of 25 (OH) D as well as the use of techniques that specifically assessed both conduit artery and microcirculatory endothelial function. At the time of designing this study, microcirculatory endothelial function had not previously been evaluated in patients with CKD and concomitant VDD in a clinical trial setting. Iontophoresis has been used in the setting of clinical trials to evaluate endothelial function. [51,52,53,54] The experimental conditions and iontophoretic protocol in the present study were standardised and changes in endothelial function were compared with baseline prior to treatment with ergocalciferol. The use of a low current iontophoresis protocol will have reduced the direct galvanic effect from the iontophoretic process on the endothelium seen when a higher current is used. [41] Therefore, any change seen in LDF after iontophoresis must be due to the direct effect of ergocalciferol itself on microvascular endothelial function.

Limitations of this study include the short follow up time and small sample size. The study duration is insufficient to detect significant differences between treatment groups in key outcome measures including CV events. Excluding patients with diabetes mellitus has limited the external validity but improved the internal validity and precision of the present study. Human aortic endothelial cells were not cultured in media consistent with the degree of CKD in the clinical trial subjects due to the complexity of establishing a culture medium that accurately reflects the earlier rather than more advanced stages of CKD. Consequently, the results from the *in vitro* experiments cannot be directly generalised to the uraemic milieu associated with CKD stage 3–4. The current study did not assess the effect of ergocalciferol on endothelial progenitor cells which are important mediators of endothelial repair and function and are reduced in patients at high risk of CVD [55]. Additional studies are required to address the effect of ergocalciferol on endothelial cells cultured in a medium more representative of the earlier stages of CKD as well as the effect of ergocalciferol on EPC number and function in CKD stage 3–4.

Conclusions

High dose ergocalciferol therapy over 6 months improved microcirculatory function and reduced tissue oxidative stress in patients with CKD stage 3–4 and concomitant vitamin D deficiency. *In vitro* studies suggest this effect is mediated through increased expression of eNOS and greater generation of nitric oxide. The primary endpoint of the study reflects global vascular health [14] and it is therefore logical to consider that the observed improvements in microcirculatory function will translate into improved clinical outcomes including a reduction in CV events.

To test this hypothesis, studies in patients with CKD and concomitant vitamin D deficiency with longer follow up and adequately powered to detect CV end points are now required to determine both if improved microcirculatory endothelial function through ergocalciferol therapy subsequently reduces CV endpoints and to determine the optimum serum level of 25 (OH) D to maximize microvascular endothelial function.

Supporting Information

Figure S1 Examples of iontophoresis dose response curves after 6 months of treatment for 2 patients after delivery of ACh demonstrating greater relative increase from baseline in flux in the ergocalciferol compared to placebo treated patient. Flux measured in arbitrary units (AU). Epoch reflects sequential dose increments of the iontophoretic protocol.

Figure S2 Percentage rise in flux from baseline after iontophoresis of ACh in patients with hypertension. Absolute values of percentage change in flux (AU): baseline - ergocalciferol 505.9, placebo 889.2 (p = NS). 1 month - ergocalciferol 853.5, placebo 1051.0 (p = NS). 3 months – ergocalciferol 519.2, placebo 1103.0 (p = NS). 6 months – ergocalciferol 671.6, placebo 1024.0 (p = NS). p values are Bonferroni post test following two way repeated measures ANOVA.

Figure S3 Percentage rise in flux from baseline after iontophoresis of SNP in patients with hypertension. Absolute values of percentage change in flux (AU): baseline - ergocalciferol 339.7, placebo 675.1 (p = NS). 1 month - ergocalciferol 866.9, placebo 724.0 (p = NS). 3 months – ergocalciferol 573.2, placebo 735.0 (p = NS). 6 months – ergocalciferol 682.2, placebo 579.0 (p = NS). p values are Bonferroni post test following two way repeated measures ANOVA.

Figure S4 Percentage rise in flux from baseline after iontophoresis of ACh in patients with glomerulonephritis. Absolute values of percentage change in flux (AU): baseline - ergocalciferol 762.9, placebo 1220.0 (p = NS). 1 month - ergocalciferol 1141.0, placebo 483.8 (p = NS). 3 months – ergocalciferol 647.7, placebo 1023.0 (p = NS). 6 months – ergocalciferol 1086, placebo 661.8 (p = NS). p values are Bonferroni post test following two way repeated measures ANOVA.

Figure S5 Percentage rise in flux from baseline after iontophoresis of SNP in patients with glomerulonephritis. Absolute values of percentage change in flux (AU): baseline - ergocalciferol 794.2, placebo 637.4 (p = NS). 1 month - ergocalciferol 690.6, placebo 708.8 (p = NS). 3 months – ergocalciferol 455.6, placebo 830.8 (p = NS). 6 months – ergocalciferol 387.3, placebo 504.1 (p = NS). p values are Bonferroni post test following two way repeated measures ANOVA.

Protocol S1 Full study protocol.

Checklist S1 Study CONSORT check list.

File S1 Full methodology. Contains Table S1, full iontophoresis protocol.

Acknowledgments

We are grateful to Amanda Smith for helpful advice on scoring SDF videos, Mawdsley Brooks UK for assistance with importing of the ergocalciferol, Alex Farrel and Jeanette Hansen for advice about dispensing the study drug, Dr Mark Westwood for advice about cMRI imaging and Dr Alex Milsom for her assistance with measuring nitrite levels. We are grateful to Dr Mavuto Mukaka for statistical advice.

Author Contributions

Conceived and designed the experiments: GD AT SH RP MJR MMY. Performed the experiments: GD SH. Analyzed the data: GD MJR MMY. Contributed reagents/materials/analysis tools: ATT SH RP MMY. Wrote the paper: GD SH MJR MMY. Conceived the original hypothesis: GD MMY Designed and executed the study: GD MJR MMY Provided scientific advice and equipment for microvascular studies: ATT RP Contributed to and have reviewed the final manuscript: GD ATT SH RP MJR MMY.

References

1. Feehally J, Griffith KE, Lamb EJ, O'Donoghue DJ, Tomson CR (2008) Early detection of chronic kidney disease. BMJ 337: a1618.
2. Li YC, Kong J, Wei M, Chen ZF, Liu SQ, et al. (2002) 1,25-Dihydroxyvitamin D(3) is a negative endocrine regulator of the renin-angiotensin system. J Clin Invest 110: 229–238.
3. Muller K, Haahr PM, Diamant M, Rieneck K, Kharazmi A, et al. (1992) 1,25-Dihydroxyvitamin D3 inhibits cytokine production by human blood monocytes at the post-transcriptional level. Cytokine 4: 506–512.
4. de Boer IH, Ioannou GN, Kestenbaum B, Brunzell JD, Weiss NS (2007) 25-Hydroxyvitamin D levels and albuminuria in the Third National Health and Nutrition Examination Survey (NHANES III). Am J Kidney Dis 50: 69–77.
5. Blair D, Byham-Gray L, Lewis E, McCaffrey S (2008) Prevalence of vitamin D [25(OH)D] deficiency and effects of supplementation with ergocalciferol (vitamin D2) in stage 5 chronic kidney disease patients. J Ren Nutr 18: 375–382.
6. LaClair RE, Hellman RN, Karp SL, Kraus M, Ofner S, et al. (2005) Prevalence of calcidiol deficiency in CKD: a cross-sectional study across latitudes in the United States. Am J Kidney Dis 45: 1026–1033.
7. Pilz S, Iodice S, Zittermann A, Grant WB, Gandini S (2011) Vitamin D status and mortality risk in CKD: a meta-analysis of prospective studies. Am J Kidney Dis 58: 374–382.

8. de Boer IH, Katz R, Chonchol M, Ix JH, Sarnak MJ, et al. (2011) Serum 25-hydroxyvitamin D and change in estimated glomerular filtration rate. Clin J Am Soc Nephrol 6: 2141–2149.
9. de Boer IH, Kestenbaum B, Shoben AB, Michos ED, Sarnak MJ, et al. (2009) 25-hydroxyvitamin D levels inversely associate with risk for developing coronary artery calcification. J Am Soc Nephrol 20: 1805–1812.
10. Chitalia N, Recio-Mayoral A, Kaski JC, Banerjee D (2012) Vitamin D deficiency and endothelial dysfunction in non-dialysis chronic kidney disease patients. Atherosclerosis 220: 265–268.
11. Recio-Mayoral A, Banerjee D, Streather C, Kaski JC (2011) Endothelial dysfunction, inflammation and atherosclerosis in chronic kidney disease—a cross-sectional study of predialysis, dialysis and kidney-transplantation patients. Atherosclerosis 216: 446–451.
12. Tatematsu S, Wakino S, Kanda T, Homma K, Yoshioka K, et al. (2007) Role of nitric oxide-producing and -degrading pathways in coronary endothelial dysfunction in chronic kidney disease. J Am Soc Nephrol 18: 741–749.
13. Pannier B, Guerin AP, Marchais SJ, Metivier F, Safar ME, et al. (2000) Postischemic vasodilation, endothelial activation, and cardiovascular remodeling in end-stage renal disease. Kidney Int 57: 1091–1099.
14. Cohn JN, Quyyumi AA, Hollenberg NK, Jamerson KA (2004) Surrogate markers for cardiovascular disease: functional markers. Circulation 109: IV31–46.
15. Teng M, Wolf M, Ofsthun MN, Lazarus JM, Hernan MA, et al. (2005) Activated injectable vitamin D and hemodialysis survival: a historical cohort study. J Am Soc Nephrol 16: 1115–1125.
16. Andress DL (2006) Vitamin D in chronic kidney disease: a systemic role for selective vitamin D receptor activation. Kidney Int 69: 33–43.
17. Shoben AB, Rudser KD, de Boer IH, Young B, Kestenbaum B (2008) Association of oral calcitriol with improved survival in nondialyzed CKD. J Am Soc Nephrol 19: 1613–1619.
18. Tentori F, Hunt WC, Stidley CA, Rohrscheib MR, Bedrick EJ, et al. (2006) Mortality risk among hemodialysis patients receiving different vitamin D analogs. Kidney Int 70: 1858–1865.
19. Wolf M, Thadhani R (2007) Vitamin D in patients with renal failure: a summary of observational mortality studies and steps moving forward. J Steroid Biochem Mol Biol 103: 487–490.
20. Santoro D, Gitto L, Ferraro A, Satta E, Savica V, et al. (2011) Vitamin D status and mortality risk in patients with chronic kidney disease. Ren Fail 33: 184–191.
21. Talmor Y, Golan E, Benchetrit S, Bernheim J, Klein O, et al. (2008) Calcitriol blunts the deleterious impact of advanced glycation end products on endothelial cells. Am J Physiol Renal Physiol 294: F1059–1064.
22. Borges AC, Feres T, Vianna LM, Paiva TB (1999) Effect of cholecalciferol treatment on the relaxant responses of spontaneously hypertensive rat arteries to acetylcholine. Hypertension 34: 897–901.
23. Wong MS, Delansorne R, Man RY, Vanhoutte PM (2008) Vitamin D derivatives acutely reduce endothelium-dependent contractions in the aorta of the spontaneously hypertensive rat. Am J Physiol Heart Circ Physiol 295: H289–296.
24. Shab-Bidar S, Neyestani TR, Djazayery A, Eshraghian MR, Houshiarrad A, et al. (2011) Regular consumption of vitamin D-fortified yogurt drink (Doogh) improved endothelial biomarkers in subjects with type 2 diabetes: a randomized double-blind clinical trial. BMC Med 9: 125.
25. Sugden J DJ, Witham M, Morris A, Struthers A (2007) Vitamin D improves endothelial function in patients with Type 2 diabetes mellitus and low vitamin D levels. Diabetic Medicine 25: 320–325.
26. Assimon MM, Salenger PV, El-Fawal HA, Mason DL (2012) Nutritional vitamin D supplementation in haemodialysis: A potential vascular benefit? Nephrology (Carlton) 17: 237–242.
27. Marckmann P, Agerskov H, Thineshkumar S, Bladbjerg EM, Sidelmann JJ, et al. (2012) Randomized controlled trial of cholecalciferol supplementation in chronic kidney disease patients with hypovitaminosis D. Nephrol Dial Transplant.
28. Clough G, Cracowski JL (2012) Spotlight issue: Microcirculation-from a clinical perspective. Microcirculation 19: 1–4.
29. Pignocchino P, Conte MR, Scarnato S, Grande A (1994) [Study of cutaneous microcirculation using the laser-Doppler method in syndrome X]. Cardiologia 39: 193–197.
30. Economides PA, Caselli A, Zuo CS, Sparks C, Khaodhiar L, et al. (2004) Kidney oxygenation during water diuresis and endothelial function in patients with type 2 diabetes and subjects at risk to develop diabetes. Metabolism 53: 222–227.
31. Tur E, Yosipovitch G, Bar-On Y (1991) Skin reactive hyperemia in diabetic patients. A study by laser Doppler flowmetry. Diabetes Care 14: 958–962.
32. Jung F, Mrowietz C, Labarrere C, Schuler S, Park JW (2001) Primary cutaneous microangiopathy in heart recipients. Microvasc Res 62: 154–163.
33. Shamim-Uzzaman QA, Pfenninger D, Kehrer C, Chakrabarti A, Kacirotti N, et al. (2002) Altered cutaneous microvascular responses to reactive hyperaemia in coronary artery disease: a comparative study with conduit vessel responses. Clin Sci (Lond) 103: 267–273.
34. McIntyre C JS, Jefferies H (2008) Advances in the cardiovascular assessment of patients with chronic kidney disease. NDT Plus 6: 383–391.
35. de Boer IH, Kestenbaum B (2008) Vitamin D in chronic kidney disease: is the jury in? Kidney Int 74: 985–987.
36. Levey AS, Bosch JP, Lewis JB, Greene T, Rogers N, et al. (1999) A more accurate method to estimate glomerular filtration rate from serum creatinine: a new prediction equation. Modification of Diet in Renal Disease Study Group. Ann Intern Med 130: 461–470.
37. (2003) K/DOQI Clinical Practice Guidelines for Bone Metabolism and Disease in Chronic Kidney Disease. Am J Kidney Dis 42: S1–S201.
38. Cupisti A, Rossi M, Placidi S, Caprioli R, Morelli E, et al. (2000) Responses of the skin microcirculation to acetylcholine and to sodium nitroprusside in chronic uremic patients. Int J Clin Lab Res 30: 157–162.
39. Cupisti A, Rossi M, Placidi S, Fabbri A, Morelli E, et al. (2000) Responses of the skin microcirculation to acetylcholine in patients with essential hypertension and in normotensive patients with chronic renal failure. Nephron 85: 114–119.
40. Morris SJ, Shore AC, Tooke JE (1995) Responses of the skin microcirculation to acetylcholine and sodium nitroprusside in patients with NIDDM. Diabetologia 38: 1337–1344.
41. Droog EJ, Henricson J, Nilsson GE, Sjoberg F (2004) A protocol for iontophoresis of acetylcholine and sodium nitroprusside that minimises nonspecific vasodilatory effects. Microvasc Res 67: 197–202.
42. Gerrits EG, Smit AJ, Bilo HJ (2009) AGEs, autofluorescence and renal function. Nephrol Dial Transplant 24: 710–713.
43. De Backer D, Hollenberg S, Boerma C, Goedhart P, Buchele G, et al. (2007) How to evaluate the microcirculation: report of a round table conference. Crit Care 11: R101.
44. Ignarro LJ, Fukuto JM, Griscavage JM, Rogers NE, Byrns RE (1993) Oxidation of nitric oxide in aqueous solution to nitrite but not nitrate: comparison with enzymatically formed nitric oxide from L-arginine. Proc Natl Acad Sci U S A 90: 8103–8107.
45. de Zeeuw D, Agarwal R, Amdahl M, Audhya P, Coyne D, et al. (2010) Selective vitamin D receptor activation with paricalcitol for reduction of albuminuria in patients with type 2 diabetes (VITAL study): a randomised controlled trial. Lancet 376: 1543–1551.
46. Molina P, Gorriz JL, Molina MD, Peris A, Beltran S, et al. (2013) The effect of cholecalciferol for lowering albuminuria in chronic kidney disease: a prospective controlled study. Nephrol Dial Transplant.
47. Thadhani R, Appelbaum E, Pritchett Y, Chang Y, Wenger J, et al. (2012) Vitamin D therapy and cardiac structure and function in patients with chronic kidney disease: the PRIMO randomized controlled trial. JAMA 307: 674–684.
48. Tarcin O, Yavuz DG, Ozben B, Telli A, Ogunc AV, et al. (2009) Effect of vitamin D deficiency and replacement on endothelial function in asymptomatic subjects. J Clin Endocrinol Metab 94: 4023–4030.
49. Rashid G, Benchetrit S, Fishman D, Bernheim J (2004) Effect of advanced glycation end-products on gene expression and synthesis of TNF-alpha and endothelial nitric oxide synthase by endothelial cells. Kidney Int 66: 1099–1106.
50. Arese M, Strasly M, Ruva C, Costamagna C, Ghigo D, et al. (1995) Regulation of nitric oxide synthesis in uraemia. Nephrol Dial Transplant 10: 1386–1397.
51. Witham MD, Adams F, Kabir G, Kennedy G, Belch JJ, et al. (2013) Effect of short-term vitamin D supplementation on markers of vascular health in South Asian women living in the UK - A randomised controlled trial. Atherosclerosis 230: 293–299.
52. Hobbs DA, Goulding MG, Nguyen A, Malaver T, Walker CF, et al. (2013) Acute ingestion of beetroot bread increases endothelium-independent vasodilation and lowers diastolic blood pressure in healthy men: a randomized controlled trial. J Nutr 143: 1399–1405.
53. Tehrani S, Mobarrez F, Lins PE, Adamson U, Wallen HN, et al. (2013) Impaired endothelium-dependent skin microvascular function during high-dose atorvastatin treatment in patients with type 1 diabetes. Diab Vasc Dis Res 10: 483–488.
54. Kaiser SE, Sanjuliani AF, Estato V, Gomes MB, Tibirica E (2013) Anti-Hypertensive Treatment Improves Microvascular Rarefaction and Reactivity in Low-Risk Hypertensive Individuals. Microcirculation.
55. Pellegatta F, Bragheri M, Grigore L, Raselli S, Maggi FM, et al. (2006) In vitro isolation of circulating endothelial progenitor cells is related to the high density lipoprotein plasma levels. Int J Mol Med 17: 203–208.

4

Maternal Vitamin D Status and Infant Outcomes in Rural Vietnam: A Prospective Cohort Study

Sarah Hanieh[1], Tran T. Ha[2], Julie A. Simpson[3], Tran T. Thuy[2], Nguyen C. Khuong[4], Dang D. Thoang[4], Thach D. Tran[2,5], Tran Tuan[2], Jane Fisher[5], Beverley-Ann Biggs[1,6*]

1 Department of Medicine, Melbourne Academic Centre, University of Melbourne at the Doherty Institute, Parkville, Victoria, Australia, **2** Research and Training Centre for Community Development (RTCCD), Hanoi, Vietnam, **3** Centre for Epidemiology and Biostatistics, Melbourne School of Population and Global Health, University of Melbourne, Parkville, Victoria, Australia, **4** Provincial Centre of Preventive Medicine, Hanam, Hanam Province, Vietnam, **5** The Jean Hailes Research Unit, School of Public Health and Preventive Medicine, Monash University, Clayton, Victoria, Australia, **6** The Victorian Infectious Diseases Service, Royal Melbourne Hospital, Parkville, Victoria, Australia

Abstract

Objective: Vitamin D deficiency affects 1 billion people globally. It has an important role in bone homeostasis, brain development and modulation of the immune system and yet the impact of antenatal vitamin D deficiency on infant outcomes is poorly understood. We assessed the association of 25- hydroxyvitamin D levels (25-OHD) in late pregnancy and early infant growth and developmental outcomes in rural Vietnam.

Design and Methods: A prospective cohort study of 960 women who had previously participated in a double-blind cluster randomized controlled trial of antenatal micronutrient supplementation in rural Vietnam was undertaken. Maternal 25-OHD concentration was measured at 32 weeks gestation, and infants were followed until 6 months of age. Main outcome measures were cognitive, motor, socio-emotional and language scores using the Bayley Scales of Infant Development, 3rd edition, and infant length-for-age z scores at 6 months of age.

Results: 60% (582/960) of women had 25-OHD levels $<$75 nmol/L at 32 weeks gestation. Infants born to women with 25-OHD deficiency ($<$37.5 nmol/L) had reduced developmental language scores compared to those born to women who were vitamin D replete ($\geq$75 nmol/L) (Mean Difference (MD) -3.48, 95% Confidence Interval (CI) -5.67 to -1.28). For every 25 nmol increase in 25-OHD concentration in late pregnancy, infant length-for-age z scores at 6 months of age decreased by 0.08 (95% CI -0.15 to -0.02).

Conclusions: Low maternal 25- hydroxyvitamin D levels during late pregnancy are of concern in rural Vietnam, and are associated with reduced language developmental outcomes at 6 months of age. Our findings strengthen the evidence for giving vitamin D supplementation during pregnancy.

Editor: Thomas H. J. Burne, University of Queensland, Australia

Funding: The original randomised trial was funded through a grant from the National Health and Medical Research Council of Australia. (Grant Number 628751). The funders had no role in study design, data collection and analysis, decision to publish, or preparation of the manuscript.

Competing Interests: The authors have declared that no competing interests exist.

* Email: babiggs@unimelb.edu.au

Introduction

Vitamin D deficiency affects more than 1 billion people [1] and is now recognised as a major public health problem [2]. Important biological functions involving growth and developmental outcomes have been attributed to vitamin D, and deficiency during pregnancy may result in important health consequences for both mother and child [3,4,5].

Maternal vitamin D readily crosses the placenta, and maternal levels strongly correlate with infant vitamin D concentration at birth [6]. The major supply of vitamin D is through synthesis in the skin, following exposure to ultraviolet light. Dietary intake makes only a small contribution to vitamin D status [3,7].

Although the current recommended dietary intake of vitamin D during pregnancy ranges from 600 to 2000 international units (IU) per day [8], a standardised definition of vitamin D deficiency during pregnancy remains controversial [4,9,10,11]. A recent meta-analysis by Aghajafari et al.[12] categorised vitamin D insufficiency for pregnancy outcomes as serum 25-OHD concentration less than 75 nmol/L, and for vitamin D insufficiency for birth outcomes, as serum 25-OHD concentration less than 37.5 nmol/L [12]. Vitamin D supplementation for the prevention of pre-eclampsia and its complications during pregnancy was recently assessed by WHO and is currently not recommended [13,14].

Adverse maternal and neonatal outcomes have previously been described in association with antenatal vitamin D deficiency, including increased risk of pre-eclampsia, gestational diabetes, caesarean section, as well as low birth weight and small for gestational age infants [15,16,17,18,19]. Vitamin D is also thought to effect bone formation and density and modulation of the

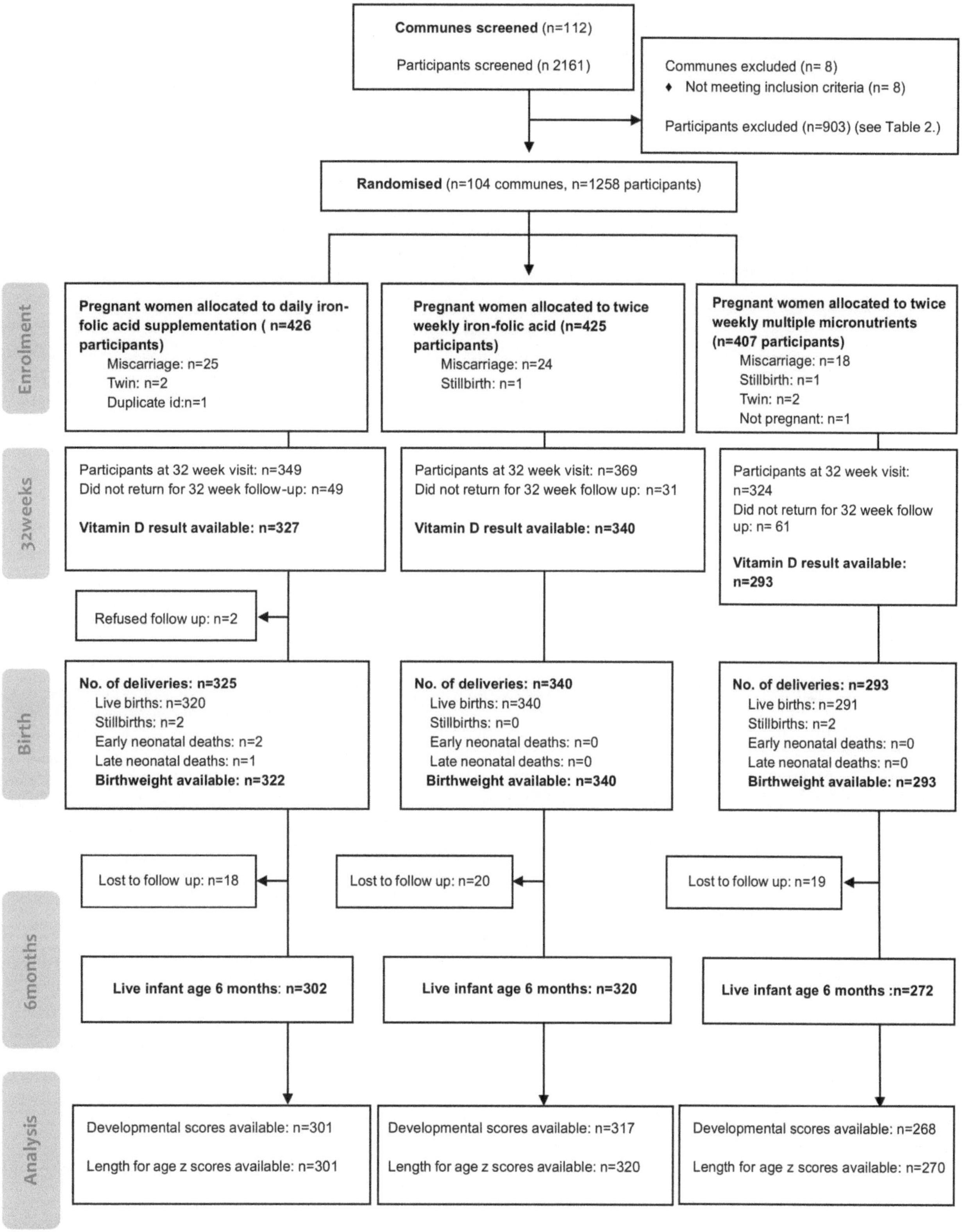

Figure 1. Flow diagram.

immune system [5,6,20,21,22,23]. More recently, maternal vitamin D deficiency has been associated with impaired infant language development in school-aged children [24], and has been suggested as a possible environmental risk factor for autism spectrum disorder, highlighting the important role of vitamin D in brain development, neuronal function and gene regulation [10,25,26].

Vitamin D insufficiency in Vietnam has previously been reported to be as high as 46% [27,28,29], however, there is limited data on the burden and consequences of vitamin D deficiency during pregnancy in this setting [17] and few studies have followed infants past the neonatal period. The role of vitamin D deficiency during pregnancy on longer term infant outcomes, particularly with regard to early childhood development is unclear.

We conducted a prospective cohort study, in a rural province representative of many areas of Vietnam, to determine the association of 25-OHD in late pregnancy with infant growth and developmental outcomes at 6 months of age. Our secondary objective was to determine whether maternal 25-OHD status was associated with infant birth outcomes.

Subjects and Methods

Study Design

This was an observational cohort study of 960 women who had previously participated in a double-blind cluster randomized controlled trial of antenatal micronutrient supplementation in rural Vietnam. Our main exposure of interest was maternal vitamin D concentration at 32 weeks gestation. Our primary outcomes of interest were infant cognitive, motor, socio-emotional and language scores using the Bayley Scales of Infant Development, 3rd Edition (BSID III), and infant length-for-age z scores at 6 months of age. Secondary outcomes were birth weight and risk of preterm delivery.

Study site and participants

The study was undertaken in Ha Nam province in northern Vietnam (latitude 20.2, climate zone- tropical) [30]. Ha Nam has a population of approximately 820,100 people, with most residents still working in subsistence agriculture. Diet consists mainly of rice, meat and vegetables. In 2010, the average annual per capita income was $USD 800 [31,32].

Participants were all women and infants previously enrolled in a cluster randomised trial, which took place between 28th September 2010 and 8th Jan 2012 (Australia New Zealand Clinical Trials Registry number: 12610000944033). For the original cluster randomised trial, women were randomised to receive either (1) one tablet of iron-folic acid (IFA) taken daily (60 mg elemental iron/0.4 mg folic acid per tablet, 7 tablets per week); (2) one capsule of IFA taken twice a week (60 mg elemental iron/1.5 mg folic acid per capsule; 2 capsules per week); or (3) one capsule of multiple micronutrients (MMN) taken twice a week (60 mg elemental iron/1.5 mg folic acid per capsule/plus zinc 20 mg, iodine 300 ug, copper 4 mg, selenium 130 ug, niacin 36 mg, folic acid 1.5 mg, Vitamins A 1.6 mg, B1 2.8 mg, B2 2.8 mg, B12 5.2 ug, C 140 mg, D 400 IU, E 20 mg;2 capsules per week.) [33].

Table 1. Screening, eligibility and enrolment, of trial participants.

Screened from Commune lists	**2161**
Not pregnant	13
Miscarried before enrollment	42
Complicated pregnancy/sickness	12
Over eligible gestational age (>16 weeks)	628
Absent at enrollment time	51
Migrated from province after screening	31
Eligible population	**1384**
Excluded at enrolment	
Work commitments, could not commit to trial protocol	90
Refused	36
Enrolled	**1258**

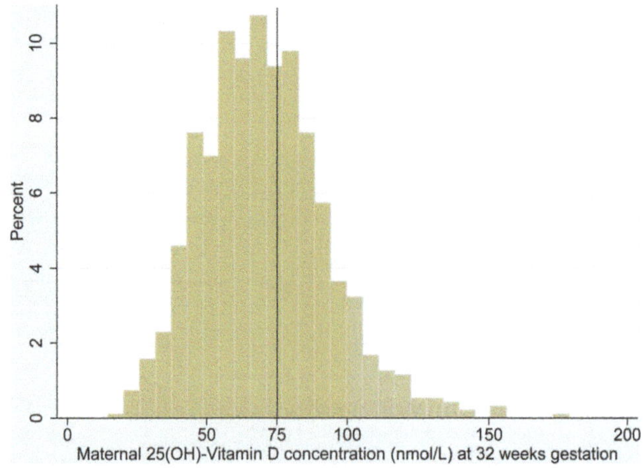

Figure 2. Maternal 25(OH)-Vitamin D concentration (nmol/L) at 32 weeks gestation.

The primary objective of the original trial was to compare the effect of twice weekly antenatal provision of a) iron-folic acid supplementation or b) multiple micronutrient supplementation with daily provision of antenatal iron-folic acid supplementation, on maternal and infant outcomes. Inclusion criteria were residence in trial communes; age >16 years, confirmed pregnancy <16 weeks gestation and registration with the commune health station. Women were excluded if they had a high-risk or multi-fetal pregnancy (confirmed on palpation or ultrasound); a significant medical condition; or if their haemoglobin concentration was <80 g/L at enrolment. In total 1258 women were enrolled into the original trial. Figure 1 summarizes the recruitment, randomization and participation of subjects in the trial. The results of this trial have been previously published [34].

Data collection and outcomes

This study was conducted between January 2011 and January 2012. Maternal serum 25-OHD was measured in women at 32 weeks gestation, and infant anthropometric and developmental measurements were performed at 6 months of age (Figure 1). Research staff who examined children at 6 months of age were blinded to maternal 25-OHD status.

Maternal characteristics

Maternal sociodemographic factors were assessed using a standardized questionnaire administered by trained research staff at enrolment. The questionnaire included information on demographics, maternal occupation, education, marital status and pregnancy history.

Birth outcomes

Gestational age at birth was calculated from estimated gestational age recorded by transabdominal ultrasound performed at the District Hospital if available, otherwise it was calculated according to the date of the last menstruation given at enrolment. Preterm delivery was defined as birth <37 weeks and low birth

Table 2. Distribution of baseline maternal sociodemographic, anthropometric characteristics, and maternal serum 25-OHD concentration (nmol/L) at 32 weeks gestation.

Maternal Characteristic	Number (%)	Mean maternal serum 25-OHD concentration nmol/L [SD]
Overall	960 (100)	70.5 [22.2]
Maternal age at enrolment (years)		
<20	37 (3.9)	70.2 [21.4]
20–24	298 (31)	72.3 [21.9]
25–29	400 (41.7)	69.1 [21.5]
30–34	152 (15.8)	69.5 [21.0]
≥35	73 (7.6)	72.6 [29.4]
Maternal height		
≥145 cm	930 (97.0)	70.3 [22.2]
<145 cm (short maternal stature)	29 (3.0)	75.8 [24.4]
Maternal body mass index		
Underweight (<18.5 kg/m^2)	251 (26.2)	70.7 [22.4]
Normal (18.5–25 kg/m^2)	655 (68.3)	69.8 [21.4]
Overweight (>25 kg/m^2)	53 (5.5)	77.4 [29.7]
Educational level		
Primary school	146 (15.2)	73.0 [23.5]
Secondary school	643 (67.0)	70.9 [22.3]
University/college	171 (17.8)	66.4 [20.2]
Occupation		
Farmer/housewife	509 (53.0)	74.1 [22.6]
Factory worker/trader	324 (33.8)	66.6 [22.1]
Government official/clerk	127 (13.2)	65.9 [18.4]
Gravidity		
Primigravida	296 (30.8)	67.7 [21.3]
Multigravida	664 (69.2)	71.7 [22.5]
Type of supplement taken during pregnancy		
Daily IFA supplements	327 (34.1)	67.8 [21.5]
Twice weekly IFA supplements	340 (35.4)	68.0 [21.5]
MMN supplements	293 (30.5)	76.3[23.8]

IFA = Iron folic acid, MMN = Multiple micronutrients, SD = Standard Deviation.

weight was defined as birth weight <2500 grams. Small for gestational age was calculated as weight below the 10th percentile for gestational age.

Infant Developmental Assessment

Measurement of infant development was performed at 6 months of age using BSID III [35]. Bayley Scales were translated in the Vietnamese language, however no questions were changed in terms of content. Questions were translated from English into Vietnamese and back-translated to English for verification. The instrument was previously pilot tested in Hanam province and found to be comprehensible and meaningful in rural Vietnam. BSID III administrators were community-based psychologists experienced in early child development assessment, and were trained by a local Vietnamese expert in BSID III following the guidelines of the BSID 3rd Edition Manual [35]. The BSID III was used to conduct direct infant developmental assessments for cognitive, language and motor domains, and rating of mothers determined the socio-emotional and adaptive behaviour scores. Individual raw scores for cognitive, language, motor, socio-emotional and adaptive behaviour were converted into composite scores based on the guidelines of the BSID 3rd Edition Manual, and used in the final analysis.

Anthropometric measurements

Maternal height was measured with a portable stadiometer (Seca 214, Hamburg, Germany), and maternal and infant weight with a mother-infant scale (Seca 872, Hamburg, Germany). Infant length was measured with a portable Shorr board (Shorr productions, USA). Infant length for age z scores were calculated using WHO Anthro (version 3.2.2, January 2011) [36]. Research staff recorded triplicate measurements of anthropometric measures, a second observer checked all measurements, and the median measurement was used for analysis. Stunting was defined as length-for-age z scores < two standard deviations below WHO growth standards. Body mass index (BMI) was calculated as weight in kilograms divided by height in metres squared [37].

Table 3. Birth outcomes associated with maternal serum 25-OHD concentration (nmol/L) at 32 weeks gestation (unadjusted and adjusted models).

		Unadjusted model		Adjusted model 1		Adjusted model 2	
Birth outcomes	**Mean [SD] or No.(%)**	**Mean difference[1,3] or Odds Ratio[2,3] (95% CI)**	**P value**	**Mean difference[1,4] or Odds Ratio[2,4] (95% CI)**	**P value**	**Mean difference[1,5] or Odds Ratio[2,5] (95% CI)**	**P value**
Birth weight (g)	3168.6 [392.3]	−11.9 (−40.0 to 16.3)	0.41	−21.0[1] (−51.2 to 9.3)	0.17	−18.9 (−49.0 to 11.3)	0.22
Birth length (cm)	49.1 [2.61]	−0.05 (−0.34 to 0.24)	0.73	−0.08[1] (−0.44 to 0.27)	0.64	−0.07 (−0.43 to 0.29)	0.70
Head circumference (cm)	32.7 [2.12]	−0.27 (−0.49 to −0.03)	**0.03**	−0.38[1] (−0.64 to −0.12)	**0.01**	−0.35 (−0.62 to −0.09)	**0.01**
Low birth weight (<2500 g)	27 (2.8%)	1.03 (0.67 to 1.59)	0.89	1.11[2] (0.77 to 1.61)	0.57	1.15 (0.74 to 1.80)	0.54
Gestational age (weeks)	39.2 [1.87]	0.07 (−0.06 to 0.20)	0.31	0.08 (−0.09 to 0.25)	0.38	0.07 (−0.10 to 0.24)	0.42
Preterm delivery (<37 weeks)	103 (10.7%)	0.78 (0.61 to 1.00)	0.054	0.60[2] (0.57 to 1.05)	0.09	0.77 (0.57 to 1.05)	0.09
Small for gestational age	50 (5.3)	1.24 (0.91 to 1.68)	0.17	1.33 (0.94 to 1.87)	0.11	1.37 (0.98 to 1.91)	0.07

[1]Values are estimated mean difference for each outcome associated with a 25 nmol/L increase in vitamin D concentration (95% confidence interval).
[2]Values are relative changes in the odds for each outcome associated with a 25 nmol/L increase in vitamin D concentration (95% confidence interval).
[3]Unadjusted model.
[4]Model adjusted for micronutrient intervention, maternal body mass index, gravidity, and clustering at commune level.
[5]Model adjusted for maternal age, education, month of sampling of maternal vitamin D, micronutrient intervention, maternal body mass index, gravidity, and clustering at commune level.
SD = standard deviation; CI = Confidence Interval.

Table 4. Developmental composite scores at 6 months of age associated with maternal serum 25-OHD concentration (nmol/L) at 32 weeks gestation.

		Unadjusted model		Adjusted model 1		Adjusted model 2	
Domain	**Mean developmental composite score [SD]**	**Mean difference[1,2] (95% CI)**	**P value**	**Mean difference[1,3] (95% CI)**	**P value**	**Mean difference [1,4] (95% CI)**	**P value**
Cognitive	104.5 [10.1]	−0.47 (−1.22 to 0.27)	0.21	−0.39 (−1.19 to 0.40)	0.30	−0.43 (−1.23 to 0.37	0.29
Language	97.8 [7.6]	−0.02 (−0.58 to 0.55)	0.96	0.04 (−0.51 to 0.59)	0.89	0.08 (−0.47 to 0.63)	0.77
Motor	110.9 [13.4]	0.03 (−0.97 to 1.03)	0.95	0.25 (−0.71 to 1.21)	0.61	0.05 (−0.92 to 0.64)	0.92
Socio-emotional	79.6 [9.8]	−0.12 (−0.85 to 0.61)	0.75	−0.06 (−0.81 to 0.70)	0.88	−0.14 (−0.92 to 0.64)	0.71

[1]Values are estimated mean difference for each outcome associated with a 25 nmol/l increase in vitamin.
D concentration (95% confidence interval).
[2]Unadjusted model.
[3]Model adjusted for micronutrient intervention, maternal education, and clustering.
[4]Model adjusted for maternal age, education, month of sampling of maternal vitamin D, micronutrient.
intervention, maternal body mass index, gravidity, post-partum depression and clustering at commune level.
SD = standard deviation, CI = Confidence Interval.

Table 5. Developmental composite scores in infants at 6 months of age according to maternal serum 25-OHD concentration levels at 32 weeks gestation.

	Unadjusted model					Adjusted model			
Domain	Vitamin D replete (≥75 nmol/L)	Vitamin D insufficient (≥37.5, <75 nmol/L)[1,2]	P value	Vitamin D deficient (<37.5 nmol/L)[1,2]	P value	Vitamin D insufficient (≥37.5, <75 nmol/L)[1,3]	P value	Vitamin D deficient (<37.5 nmol/L)[1,3]	P value
Cognitive	Reference	0.86 (−1.07 to 2.79)	0.38	−0.22 (−3.35 to 2.92)	0.89	0.58 (−1.24 to 2.40)	0.53	−0.44 (−3.21 to 2.33)	0.75
Language	Reference	1.14 (−0.31 to 2.58)	0.12	−3.14 (−5.49 to −0.79)	**0.01**	0.98 (−0.47 to 2.42)	0.18	−3.48 (−5.52 to −1.44)	**0.01**
Motor	Reference	0.11 (−2.46 to 2.69)	0.93	−0.49 (−4.68 to 3.71)	0.82	−0.27 (−2.76 to 2.23)	0.83	−0.57 (−5.21 to 4.07)	0.81
Socio-emotional	Reference	0.35 (−1.53 to 2.24)	0.71	−0.56 (−3.63 to 2.51)	0.72	0.14 (−0.1.56 to 1.85)	0.89	−0.45 (−3.7 to 2.8)	0.79

[1]Values are estimated mean difference (95% confidence interval).
[2]Unadjusted model.
[3]Model adjusted for maternal age, education, month of sampling of maternal vitamin D, micronutrient intervention, maternal body mass index, gravidity, maternal depression and clustering.

Vitamin D Analyses

Five mls of venous blood was collected from each pregnant woman at 32 weeks gestation, and one ml of venous blood was collected from each infant at 6 months of age. Serum samples were frozen at −20°C and transported to the Alfred Hospital, Melbourne, and analysis for vitamin D was performed on those with a sufficient volume of blood. Solid Phase Extraction (SPE) using Waters Oasis uElution SPE plates was used as a pre-treatment step to release 25-OHD binding protein. Extracted patient samples were then analysed using a WatersACQUITY UPLC with an ACQUITY BEH Phenyl column (2.1×50 mm) with a water/methanol/ammonium acetate gradient. A Waters TQD mass spectrometer was used to quantify 25-OHD2 and 25-OHD3. The coefficient of variation for 25-OHD3 was 9.9% at 42 nmol/L and 9.6% at 96 nmol/L. The coefficient of variation for 25-OHD2 was 12% at 42 nmol/L and 8.8% at 94 nmol/L. Vitamin D levels were categorized as replete (≥ 75 nmol/L), insufficient (≥37.5 nmol/and<75 nmol/L) or deficient (<37.5 nmol/L) [12]. (1 nmol/L 25-OHD = 0.4 ng/ml 25-OHD).

Ethics statement

The study was approved by the Melbourne Health Human Research Ethics Committee and the Hanam Provincial Human Research Ethics Committee. The original cluster randomised trial is registered in the Australia New Zealand Clinical Trials Registry: 12610000944033. Written informed consent was collected from all participants prior to enrolment and permission was obtained from the Ministry of Health to transport biological samples across an international border.

Statistical methods

Data were analysed using Stata, Version 12 (StataCorp, College Station, TX, USA). Categorical data are presented as percentages with frequency and continuous data are presented as mean and standard deviation (SD). Multivariable linear regression was performed to derive estimates of mean differences (95% confidence intervals (CI)) of the continuous outcome data (developmental composite scores of the infant at 6 months, gestational age and anthropometric measurements) associated with maternal vitamin D concentrations at 32 weeks, and multivariable logistic regression was used to assess the associations between maternal vitamin D concentrations and the binary outcomes (preterm delivery, low birth weight, small for gestational age and infant stunting). The association between maternal vitamin D concentrations and each of the outcome variables was assessed for linearity both visually and by comparing regression models with a categorized and pseudo-continuous form of maternal vitamin D concentrations (quintile groupings) using the likelihood ratio test. Confounders adjusted for in the multivariable regression analyses were determined a priori and included maternal age, education, gravidity, maternal body mass index (as a continuous variable), month of sampling of and micronutrient intervention. Maternal depression was also included in the analyses for infant developmental outcomes.

To account for clustering at the commune level, robust standard errors were calculated using the Huber-White Sandwich estimator. To further investigate the presence of a potential threshold effect of vitamin D concentration on infant developmental outcomes [24], secondary statistical analyses were performed on maternal vitamin D concentration categorized as deficient (<37.5 nmol/L), insufficient(≥37.5 nmol/L and <75 nmol/L) or replete (≥75 nmol/L). The level of statistical significance was 0.05.

Table 6. Infant anthropometric outcomes at 6 months of age associated with maternal serum 25-OHD concentration (nmol/L) at 32 weeks gestation.

		Unadjusted model		Adjusted model	
Infant anthropometric outcomes	**Mean [SD] or number(%)**	**Mean difference[1,3] or Odds Ratio[2,3] (95% CI)**	**P value**	**Mean difference[1,4] or Odds Ratio[2,4] (95% CI)**	**P value**
Length (cm)	66.0 [2.28]	−0.10 (−0.27 to 0.06)[1]	0.23	−0.11 (−0.26 to 0.05) [1]	0.19
Weight (kg)	7.71 [0.98]	−0.02 (−0.09 to 0.05) [1]	0.61	−0.03 (−0.10 to 0.04) [1]	0.45
Head circumference (cm)	42.6 [1.43]	0.003 (−0.10 to 0.11) [1]	0.95	−0.01 (−0.10 to 0.11) [1]	0.95
HAZ	−0.57 [0.91]	−0.09 (−0.15 to −0.02)[1]	**0.02**	−0.09 (−0.12 to −0.02)[1]	**0.02**
Stunted	55/891 (6.2)	0.92 (0.68 to 1.26) [2]	0.62	0.89 (0.59 to 1.32) [2]	0.52

[1]Values are estimated mean difference for each outcome associated with a 25 nmol/L increase in vitamin D.
concentration (95% confidence interval).
[2]Values are relative changes in the odds for each outcome associated with a 25 nmol/L increase in vitamin D concentration (95% confidence interval).
[3]Unadjusted model.
[4]Model adjusted for maternal age, education, month of sampling of maternal vitamin D, micronutrient intervention, maternal body mass index, gravidity, and clustering.

Results

The study profile is presented in Figure 1. A total of 2161 women were screened and 1258 pregnant women were enrolled into the original cluster randomised trial (Table 1). Serum 25-OHD results were available for 960 (92%) of the 1042 women who presented at the 32 week follow up visit. Baseline maternal sociodemographic and anthropometric characteristics are presented in Table 2. Sixty percent (582/960) of women had vitamin D concentrations less than 75 nmol/L in late pregnancy. Figure 2 shows the distribution of vitamin D concentration among pregnant women at 32 weeks gestation.

Maternal vitamin D and birth outcomes

Table 3 summarizes birth outcomes related to maternal vitamin D in late pregnancy. A trend towards an association with preterm delivery (Odds Ratio (OR) 0.77 per 25 nmol/L increase in vitamin D concentration, 95% CI 0.57 to 1.05) and small for gestational age (Odds Ratio (OR) 1.37 per 25 nmol/L increase in vitamin D concentration, 95% CI 0.98 to 1.91) was observed. For the 49.5% of infants with a measurement of head circumference, there was an inverse relationship between infant head circumference at birth and maternal 25-OHD (MD of −0.35 cm per 25 nmol/L increase in vitamin D concentration, 95% CI −0.62 to −0.09).

Maternal vitamin D concentration and infant development at 6 months of age

No association between overall maternal vitamin D concentration and developmental composite scores was observed (Table 4). However, lower language composite scores were seen in infants born to women with vitamin D deficiency (<37.5 nmol/L) compared to those born to women who were vitamin D replete (≥75 nmol/L) (MD −3.48, 95% CI −5.52 to −1.44) (Table 5).

Maternal vitamin D and anthropometric measurements at six months of age

An inverse association between maternal 25-OHD and infant length-for-age z scores at 6 months of age was demonstrated (MD −0.09 per 25 nmol/L increase in vitamin D concentration, 95% CI −0.12 to −0.02) (Table 6).

Discussion

These results indicate that there is a high prevalence of vitamin D insufficiency in pregnant women residing in rural Ha Nam Province, Vietnam. Our findings show that low vitamin D levels in late pregnancy (<37.5 nmol/L) are associated with reduced infant language development at six months of age.

An association between low maternal vitamin D concentration and language impairment has previously been suggested by Whitehouse et al. in a study involving a cohort of pregnant women and school-aged children in Australia. They reported that the risk of having a child with language difficulties at 5 and 10 years of age increased by two-fold in women with an antenatal vitamin D concentration ≤46 nmol/L [24]. In this study, vitamin D concentration was measured early, at 18 weeks gestation, and receptive language was assessed using the Peabody Picture Vocabulary Test. Gale et al., measured maternal vitamin D concentration during the third trimester and assessed infants using the Weschler Abbreviated Scale of Intelligence (n = 178), and found no association between maternal vitamin D levels and full scale, verbal or performance IQ at 9 years of age [38].

In our previous publication [34], no significant differences in infant language or developmental outcomes were observed in infants born to women who received twice weekly multiple micronutrients compared to those who received daily iron folic acid. Although vitamin D concentration was significantly higher in the twice weekly multiple micronutrient group compared to daily iron folic acid group, (mean [SD] of 76.3 [23.8] versus 67.8 [20.6] nmol/L), the prevalence of vitamin D deficiency (<37.5 nmol/L) was similar (4.9% (16/326) versus 3.1% (9/293). Our finding of an association between maternal vitamin D and infant language composite scores, that was only observed when maternal vitamin D levels fell below 37.5 nmol/L in late pregnancy, raises the possibility that there is a threshold effect, and that language impairment is a feature of more marked vitamin D deficiency. The observed association between antenatal vitamin D concentration and infant development is plausible as vitamin D has an important role in neurodevelopment through cell differentiation, cytokine regulation, neurotransmitter synthesis and anti-oxidant activity, and it is has been suggested that *in utero* exposure to vitamin D deficiency during the second and third trimesters may affect the development of the Perisylvian structures, which are responsible for language in children [24,39].

There has also been interest in the link between autism and vitamin D deficiency. Recent research suggests that vitamin D deficiency during pregnancy or early childhood may be an environmental trigger for autism spectrum disorder in infants genetically predisposed to autism, either through its effect on neuronal function and brain development, or through gene interaction and regulation. However larger, high quality trials are required [10,25,26].

We observed an inverse relationship between length-for-age z scores at 6 months of age and overall maternal vitamin D concentration, although the estimated magnitude of change associated with an increase in vitamin D of 25 nmol/L was small. Several studies have found an association between maternal vitamin D status and post-natal growth, but results are inconsistent and the majority are observational studies that have been carried out in developed countries. Previous authors have suggested that accelerated growth in length may occur during an infant's first year of life in infants born to mothers with vitamin D <30 nmol/L, as infant vitamin D levels increase postnatally, through post-natal vitamin D supplementation [5]. Other studies have shown no differences in weight or height across quartiles of vitamin D status during infancy [40].

We found increasing maternal vitamin D concentration showed a trend towards a reduced risk of preterm delivery. A positive association between maternal vitamin D concentration and gestational duration has previously been described [41,42], and Morley et al. [43] demonstrated a significantly shorter gestation (0.7 weeks) among women with 25-OHD <28 nmol/L living in Australia, compared to those with higher levels. A pooled analyses of two previous studies [17] showed no significant link between vitamin D supplementation and preterm delivery, however the two studies had small sample sizes (350 and 180 participants) [4,44], with relatively large loss to follow up (30%). One potential explanation for the association with preterm birth, is an increased risk of vaginal infection with low antenatal Vitamin D concentration, as bacterial vaginosis is a known risk factor for preterm birth. The association between vitamin D concentration and vaginal infection has previously been described by several authors [45,46,47].

We found no association between vitamin D deficiency and infant birth weight, low birth weight and birth length. This is in keeping with a Cochrane review of data from three trials showing that vitamin D supplementation during pregnancy did not affect birth weight or birth length [13]. An inverse association between birth head circumference and maternal vitamin D was observed, however this finding did not persist at 6 months of age. This result needs to be interpreted with caution, as head circumference at birth was recorded in less than half the infants. These findings are in contrast to Aghajafari et al. [12] who assessed the effect of 25-OHD levels on pregnancy outcomes and birth variables in a systematic review of four studies, and found no significant difference in head circumference in infants born to women with 25-OHD concentrations less than 37.5 nmol/L during pregnancy. Our findings need to be interpreted with caution, as head circumference at birth was recorded in less than half the infants. Further exploration is required.

There are no standardised definitions for vitamin D thresholds in pregnancy (deficiency, insufficiency and sufficiency), however a recent meta-analysis defined insufficiency for pregnancy outcomes as less than 75 vnmol/L, and insufficiency for birth variables as less than 37.5 nmol/L [12]. The reported prevalence and definitions of vitamin D insufficiency/deficiency in Vietnamese women has varied in previous studies, ranging from 7% to 46% [27,28,29]. In our trial, even though the majority of women worked as farmers, we observed a very high prevalence (60%) of women with vitamin D levels less than 75 nmol/L. This is likely to be the result of cultural influences, with the common use of face masks and long sleeved gloves, and the perception that white skin is 'attractive', leading to restricted exposure to sunlight [28]. Some authors have also suggested that the cut off for sufficient vitamin D levels during pregnancy should be as high as 100–150 nmo/L [10,11], and therefore the problem of vitamin D deficiency in Vietnam and other South East Asian countries may be even more widespread than previously thought.

To our knowledge, our study is the largest and most comprehensive study on maternal vitamin D status to be conducted in Vietnam. Our study was conducted in a rapidly developing rural area, which is representative of many other areas of Vietnam. The large sample size and rigorous trial design of the original cluster randomised controlled trial also allowed us to follow the cohort of infants past the neonatal period into infancy, to document important growth and developmental outcomes within the first 6 months of life.

A limitation of our study was that we investigated several outcome measures and therefore the evidence against the null hypothesis observed for language development may be due to Type I error. However, similar findings in previous studies [24,38,41,42,43] and the increasing evidence for vitamin D deficiency as a potential environmental risk factor for autism [10,25,26] suggest that these associations should not be discounted. The differences we observed were also of magnitudes of clinical importance; thus further exploration in larger cohorts, preferably in non-western settings, is indicated.

Conclusions

Our study indicates that low levels of vitamin D during pregnancy are of concern in rural Vietnam, and are associated with impaired language development at 6 months of age. Our results strengthen the evidence for giving vitamin D supplementation during pregnancy and highlight the need for further research to explore the impact of supplementation on longer term child growth and developmental outcomes, particularly with regard to language.

Acknowledgments

We thank the participants and health workers in Hanam province, the Hanam Provincial Centre of Preventive Medicine, Ministry of Health, RTCCD; Alfred Pathology; Beth Hilton-Thorp, and Christalla Hajisava.

Author Contributions

Conceived and designed the experiments: SH BB JF T. Tuan JAS. Performed the experiments: TTH TTT NCK. Analyzed the data: SH TTT JAS. Contributed reagents/materials/analysis tools: DT T. Tuan T. Tran. Wrote the paper: SH BB.

References

1. Holick MF (2011) Vitamin D: evolutionary, physiological and health perspectives. Curr Drug Targets 12: 4–18.
2. Mithal A, Wahl DA, Bonjour JP, Burckhardt P, Dawson-Hughes B, et al. (2009) Global vitamin D status and determinants of hypovitaminosis D. Osteoporos Int 20: 1807–1820.

3. Wagner CL, Taylor SN, Dawodu A, Johnson DD, Hollis BW (2012) Vitamin D and its role during pregnancy in attaining optimal health of mother and fetus. Nutrients 4: 208–230.
4. Yu CK, Sykes L, Sethi M, Teoh TG, Robinson S (2009) Vitamin D deficiency and supplementation during pregnancy. Clin Endocrinol (Oxf) 70: 685–690.
5. Leffelaar ER, Vrijkotte TG, van Eijsden M (2010) Maternal early pregnancy vitamin D status in relation to fetal and neonatal growth: results of the multi-ethnic Amsterdam Born Children and their Development cohort. Br J Nutr 104: 108–117.
6. Greer FR (2008) 25-Hydroxyvitamin D: functional outcomes in infants and young children. Am J Clin Nutr 88: 529S–533S.
7. Lips P (2010) Worldwide status of vitamin D nutrition. J Steroid Biochem Mol Biol 121: 297–300.
8. Institute of Medicine (2010) Dietary Reference Intakes for Calcium and Vitamin D. Washington DC: National Academy Press.
9. Dror DK, Allen LH (2010) Vitamin D inadequacy in pregnancy: biology, outcomes, and interventions. Nutr Rev 68: 465–477.
10. Grant WB, Cannell JJ (2013) Autism prevalence in the United States with respect to solar UV-B doses: An ecological study. Dermatoendocrinol 5: 159–64.
11. Hollis BW, Wagner CL (2011) Vitamin D requirements and supplementation during pregnancy. Curr Opin Endocrinol Diabetes Obes 18: 371–375.
12. Aghajafari F, Nagulesapillai T, Ronksley PE, Tough SC, O'Beirne M, et al. (2013) Association between maternal serum 25-hydroxyvitamin D level and pregnancy and neonatal outcomes: systematic review and meta-analysis of observational studies. BMJ 346: f1169.
13. De-Regil LM, Palacios C, Ansary A, Kulier R, Pena-Rosas JP (2012) Vitamin D supplementation for women during pregnancy. Cochrane Database Syst Rev 2: CD008873.
14. WHO (2012) Vitamin D supplementation during pregnancy for the prevention and treatment of pre-eclampsia and eclampsia. Available: http://www.who.int/elena/titles/vitamind_pregnancy/en/. Accessed Jan 2013.
15. Dror DK (2011) Vitamin D status during pregnancy: maternal, fetal, and postnatal outcomes. Curr Opin Obstet Gynecol 23: 422–426.
16. Soheilykhah S, Mojibian M, Rashidi M, Rahimi-Saghand S, Jafari F (2010) Maternal vitamin D status in gestational diabetes mellitus. Nutr Clin Pract 25: 524–527.
17. Thorne-Lyman A, Fawzi WW (2012) Vitamin D during pregnancy and maternal, neonatal and infant health outcomes: a systematic review and meta-analysis. Paediatr Perinat Epidemiol 26 Suppl 1: 75–90.
18. Bodnar LM, Catov JM, Simhan HN, Holick MF, Powers RW, et al. (2007) Maternal vitamin D deficiency increases the risk of preeclampsia. J Clin Endocrinol Metab 92: 3517–3522.
19. Merewood A, Mehta SD, Chen TC, Bauchner H, Holick MF (2009) Association between vitamin D deficiency and primary cesarean section. J Clin Endocrinol Metab 94: 940–945.
20. Javaid MK, Crozier SR, Harvey NC, Gale CR, Dennison EM, et al. (2006) Maternal vitamin D status during pregnancy and childhood bone mass at age 9 years: a longitudinal study. Lancet 367: 36–43.
21. Pawley N, Bishop NJ (2004) Prenatal and infant predictors of bone health: the influence of vitamin D. Am J Clin Nutr 80: 1748S–1751S.
22. Mullins RJ, Camargo CA Jr (2011) Shining a light on vitamin D and its impact on the developing immune system. Clin Exp Allergy 41: 766–768.
23. Camargo CA, Jr., Ingham T, Wickens K, Thadhani R, Silvers KM, et al. (2011) Cord-blood 25-hydroxyvitamin D levels and risk of respiratory infection, wheezing, and asthma. Pediatrics 127: e180–187.
24. Whitehouse AJ, Holt BJ, Serralha M, Holt PG, Kusel MM, et al. (2012) Maternal serum vitamin D levels during pregnancy and offspring neurocognitive development. Pediatrics 129: 485–493.
25. Kocovska E, Fernell E, Billstedt E, Minnis H, Gillberg C (2012) Vitamin D and autism: clinical review. Res Dev Disabil 33: 1541–1550.
26. Mostafa GA, Al-Ayadhi LY (2012) Reduced serum concentrations of 25-hydroxy vitamin D in children with autism: relation to autoimmunity. J Neuroinflammation 9: 201.
27. Ho-Pham LT, Nguyen ND, Lai TQ, Eisman JA, Nguyen TV (2011) Vitamin D status and parathyroid hormone in a urban population in Vietnam. Osteoporos Int 22: 241–248.
28. Nguyen HT, von Schoultz B, Nguyen TV, Dzung DN, Duc PT, et al. (2012) Vitamin D deficiency in northern Vietnam: Prevalence, risk factors and associations with bone mineral density. Bone 51: 1029–1034.
29. Hien VT, Lam NT, Skeaff CM, Todd J, McLean JM, et al. (2012) Vitamin D status of pregnant and non-pregnant women of reproductive age living in Hanoi City and the Hai Duong province of Vietnam. Matern Child Nutr 8: 533–539.
30. Ha Nam Vietnam, Satellite View. Available: http://www.satelliteviews.net/cgi-bin/w.cgi?c = vm&UF = -3714931&UN = -4937507&AF = P_H. Accessed March 2013.
31. Viet Nam Academy of Social Science (2006) Vietnam poverty update: poverty and poverty reduction in Vietnam 1993–2004. Hanoi: Viet Nam Academy of Social Science.
32. General Statistics Office of Vietnam (2011) Statistical year book of Vietnam. Hanoi: Statistical Publishing House.
33. UNICEF/WHO/UNU (1999) Composition of a Multi-Micronutrient Supplement to be used in Pilot Programmes among Pregnant Women in Developing Countries. Report of a UNICEF/WHO/UNU Workshop. New York: United Nations Children's Fund.
34. Hanieh S, Ha TT, Simpson JA, Casey GJ, Khuong NC, et al. (2013) The effect of intermittent antenatal iron supplementation on maternal and infant outcomes in rural Viet Nam: a cluster randomised trial. PLoS Med 10(6): e1001470. doi:10.1371/journal.pmed.1001470.
35. Bayley N. (2006) Bayley Scales of Infant and Toddler Development–Third Edition. San Antonio: TX: Harcourt Assessment Bayley N (2006) Bayley Scales of Infant and Toddler Development.: PsychCorp.
36. WHO (2011) WHO Anthro, version 3.2.2 [computer program]. Geneva: World Health Organization.
37. WHO (2012) The WHO Child Growth Standards. Geneva: World Health Organization.
38. Gale CR, Robinson SM, Harvey NC, Javaid MK, Jiang B, et al. (2008) Maternal vitamin D status during pregnancy and child outcomes. Eur J Clin Nutr 62: 68–77.
39. Webster RI, Shevell MI (2004) Neurobiology of specific language impairment. J Child Neurol 19: 471–481.
40. Prentice A, Jarjou LM, Goldberg GR, Bennett J, Cole TJ, et al. (2009) Maternal plasma 25-hydroxyvitamin D concentration and birthweight, growth and bone mineral accretion of Gambian infants. Acta Paediatr 98: 1360–1362.
41. Shibata M, Suzuki A, Sekiya T, Sekiguchi S, Asano S, et al. (2011) High prevalence of hypovitaminosis D in pregnant Japanese women with threatened premature delivery. J Bone Miner Metab 29: 615–620.
42. Dawodu A, Nath R (2011) High prevalence of moderately severe vitamin D deficiency in preterm infants. Pediatr Int 53: 207–210.
43. Morley R, Carlin JB, Pasco JA, Wark JD (2006) Maternal 25-hydroxyvitamin D and parathyroid hormone concentrations and offspring birth size. J Clin Endocrinol Metab 91: 906–912.
44. Hollis BW, Johnson D, Hulsey TC, Ebeling M, Wagner CL (2011) Vitamin D supplementation during pregnancy: double-blind, randomized clinical trial of safety and effectiveness. J Bone Miner Res 26: 2341–2357.
45. Bodnar LM, Krohn MA, Simhan HN (2009) Maternal vitamin D deficiency is associated with bacterial vaginosis in the first trimester of pregnancy. J Nutr 139: 1157–1161.
46. Hensel KJ, Randis TM, Gelber SE, Ratner AJ (2011) Pregnancy-specific association of vitamin D deficiency and bacterial vaginosis. Am J Obstet Gynecol 204: 41 e41–49.
47. Davis LM, Chang SC, Mancini J, Nathanson MS, Witter FR, et al. (2010) Vitamin D insufficiency is prevalent among pregnant African American adolescents. J Pediatr Adolesc Gynecol 23: 45–52.

5

Mechanisms Involving Ang II and MAPK/ERK1/2 Signaling Pathways Underlie Cardiac and Renal Alterations during Chronic Undernutrition

Paulo A. Silva[1,2]⁹, Gustavo Monnerat-Cahli[1,2]⁹, Amaury Pereira-Acácio[1,2], Ricardo Luzardo[1,2], Luzia S. Sampaio[1,2], Marcia A. Luna-Leite[1], Lucienne S. Lara[2,3], Marcelo Einicker-Lamas[1,2], Rogério Panizzutti[2,3], Caroline Madeira[2,3], Leucio D. Vieira-Filho[2,4], Carmen Castro-Chaves[2,4], Valdilene S. Ribeiro[2,4], Ana D. O. Paixão[2,4], Emiliano Medei[1,2], Adalberto Vieyra[1,2]*

1 Carlos Chagas Filho Institute of Biophysics, Federal University of Rio de Janeiro, Rio de Janeiro, Brazil, **2** National Institute of Science and Technology for Structural Biology and Bioimaging, Rio de Janeiro, Brazil, **3** Institute of Biomedical Sciences, Federal University of Rio de Janeiro, Rio de Janeiro, Brazil, **4** Department of Physiology and Pharmacology, Federal University of Pernambuco, Recife, Brazil

Abstract

Background: Several studies have correlated protein restriction associated with other nutritional deficiencies with the development of cardiovascular and renal diseases. The driving hypothesis for this study was that Ang II signaling pathways in the heart and kidney are affected by chronic protein, mineral and vitamin restriction.

Methodology/Principal Findings: Wistar rats aged 90 days were fed from weaning with either a control or a deficient diet that mimics those used in impoverished regions worldwide. Such restriction simultaneously increased ouabain-insensitive Na^+-ATPase and decreased (Na^++K^+)ATPase activity in the same proportion in cardiomyocytes and proximal tubule cells. Type 1 angiotensin II receptor (AT_1R) was downregulated by that restriction in both organs, whereas AT_2R decreased only in the kidney. The PKC/PKA ratio increased in both tissues and returned to normal values in rats receiving Losartan daily from weaning. Inhibition of the MAPK pathway restored Na^+-ATPase activity in both organs. The undernourished rats presented expanded plasma volume, increased heart rate, cardiac hypertrophy, and elevated systolic pressure, which also returned to control levels with Losartan. Such restriction led to electrical cardiac remodeling represented by prolonged ventricular repolarization parameters, induced triggered activity, early after-depolarization and delayed after-depolarization, which were also prevented by Losartan.

Conclusion/Significance: The mechanisms responsible for these alterations are underpinned by an imbalance in the PKC- and PKA-mediated pathways, with participation of angiotensin receptors and by activation of the MAPK/ERK1/2 pathway. These cellular and molecular alterations culminate in cardiac electric remodeling and in the onset of hypertension in adulthood.

Editor: Krisztian Stadler, Pennington Biomedical Research Center, United States of America

Funding: This work was funded by the Brazilian National Research Council (grants 302513/2008-6 to A.V., 474712/2010-9 to E.M., and 470740/2010/8 to A.D.P.), the Carlos Chagas Filho Rio de Janeiro State Research Foundation (grant E-26/102.764/2008 to A.V.), the Pernambuco State Research Foundation (grant IBPG-1228-2.07/08 to A.D.O.P.), the Ministry of Science and Technology/CNPq-Department of Science and Technology/Ministry of Health (grant 552162/2005-1 to A.V.), the Brazilian Federal Agency for Support and Evaluation of Graduate Education (grant 00852NF), and the National Institute of Science and Technology for Structural Biology and Bioimaging (grant 573767/2008-4), Brazil. The funders had no role in study design, data collection and analysis, decision to publish, or preparation of the manuscript.

Competing Interests: The authors have declared that no competing interests exist.

* Email: avieyra@biof.ufrj.br

⁹ These authors contributed equally to this work.

Introduction

Chronic undernutrition (with severe protein restriction) is a worldwide public health problem, especially in developing countries [1], where young people are particularly vulnerable to the consequences of food restriction, including the development of different diseases in later life (adulthood) [2]. Some developmental changes lead to the onset of hypertension [3], heart disease [4], and kidney disease [5].

Many experimental studies designed to elucidate the mechanisms by which chronic undernutrition provokes functional and morphological alterations in various human systems – including cardiac and renal Na^+ transport systems – have focused on the prenatal and lactation periods [6–8]. However, chronic undernutrition provoked by protein restriction associated with other dietary deficiencies is not confined to early life; it is a widespread lifelong condition frequently imposed from conception, persisting through growth and development into adult life [9].

The cardiovascular system and the kidneys are special targets of protein restriction (for classical reports concerning clinical and experimental data see refs. [10], [11]). As an example of combined vascular and renal alterations, early studies demonstrated that an isocaloric-hypoproteic diet in rats led to hemodynamic alterations, in which increased afferent and efferent arteriolar resistance was responsible for a decline in both glomerular filtration rate and renal blood flow [12]. In humans, some epidemiological studies have indicated a low incidence of hypertension under conditions of chronic undernutrition [13], [14]; but the opposite trend was found in other studies [15]. These differences could be ascribed to the differing proportions of nutrients in deficient diets.

Common mechanisms seem to underlie cardiovascular and renal alterations, including those that share common modifications in the reactivity and participation of the systemic and local renin angiotensin system (RAS). Cardiovascular and renal changes occurring over short periods of protein restriction in adult rats correlate with altered responsiveness to angiotensin II (Ang II) [10], [16], but no studies seem to have focused on the relationships among different transport/signaling systems that are crucial for cardiac and renal functions.

The driving hypothesis for the present work was that Ang II-signaling pathways linked to Na^+ pumps in heart and kidney are affected by chronic administration of a low-protein multideficient diet, promoting electric cardiac remodeling and other renovascular alterations, which could culminate in the onset of hypertension. To test the hypothesis that angiotensin II type 1 receptors (AT_1R) are involved in the cardiorenal alterations, we analyzed the effect of simultaneous administration of the receptor blocker Losartan (Los). We used a diet prepared according to data from food consumption surveys in different geographic zones of Northeast Brazil (the Basic Regional Diet/BRD) [17]. This diet mimics other deficient diets that are consumed in many parts of the world.

Materials and Methods

Ethical considerations

All experimental procedures were approved by the Committee for Ethics in Animal Experimentation of the Federal University of Rio de Janeiro (protocol N° IBCCF 104), and were carried out in accordance with the Committee's guidelines, which follow the Uniform Requirements for Manuscripts Submitted to Biomedical Journals.

Animals and experimental groups

The experimental groups consisted of male Wistar rats (Biocampo and Fiocruz) that were kept at 23±2°C in a 12 h/12 h light/dark cycle. The animals were divided into four groups: (i) control (CTR) rats, with free access to standard chow (Purina Agribands) and water from weaning (21 days after birth) to 90 days of age; (ii) rats chronically subjected to the basic regional diet (BRD), with free access to the deficient diet and water from weaning to 90 days of age; (iii) CTR Los, control rats receiving Los (Merck) by gavage (30 mg/kg body mass) from weaning (21 days after birth) to 90 days of age; and (iv) BRD Los, BRD rats receiving the same treatment with Los. Several series of successive breedings using 3-month old female rats (~250 g) and male rats in a 3:1 ratio gave the number of pups from different litters required for isolation of adequate membrane preparations, and for the *in vivo* experiments (chronic administration of the AT_1 receptor antagonist, Los, measurement of plasma volume, arterial pressure and heart recording, food and water intake assessment, blood collection for plasma amino acid analyses). The female pups were humanely killed by decapitation in accordance with the guidelines mentioned above. All series gave consistent biochemical/immunochemical results with no differences within the same class of experiment. Litter effects were avoided by randomly assigning male offspring from the same litters to the four conditions to which they were subjected after weaning.

Number of animals

At the start, the number of rats in a typical experimental set was 10–15 for the CTR and CTR Los groups, and 20–25 for the BRD and BRD Los groups. The larger number of initially undernourished rats compared with the normonourished groups was due to the shorter lifespan of the former (at 90 days of age) (some rats from the undernourished groups do not live 90 days). These runs were repeated 4 times. For the *in vivo* experiments, the number of rats from each group (see the corresponding figure legends) includes animals from the different runs. For arterial pressure measurements, the number of rats in each group ($n = 7$) corresponds to recordings obtained in 6 animals from 3 different litters (2 for each) and 1 animal (from 1 run), due to the special conditions required to obtain accurate readings quickly and in the same time of the day (between 02:00 and 06:00 pm).

Five rats from the CTR and CTR Los groups and 7 rats from the BRD and BRD Los groups were used to isolate the plasma membranes from cardiomyocytes and proximal tubule cells, and to obtain pooled membrane preparations for the *in vitro* experiments. The number of pooled samples ranged from 5 to 7. Due to the limited amount of protein and the wide variation in the experiments, a larger number of experiments were carried out when the determinations showed high variability, as in the case of PKA. The number of membrane preparations used in each class of experiment is given in the corresponding figure and table legends. For the electrophysiological studies, small fragments of the left ventricle were removed isolated from different rats prior homogenization of the rest of the organ.

Diets

The deficient diet contained the following ingredients (g/g%): beans, 18.3; manioc flour, 64.8; jerked meat, 3.7; and sweet potatoes, 12.8 [17]. The ingredients were cooked, dehydrated at 60°C and pulverized. This diet provides the following percentage composition (g/g%): protein, 8; carbohydrate, 69; lipid, 0.8; Na^+, 0.2; fiber, 8. Besides the lower percent, the diet is deficient in the quality of proteins, since >90% is provided by beans and <10% by meat. Even though the adequacy of energy supply is slightly higher (~316 kcal/100 g dry weight) than the control diet (~280 kcal/100 g), only a small fraction is provided by fats, corresponding to ~1% of the dry mass in contrast to ~9% in the control diet. Most of the calories come from carbohydrates (sweet potatoes and manioc flour). BRD has only ~30% of the total mineral salts present in the control diet, with important differences regarding its specific components. Ca^{2+} (0.04 g/g%), K^+ (0.3 g/g%), and iron (0.007 g/g%) contents are much below those in the control diet (1.8, 0.9 and 0.018, respectively) [18]. Na^+ oscillates in the control range (0.2–0.4 g/g% according to repeated measurements in samples taken at random). Several vitamins (ascorbic acid, retinol, biotin, thiamin, riboflavin, niacin, para-aminobenzoic acid, pyridoxine, inositol, cyanocobalamine, choline) are extremely low, as previously calculated by Teodósio et al. [17] from the vitamin content of the components of BRD [19]. The nutrient contents in the control diet (regular chow diet from Purina Agriband) were (g/g%): protein, 23; carbohydrate, 50; lipid, 9; and Na^+, 0.3, which gives a total of 280 kcal/100 g dry weight. This was supplemented with vitamins to meet AIN-93G requirements [20], whereas the deficient diet was not supplemented.

Plasma volume, systolic arterial pressure, heart rate and plasma amino acids, determinations

Plasma volume, arterial pressure and heart rate were assessed at 90 days. Plasma volume was assessed using Evans Blue Dye. After the rats had been anesthetized with pentobarbital (60 mg/kg), a femoral artery was catheterized and a 1 ml basal blood sample was collected. Evans Blue dye (Sigma-Aldrich; 0.1% in 150 mM NaCl) was then administered (100 µg/100 g body weight) through the catheter. The catheter was filled with physiological saline to push all the injected dye into the animal. After 7.5 min, the NaCl solution inside the catheter was discarded and 1 ml of blood was collected in a heparinized syringe. The concentration of the Evans Blue dye was measured spectrophotometrically at 610 nm and compared to a standard curve obtained with known dilutions of the dye in the basal plasma (before dye injection).

Systolic arterial pressure and heart rate were measured using the tail cuff method, which allows repeated and reliable non-invasive measurements to be made over a short period in conscious animals [21], [22]. A Letica LE 5000 pletismograph was used (Panlab). Animals from different litters (see above) were acclimated by placing them for 10–15 min each day for a week in the chamber at 30–32°C before taking recorded measurements. On the day of measurements, the rats were held for 10 min to carefully checked that they had stopped moving before starting the recording. If any movement was detected, another attempt was made after a further 10 min period. Three successive determinations were made for each animal and the procedure was repeated on 3 consecutive days. A typical data acquisition lasted ~30 min. Two criteria were used to assess that the readings were correct: (i) the intra-assay coefficient of variation among the 3 different determinations, which were always <5% (ranging from 2.3 for CTR to 3.4% for BRD); (ii) the stability of heart rhythm after the 10 min preparation period.

Blood samples for determining plasma amino acids were collected at 85 days of age and EDTA was added. After separation of the cells by centrifugation, the plasma was analyzed by high performance liquid chromatography (HPLC) as described in [23], [24].

Food and water intake

Food and water intake was assessed in metabolic cages, as previously described [22], [25].

ECG and action potentials recording

Electrocardiograms were recorded from anesthetized animals (Xylazine and Ketamine, 15 and 80 mg/kg ip, respectively). Electrodes were positioned in DI derivation and connected by flexible cables to a differential AC amplifier (model 1700, A-M Systems), with signals low-pass filtered at 1 kHz and digitized at a 2–10 kHz sample rate by a 16-bit A/D converter (Minidigi 1-D, Axon Instruments) using Axoscope 9.0 software (Axon Instruments). Data were stored in a PC for offline processing.

Both right and left endocardial ventricle preparations were used to assess the action potential profile [26]. Muscle strips (approximately 0.5 cm×0.5 cm×0.1 cm) were obtained and pinned in order to expose the endocardial side above the bottom of a tissue bath. The preparations were superfused with an oxygenated (95% O_2, 5% CO_2) Tyrode's solution containing (in mM) 150.8 NaCl, 5.4 KCl, 1.8 $CaCl_2$, 1.0 $MgCl_2$, 11.0 D-glucose, 10.0 HEPES (pH 7.4 adjusted with NaOH at 37±0.5°C) at a flow of 5 ml/min (Gilson Miniplus 3). The tissue was stimulated at four different basic cycle lengths (BCL) (1000, 800, 500 and 300 ms) using field stimulation. The transmembrane potential was recorded using glass microelectrodes (10–40 MΩ DC resistance) filled with 2.7 M KCl connected to a high input impedance microelectrode amplifier (MEZ7200, Nihon Kohden). Amplified signals were digitized (1440 digidata A/D interface and Axotape software, Axon Instrument, Inc.) and stored in a personal computer for later analysis using the software Clampfit 10.2 (Axon Instrument, Inc.). The following action potential parameters were analyzed: resting membrane potential (RMP), action potential amplitude (APA) and action potential duration at 90% (APD_{90}), 50% (APD_{50}) and 30% (APD_{30}) repolarization. The Maximum Negative Slope (MaxNeg-Slope) was calculated by the steepest downhill slope starting 5 ms after the peak using a linear regression during a window of 4 ms. The AP triangulation was calculated by subtracting APD_{40} from APD_{90}. To assess the presence of arrhythmic events, a 10 beat train pulse followed by a pause was applied at three different BCLs (200, 150 and 100 ms).

Isolation of cardiomyocyte plasma membranes

Plasma membranes from cardiomyocytes were prepared by differential centrifugation as in [27].The hearts were removed together with the kidneys after decapitation of the rats at 90 days of age, placed on ice and carefully dissected to obtain the left ventricle and the septum, which were first minced into small fragments to obtain, with slight modifications, a membrane preparation that was previously shown to be adequate for assays of (Na^++K^+)ATPase activity with ^{3}H-ouabain and immunoassays for (Na^++K^+)ATPase [27]. Briefly, the fragments obtained from 5–7 hearts from each experimental group (see "number of animals" above) were suspended in an isotonic solution containing 250 mM sucrose, 1 mM imidazole (pH adjusted to 7.6 with Tris) and 1 mM EDTA to obtain pooled preparations. These were mechanically homogenized at 4°C using a Potter Elvejhem homogenizer fitted with a Teflon pestle (five periods of 1 min at 1,700 rpm). The preparation was centrifuged at 1,669×*g* and the resulting supernatant was centrifuged again at 115,000×*g*; the final sediment was suspended in 250 mM sucrose and stored under liquid N_2. Five to 7 pooled cardiac membrane preparations were thus obtained for biochemical determinations (see below). The protein concentration was measured by the Folin method [28]. The small pieces of left ventricle taken for electrophysiological measurements were homogenized and used immediately.

Isolation of proximal tubule cell membranes

Plasma membranes from proximal tubule cells were also prepared by differential centrifugation as in [29]. The kidneys were placed in an isotonic solution containing 250 mM sucrose, 10 mM Hepes-Tris (pH 7.4), 2 mM EDTA and 0.15 mg/ml trypsin inhibitor type II-S (Sigma-Aldrich) (1 g tissue/4 ml solution). Membranes from different rats (see "number of animals" above) were prepared from the outer region of the cortex (*cortex corticis*) as described elsewhere [30], where the predominant cell population is proximal tubule cells [31]. Controls for enrichment with basolateral membranes (3–4 fold with respect to the total homogenate using (Na^++K^+)ATPase as a marker) and for minimal residual contamination with intracellular membranes and cytosol were as described in [29], [30]. No attempt at further enrichment was made in this case, as the (Na^++K^+)ATPase and the ouabain-resistant Na^+-ATPase are exclusively located in the basolateral membranes of epithelial cells [32], and a low yield of purified basolateral membranes was obtained using the Percoll gradient method with the minimum number of animals recommended by the Committee for Ethics in Animal Experimentation. The plasma membrane fraction was stored under liquid N_2. The protein concentration was also measured by the Folin reagent method [28].

Measurement of ouabain-insensitive Na^+-ATPase and of (Na^++K^+)ATPase activities

Ouabain-resistant, furosemide-sensitive Na^+-ATPase and (Na^++K^+)ATPase activities were measured as in [8], [22]. Ouabain-resistant, furosemide-sensitive Na^+-ATPase activity was measured as the difference in $^{32}P_i$ released from (γ-^{32}P)ATP in the absence and presence of 2 mM furosemide (Sigma-Aldrich) (with 2 mM ouabain throughout), as described elsewhere [8], [22], [30]. (γ-^{32}P)ATP was prepared as per Maia et al. [33], using radioactive orthophosphate ($^{32}P_i$) purchased from the São Paulo Institute of Nuclear and Energetic Research. The cardiac and renal membranes (0.2 mg protein/ml) were also preincubated with ouabain for 10 min at 37°C in a medium containing 20 mM Hepes-Tris (pH 7.0), 10 mM $MgCl_2$ and 120 mM NaCl. The reaction was started by adding (γ-^{32}P)ATP (5 mM, specific activity ~1 μCi/μmol; final concentration). After 10 min at 37°C, the reaction was stopped with charcoal. The released $^{32}P_i$ was quantified by liquid scintillation counting in an aliquot of the supernatant obtained after centrifugation of the charcoal suspension (1,500×*g* for 5 min).

(Na^++K^+)ATPase activity was determined by measuring P_i release from ATP (Sigma-Aldrich) in the absence or presence of 2 mM ouabain (Sigma-Aldrich) as previously described [8], [22], [30]. The cardiac or renal membranes (0.05 mg protein/ml) were preincubated with ouabain for 10 min at 37°C in a medium containing 50 mM Bis-Tris-propane (pH 7.4), 0.2 mM EDTA, 5 mM $MgCl_2$ and 120 mM NaCl. The reaction was started by adding a mixture of KCl and ATP (20 and 5 mM, respectively; final concentrations), and stopped after 10 min with 2 volumes of activated charcoal in 0.1 M HCl. The released P_i was quantified colorimetrically [34].

To investigate the possible involvement of the MAPK/ERK pathway in modulating the ouabain-insensitive Na^+-ATPase activity in cardiac and renal membranes of undernourished rats, a series of assays were performed as above using 30 μM PD098059 (InvivoGen), a selective inhibitor of MAPK [35], to prevent phosphorylation of ERK1/2. The membranes were preincubated with the inhibitor for 10 min before addition of ATP.

SDS-PAGE and immunoblotting

SDS-PAGE and imunoblotting for AT_1R, AT_2R, ERK1 and phospho-ERK1/2 were carried out as in [8], [36] using the specific antibodies. Briefly, the proteins of renal proximal tubule cells and cardiomyocytes were separated on 10% SDS-PAGE [37] and transferred to nitrocellulose membranes. Non-specific binding was prevented by incubating the membranes with 5% non-fat milk in Tris-buffered NaCl (TBS, pH 7.6) for 1 h. The membranes were probed with the corresponding primary antibodies against: AT_1R or AT_2R (1:500, Santa Cruz Biotechnology in both cases); ERK1 (1:1,000) or phospho-ERK1/2 (1:500) (Cell Signaling in both cases); β-actin (1:5,000, Sigma-Aldrich) for 1 h at room temperature with gentle stirring. Then, they were washed three times with TBS containing 0.1% Tween 20 (TBS-T), exposed to the secondary fluorescent antibodies (anti-rabbit, Li-Cor, IRDye 680RD, 1:20,000 for AT_1R, AT_2R, ERK1 and phospho-ERK1/2; anti-mouse, Li-Cor, IRDye 800CW, 1:20,000 for β-actin),and washed again. Immunoreactivity was detected using the Odyssey system (Li-Cor) for infrared imaging recording, and the band intensities quantified using Scion Image software. The β-actin immunosignal from the corresponding lane was used to normalize the immunosignals of AT_1R, AT_2R, ERK1 and p-ERK1/2 for protein loading. Duplicates for each analyzed protein – from heart or kidney membranes – corresponding to the four experimental conditions (CTR, BRD, CTR Los and BRD Los) were analyzed in the same gel, and the results were expressed as a percentage of the corresponding CTR value (taken as 100%). Each of these assays was repeated using different preparations (see "n" values in the corresponding figure legends). The Scion Image software was used to quantify the band intensities. In preliminary experiments, the nitrocellulose membranes were stained with *Ponceau Red* to assess protein loading.

Herrera et al. [38] demonstrated that several anti-Ang II receptors antibodies available from commercial sources display nonspecific binding in kidney and in other tissues. In the present work, the specificities of the primary antibodies against AT_1R and AT_2R were confirmed in the present study by preadsorption experiments using a matrix of human Ang II type 2 receptor recombinant full-length protein (amino acids 1–363, ab157871, Abcam), as in [39] for the anti-renin antibody. A three-fold mass of the immunizing peptide was incubated with the antibodies: (i) sc1173 Santa Cruz, anti-AT_1R raised against a peptide mapping an N-terminal extracellular domain of AT_1R (human); or (ii) sc-9040 Santa Cruz, anti-AT_2R raised against amino acids 221–363 of AT_2R (human). After centrifugation and dilution of the supernatants (1:500), immunostaining demonstrated the presence of the AT_1R band in renal membranes using the AT_1R-containing solution, whereas no signal appeared when the AT_2R-containing solution was used (Figure 1). These antibodies against AT_1R and AT_2R were those used in the immunoassays described above.

Protein kinase C (PKC) and cyclic AMP-dependent protein kinase (PKA) activities

The activities of PKC and PKA were measured as in [8], [36].The activities of PKC and PKA associated with the isolated membranes of renal and cardiac origin were measured by

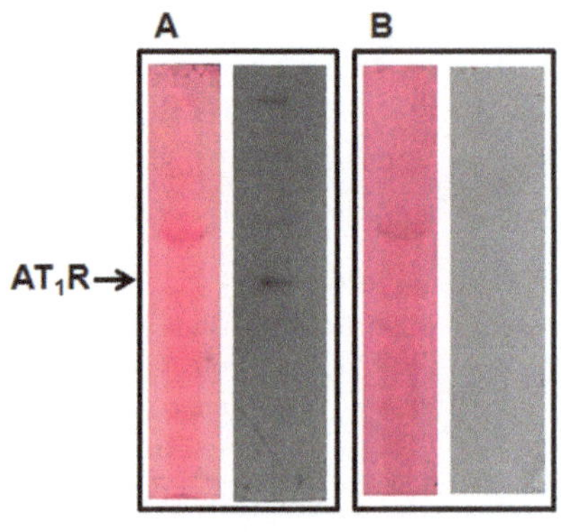

Figure 1. Specificity of the Ang II receptor antibodies. Electrophoresis of renal membranes was carried out as described in the Materials and Methods section, using 80 μg of total protein. The specificity of the antibodies was confirmed by a preadsorption experiment using full-length human Ang II type 2 receptor recombinant protein as a matrix. The samples were incubated for 72 h at 4°C with gentle stirring and then centrifuged at 18,000×*g* for 1 min. The secondary antibody was a polyclonal anti-rabbit (NIF824, GE; 1:2,500). See additional details in the Materials and Methods section. A: Ponceau red-stained nitrocellulose membrane (left) and immunosignal obtained after incubation of the AT_1R antibody with the full-length AT_2R recombinant protein (right). B: Ponceau red-stained nitrocellulose membrane (left) with no signal when the AT_2R antibody was preadsorbed on to the full-length AT_2R recombinant protein (right).

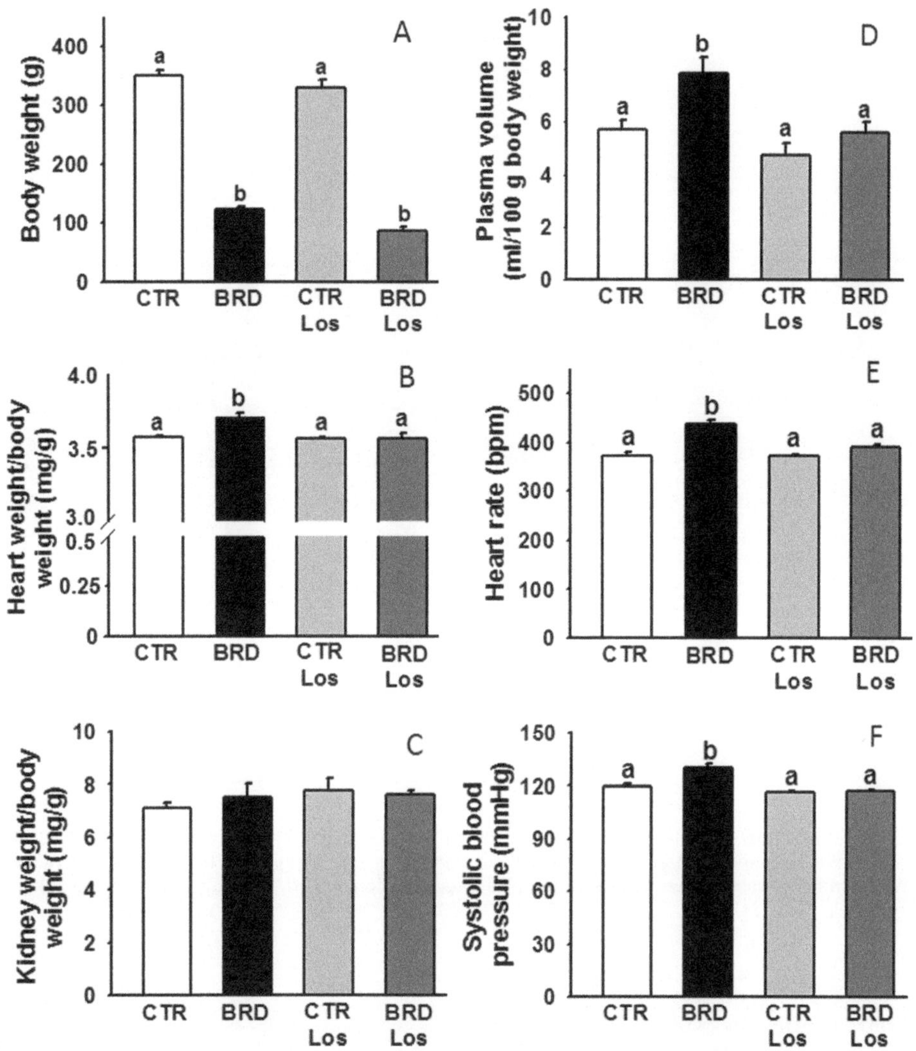

Figure 2. Alterations in body weight, cardiac index and renal index (A–C), and expanded plasma volume, accelerated heart rate and increased systolic pressure (D–F), in rats subjected to protein restriction (aged 90 days). The animal groups were: control (CTR); fed with the deficient diet after weaning (BRD); control receiving Losartan (CTR Los); and BRD receiving Losartan (BRD Los) (A–C, n = 7; D, n = 13 in CTR and CTR Los groups; n = 5 in BRD and BRD Los groups; E, n = 23 in CTR and CTR Los groups; n = 8 in BRD and BRD Los groups; F, n = 7 in all groups). Histograms show mean ± SEM. Different lower-case letters above the bars indicate statistically significant differences in mean values within the corresponding panel ($P<0.05$).

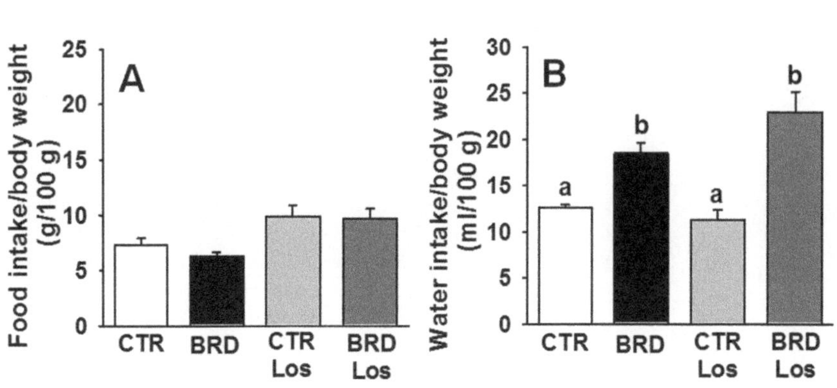

Figure 3. Food and water intake. Food and water ingestion was recorded one day before sacrifice at 90 days of age at the end of a 24 h period. The animal groups were those described in the legend to Figure 2. The rats were maintained in individual metabolic cages in the same conditions of light and temperature described in the Methods section of the main text. Simultaneous recording of body weight at the end of the period allowed correction of the data, as shown on the *abscissae*. Different lowercase letters above the bars indicate statistically different mean values in panel B ($P< 0.05$; n = 5).

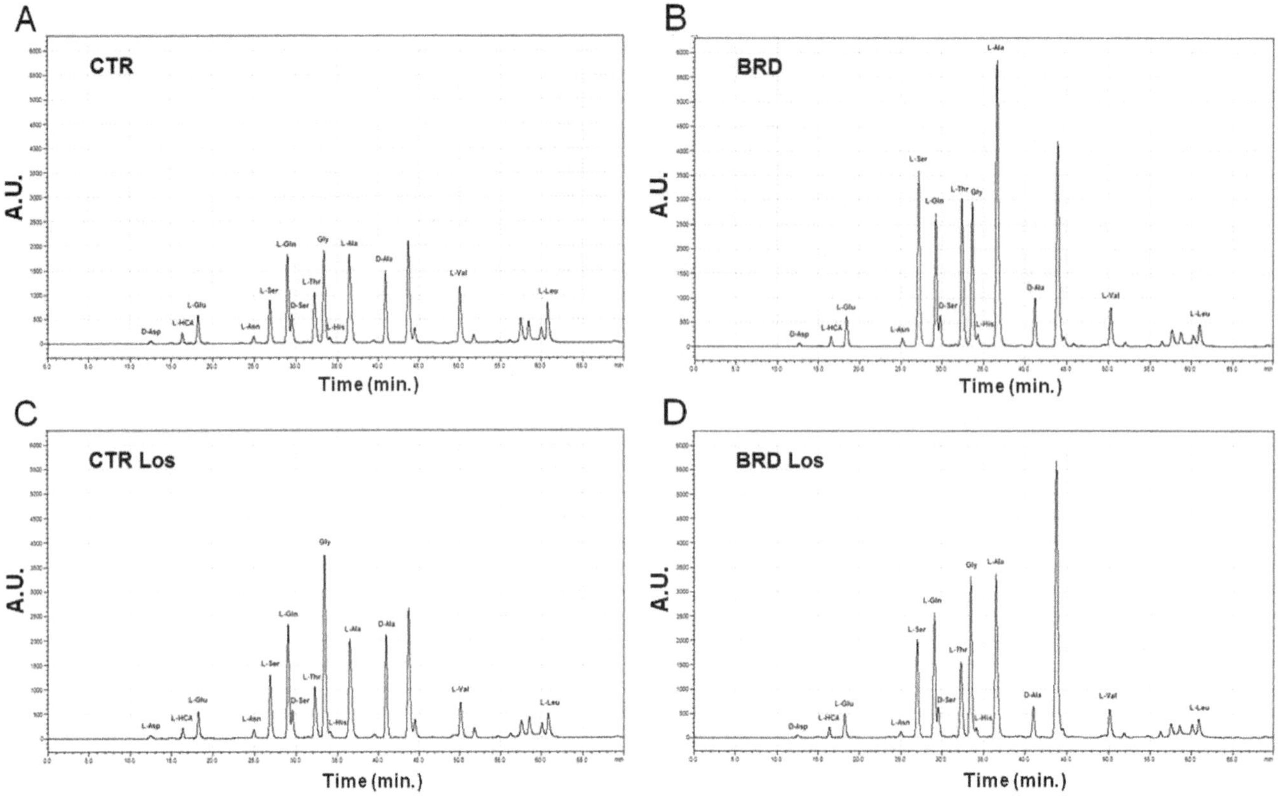

Figure 4. Representative plasma amino acids analysis. The plasma was analyzed by high performance liquid chromatography (HPLC) as described in Materials and Methods. Abbreviations of the experimental groups are those defined in the legend to Figure 2. The peaks were identified using individual amino acid standards that were run immediately after the plasma samples. Quantification and statistical analysis of the peaks are presented in Figures 5 and 6.

incorporation of the γ-phosphoryl group of (γ-^{32}P)ATP into histone in the absence and presence of their respective inhibitors: 10 nM calphostin C (Calbiochem) for PKC, 10 nM PKAi$_{(5-24)}$ peptide (Sigma-Aldrich) for PKA [8], [30], [36]. The reaction was started by adding (γ-^{32}P)ATP (10 μM; specific activity ~4.5 μCi/nmol) to the reaction medium (0.1 ml) containing 20 mM Hepes-Tris (pH 7.0), 4 mM $MgCl_2$, 1.5 mg/ml histone 2S (Sigma-Aldrich) and 0.7 mg/ml membrane protein. After 2 min, the reaction was stopped by adding 0.1 ml 40% (w/v) TCA and the samples were immediately placed on ice. After intense stirring, an aliquot of 0.1 ml was filtered through a Millipore filter (0.45 μm pore size) and successively washed with ice-cold 20% (w/v) TCA and 0.1 M phosphate buffer (pH 7.0). The radioactivity was quantified in a liquid scintillation counter.

Statistical analysis

The data are shown as mean values ± SEM. The differences between the groups were analyzed by one-way ANOVA followed by a Tukey test or by one-way ANOVA followed by a Bonferroni test for selected pairs. Intra-assay coefficients of variation ((standard deviation/mean of 3 determinations)×100) per run were calculated for the arterial pressure recordings (see above). Intra-assay coefficients of variation for the immunosignals corresponding to each protein (AT_1R, AT_2R, ERK1 and phospho-ERK1/2 in the four experimental conditions), which were detected using the Odyssey system, were always less than 10% (see above).

Results

General data

Dietary restriction led to an accentuated decrease in the rate of body weight gain in both the BRD and BRD Los groups compared with the CTR- and CTR Los-matched groups. The lighter body weight at 90 days (Figure 2A) was accompanied by a significant, though small, increase in the heart index of the BRD rats (Figure 2B), which was prevented in the group treated with Los (BRD Los). The decrease in kidney weight paralleled the reduction in body weight and Los had no observable effect (Figure 2C). Also as expected, the same profile was seen when plasma volume, heart rate and systolic blood pressure were investigated: all increased in the BRD group (Figure 2D–F). Administration of Los to rats that had received the deficient diet restored all the altered values to the levels found in the control group. Food and water intake is presented in Figure 3. There was no difference in food intake among the four groups; but water intake was significantly increased in BRD rats. The AT_1R antagonist Los did not influence this last parameter in both groups.

Besides its accentuated lower protein level, the poor quality of the proteins (90% from beans, only 10% from meat) reflects on the amino acid content, with low levels of most essential and non-essential amino acids [17]. Thus, it was hypothesized that plasma amino acids in the BRD group could have suffered from quantitative/qualitative alterations. Quantification of aminograms shown (for a representative aminogram see Figure 4) corroborates this hypothesis; changes in dietary amino acid content were reflected in the plasma amino acids of the BRD group with an

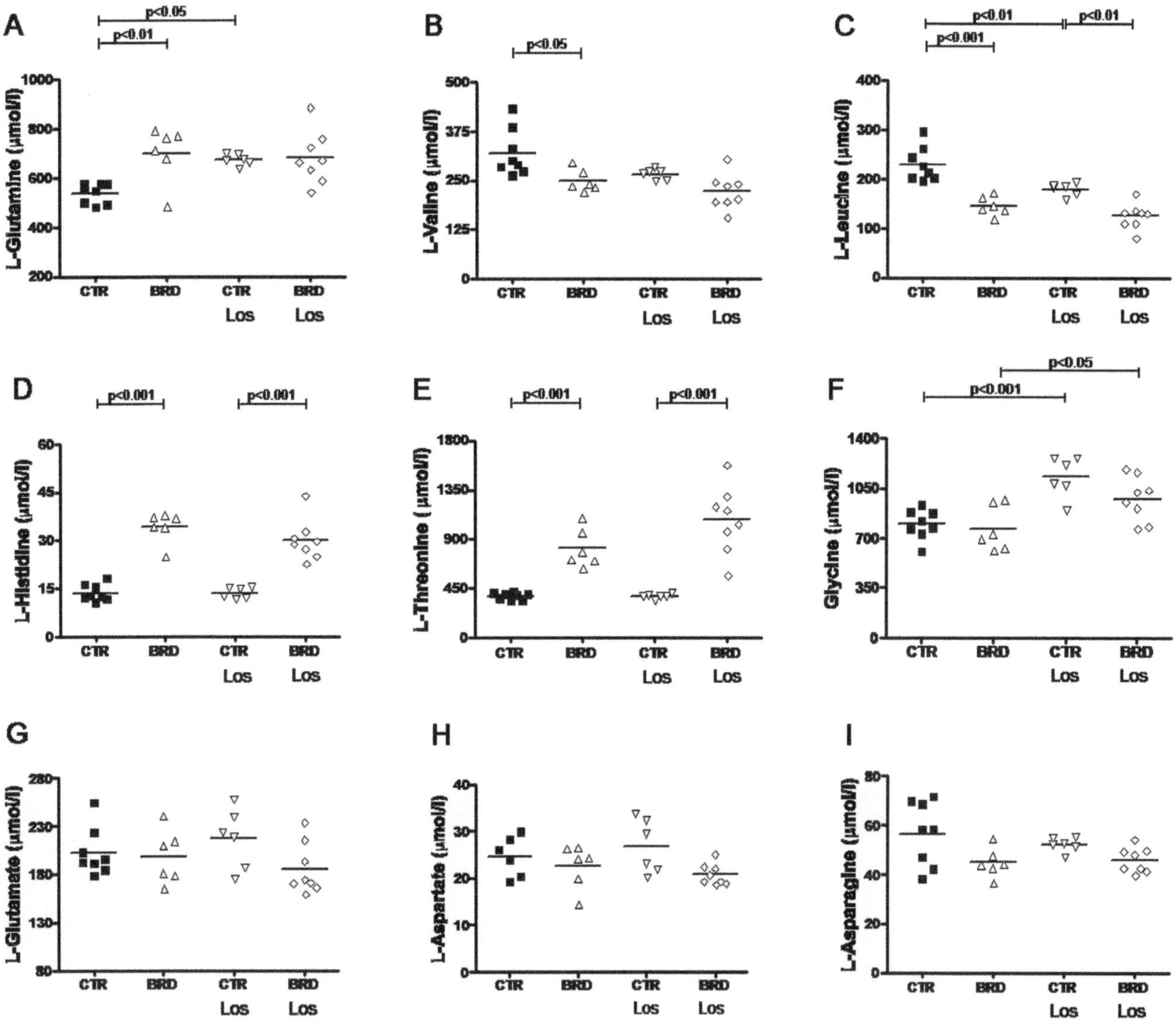

Figure 5. Changes in the plasma levels of L-amino acids and glycine. Panels show values for each animal. Horizontal lines represent mean values (n = 5–8 blood samples from different rats of each group). Statistical differences were assessed by one-way ANOVA followed by Bonferroni adjustment for CTR vs. BRD, CTR vs. CTR Los, BRD vs. BRD Los, and CTR Los vs. BRD Los, as indicated.

unexpected profile (Figures 5 and 6). BRD rats presented with increased levels of L-serine, L-Glutamine, L-Threonine, L-Histidine, L-Alanine and decreased levels of L-Valine and L-Leucine. Also interesting was the decrease in D-Serine and D-Alanine (Figure 6).

Cardiac electrical remodeling and increased risk of arrhythmias in the BRD group

The next step in understanding the effect of chronic protein restriction associated with deficiency of other nutrients was to study the cardiac electric activity, which could be associated with structural remodeling (higher heart index). The BRD group presented an expressive ventricular repolarization dysfunction, as indicated by a significantly longer QT interval than in the CTR group (Figure 7A and upper panel in Figure 7B). When this prolongation was corrected by Bazett's formula, no dependence on the heart rate could be seen (QTc, Figure 7B, middle panel). In addition, the Tpeak-Tend interval in the BRD group was longer than in the CTR group (Figure 7B, lower panel). Like the cardiovascular parameters (Figure 2D–E), all the abnormal ventricular repolarization parameters in ECG records regained normal profiles after Los treatment. The Los group revealed no difference in ECG tracings from the CTR group (Figure 7B), as expected from the hypothesis of a selective effect of chronic undernutrition on the AT_1R-linked pathway.

The next step was to investigate whether the *in vivo* repolarization profile demonstrated by ECG correlated with the cardiac action potential, raising the possibility that BRD could affect the left ventricle selectively. The two aspects of this hypothesis were investigated by performing the experiments depicted in Figure 7C. The cardiac action potential (AP) tracing revealed that BRD provoked prolongation in the left but not the right ventricular tissue, and this was prevented by Los (Figure 7C). Figure 7D indicates that the longer AP duration at 90% of repolarization (APD_{90}) in the BRD group was not dependent on stimulation frequency. This picture, intended to elucidate the electric

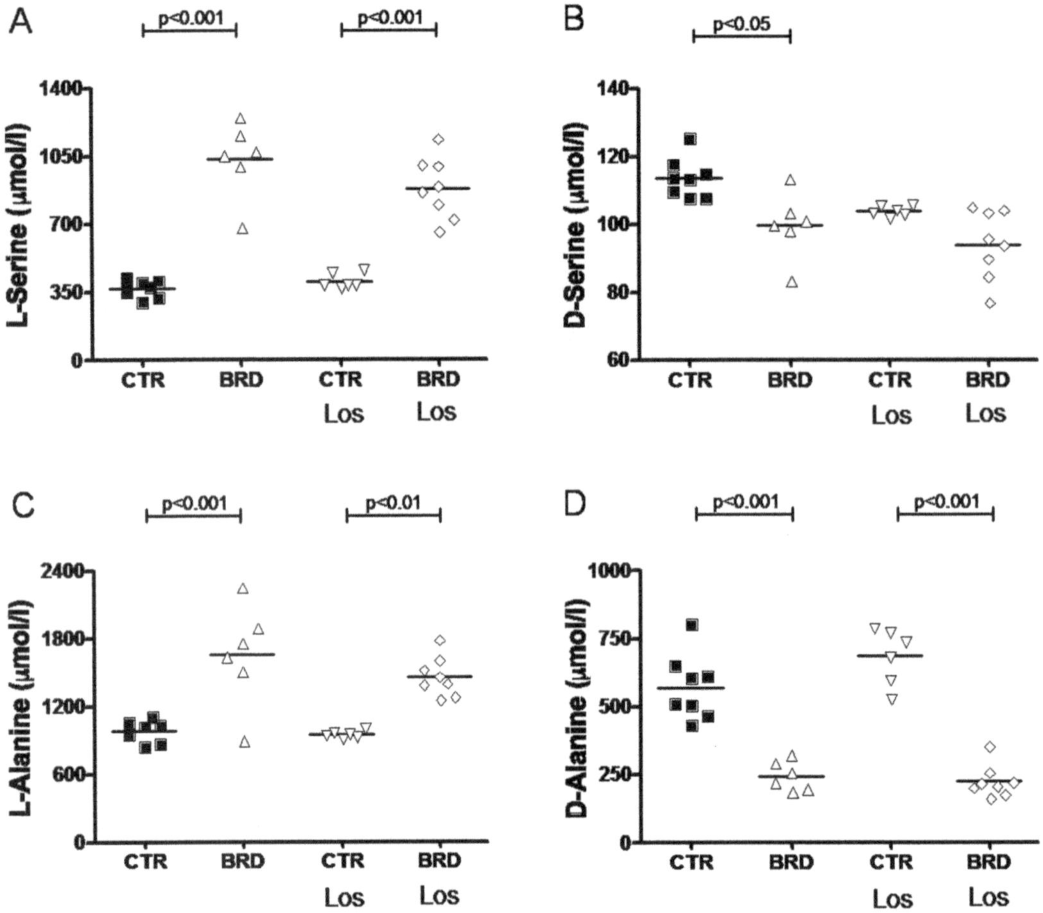

Figure 6. BRD induces increase in plasma levels of L-Serine and L-Alanine with simultaneous decrease in D-Serine and D-Alanine. Panels show values for each animal. Horizontal lines represent mean values (n = 6–8 blood samples from different rats of each group). Statistical differences were assessed by one-way ANOVA followed by Bonferroni adjustment for CTR vs. BRD, CTR vs. CTR Los, BRD vs. BRD Los, and CTR Los vs. BRD Los, as indicated.

parameters affected by BRD, was completed by the observation that proarrythmic markers, maximal negative slope (MaxNeg-Slope), and triangulation in AP were significantly different in BRD from the other three groups; however, no differences were observed among groups in the other AP parameters analyzed (Tables 1 and 2).

From the above results emerged the hypothesis that triggered activity, early after depolarization (EAD) and/or delayed after depolarization (DAD) could be present. To test this, trains of 10 beats at basic cycle lengths (BCLs) of 200, 150, and 100 ms followed by a pause were applied (Figure 8A–D). The most remarkable observation was the presence, in the BRD group, of a rate-dependent triggered activity during the pause in four out of five left ventricle endocardial preparations at BCLs of 150 ms and 100 ms (representatives in Figure 8C), also prevented by Los (Figure 8D) and not observed in the right ventricle (not shown). Late phase 3 EAD and DAD appeared spontaneously in two out of five right ventricle endocardial preparations only in the BRD group at a BCL of 1000 ms (Figure 8E).

Contrasting effects on ouabain-resistant Na^+-ATPase and $(Na^+ + K^+)$ATPase activities

Expansion of plasma volume, and the rich constellation of signs of cardiac remodeling, were then associated with dysfunctions in the active transport of Na^+ (among others not considered in the present study). This plausible view is demonstrated in Figure 9. Chronic dietary restriction affected both Na^+ active transporters similarly in left heart cardiomyocytes and renal proximal tubule cells, although the effect differed depending on the pump. There was a huge activation (more than 100%) of ouabain-resistant Na^+-ATPase activity in cardiac and renal membranes, which was no longer hyperactive in the BRD rats treated with Los (Figure 9A and 9B). Administration of Los to the CTR rats did not modify the Na^+-ATPase. $(Na^+ + K^+)$ATPase activity decreased in BRD animals (Figure 9C and 9D) but the decrease was not modified by Los. In the CTR rats, chronic administration of Los also led to a comparable degree of inhibition.

Altered density of Ang II receptors in membranes from left heart cardiomyocytes and proximal cells

AT_1R and AT_2R are the first components of a complex and interactive kinase-mediated signaling network that culminates in modulation of the renal Na^+-ATPase by Ang II [40], [41]. Owing to the striking effect of chronic undernutrition on this pump and its reversal by Los, investigation of this network was started by examining AT_1R and AT_2R densities in cardiac and renal membranes. Expression of AT_1R was decreased in the cardiomyocytes and proximal tubule cells from BRD rats (Figure 10A and

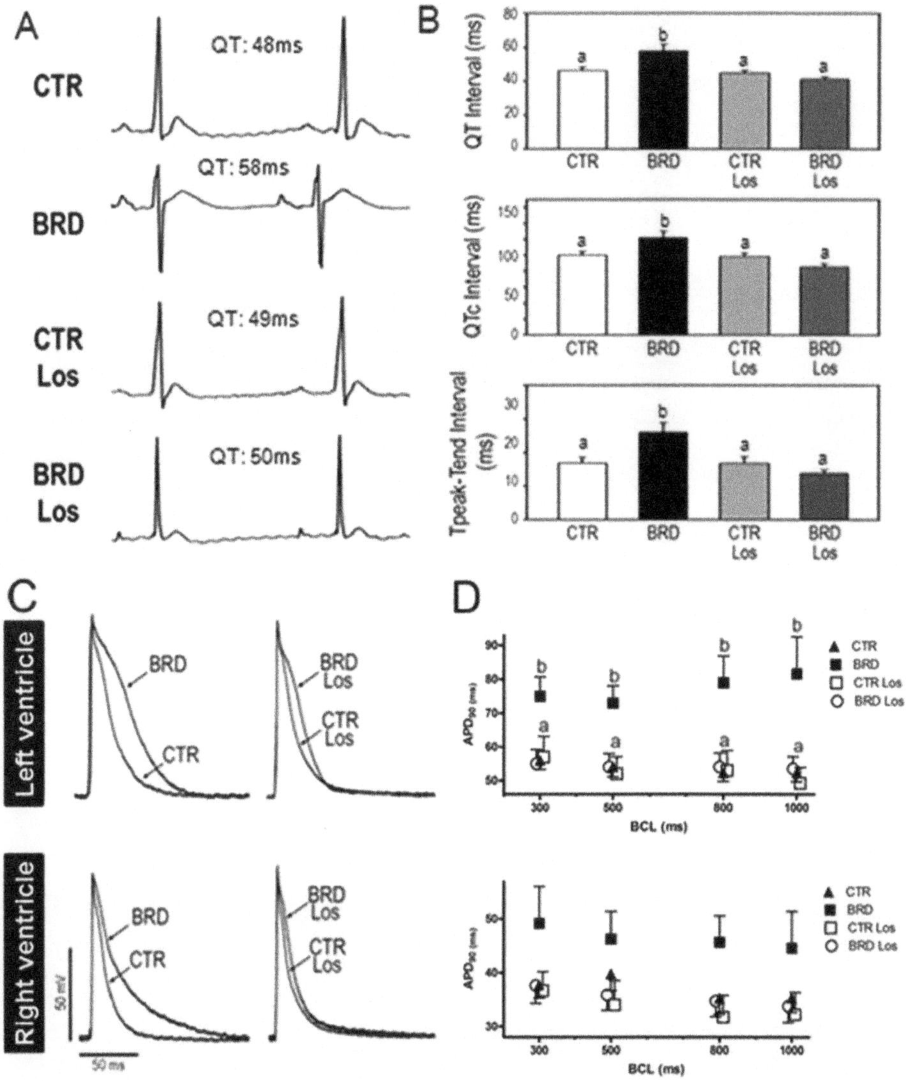

Figure 7. BRD induced longer QT, QTc, Tpeak-Tend and action potential duration. The animal groups were as described for Figure 2. (A) Representative traces of electrocardiograms show longer QT in the BRD group. (B) BRD induced ventricular repolarization disturbances, as summarized in the bar graph. Histograms show mean ± SEM. (C) Representative traces show longer left, but not right, ventricular action potential in BRD. (D) Longer ventricular action potential duration at 90% repolarization (APD_{90}) in the BRD group under different basic cycle lengths (BCL), as shown on the abscissae (panels B and D, n = 6–10). Different lowercase letters above the bars indicate statistically different mean values within the corresponding panel ($P<0.05$).

10B), thus confirming that they are relevant targets in cardiorenal dysfunction resulting from chronic undernutrition. However, the picture was not identical for AT_2R or for the influence of Los. AT_2R remained unmodified in cardiomyocytes (Figure 10 C) and in tubules from the BRD and CTR Los groups (Figure 10D). Los promoted an accentuated upregulation of both classes of receptors in the kidneys of rats submitted to BRD and downregulation of AT_1R from the CTR group (Figure 10B and 10D). In cardiomyocytes, downregulation of AT_1R was cancelled by Los (Figure 10A).

Effects on PKC and PKA: imbalance in the PKC/PKA ratio

This scrutiny of the effect of the BRD diet on Ang II signaling pathways was followed by an investigation of PKC and PKA activities. PKC activity in heart membranes was not affected in all experimental groups (Figure 10E); conversely, BRD led to a significant increase of PKC (about 100%) in kidney membranes, which returned to control values in the Los-treated animals (Figure 10F). Contrasting effects on PKA activities in heart and kidney were also revealed (Figure 10G and 10H). While BRD strongly downregulated cardiac PKA activity, the diet induced no change in this kinase in the kidney. Moreover, the set of experiments with Los-treated animals revealed that the AT_1R antagonist: (i) prevented the downregulation of cardiac PKA, (ii) had no effect on heart membranes from the CTR group, and (iii) upregulated PKA activity in kidney membranes from both CTR and BRD rats (Figure 10G and 10H). Since an imbalance between these two kinases is associated with alterations in renal active Na^+ transporters promoted by perinatal programming with the same diet [8], we determined the ratio between them. This imbalance is clearly seen in Figure 10I and 10J: BRD strongly increased the PKC/PKA ratio in both organs, an effect that was reversed by Los.

Table 1. Action potential parameters recorded in left endocardial ventricle preparation.

Variables	Groups			
	CTR	BRD	CTR Los	BRD Los
RMP (mV)	−69.4±2.8	−59.5±3.9	−63.4±4.6	−67.6±1.6
APA (mV)	83.9±3.3	76.3±5.5	75.3±7.7	78.8±2.9
MaxNegSlope (mV/s)	2722±144	1707±180*,#	2624±133	2252±172
Triangulation (ms)	32.5±2.8	55.7±10.1*,#,†	32.2±2.1	26.7±2.1
APD30 - 1000 (ms)	16.5±0.6	20.7±1.7	15.2±2.6	21.4±1.9
APD30 - 800 (ms)	16.9±0.6	20.9±1.7	15.2±2.9	21.7±1.7
APD30 - 500 (ms)	17.5±0.6	21.2±1.3	14.6±2.9	22.5±1.6
APD30 - 300 (ms)	18.0±0.8	22.0±1.4	15.7±3.2	23.4±1.8
APD50 - 1000 (ms)	23.1±0.7	31.3±2.4	20.1±2.9	30.5±2.2
APD50 - 800 (ms)	23.4±0.7	30.5±2.4	22.4±3.6	29.6±1.9
APD50 - 500 (ms)	24.5±0.8	31.7±2.1	21.8±3.5	30.7±1.9
APD50 - 300 (ms)	25.3±1.1	32.3±2.2	23.8±3.7	31.9±2.1
APD90 - 1000 (ms)	52.4±2.6	81.7±10.8*,#,†	49.2±4.6	53.5±3.5
APD90 - 800 (ms)	52.3±2.5	79.3±7.9*,#,†	53.7±5.8	54.1±4.1
APD90 - 500 (ms)	54.1±3.0	73.6±5.1*,#,†	52.2±5.0	54.8±3.9
APD90 - 300 (ms)	56.1±2.7	75.4±5.7*	57.4±6.1	55.9±4.1

RMP: Resting membrane potential; APA: Action potential amplitude; APD: Action potential duration. The results are expressed as mean ± SEM; n = 6 (CTR), n = 5 (BRD), n = 4 (CTR Los), n = 5 (BRD Los). Statistical significance: * $P<0.05$ *vs.* CTR, #$P<0.05$ *vs.* CTR Los, †$P<0.05$ *vs.* BRD Los.

Table 2. Action potential parameters recorded in right endocardial ventricle preparation.

Variables	Groups			
	CTR	BRD	CTR Los	BRD Los
RMP (mV)	−61.4±1.0	−64.2±2.9	−60.7±2.8	−70.1±1.8
APA (mV)	76.3±2.2	81.1±5.1	70.3±5.5	88.0±3.0
MaxNegSlope (mV/s)	3822±258	3152±274	3691±445	4456±607
Triangulation (ms)	27.0±3.1	30.2±5.3	23.1±2.8	21.4±1.3
APD_{30} - 1000 (ms)	8.6±0.7	11.7±1.4	7.6±1.3	10.4±1.6
APD_{30} - 800 (ms)	9.1±0.5	12.0±0.5	7.3±1.2	11.1±1.6
APD_{30} - 500 (ms)	10.6±1.0	12.1±1.1	8.1±1.4	11.5±1.7
APD_{30} - 300 (ms)	10.9±0.6	14.2±1.9	8.8±1.3	12.4±1.9
APD_{50} - 1000 (ms)	13.3±0.9	17.2±2.0	11.3±1.9	14.6±2.2
APD_{50} - 800 (ms)	13.5±0.9	17.5±1.0	11.1±1.7	15.3±2.2
APD_{50} - 500 (ms)	16.0±1.7	17.7±1.7	12.2±2.0	16.1±2.3
APD_{50} - 300 (ms)	16.1±1.0	20.6±2.9	13.32±1.7	17.1±2.5
APD_{90} - 1000 (ms)	35.4±2.7	44.6±6.7	32.3±4.1	33.8±3.0
APD_{90} - 800 (ms)	35.3±2.9	45.7±4.8	31.8±4.0	34.8±2.8
APD_{90} - 500 (ms)	39.8±3.1	46.3±5.1	34.1±4.5	35.9±2.8
APD_{90} - 300 (ms)	37.8±2.4	49.2±6.8	36.7±3.4	37.7±3.3

RMP: Resting membrane potential. APA: Action potential amplitude; APD: Action potential duration. The results are expressed as mean ± SEM; n = 6 (CTR), n = 5 (BRD), n = 4 (CTR Los), n = 5 (BRD Los). No statistical differences were found among groups.

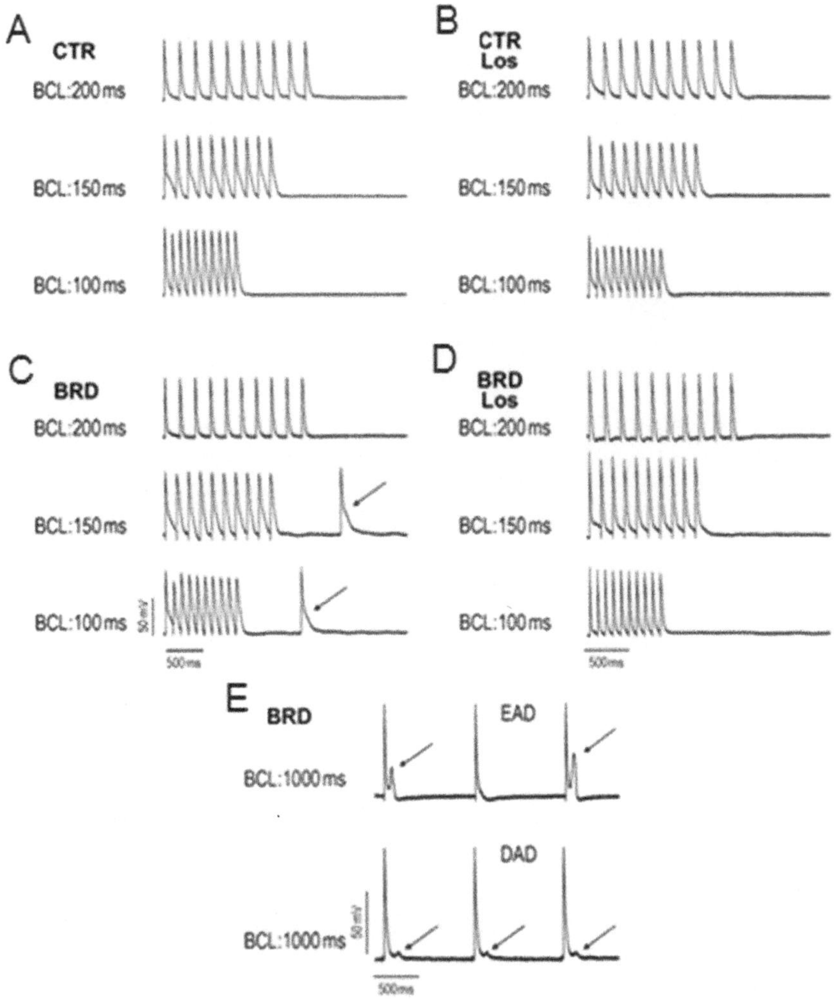

Figure 8. Triggered activity, early after depolarization (EAD) and delayed after depolarization (DAD), was induced by chronic BRD intake. (A–D) Representative action potential traces after a train of 10 beats at BCLs of 200, 150 and 100 ms followed by a pause in the left ventricle of all studied groups. (C) Representative action potential traces from the BRD group show rate-dependent triggered activity during a pause (arrows) after a train of 10 beats at BCLs of 150 and 100 ms followed by a pause protocol. (D) Los prevented the appearance of BRD-induced triggered activity. (E) In right ventricle BRD induced late-phase 3 EAD and DAD at BCL 1000 ms (arrows).

The MAPK/ERK1/2 network participates in the chronic undernutrition-induced activation of Na^+-ATPase in cardiomyocytes and proximal tubule cells

Recently, Gildea et al., demonstrated crosstalk between the AT_1R and the MAPK/ERK1/2 pathway in proximal tubules [42].To elaborate the view that other mechanisms could be involved in the modifications of the Na^+ pumps, we first investigated the effect of PD098059, a specific inhibitor of MAPK. The enormous increase in Na^+-ATPase activity in cardiomyocytes and in proximal tubule cell membranes from BRD rats was completely cancelled when PD098059 was added to the reaction medium (Figure 11A and 11B). The inhibitor had no effect on the activity measured in the other three groups, evidence of influence on a pathway that was selectively affected by BRD in rats not treated with Los. The influence of the inhibitor upon the (Na^++ K^+)ATPase was not assessed because, in contrast to the Na^+-ATPase, it needs key cytosolic Ang II-linked regulatory components [43] that are not retained in the purified plasma membranes. The extent to which the expression of ERK1 and phospho-ERK1/2 is constitutive was compared among the four groups (Figure 11C–F). The most striking finding was the upregulation of phospho-ERK1/2 in the BRD group treated with Los, in both heart and renal membranes, with increase and preservation of the phospho-ERK1/2:ERK1 ratio in heart and kidney, respectively (Figure 11G and 11H).

Discussion

Long-term general impact of dietary restriction

In this study we present evidence that chronic protein, mineral and vitamin restriction, a systemic pathological state that affects about one billion people across the world, simultaneously affects heart and kidney functions in young adult rats, leading to heart hypertrophy, electric cardiac remodeling, expanded plasma volume and the onset of hypertension in young adult rats. The driving hypothesis of this study was that chronic undernutrition affects cardiac and renal function at an early age (90 days). Moreover, the deficient diet, which mimics those used in vast impoverished regions of the world, is too drastic, such that survival decreases after 100 days of age. The lighter body weight – and the increase in systolic pressure – was accompanied by a phenotype

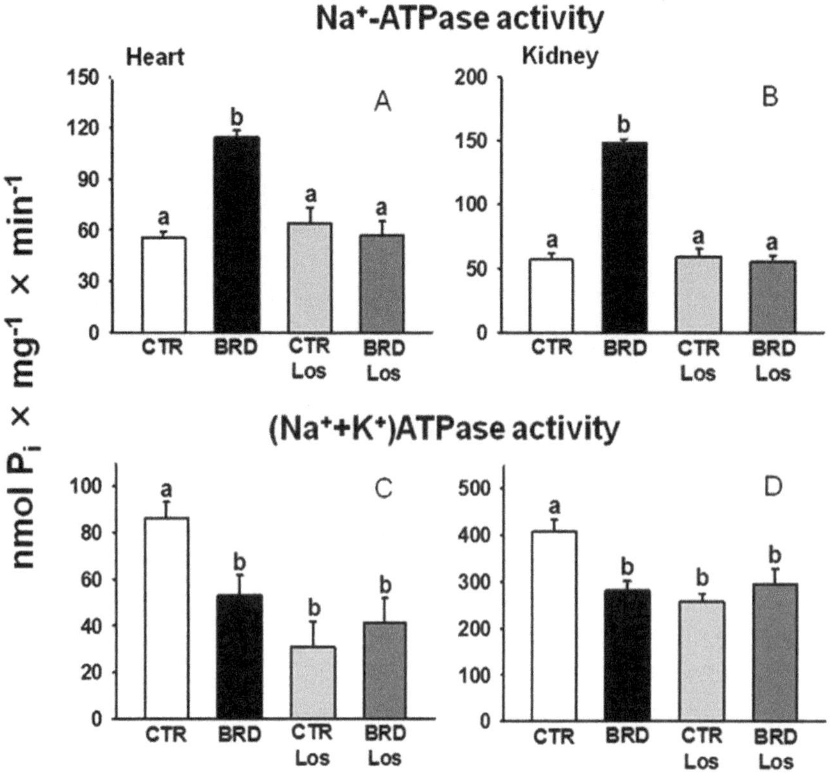

Figure 9. The increment of ouabain-resistant Na^+-ATPase and the decrease of (Na^++K^+)ATPase activities were similar in cardiomyocytes and renal proximal tubule cells of BRD rats, but the pumps were differentially modulated by Los. Upper: ouabain-insensitive Na^+-ATPase (A, heart, n = 5; B, kidney, n = 5). Lower: (Na^++K^+)ATPase (C, heart, n = 5; D, kidney, n = 5). Histograms show mean ± SEM. Different lowercase letters above the bars indicate statistically different mean values within the corresponding panel ($P<0.05$), assessed by one-way ANOVA followed by Tukey test for multiple comparisons.

resembling that found in marked and stable hypertension, including cachexia and severe lethargy, as seen by others [17]. This phenotype, therefore, can be considered a predictive marker for a reduced lifespan under huge chronic undernutrition that severely impacts on the cardio-renal axis. The hypothesis is that blocking AT_1R increases lifespan (currently under investigation). As a central finding, the present report addresses unknown mechanisms regarding the modulation during protein restriction, and the activities in heart and kidney of the recently cloned and purified ouabain-insensitive Na^+-ATPase [32], [44], the machinery responsible for fine-tuning Na^+ transport across the plasma membrane [45].

Role of Na^+-ATPase: possible mechanisms underlying electric cardiac remodeling

In the kidney, the huge increase in ouabain-insensitive Na^+-ATPase activity can explain the expanded plasma volume in chronically undernourished rats *via* an increase in Na^+ flux from the lumen to the renal interstitium, leading to simultaneous increments in heart rate, systolic pressure, and heart weight/body weight ratio. To date, no reports have indicated the physiological influence of the ouabain-resistant Na^+ in cardiomyocytes, which was described in rabbit cardiac sarcolemma several years ago [46]. On the basis of the findings presented here, it can be proposed that restoration of the normal level of this pumping activity by Los, together with the direct influence of the drug mentioned above, could make a key contribution to the prevention of cardiac electric remodeling in the BRD Los rats, thus counteracting the proarrhythmia risk consequent on (Na^++K^+)ATPase downregulation.

The mechanisms described above involving the two modes of active Na^+ flux can, therefore, help to explain mechanistically why BRD rats present electrocardiograph modifications, increasing the risk of cardiac arrhythmias and sudden death. Moreover, the risk of cardiac electrical disturbances could be partially explained by the presence of beat-dependent triggered activities and of EAD and DAD events. A plausible mechanism for the genesis of EAD and increased APD could involve the increment of I_{Na} with no increase in peak I_{Na}, a disorder that is associated with abnormal cellular Na^+ handling, as recently suggested for rat cardiomyocytes [47].

Participation of RAS and kinase-mediated phosphorylations

Blocking of AT_1R completely abolishes the activation of Na^+-ATPase provoked by BRD, thus confirming the hypothesis of a central effect on the RAS, alterations in which could arise from a direct influence of the low-protein BRD – and possibly of an altered plasma amino acid composition – on tissue Ang II. Protein restriction during gestation programmed the downregulation of signaling components of the RAS with effects on blood pressure [7], [48], and this seems also to be the case for chronic protein deprivation through eating BRD after weaning. It has been demonstrated that RAS is important in the pathological heart hypertrophy [49], [50] that is counteracted by blocking AT_1R [51] with simultaneous prevention of cardiac electric remodeling [52].

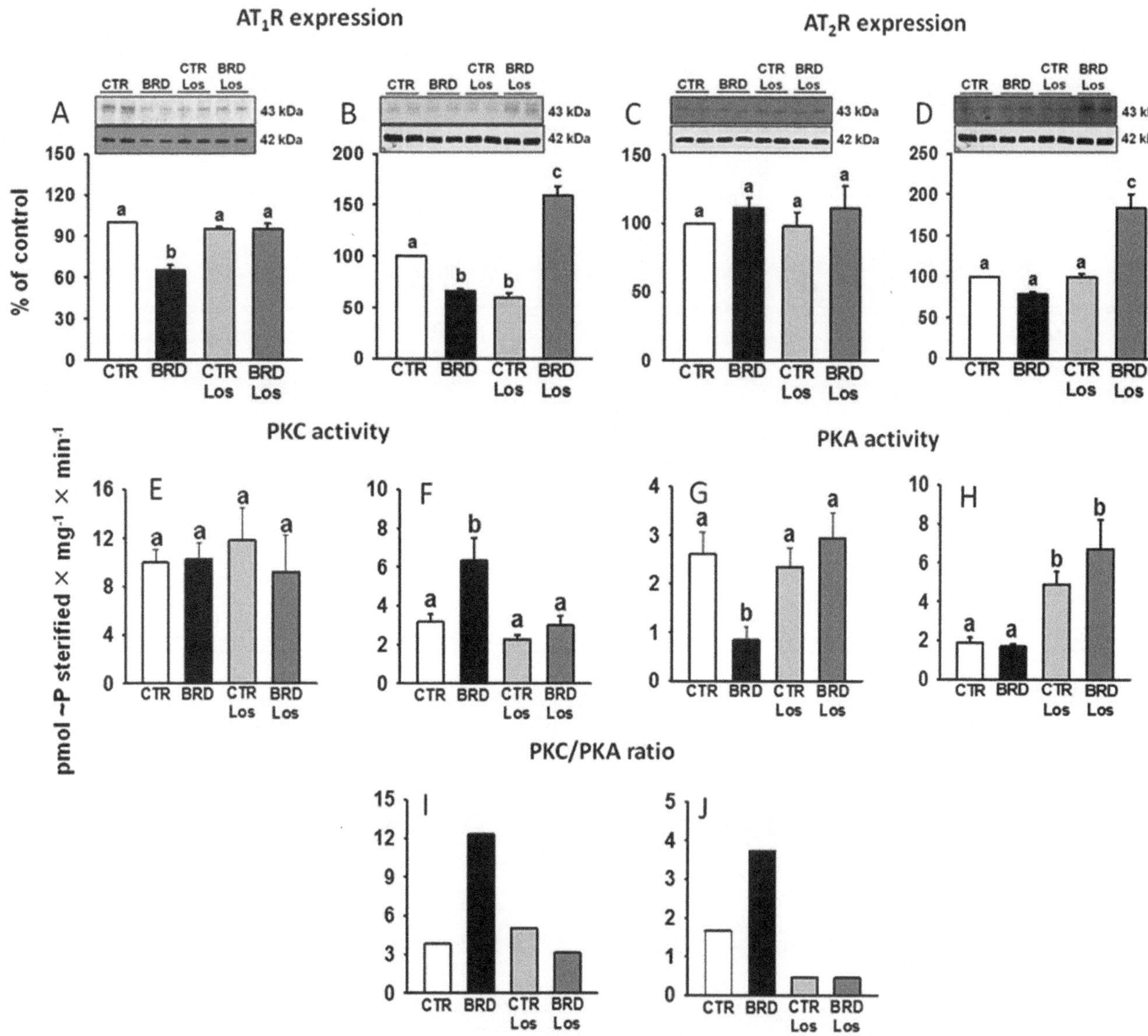

Figure 10. Chronic BRD intake altered Ang II receptor density in membranes and PKC and PKA activities. (A–D) AT_1R and AT_2R density. Upper panels: representative immunostainings (duplicates for each experimental condition) and densitometric representations (lower panels) of 7–12 experiments in duplicate corrected for protein loading (β-actin immunosignals in the corresponding lane, middle panels), which were carried out using different membrane preparations (left panels: heart; right panels: kidney). Different lowercase letters above the bars indicate statistically different mean values within the corresponding panel, assessed by one-way ANOVA followed by Tukey test for multiple comparisons. P values for AT_1R comparisons: $P<0.001$ (BRD against the other three groups in heart, $P=0.607–1.000$ when the other groups were compared among them); $P<0.001$ (BRD and CTR Los against the other two groups in kidney, $P<0.001$ BRD Los against the other three groups, $P=0.811$ BRD versus CTR Los). P values for AT_2R comparisons: $P=0.686$ (heart, where differences among the four groups were not found and Tukey test was not carried out); $P<0.001$ (BRD against the other three groups in kidney, $P=0.317–1.000$ when the other groups were compared among them). (E–J) PKC and PKA activities ($n=5–7$), and PKC/PKA ratio (left panels: heart; right panels: kidney). Different lowercase letters above the bars indicate statistically different mean values within the corresponding panel, also assessed by one-way ANOVA followed by Tukey test.

The view that kidney receptors are associated with heart receptors in the cardiac structural and electric remodeling receives further support from the observation that elimination of AT_1R in mice reduces cardiac hypertrophy and the risk of hypertension [49], and also from the observation that primary renal dysfunction in rats is associated with an augmented risk of congestive cardiac failure in simultaneous alterations that constitute a cardiorenal syndrome [53].

The consequences of BRD, which are similar in heart and kidney in terms of Na^+ pumping activities and can explain the integration of pathophysiological events, are partially distinct in terms of Ang II receptors and protein kinases. The different profiles of Ang II receptors expression and PKC and PKA activities can shed light on their tissue-specific participation in the alterations of electric activity (heart) and fluid handling (kidney). The decrease in AT_1R combined with an imbalance between PKC and PKA (increased PKC/PKA ratio in BRD rats) could contribute to both upregulation of Na^+-ATPase activity and decreased (Na^++K^+)ATPase activity in both organs. It has been demonstrated that normal balance between these kinases is

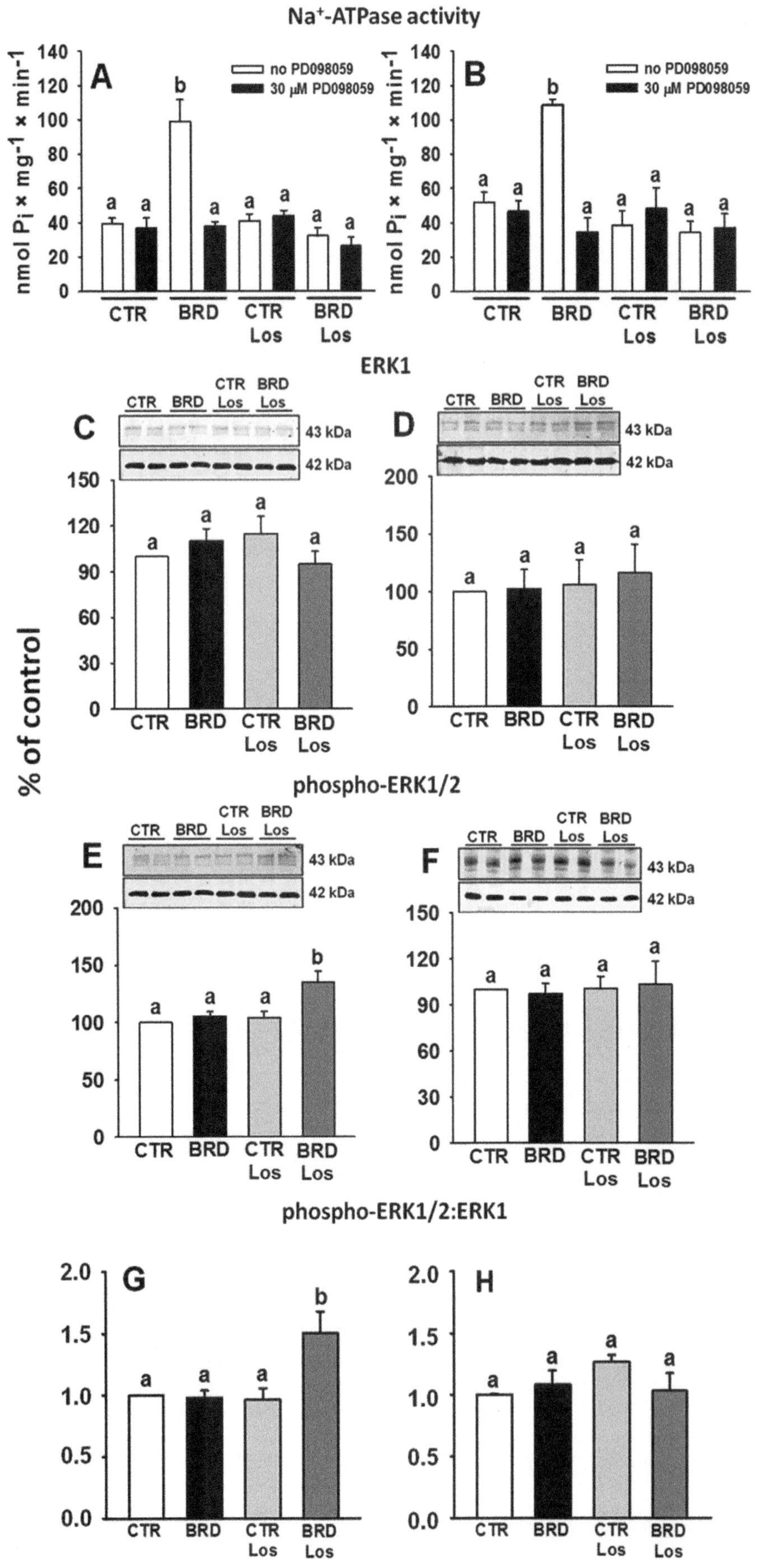

Na+-ATPase activity
A
B
no PD098059
30 μM PD098059
nmol Pi × mg-1 × min-1
CTR
BRD
CTR Los
BRD Los
ERK1
C
D
43 kDa
42 kDa
% of control
phospho-ERK1/2
E
F
phospho-ERK1/2:ERK1
G
H

Figure 11. Na^+-ATPase activity and MAPK pathway in heart (left panels) and kidney (right panels). (A, B) Na^+-ATPase activity was measured in the four experimental groups in the absence or presence of 30 μM PD098059, as indicated. Results are mean ± SEM (n = 5) in assays carried out using different membrane preparations. (C, D) Representative immunoblottings of ERK1 in duplicate (upper panels), β-actin loading-controls for each blotting (middle panels) and densitometric representations (n = 8–10) (lower panels). (E, F) Representative immunoblottings of phospho-ERK1/2 in duplicate (upper panels), β-actin loading controls for each blotting (middle panels) and densitometric representations (n = 8–10) (lower panels). (G, H) phospho-ERK1/2:ERK1 ratio (n = 8–10). Each phospho-ERK1/2:ERK1 ratio value was calculated using the corresponding densitometric value obtained from the same lane. Different lowercase letters above the bars indicate statistically different mean values within the corresponding panel, assessed by one-way ANOVA followed by Tukey test. P values for ERK1 comparisons: P = 0.302 and 0.968 (heart and kidney, respectively, where no statistical differences were found among the four groups and Tukey test was not carried out). P values for phospho-ERK1/2 comparisons: P = 0.001–0.007 (heart, BRD Los against the other three groups, P = 0.928–0.999 for the comparisons among the other groups); P = 0.928 (kidney, where no statistical differences were found among the four groups and Tukey test was not carried out). P values for phospho-ERK1/2:ERK1 ratio comparisons: P = 0.004–0.007 (heart, BRD Los against the other four groups, P = 0.995–0.999 for the comparisons among the other groups); P = 0.977 (kidney, no differences among the four groups).

essential for the modulation of Na^+-ATPase [40], [41]. Thus, the Los-induced decrease in the PKC/PKA ratio could contribute to restoration of the Na^+-ATPase activity upregulated in BRD rats by the simultaneous increase in PKC and decrease in PKA. The Los-induced recovery of the PKC/PKA ratio in cardiomyocytes could be also a key mechanism in the prevention of electric cardiac remodeling. Increased expression of both AT_1R and AT_2R in renal membranes of the BRD group treated with Los could be explained by modifications in the association of the two classes of receptors that perturb their mutual signaling exchange [54] or by stimulation of intracellular partners that facilitates their insertion into the membranes, as proposed for AT_2R [55]. Possibly, the Los-induced decreased abundance of renal AT_1R in CTR rats relies on the same complex and not completely elucidated pathway interactions in proximal kidney tubules [42].

Involvement of the MAPK/ERK1/2 pathway

The MAPK/ERK1/2 signaling routes seem to be crucial for regulating cardiac physiological and pathological events [56–60]. In the present study, the combined effects of Los administration, the recovery of control values of ouabain-insensitive Na^+-ATPase when the MAPK inhibitor PD098059 was present in the assays, and the normal values of Na^+-ATPase activity from non-Los BRD rats when MAPK was blocked, help to elucidate – at least in part – the interrelated mechanisms on which rest the simultaneous cardiac and renal alterations induced by BRD. The proposal of crosstalk between the Ang II and MAPK/ERK1/2 cascades finds support in the observations that (i) Ang II phosphorylates cardiac ERK1/2 *in vivo* [60]; (ii) Ang II phosphorylates ERK1/2 from proximal tubule cells *in vitro* [61] in events that involve Ang II receptors [62]; (iii) Ang II receptor signaling modulates the phosphorylation of ERK1/2 in renal proximal tubules [42]. Since there was no additive action on Na^+-ATPase when AT_1R are blocked or when MAPK is blocked, it is likely that the wrong signals induced by BRD interact with different kinases and, ultimately, converge on that key target for Na^+-handling. These proposed interactions are outlined in Figure 12.

It is possible that undernutrition-induced stress [7], [8], [18], [22], [63] evokes abnormal constitutive modifications in MAPK leading directly to modifications in ERK1/2 activity, irrespective of signals from AT_1R. As in the case of Ang II receptors densities, the modifications in the phospho-ERK1/2:ERK1 ratio in heart and kidney from the BRD Los group exhibit different images (increase and preservation, respectively), thus pointing to a tissue-specific outcome of protein restriction, despite the final common effect on Na^+-ATPase. Finally, the lack of influence of PD098059

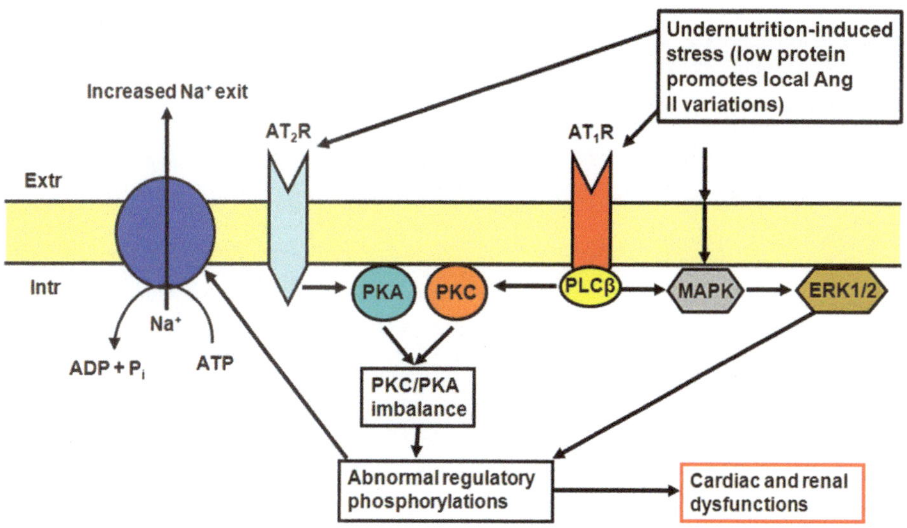

Figure 12. Proposed interactions among Ang II receptors, PKC/PKA, MAPK and ERK1/2 in heart and kidney from BRD rats, ultimately targeting the ouabain-insensitive Na^+-ATPase and therefore the fine tuning of Na^+ extrusion. Extracellular-induced stress (low protein and altered local Ang II levels) can induce wrong signaling in the branches linked to AT_1R and AT_2R as well as increase of MAPK/ERK1/2 turnover. The resulting imbalance (increase) in PKC activity/PKA activity ratio, together with modified ERK1/2 activity, would result in abnormal regulatory phosphorylation(s) of the ouabain-insensitive Na^+-ATPase and culminate in the accelerated Los- and PD98059-sensitive turnover of the pump (Figure 9A and 9B). The representation also indicates a possible link between AT_1R and MAPK/ERK1/2 according to ref. [42].

upon Na^+-ATPase in Los-treated rats is consistent with the proposal that PKC exerts a permissive action in the catalysis by phospho-ERK1/2 [64].

Although this model could provide a step towards elucidating the complex cardiorenal alterations induced by chronic protein restriction associated with other dietary deficiencies, it is clearly far from complete. Ang II in serum and left ventricle/kidney cortical tissues was not measured. However, two observations support the link between protein restriction and altered local Ang II levels. First, Ceravolo et al. [63] demonstrated that intrauterine undernourished rats presented at 16 weeks with moderate hypertension, and increased mesenteric vascular reactivity *in vivo-in situ* to Ang II, with both alterations being normalized by Los. These findings strongly support an increased local activation of the AT_1R-mediated pathway, as proposed in Figure 12. Second, we recently demonstrated using the same diet that adult offspring from dams undernourished during pregnancy gradually develop hypertension with age, a process that is concomitant with an increase in Na^+-ATPase activity and an augmented number of Ang II-positive cells in the kidney cortex [65]. Thus, even though the window of exposure to the deficient diet was different in this parallel study (gestation), the increased Ang II local levels in proximal tubule cells seems indicative that protein restriction at different periods of development could be a key stress factor that activates the AT_1R-mediated pathway in different tissues.

It is also plausible that other axes of plasma volume regulation – and therefore, of arterial pressure – are affected by dietary restriction, especially in the kidney and its proximal tubules, as focused upon in this study. Cornock and et al. [66] showed that pregnant rats fed a low-protein diet downregulated aquaporin 2 – the water channel in the apical membrane of collecting ducts – in conjunction with a significantly lower expression of AT_2R. These observations point to an additional effect of undernutrition on the handling of renal fluid in distal segments and possibly the disruption of the delicate balance between proximal and distal transport processes.

Finally, the important alterations in plasma amino acids and in the overall nutritional status could also have important implications for the observed alterations in Na^+ pumping activities. The huge increases of L-Serine, L-Threonine, L-Histidine and L-Alanine that accompany that of L-Glutamine – the key amino acid for renal cortex metabolism – with simultaneous decrease of L-Valine and L-Leucine, suggest that chronic BRD administration led to tissue proteolysis in an attempt to compensate for the poor quality of the ingested protein. The mirror images L-Serine/D-Serine and of L-Alanine/D-Alanine also indicates BRD-induced racemization. The alterations in these plasma amino acids could be sensed by intracellular receptors involved in adaptations to the availability of nutrients, such as mTOR, as recently demonstrated [67], with subsequent effects on signaling pathways and pumps. Moreover, signals coming from the altered levels of (Na^+-K^+)ATPase – possibly as a result of the altered plasma amino acids – can in turn influence the kinase pathways, including the mTOR pathway, in a cell-specific manner, as demonstrated in [68].

Acknowledgments

We thank Gloria Costa Sarmento and Alexandre Abrantes for their technical assistance. Required correction of the English style of the revised manuscript by BioMedES (UK) is acknowledged.

Author Contributions

Conceived and designed the experiments: PAS GMC LSL ME-L RP LV-F CC-C ADOP EM AV. Performed the experiments: PAS GMC AP-A RL LSS MAL-L LSL CM LV-F VSR EM. Analyzed the data: PAS GMC AP-A RL LSS MAL-L LSL ME-L RP CM LV-F CC-C VSR ADOP EM AV. Contributed reagents/materials/analysis tools: LSL ME-L RP CC-C ADOP EM AV. Wrote the paper: PAS GMC CC-C ADOP EM AV.

References

1. Monteiro CA, Benicio MH, Konno SC, Silva AC, Lima AL, et al. (2009) Causes for the decline in child under-nutrition in Brazil, 1996–2007. Rev Saude Publica 43: 35–43.
2. Fowden AL, Giussani DA, Forhead AJ (2006) Intrauterine programming of physiological systems: causes and consequences. Physiology (Bethesda) 21: 29–37.
3. Law CM, de Swiet M, Osmond C, Fayers PM, Barker DJ, et al. (1993) Initiation of hypertension in utero and its amplification throughout life. BMJ 306: 24–27.
4. Fernandez-Twinn DS, Ekizoglou S, Wayman A, Petry CJ, Ozanne SE (2006) Maternal low-protein diet programs cardiac beta-adrenergic response and signaling in 3-mo-old male offspring. Am J Physiol Regul Integr Comp Physiol 291: R429–436.
5. Langley-Evans SC, Welham SJ, Jackson AA (1999) Fetal exposure to a maternal low protein diet impairs nephrogenesis and promotes hypertension in the rat. Life Sci 64: 965–974.
6. Alwasel SH, Ashton N (2009) Prenatal programming of renal sodium handling in the rat. Clin Sci (Lond) 117: 75–84.
7. Mesquita FF, Gontijo JA, Boer PA (2010) Maternal undernutrition and the offspring kidney: from fetal to adult life. Braz J Med Biol Res 43: 1010–1018.
8. Vieira-Filho LD, Lara LS, Silva PA, Santos FT, Luzardo R, et al. (2011) Placental malnutrition changes the regulatory network of renal Na-ATPase in adult rat progeny: Reprogramming by maternal α-tocopherol during lactation. Arch Biochem Biophys 505: 91–97.
9. Hoppe CC, Evans RG, Moritz KM, Cullen-McEwen LA, Fitzgerald SM, et al. (2007) Combined prenatal and postnatal protein restriction influences adult kidney structure, function, and arterial pressure. Am J Physiol Regul Integr Comp Physiol 292: R462–469.
10. Benabe JE, Fernández-Repollet E, Tapia E, Luo C, Martinez-Maldonado M (1993) Angiotensin II and catecholamines interaction in short-term low protein feeding. Kidney Int 44: 285–293.
11. Benabe JE, Martinez-Maldonado M (1998) The impact of malnutrition on kidney function. Miner Electrolyte Metab 24: 20–26.
12. Ichikawa I, Purkerson ML, Klahr S, Troy JL, Martinez-Maldonado M, et al. (1980) Mechanism of reduced glomerular filtration rate in chronic malnutrition. J Clin Invest 65: 982–988.
13. He J, Klag MJ, Whelton PK, Chen JY, Qian MC, et al. (1994) Body mass and blood pressure in a lean population in southwestern China. Am J Epidemiol 139: 380–389.
14. Kaufman JS, Owoaje EE, Rotimi CN, Cooper RS (1997) Blood pressure change in Africa: case study from Nigeria. Hum Biol 71: 641–657.
15. Beilin LJ, Puddey IB, Burke V (1999) Lifestyle and hypertension Am J Hypertens 12: 934–945.
16. Martinez-Maldonado M, Benabe JE, Wilcox JN, Wang S, Luo C (1993) Renal renin, angiotensinogen, and ANG I-converting-enzyme gene expression: influence of dietary protein. Am J Physiol 264: F981–988.
17. Teodósio NR, Lago ES, Romani SA, Guedes RC (1990) A regional basic diet from northeast Brazil as a dietary model of experimental malnutrition. Arch Latinoam Nutr 40: 533–547.
18. Vieira-Filho LD, Lara LS, Silva PA, Luzardo R, Einicker-Lamas M, et al. (2009) Placental oxidative stress in malnourished rats and changes in kidney proximal tubule sodium ATPases in offspring. Clin Exp Pharmacol Physiol 36: 1157–1163.
19. Sebrell WH Jr, RS Harris (1954) The Vitamins. New York, NY. Academic Press.
20. Reeves PG, Nielsen FH, Fahey GC Jr (1993) AIN−93 Purified diets for laboratory rodents: final report of the American Institute of Nutrition Ad Hoc writing committee on the reformulation of the AIN−76A rodent diet. J Nutr 123: 1939–1951.
21. Ikeda K, Nara Y, Yamori Y (1991) Indirect systolic and mean blood pressure determination by a new tail cuff method in spontaneously hypertensive rats. Lab Anim 25: 26–29.
22. Costa-Silva JH, Silva PA, Pedi N, Luzardo R, Einicker-Lamas M, et al. (2009) Chronic undernutrition alters renal active Na^+ transport in young rats: potential hidden basis for pathophysiological alterations in adulthood? Eur J Nutr 48: 437–445.
23. Hashimoto A, Nishikawa T, Oka T, Takahashi K (1992) Determination of free amino acids enatiomers in rat brain and serum high-performance liquid chromatography after derivatization with N-tert.-butyloxycarbonyl-L-cysteine and o-phthaldialdehyde. J Chromatogr 582: 41–48.
24. Calcia MA, Madeira C, Alheira FV, Silva TC, Tannos FM, et al. (2012) Plasma levels of D-serine in Brazilian individuals with schizophrenia. Schizophr Res 142: 83–87.

25. Cardoso HD, Cabral EV, Vieira-Filho LD, Vieyra A, Paixão AD (2009) Fetal development and renal function in adult rats prenatally subjected to sodium overload. Pediatr Nephrol 24: 1959–1965.
26. Medei E, Marocolo M, Rodrigues DC, Arantes PC, Takiya CM, et al. (2010) Chronic treatment with anabolic steroids induces ventricular repolarization disturbances: cellular, ionic and molecular mechanism. J Mol Cell Cardiol 49: 165–175.
27. Dostanic I, Schultz JEJ, Lorenz JN, Lingrel JB (2004) The alpha 1 isoform of Na,K-ATPase regulates cardiac contractility and functionally interacts and co-localizes with the Na/Ca exchanger in heart. J Biol Chem 279: 54053–54061.
28. Lowry OH, Rosebrough NJ, Farr AL, Randall RJ (1951) Protein measurement with the Folin phenol reagent. J Biol Chem 193: 265–275.
29. Vieyra A, Nachbin L, de Dios-Abad E, Goldfeld M, Meyer-Fernandes JR, et al. (1986) Comparison between calcium transport and adenosine triphosphatase activity in membrane vesicles derived from rabbit kidney proximal tubules. J Biol Chem 261: 4247–4255.
30. Luzardo R, Silva PA, Einicker-Lamas M, Ortiz-Costa S, do Carmo MaG (2011) Metabolic programming during lactation stimulates renal Na^+ transport in the adult offspring due to an early impact on local angiotensin II pathways. PLoS One 6: e21232.
31. Whittembury G, Proverbio F (1970) Two modes of Na extrusion in cells from guinea pig kidney cortex slices. Pflugers Arch 316: 1–25.
32. Rocafull MA, Thomas LE, del Castillo JR (2012) The second sodium pump: from the function to the gene. Pflügers Arch 463: 755–777.
33. Maia JCC, Gomes SL, Juliani MH (1983) Preparation of (gamma-^{32}P) and (alpha-^{32}P)-nucleoside triphosphates with high specific activity. In: Morel CM, ed. Genes and antigens of parasites – a laboratory manual proceedings. Rio de Janeiro: Fundação Oswaldo Cruz. pp. 146–157.
34. Taussky HH, Shorr E (1953) A microcolorimetric method for the determination of inorganic phosphorus. J Biol Chem 202: 675–685.
35. Alessi DR, Cuenda A, Cohen P, Dudley DT, Saltiel AR (1995) PD 098059 is a specific inhibitor of the activation of mitogen-activated protein kinase kinase in vitro and in vivo. J Biol Chem 270: 27489–27494.
36. Cabral LM, Wengert M, Almeida FG, Caruso-Neves C, Vieyra A (2010) Ceramide-activated protein kinases A and C zeta inhibit kidney proximal tubule cell Na^+-ATPase. Arch Biochem Biophys 498: 57–61.
37. Laemmli UK (1970) Cleavage of structural proteins during the assembly of the head of bacteriophage T4. Nature 227: 680–685.
38. Herrera M, Sparks MA, Alfonso-Pecchio AR, Harrison-Bernard LM, Coffman TM (2013) Lack of specificity of commercial antibodies leads to misidentification of angiotensin type 1 receptor protein. Hypertension 61: 253–8.
39. Liu L, Gonzalez AA, McCormack M, Seth DM, Kobori H, et al. (2011) Increased renin excretion is associated with augmented urinary angiotensin II levels in chronic angiotensin II-infused hypertensive rats. Am J Physiol Renal Physiol 301: F1195–F1201.
40. Rangel LB, Lopes AG, Lara LS, Carvalho TL, Silva IV, et al. (2005) PI-PLCβ is involved in the modulation of the proximal tubule Na^+-ATPase by angiotensin II. Regul Pept 127: 177–182.
41. Lara LS, Vives D, Correa JS, Cardozo FP, Marques-Fernandes MF, et al. (2010) Arch Biochem Biophys 496: 117–122.
42. Gildea JJ, Wang X, Shah N, Tran H, Spinosa M, et al.(2012) Dopamine and angiotensin type 2 receptors cooperatively inhibit sodium transport in human renal proximal tubule cells. Hypertension 60: 396–403.
43. Aperia A, Holtbäck U, Syrén ML, Svensson LB, Fryckstedt J, et al. (1994) Activation/deactivation of renal Na^+,K^+-ATPase: a final common pathway for regulation of natriuresis. FASEB J 8: 436–439.
44. Rocafull MA, Romero FJ, Thomas LE, del Castillo JR (2011) Isolation and cloning of the K^+-independent, ouabain-insensitive Na^+-ATPase. Biochim Biophys Acta 1808: 1684–700.
45. Bełtowski J, Borkowska E, Wójcicka G, Marciniak A (2007) Regulation of renal ouabain-resistant Na^+-ATPase by leptin, nitric oxide, reactive oxygen species, and cyclic nucleotides: implications for obesity-associated hypertension. Clin Exp Hypertension 29: 189–207.
46. Camejo JL, Proverbio T, Proverbio F (1995) Ouabain-insensitive, Na^+-stimulated ATPase activity in rabbit cardiac sarcolemma. Comp Biochem Physiol B Biochem Mol Biol 110: 345–348.
47. Auerbach DS, Grzda KR, Furspan PB, Sato PY, Mironov S, et al. (2011) Structural heterogeneity promotes triggered activity, reflection and arrhythmogenesis in cardiomyocyte monolayers. J Physiol 2011 589: 2363–2381.
48. Vehaskari VM, Aviles DH, Manning J (2001) Prenatal programming of adult hypertension in the rat. Kidney Int 59: 238–245.
49. Crowley SD, Gurley SB, Herrera MJ, Ruiz P, Griffiths R, et al. (2006) Angiotensin II causes hypertension and cardiac hypertrophy through its receptors in the kidney. Proc Natl Acad Sci USA 103: 17985–17990.
50. Cleal JK, Poore KR, Boullin JP, Khan O, Chau R, et al.(2007) Mismatched pre- and postnatal nutrition leads to cardiovascular dysfunction and altered renal function in adulthood. Proc Natl Acad Sci USA 104: 9529–9533.
51. Tanaka Y, Tamura K, Koide Y, Sakai M, Tsurumi Y, et al. (2005) The novel angiotensin II type 1 receptor (AT_1R)-associated protein ATRAP downregulates AT_1R and ameliorates cardiomyocyte hypertrophy. FEBS Lett 579: 1579–1586.
52. Sicouri S, Cordeiro JM, Talarico M, Antzelevitch C (2011) Antiarrhythmic effects of losartan and enalapril in canine pulmonary vein sleeve preparations. J Cardiovasc Electrophysiol 22: 698–705.
53. Szymanski MK, Buikema JH, van Veldhuisen DJ, Koster J, van der Velden J, et al. (2012) Increased cardiovascular risk in rats with primary renal dysfunction; mediating role for vascular endothelial function. Basic Res Cardiol 107: 242.
54. Miura S, Matsuo Y, Kiya Y, Karnik SS, Saku K (2010) Molecular mechanisms of the antagonistic action between AT_1 and AT_2 receptors. Biochem Biophys Res Commun 391: 85–90.
55. Rodrigues-Ferreira S, Nahmias C (2010) An ATIPical family of angiotensin II AT_2 receptor-interacting proteins. Trends Endocrinol Metab 21: 684–690.
56. Fryer RM, Pratt PF, Hsu AK, Gross GJ (2001) Differential activation of extracellular signal regulated kinase isoforms in preconditioning and opioid-induced cardioprotection. J Pharmacol Exp Ther 296: 642–649.
57. Kovacs K, Hanto K, Bognar Z, Tapodi A, Bognar E, et al. (2009) Prevalent role of Akt and ERK activation in cardioprotective effect of Ca^{2+} channel- and beta-adrenergic receptor blockers. Mol Cell Biochem 321: 155–164.
58. Rose BA, Force T, Wang Y (2010) Mitogen-activated protein kinase signaling in the heart: angels versus demons in a heart-breaking tale. Physiol Rev 90: 1507–1546.
59. Wu W, Muchir A, Shan J, Bonne G, Worman HJ (2011) Mitogen-activated protein kinase inhibitors improve heart function and prevent fibrosis in cardiomyopathy caused by mutation in lamin A/C gene. Circulation 123: 53–61.
60. Lo J, Patel VB, Wang Z, Levasseur J, Kaufman S, et al. (2012) Angiotensin Converting Enzyme 2 antagonizes Ang II-induced pressor response and NADPH oxidase activation in WKY rats and in SHR model. Exp Physiol 98: 109–122.
61. Li XC, Zhuo JL (2011) Phosphoproteomic analysis of AT1 receptor-mediated signaling responses in proximal tubules of angiotensin II-induced hypertensive rats. Kidney Int 80: 620–632.
62. Li XC, Hopfer U, Zhuo JL (2012) Novel signaling mechanisms of intracellular angiotensin II-induced NHE3 expression and activation in mouse proximal tubule cells. Am J Physiol Renal Physiol 303: F1617–F1628.
63. Ceravolo GS, Franco MC, Carneiro-Ramos MS, Barreto-Chaves MLM, Tostes RCA et al. (2007) Enalapril and Losartan restored blood pressure and vascular reactivity in intrauterine undernourished rats. Life Sci 80: 782–787.
64. Schönwasser DC, Marais RM, Marshall CJ, Parker PJ (1998) Activation of the mitogen-activated protein kinase/extracellular signal-regulated kinase pathway by conventional, novel, and atypical protein kinase C isotypes. Mol Cell Biol 18: 790–798.
65. Vieira-Filho LD, Cabral EV, Farias JS, Silva PA, Muzi-Filho H et al. (2014) Renal Molecular mechanisms underlying altered Na^+ handling and genesis of hypertension during adulthood in prenatally undernourished rats. Br J Nutr: DOI 10.1017/S0007114513004236.
66. Cornock R, Langley-Evans SC, Mobasheri A, Mcmullen S (2010) The impact of maternal protein restriction during rat pregnancy upon renal expression of angiotensin receptors and vasopressin-related aquaporins. Reprod Biol Endocrinol 8: 105–110.
67. Cang C, Zhou Y, Navaro B, Seo Y, Aranda K, et al. (2013) mTOR regulates lysosomal ATP-sensitive two-pore Na^+ channels to adapt to metabolic state. Cell 152: 778–790.
68. Tian J, Li X, Liang M, Liu L, Xie JX, et al. (2009) Changes in sodium pump expression dictate the effects of ouabain on cell growth. J Biol Chem 284: 14921–14929.

Cord Blood 25(OH)-Vitamin D Deficiency and Childhood Asthma, Allergy and Eczema: The $COPSAC_{2000}$ Birth Cohort Study

Bo L. Chawes[1], Klaus Bønnelykke[1], Pia F. Jensen[1], Ann-Marie M. Schoos[1], Lene Heickendorff[2], Hans Bisgaard[1]*

1 Copenhagen Prospective Studies on Asthma in Childhood, Health Sciences, University of Copenhagen, Danish Pediatric Asthma Center, Copenhagen University Hospital, Gentofte, Denmark, **2** Department of Clinical Biochemistry, Aarhus University Hospital, Aarhus, Denmark

Abstract

Background: Epidemiological studies have suggested an association between maternal vitamin D dietary intake during pregnancy and risk of asthma and allergy in the offspring. However, prospective clinical studies on vitamin D measured in cord blood and development of clinical end-points are sparse.

Objective: To investigate the interdependence of cord blood 25-hydroxyvitamin D (25(OH)-Vitamin D) level and investigator-diagnosed asthma- and allergy-related conditions during preschool-age.

Methods: Cord blood 25(OH)-Vitamin D level was measured in 257 children from the Copenhagen Prospective Studies on Asthma in Childhood ($COPSAC_{2000}$) at-risk mother-child cohort. Troublesome lung symptoms (TROLS), asthma, respiratory infections, allergic rhinitis, and eczema, at age 0–7 yrs were diagnosed exclusively by the COPSAC pediatricians strictly adhering to predefined algorithms. Objective assessments of lung function and sensitization were performed repeatedly from birth.

Results: After adjusting for season of birth, deficient cord blood 25(OH)-Vitamin D level (<50 nmol/L) was associated with a 2.7-fold increased risk of recurrent TROLS (HR = 2.65; 95% CI = 1.02–6.86), but showed no association with respiratory infections or asthma. We saw no association between cord blood 25(OH)-Vitamin D level and lung function, sensitization, rhinitis or eczema. The effects were unaffected from adjusting for multiple lifestyle factors.

Conclusion: Cord blood 25(OH)-Vitamin D deficiency associated with increased risk of recurrent TROLS till age 7 years. Randomized controlled trials of vitamin D supplementation during pregnancy are needed to prove causality.

Editor: Yungling Leo Lee, National Taiwan University, Taiwan

Funding: COPSAC is funded by private and public research funds listed on www.copsac.com. The Lundbeck Foundation; The Danish Strategic Research Council; the Pharmacy Foundation of 1991; Augustinus Foundation; the Danish Medical Research Council and The Danish Pediatric Asthma Centre provided the core support for COPSAC research center. No pharmaceutical company was involved in the study. The funders had no role in study design, data collection and analysis, decision to publish, or preparation of the manuscript.

Competing Interests: The authors have declared that no competing interests exist.

* E-mail: bisgaard@copsac.com

Introduction

Vitamin D deficiency caused by adaption of a more sedentary indoor lifestyle and changing dietary habits has become a common health problem in developed and developing countries worldwide[1] which has occurred in parallel with the "asthma epidemic"[2]. It is now evident that vitamin D possesses a panoply of immune-regulatory functions that may protect against asthma and allergy [3] and recent findings also suggest a role of vitamin D for fetal lung cell maturation and subsequent lung function development [4]. These findings lend support to the hypothesis that fetal vitamin D deficiency may promote a trajectory to develop asthma and allergy [5]. A growing amount of studies have attempted to prove this hypothesis but with inconsistent findings.

Some epidemiological studies have shown an association between low maternal vitamin D intake during pregnancy and increased risk of wheezy phenotypes in the offspring [6,7] whereas others showed association with lower respiratory tract infections but not with wheezy symptoms [8] or asthma [8,9]. Likewise, some studies have shown that fetal vitamin D deficiency increases the risk of food allergy [10] and eczema [11,12] whereas others found no association with allergic sensitization [12]. Thus, it remains uncertain whether fetal vitamin D deficiency contributes to the development of childhood asthma, allergy and eczema. This may be a result from the inaccuracy of determining fetal Vitamin D exposure by questionnaire-based estimations of maternal dietary intake of vitamin D and/or poorly defined case definitions.

The aim of the current study was to investigate the programming effect of cord blood vitamin D deficiency on the subsequent development of troublesome lung symptoms (TROLS), asthma, lower respiratory tract infections, lung function, allergy, and eczema during preschool age. We studied these aspects in the children from the Copenhagen Prospective Study on Asthma in Childhood ($COPSAC_{2000}$) high-risk birth cohort [13–15] with longitudinal clinical data determined from strict predefined algorithm-based clinical case definitions and repeated objective assessments of intermediary end-points.

Materials and Methods

Study Design

The $COPSAC_{2000}$ birth cohort is a single-center prospective clinical study of 411 children born to mothers with physician verified asthma recruited between 1998 and 2001 as previously described [13–15]. The children were enrolled at one month of age and subsequently attended the clinical research unit for scheduled clinical investigations at six-monthly intervals as well as immediately upon onset of any respiratory-, allergy- or skin-related symptom. The pediatricians employed at the clinical research unit (not the family practitioners) were solely responsible for diagnosis and treatment of asthma, allergy, and eczema. At every visit a full physical examination was performed including lung function testing and history was obtained by parental interviews using predefined questions with closed response categories. History information was collected online during the visits and the objective measurements were double checked against source data and subsequently locked.

The study was conducted in accordance with the Declaration of Helsinki and was approved by The Copenhagen Ethics Committee (KF 01-289/96) and The Danish Data Protection Agency (2008-41-1754). Written informed consent was obtained from both parents before enrollment.

Cord Blood Vitamin D Measurement

Cord blood was collected by the midwives by needle puncture from the umbilical cord vein obtaining an aliquot of approximately 14 mL which was subsequently sent to the COPSAC research unit, centrifuged for 10 min at 4300 rpm to separate serum, and thereafter frozen at −80°C until analysis.

The serum samples were transported on dry ice for duplicate analyses for 25-hydroxyvitamin D2 (25(OH)-Vitamin D2) and 25(OH)-Vitamin D3 at the Dept. of Clinical Biochemistry, Aarhus University Hospital, Denmark. Serum 25-hydroxyvitamin D levels were analyzed by isotope dilution liquid chromatography-tandem mass spectrometry (LC-MS/MS) [16,17]. Calibrators traceable to NIST SRM 972 (Chromsystems, DE) were used. Mean coefficients of variation (CV) for 25(OH)-Vitamin D3 were 6.4% and 9.1% at levels of 66.5 and 21.1 nmol/L and for 25(OH)-Vitamin D2 the CV values were 8.8% and 9.4% at levels of 41.2 and 25.3 nmol/L. The average of the combined 25(OH)-Vitamin D values was calculated and used in the analysis. If both 25(OH)-Vitamin D2 and 25(OH)-Vitamin D3 were under the detection level, the combined value was defined as equal to 10 nmol/L.

Clinical Investigator-diagnosed End-points

Troublesome lung symptoms (TROLS) were defined as significant cough or wheeze or dyspnea and were explained to the parents as wheeze or whistling sounds, breathlessness, or recurrent troublesome cough severely affecting the well-being of the child and were recorded by the parents in a day-to-day diary chart as a dichotomized daily score (yes/no) from birth till age 7 yrs [18]. **Recurrent TROLS** was defined from the diaries at the scheduled or acute visits to the research clinic as five episodes within 6 months, each episode lasting at least three consecutive days, or daily symptoms for four consecutive weeks [19,20]. Children meeting these criteria were prescribed a 3-month trial of budesonide 200 mcg bid increasing to 6 and 12 months at subsequent relapses.

Asthma at age 7 yrs was diagnosed according to international guidelines and was based on recurrent TROLS as defined above, symptoms judged by the COPSAC pediatricians to be typical of asthma (e.g. exercise induced symptoms, prolonged nocturnal cough, recurrent cough outside common cold, symptoms causing wakening at night); in need of intermittent rescue use of inhaled β_2-agonist; responding to a 3-month trial of inhaled corticosteroids and relapsing when stopping treatment [14,15].

Lower respiratory tract infections (LRTI) included occurrence of pneumonia and/or acute bronchiolitis at age 0–3 yrs where such disorders are most prevalent. The diagnoses were established at the acute visits to the clinic by the research pediatricians based on clinical appearance regardless of identified pathogen(s) in accordance with predefined standard procedures [21] or if the child had been hospitalized for such disorders.

Allergic rhinitis was diagnosed at age 7 yrs based on clinical interviews of the parents on history of symptoms in the child's 7th year of life [22–24]. Rhinitis was defined as troublesome sneezing or blocked or runny nose in the past 12 months in periods without accompanying cold or flu [25].

Eczema was diagnosed utilizing the Hanifin-Rajka criteria as previously detailed [26,27] obtaining age at onset data. Skin lesions were described at both scheduled and acute visits according to pre-defined morphology and localization.

Lung Function

Infant spirometry was performed during sedation at age 1 month by applying the raised volume rapid thoraco-abdominal compression technique as previously detailed [28–30]. The forced expiratory volume at 0.5 seconds ($FEV_{0.5}$) and forced expiratory flow at 50% of the forced vital capacity (FEF_{50}) were used as lung function indices.

Spirometry at age 7 yrs was performed as previously detailed [31] using a pneumotachograph Masterscope Pneumoscreen, system 754,916 spirometer (Erich Jaeger, Wurtzburg, Germany) for assessing FEV_1 and maximal mid-expiratory flow (MMEF).

Bronchial responsiveness at age 1 month was assessed as previously detailed [29] by continuous measurements of transcutaneous oxygen saturation ($PtcO_2$) during quadrupling methacholine dose-steps and was defined as the provocative dose causing a 15% drop in $PtcO_2$ (PD_{15}). Bronchial responsiveness at age 7 yrs was defined as the provocative dose of methacholine causing a 20% drop in FEV_1 from baseline (PD_{20}) [31].

Allergy Intermediary End-points

Specific-IgE was measured at age ½, 1½, 4, and 6 yrs against 16 common inhalant and food allergens (cat, dog, horse, birch, timothy grass, mugwort, house dust mites, moulds, hen's egg, cow's milk, fish, wheat, peanut, soybean, or shrimp) by ImmunoCAP assay (Pharmacia Diagnostics AB, Uppsala, Sweden). Allergic sensitization was defined as specific-IgE ≥0.35 kU/L [32,33] for (1) any of the tested allergens, (2) any inhaled allergen, and (3) any food allergen.

Total-IgE was measured at age ½, 1½, 4, and 6 yrs by ImmunoCAP (Pharmacia Diagnostics AB, Uppsala, Sweden) with a detection limit of 2 kU/L [33].

Covariates

Blood sampling season was categorized as: winter (Dec-Feb), spring (March-May), summer (June-Aug) and fall (Sep-Nov). *Demographics* included child gender, birth BMI, maternal age at birth of proband, and household income (low: <50,000€, medium: 50,000–80,000€, high>80,000€). **Postnatal exposures** were older siblings (yes/no), length of solely breastfeeding, age at start in daycare, and environmental tobacco exposure measured objectively as hair nicotine level at age 1 yr [34].

Statistical Analysis

The combined cord blood 25(OH)-Vitamin D value was analyzed as a continuous variable per 100 nmol/L decrease as well as categorized as: deficient (<50 nmol/L), insufficient (50–75 nmol/L), sufficient (>75 nmol/L), based on biologically relevant levels according to recent studies on multiple health outcomes [1].

Distribution of baseline characteristics within the study group and the drop-out analysis was done with univariable parametric and non-parametric tests such as χ^2, Fischer's exact test, t-test, and Kruskal-Wallis rank sum test.

The association of cord blood 25(OH)-Vitamin D level with age at onset end-points (recurrent TROLS, LRTI, eczema) was estimated as hazard ratios by Cox regression and visualized by Kaplan-Meier curves for the categorized 25(OH)-Vitamin D levels. The effect of 25(OH)-Vitamin D level on the cross-sectional end-points, e.g. asthma and allergic rhinitis, was estimated as odds ratios by logistic regression. The association between 25(OH)-Vitamin D and cross-sectional continuous outcomes such as lung function incentives was explored by general linear models (GLM). The effect on outcome measures with repetitive assessments (allergic sensitization, total-IgE) was modeled using general estimating equations (GEE) applied to compute the overall odds ratio utilizing compiled data from all four time points (½, 1½, 4, 6 yrs). PD_{15}, PD_{20} and total-IgE were log-transformed and z-scores were calculated for $FEV_{0.5}$, FEV_1, FEF_{50} and MMEF prior to analyses.

Additional adjusted effect estimates were calculated with multivariable models including all covariates significantly associated with cord blood 25(OH)-Vitamin D level ($p \leq 0.05$) in the models. All analyses were adjusted for blood sampling season [12]. Results are reported with 95% confidence intervals (CI) in brackets, a p-value≤0.05 is considered significant. Analyses were done using SAS version 9.2 (SAS Institute, Cary, NC).

The core data of the manuscript is available online in **Data S1**.

Results

Baseline Characteristics

Cord blood was available for 25(OH)-Vitamin D analysis in 257 (63%) of the 411 children in the $COPSAC_{2000}$ cohort. Characteristics of the children with and without available cord blood samples are given in Table 1. Children in the drop-out group without available cord blood came from families with significantly lower household income ($p = 0.01$), but did not differ from the study group in any other baseline characteristics studied.

The median cord blood 25(OH)-Vitamin D level in the study group was 47.6 nmol/L (range, 10–145 nmol/L). The distribution of cord blood 25(OH)-Vitamin D concentrations was: 132 (53%) children with deficient levels, 82 (32%) with insufficient, and 39 (15%) with sufficient levels. Concentration of cord blood 25(OH)-Vitamin D varied significantly with season of birth ($p<0.01$) with most 25(OH)-Vitamin D deficient children born during winter and most sufficient children born during summer. Children with deficient vs. sufficient levels were born to younger mothers (median age at birth, 29.5 yrs vs. 30.8 yrs; $p = 0.02$), had fewer siblings (children with older siblings, 44% vs. 50%; $p = 0.02$), and had a higher exposure to environmental tobacco smoke (median hair nicotine level at age 1 yr, 0.84 vs. 0.47 ng/mg; $p = 0.03$).

Cord Blood 25(OH)-Vitamin D Level vs. Asthma-related Outcomes and LRTI

Recurrent TROLS was diagnosed in 24% (N = 61) of the children at age 0–7 yrs. The cumulative prevalence rates were 4% (N = 11) at age 0–1 yrs, 14% (N = 35) at 0–2 yrs, 16% (N = 42) at 0–3 yrs, 19% (N = 50) at 0–4 yrs, 22% (N = 57) at 0–5 yrs, and 23% (N = 59) at 0–6 yrs. Cord blood 25(OH)-Vitamin D levels were lower in children developing recurrent TROLS as illustrated in Figure 1. Having deficient vs. sufficient cord blood 25(OH)-Vitamin D level was associated with a 2.7-fold increased risk of recurrent TROLS (hazard ratio (HR), 2.65; 95% CI = 1.02–6.86; **p = 0.04**). The association was borderline significant when adjusting for multiple confounding factors but with unchanged effect estimates (aHR, 2.50; 95% CI, 0.95–6.57; $p = 0.06$).

Asthma at age 7 yrs was diagnosed in 16% (N = 34) of the children. 25(OH)-Vitamin D levels in cord blood showed no association with asthma at age 7 yrs (**Table 2**). In addition, cord blood 25(OH)-Vitamin D level was not suppressed in the subgroup of children experiencing recurrent TROLS who were subsequently diagnosed with asthma at age 7 yrs (N = 31): OR 2.25 (95% CI, 0.60–8.49; $p = 0.21$) for deficient vs. sufficient levels.

LRTI occurred in 56% (N = 119) of the study group with a mean of 1.2 (SD, 1.6) episodes per child till age 3 yrs. Cord blood 25(OH)-Vitamin D deficiency did not modify time to first LRTI (**Figure 2**) nor was the number of episodes affected by cord blood 25(OH)-Vitamin D level (**Table 2**).

Association between Cord Blood 25(OH)-Vitamin D Level and Lung Function

Cord blood 25(OH)-Vitamin D level was not associated with forced flows assessed at age 1mo ($FEV_{0.5}$, FEF_{50}) or 7 yrs (FEV_1, MMEF) nor bronchial responsiveness to methacholine at any age point (PD_{15}, PD_{20}) (Table 2).

Relationship between Cord Blood 25(OH)-Vitamin D and Allergic Outcomes (Table 3)

Specific-IgE. Allergic sensitization at any of the four measuring points (½, 1½, 4, 6 yrs) was present in 35% (N = 88) for any of the investigated allergens, in 26% (N = 64) for any food allergens, and in 21% (N = 52) for any inhaled allergen. There was no significant association between cord blood 25(OH)-Vitamin D level and allergic sensitization throughout childhood although there was a tendency of Vitamin D deficiency being associated with decreased risk of sensitization.

Total-IgE. Cord blood 25(OH)-Vitamin D level was not associated with level of total-IgE throughout childhood.

Allergic rhinitis was diagnosed in 12% (N = 23) at age 7 yrs. Deficient vs. sufficient cord blood 25(OH)-Vitamin D level seemed to be associated with a reduced risk of allergic rhinitis at age 7 yrs but this was not significant.

Table 1. Baseline characteristics of children with and without available cord blood for 25(OH)-Vitamin D analysis.

	Cord blood 25(OH)-Vitamin D (nmol/l), N = 257				No cord blood available, N = 154	
	Deficient: <50	**Insufficient: 50–75**	**Sufficient:>75**	**P***		**P****
Vitamin D cord blood (N)	53% (136)	32% (82)	15% (39)	-	-	-
DEMOGRAFICS						
Maternal age at birth[1], median (range)	29.5 yrs (20.9–38.9)	29.2 yrs (22.6–41.1)	30.8 yrs (22.1–37.8)	**0.02**	30.0 (19.2–41.2)	0.31
Household income[2] (N)				0.25		**0.01**
Low, <50.000E	28% (35)	25% (19)	13% (5)		37% (53)	
Medium, 50.000–80.000E	52% (65)	55% (42)	53% (20)		38% (55)	
High, >80.000E	21% (26)	20% (15)	34% (13)		25% (36)	
Boy[2] (N)	45% (61)	55% (45)	46% (18)	0.34	51% (79)	0.55
Birth BMI1, median (range)	12.8 kg/m^2 (7.0–16.3)	12.7 kg/m^2 (10.0–16.6)	12.8 kg/m^2 (9.6–15.1)	0.98	12.6 kg/m^2 (8.4–16.5)	0.35
Birth season[1] (N)				**<0.01**		0.39
Winter	30% (41)	15% (12)	18% (7)		23% (35)	
Spring	24% (33)	21% (17)	15% (6)		19% (30)	
Summer	21% (28)	33% (27)	49% (19)		24% (37)	
Fall	25% (34)	32% (26)	18% (7)		34% (52)	
POSTNATAL EXPOSURES						
Older siblings[2] (N)	44% (55)	26% (20)	50% (19)	**0.02**	40% (58)	0.87
Breastfeeding[3+4], median (range)	123 (0–243)	121 (0–274)	137 (0–266)	0.14	120 (0–244)	0.14
Daycare[4+5], median (range)	339 (140–1074)	308 (156–674)	286 (179–578)	0.46	355 (127–1003)	0.16
Nicotine in hair 1 yr[4], median (range)	0.84 ng/mg (0.06–30.9)	0.53 ng/mg (0.03–43.5)	0.47 ng/mg (0.1–12.9)	**0.03**	0.95 (0.03–103.9)	0.14

*P-value for the distribution of characteristics within the groups of 25(OH)-Vitamin D.
**P-value for the distribution of characteristics between children with and without available 25(OH)-Vitamin D data.
[1]Linear regression; [2]Chi-Square test; [3]Days solely breastfed; [4]Kruskal-Wallis rank sum test; [5]Age at start in daycare.

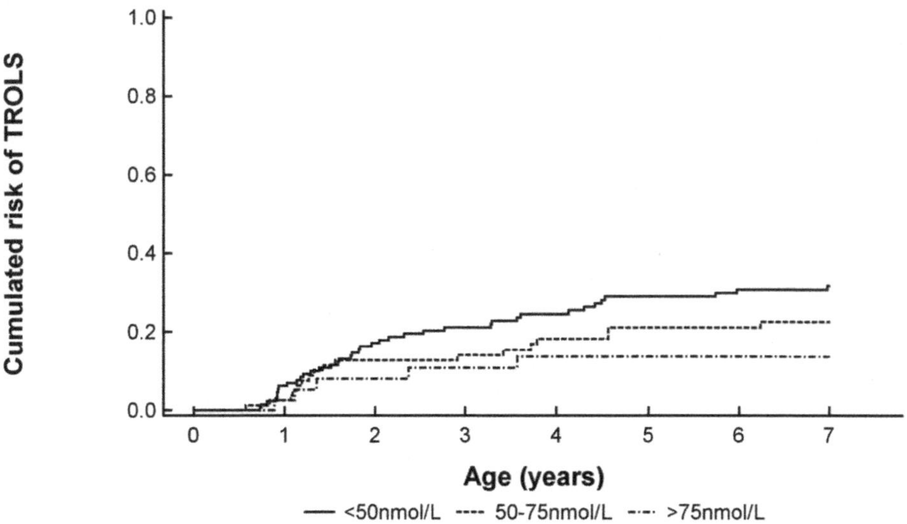

<50nmol/L	136	132	122	115	105	97	94	90	86	81	80	80	78	77	76	0
50-75nmol/L	82	79	77	69	66	66	65	62	58	56	54	54	54	53	53	0
>75nmol/L	39	39	38	34	33	32	32	30	28	28	28	28	28	28	28	0

Figure 1. Kaplan Meier survival curve showing the risk of developing recurrent troublesome lung symptoms (TROLS) at age 0–7 yrs stratified by cord blood 25(OH)-Vitamin D level.

Table 2. Cord blood 25(OH)-Vitamin D vs. asthma-related outcomes, lower respiratory tract infections and lung function.

	Cord blood 25(OH)-Vitamin D							
	<50 vs >75 nmol/L	P	<50 vs >75 nmol/L Adjusted*	P	Per 100 nmol/L decrease	P	Per 100 nmol/L decrease Adjusted*	P
Asthma-related outcomes								
Recurrent TROLS, 0–7 yrs[1+2]	**2.65 (1.02 to 6.86)**	**0.04**	**2.50 (0.95 to 6.57)**	**0.06**	**2.65 (0.83 to 8.50)**	**0.10**	2.27 (0.65 to 7.90)	0.20
Asthma, 7 yrs[3]	1.60 (0.49 to 5.22)	0.31	1.63 (0.47 to 5.61)	0.38	1.18 (0.25 to 5.58)	0.84	1.01 (0.18 to 5.80)	0.99
LRTI[4]								
Time to first LRTI, 0–3 yrs	1.08 (0.63 to 1.85)	0.78	1.08 (0.62 to 1.87)	0.79	1.17 (0.54 to 2.52)	0.69	1.05 (0.46 to 2.39)	0.91
No. of LRTI, 0–3 yrs[5]	1.07 (0.66 to 1.75)	0.78	0.94 (0.57 to 1.55)	0.81	1.08 (0.53 to 2.20)	0.83	0.75 (0.35 to 1.58)	0.69
Lung function								
z-FEV0.5, 1mo[6+7]	0.02 (−0.10 to 0.15)	0.73	−0.01 (−0.14 to 0.13)	0.94	0.01 (−0.02 to 0.04)	0.40	0.01 (−0.02 to 0.04)	0.70
z-FEV1, 7 yrs	0.04 (−0.09 to 0.18)	0.54	0.07 (−0.08 to 0.22)	0.37	0.02 (−0.02 to 0.06)	0.28	0.02 (−0.01 to 0.06)	0.24
z-FEF50, 1mo	−0.03 (−0.15 to 0.09)	0.63	−0.06 (−0.18 to 0.07)	0.38	0.01 (−0.02 to 0.04)	0.42	0.00 (−0.03 to 0.03)	0.82
z-MMEF, 7 yrs	−0.04 (−0.17 to 0.09)	0.55	−0.05 (−0.18 to 0.09)	0.50	0.00 (−0.03 to 0.03)	0.90	−0.01 (−0.04 to 0.02)	0.62
logPD15, 1mo[8]	0.02 (−0.05 to 0.09)	0.62	0.01 (−0.07 to 0.03)	0.92	0.01 (−0.01 to 0.02)	0.66	0.00 (−0.01 to 0.02)	0.82
logPD20, 7 yrs[9]	0.02 (−0.08 to 0.12)	0.68	0.03 (−0.07 to 0.14)	0.52	0.01 (−0.02 to 0.04)	0.41	0.01 (−0.02 to 0.04)	0.40

*Adjusted for mother's age at birth, blood sampling season, older siblings, and hair nicotine level at age 1 yr.

[1]TROLS = Troublesome lung symptoms; [2]Cox regression: hazards ratio (95% CI); [3]Logistic regression: odds ratio (95% CI); [4]Lower respiratory tract infections; [5]Poisson regression: incidence risk ratio (95% CI); [6]All lung function analyses are done with general linear models: β-coefficents (95% CI); [7]z refers to the calculated z-score; [8]PD_{15} refers to the provocative dose of methacholine resulting in a 15% decrease in transcutaneuos oxygen saturation ($PtcO_2$) from baseline; [9]PD_{20} refers to the provocative dose of methacholine resulting in a 20% decrease in FEV_1 from baseline.

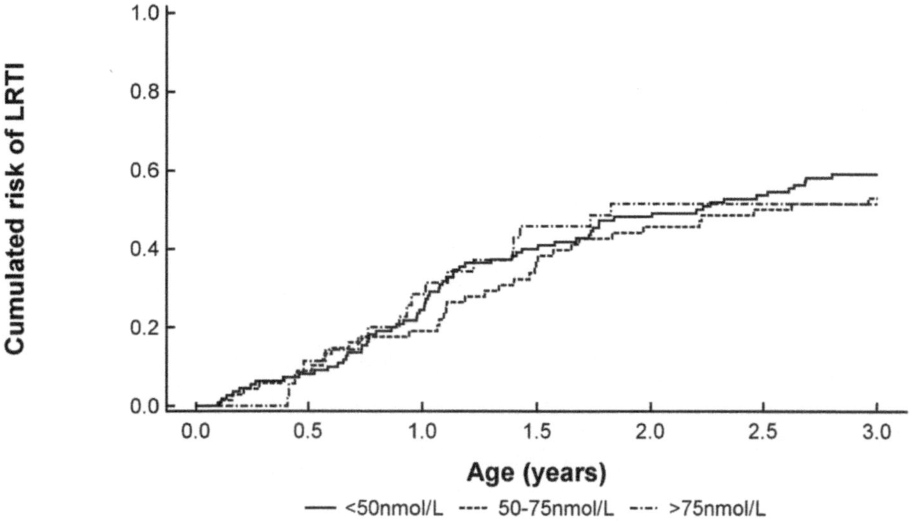

<50nmol/L	110	101	83	66	57	51	45
50-75nmol/L	68	62	55	43	37	34	32
>75nmol/L	35	31	25	19	17	17	17

Figure 2.Kaplan Meier survival curve showing the risk of developing lower respiratory tract infections (LRTI) at age 0–3 yrs stratified by cord blood 25(OH)-Vitamin D level.

Cord Blood 25(OH)-Vitamin D Level and Risk of Eczema

Eczema was diagnosed in 42% (N = 109) of the study group. Cord blood 25(OH)-Vitamin D level was not significantly associated with the risk of eczema during preschool age although the effect estimates suggested an increased risk by deficient cord blood levels (See Table 3 and Figure 3).

Discussion

Principal Findings

Deficient cord blood 25(OH)-Vitamin D level was associated with a more than doubled risk of developing TROLS during preschool age in children of the Danish $COPSAC_{2000}$ high-risk birth cohort study. This finding supports the theory that deficient 25(OH)-Vitamin D exposure in utero has a programming effect on the immune maturation thus predisposing to development of chronic inflammation.

Strengths and Limitations of the Study

The primary strength of the study is the seven years of clinical assessments of our birth cohort with longitudinal clinical deep phenotyping and standardized diagnoses solely performed by the COPSAC research pediatricians. Repeated objective measurements along with day-to-day respiratory symptom diary recordings through the first seven years of life provided strong age at onset data which is a major advantage compared to studies using cross-sectional unspecific community-based diagnoses [6,7,11].

Another significant strength is the objective assessment of fetal 25(OH)-Vitamin D exposure by measuring the concentration in the cord blood. Even though cord blood 25(OH)-Vitamin D level primarily reflects recent exposure during 3rd trimester and may be contaminated by maternal blood, this biological measure is a more accurate estimate of fetal 25(OH)-Vitamin D exposure compared to approximations from questionnaires on maternal dietary and supplementary intake since only 10% of vitamin D is obtained through diet [35].

It is also a strength of the analyses that environmental exposure assessments were comprehensive including hair nicotine level [34] as a validated objective measure of tobacco smoke exposure allowing for robust confounder adjustment. In agreement with other studies we found a marked seasonal variation in cord blood 25(OH)-Vitamin D level [12] as well as significant influence of various lifestyle factors such as passive smoking, maternal age at delivery, and older siblings [6,7]. We adjusted for season of blood sampling (i.e. sunlight exposure) which is a major determinant of serum 25(OH)-Vitamin D level [12]. We did not adjust our analyses for ethnicity [1] as 98% of the study group is of Caucasian origin.

The study is limited from the at-risk nature of the cohort as all mothers have a history of asthma which may limit the generalizability of our findings to other populations. However, this should not affect our ability to analyze the relationship between 25(OH)-Vitamin D levels and development of asthma and allergy-related traits within the cohort, and our findings are in line with studies of unselected populations [7,11].

We expected to see the largest effects in children with deficient compared to sufficient cord blood 25(OH)-Vitamin D levels. An essential limitation of the study is therefore the study sample size as only 15% had sufficient cord blood levels, equivalent to 39 participants, which results in lack of statistical power and a likelihood of overlooking the true effect of 25(OH)-Vitamin D exposure in fetal life on development of childhood asthma and allergy.

Interpretation

Our finding that deficient cord blood 25(OH)-Vitamin D level was associated with a more than doubled risk of developing recurrent TROLS during preschool age is in line with a range of epidemiological studies utilizing maternal dietary vitamin D intake during pregnancy as a surrogate measure of fetal vitamin D exposure [6,7,36]. However, studies of cord blood 25(OH)-Vitamin D are still sparse [9,11,12] and our study is the only one with a full clinical follow-up till age 7 yrs at a single research

Table 3. Cord blood 25(OH)-Vitamin D vs. allergic outcomes and eczema at 0–7 yrs.

	Cord blood 25(OH)-Vitamin D							
	<50 vs >75 nmol/L	P	<50 vs >75 nmol/L Adjusted*	P	Per 100 nmol/L decrease	P	Per 100 nmol/L decrease Adjusted*	P
Allergic outcomes								
Any sensitization, spec-IgE, 0–6 yr[1+2]	0.96 (0.43–2.16)	0.93	0.96 (0.64–2.31)	0.93	0.52 (0.17–1.52)	0.23	0.64 (0.19–2.12)	0.47
Food sensitization, spec-IgE, 0–6 yr[2]	0.86 (0.34–2.18)	0.74	0.94 (0.35–2.53)	0.91	0.47 (0.13–1.68)	0.25	0.63 (0.16–2.57)	0.53
Inhaled sensitization, spec-IgE, 0–6 yr[2]	0.97 (0.47–2.01)	0.94	1.20 (0.54–2.67)	0.65	0.36 (0.09–1.55)	0.17	0.43 (0.09–2.05)	0.29
Total-IgE, 0–6 yr[2]	0.98 (0.66–1.45)	0.91	0.98 (0.65–1.48)	0.93	0.86 (0.46–1.60)	0.63	0.83 (0.42–1.65)	0.60
Allergic rhinitis, 7 yr[3]	0.40 (0.12–1.26)	0.32	0.44 (0.13–1.49)	0.47	0.33 (0.06–1.92)	0.22	0.29 (0.04–2.14)	0.23
Eczema								
Time to eczema, 0–7 yr[4]	0.97 (0.56–1.69)	0.97	1.13 (0.63–2.01)	0.69	0.88 (0.41–1.92)	0.76	1.04 (0.44–2.41)	0.94
Eczema, 7 yr[3]	1.80 (0.56–5.79)	0.68	2.00 (0.59–6.76)	0.94	1.39 (0.33–5.82)	0.65	1.25 (0.27–5.82)	0.78

*Adjusted for mother's age at birth, blood sampling season, older siblings, and hair nicotine level at age 1 yr.
[1]Specific-IgE≥0.35 kU/mL against any of: dog, cat, horse, birch, timothy grass, mugwort, house dust mites, molds, milk, egg, wheat, soya bean, cod and peanut; [2]GEE model including data from age ½, 1½, 4 and 6 yrs: OR (95% CI); [3]Logistik regression: odds ratio (95% CI); [4]Cox regression: hazard ratio (95% CI).

unit employed solely with research pediatricians. Among available cord blood studies, one study found no association with recurrent wheeze [12], but only assessed the children at age 1 yr where such a diagnosis is quite infrequent in an unselected population. In line with our findings, an increased risk of deficient levels has been reported for early transient wheeze [11] and for development of wheeze till age 5 yrs [9].

It has been speculated that deficient neonatal vitamin D level mainly increases the risk of early transient wheezing exerting the effect through immune-modulatory mechanisms [3] which increase the frequency of respiratory tract infections and thus virus-induced wheezing [8,9]. We found that low cord blood level was associated with a significantly increased risk of early recurrent TROLS, but saw no association with occurrence of early childhood respiratory infections.

We found no significant association between cord blood 25(OH)-Vitamin D level and subsequent development of allergic sensitization or allergic rhinitis although the effect estimates showed a trend of decreased risk of allergic outcomes by deficient Vitamin D levels which has also been suggested by others [37].

We did not see any significant association between fetal vitamin D exposure and development of eczema although low cord blood levels seemed to associate with an increased risk. This finding is supported by other cord blood studies demonstrating that deficient vitamin D levels increase the risk of eczema both physician diagnosed and questionnaire-based [11,12].

The immune-regulatory properties of vitamin D exerted through e.g. promotion of pro-inflammatory cytokines and induction of regulatory T cells include an ability to shift the Th1/Th2 balance with capacity to inhibit both Th1 and Th2-type responses leading to opposite effects on disease development, i.e. enhancing vs. reducing the risk [38]. The complex interplay between the genetic makeup, the early life milieu, and the timing of sufficient vitamin D exposure during maturation of the immature immune system may determine the direction of the immune-modulatory properties of Vitamin D. Additional programming effects of fetal vitamin D exposure apart from immune-modulation might be alterations of the airway microbiome from e.g. induction of the endogenous antimicrobial peptide cathelicidin in bronchial epithelial cells [39].

Overall, our study suggests an association between deficient fetal 25(OH)-Vitamin D exposure and development of recurrent TROLS during preschool age with a sizable effect estimate. However, despite the rigorously clinically determined diagnoses in this study and the objective assessment of cord blood 25(OH)-Vitamin D, the question of causality cannot be answered by an observational study. Thus, acknowledging that and the possibility of residual lifestyle confounding, this study prompts the performance of randomized controlled trials of maternal supplementation of vitamin D during pregnancy to shed light on the possible causative and thus modifiable effect of fetal vitamin D deficiency for development of asthma, allergy and eczema. Several randomized controlled trials are currently being conducted by our group and others (clinicalTrials.gov identification numbers: NCT00856947, NCT00920621).

Conclusion

This study shows an interdependence of 25(OH)-Vitamin D deficiency in fetal life and occurrence of recurrent TROLS during preschool in children of the at-risk $COPSAC_{2000}$ cohort. Further research is required to establish whether vitamin D supplementation during pregnancy can prevent development and severity of such disorders.

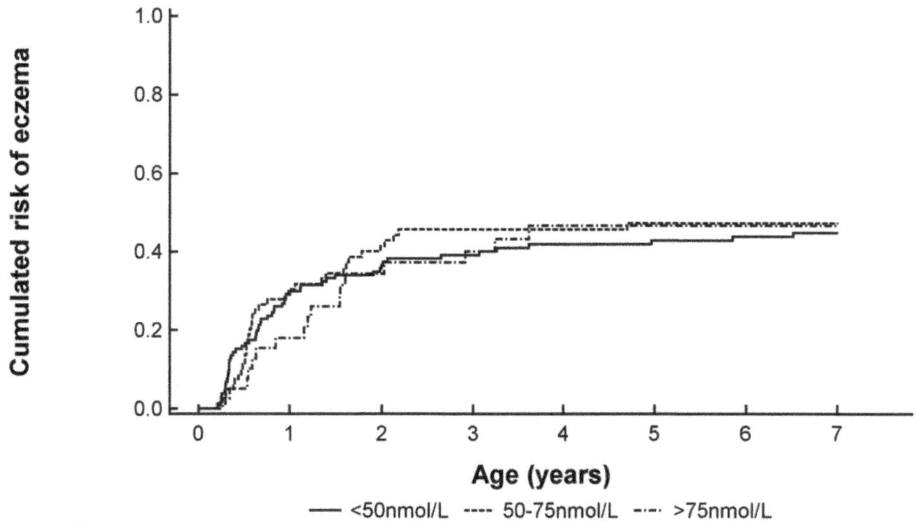

<50nmol/L	136	110	88	81	76	70	69	64	60	60	59	59	58	58	57	0
50-75nmol/L	82	70	54	49	42	39	38	38	37	35	34	34	33	33	33	0
>75nmol/L	39	37	32	27	23	22	21	17	16	16	16	16	16	16	16	0

Figure 3. Kaplan Meier survival curve showing the risk of developing eczema at age 0–7 yrs stratified by cord blood 25(OH)-Vitamin D level.

Acknowledgments

We gratefully express our gratitude to the children and families of the $COPSAC_{2000}$ cohort study for all their support and commitment. We acknowledge and appreciate the unique efforts of the COPSAC research team.

Author Contributions

Conceived and designed the experiments: BLC KB HB. Performed the experiments: BLC KB PFJ AMS. Analyzed the data: BLC KB PFJ AMS HB. Contributed reagents/materials/analysis tools: LH. Wrote the paper: BLC KB PFJ AMS LH HB. The guarantor of the study who has been responsible for the integrity of the work as a whole, from conception and design to conduct of the study and acquisition of data, analysis and interpretation of data and writing of the manuscript: HB. Responsible for data analysis, interpretation and writing the manuscript: BLC KB PFJ AMS LH. Wrote the first draft of the manuscript: BC. No honorarium, grant, or other form of payment was given to anyone to produce the manuscript. All co-authors have contributed substantially to the analyses and interpretation of the data, and have provided important intellectual input and approval of the final version of the manuscript.

References

1. Holick MF (2007) Vitamin D deficiency. N Engl J Med 357: 266–281.
2. Eder W, Ege MJ, von ME (2006) The asthma epidemic. N Engl J Med 355: 2226–2235.
3. Hollams EM (2012) Vitamin D and atopy and asthma phenotypes in children. Curr Opin Allergy Clin Immunol 12: 228–234.
4. Zosky GR, Berry LJ, Elliot JG, James AL, Gorman S, et al. (2011) Vitamin D deficiency causes deficits in lung function and alters lung structure. Am J Respir Crit Care Med 183: 1336–1343.
5. Litonjua AA, Weiss ST (2007) Is vitamin D deficiency to blame for the asthma epidemic? J Allergy Clin Immunol 120: 1031–1035.
6. Camargo CA, Jr., Rifas-Shiman SL, Litonjua AA, Rich-Edwards JW, Weiss ST, et al. (2007) Maternal intake of vitamin D during pregnancy and risk of recurrent wheeze in children at 3 y of age. Am J Clin Nutr 85: 788–795.
7. Devereux G, Litonjua AA, Turner SW, Craig LC, McNeill G, et al. (2007) Maternal vitamin D intake during pregnancy and early childhood wheezing. Am J Clin Nutr 85: 853–859.
8. Morales E, Romieu I, Guerra S, Ballester F, Rebagliato M, et al. (2012) Maternal vitamin D status in pregnancy and risk of lower respiratory tract infections, wheezing, and asthma in offspring. Epidemiology 23: 64–71.
9. Camargo CA, Jr., Ingham T, Wickens K, Thadhani R, Silvers KM, et al. (2011) Cord-blood 25-hydroxyvitamin D levels and risk of respiratory infection, wheezing, and asthma. Pediatrics 127: e180–e187.
10. Liu X, Arguelles L, Zhou Y, Wang G, Chen Q, et al. (2013) Longitudinal trajectory of vitamin D status from birth to early childhood in the development of food sensitization. Pediatr Res 74: 321–326.
11. Baiz N, rgent-Molina P, Wark JD, Souberbielle JC, nnesi-Maesano I (2013) Cord serum 25-hydroxyvitamin D and risk of early childhood transient wheezing and atopic dermatitis. J Allergy Clin Immunol.
12. Jones AP, Palmer D, Zhang G, Prescott SL (2012) Cord blood 25-hydroxyvitamin D3 and allergic disease during infancy. Pediatrics 130: e1128–e1135.
13. Bisgaard H (2004) The Copenhagen Prospective Study on Asthma in Childhood (COPSAC): design, rationale, and baseline data from a longitudinal birth cohort study. Ann Allergy Asthma Immunol 93: 381–389.
14. Bisgaard H, Hermansen MN, Loland L, Halkjaer LB, Buchvald F (2006) Intermittent inhaled corticosteroids in infants with episodic wheezing. N Engl J Med 354: 1998–2005.
15. Bisgaard H, Hermansen MN, Buchvald F, Loland L, Halkjaer LB, et al. (2007) Childhood asthma after bacterial colonization of the airway in neonates. N Engl J Med 357: 1487–1495.
16. Maunsell Z, Wright DJ, Rainbow SJ (2005) Routine isotope-dilution liquid chromatography-tandem mass spectrometry assay for simultaneous measurement of the 25-hydroxy metabolites of vitamins D2 and D3. Clin Chem 51: 1683–1690.
17. Hojskov CS, Heickendorff L, Moller HJ (2010) High-throughput liquid-liquid extraction and LCMSMS assay for determination of circulating 25(OH) vitamin D3 and D2 in the routine clinical laboratory. Clin Chim Acta 411: 114–116.
18. Bisgaard H, Pipper CB, Bonnelykke K (2011) Endotyping early childhood asthma by quantitative symptom assessment. J Allergy Clin Immunol.
19. Bisgaard H, Bonnelykke K, Sleiman PM, Brasholt M, Chawes B, et al. (2009) Chromosome 17q21 gene variants are associated with asthma and exacerbations but not atopy in early childhood. Am J Respir Crit Care Med 179: 179–185.
20. Chawes BL, Buchvald F, Bischoff AL, Loland L, Hermansen M, et al. (2010) Elevated Exhaled Nitric Oxide in High-risk Neonates Precedes Transient Early but not Persistent Wheeze. Am J Respir Crit Care Med 182: 138–142.

21. Vissing NH, Chawes BL, Bisgaard H (2013) Increased risk of pneumonia and bronchiolitis after bacterial colonization of the airways as neonates. Am J Respir Crit Care Med 188: 1246–1252.
22. Chawes BL, Kreiner-Moller E, Bisgaard H (2009) Objective assessments of allergic and nonallergic rhinitis in young children. Allergy 64: 1547–1553.
23. Chawes BL, Kreiner-Moller E, Bisgaard H (2010) Upper and Lower Airway Patency are Associated in Young Children. Chest 137: 1332–1337.
24. Chawes BL, Bonnelykke K, Kreiner-Moller E, Bisgaard H (2010) Children with allergic and nonallergic rhinitis have a similar risk of asthma. J Allergy Clin Immunol 126: 567–573.
25. Braun-Fahrlander C, Wuthrich B, Gassner M, Grize L, Sennhauser FH, et al. (1997) Validation of a rhinitis symptom questionnaire (ISAAC core questions) in a population of Swiss school children visiting the school health services. SCARPOL-team. Swiss Study on Childhood Allergy and Respiratory Symptom with respect to Air Pollution and Climate. International Study of Asthma and Allergies in Childhood. Pediatr Allergy Immunol 8: 75–82.
26. Bisgaard H, Simpson A, Palmer CN, Bonnelykke K, McLean I, et al. (2008) Gene-environment interaction in the onset of eczema in infancy: filaggrin loss-of-function mutations enhanced by neonatal cat exposure. PLoS Med 5: e131.
27. Halkjaer LB, Loland L, Buchvald FF, Agner T, Skov L, et al. (2006) Development of atopic dermatitis during the first 3 years of life: the Copenhagen prospective study on asthma in childhood cohort study in high-risk children. Arch Dermatol 142: 561–566.
28. Chawes BL, Poorisrisak P, Johnston SL, Bisgaard H (2012) Neonatal bronchial hyperresponsiveness precedes acute severe viral bronchiolitis in infants. J Allergy Clin Immunol 130: 354–361.
29. Loland L, Buchvald FF, Halkjaer LB, Anhoj J, Hall GL, et al. (2006) Sensitivity of bronchial responsiveness measurements in young infants. Chest 129: 669–675.
30. Loland L, Bisgaard H (2008) Feasibility of repetitive lung function measurements by raised volume rapid thoracoabdominal compression during methacholine challenge in young infants. Chest 133: 115–122.
31. Bisgaard H, Jensen SM, Bonnelykke K (2012) Interaction between Asthma and Lung Function Growth in Early Life. Am J Respir Crit Care Med.
32. Ballardini N, Nilsson C, Nilsson M, Lilja G (2006) ImmunoCAP Phadiatop Infant—a new blood test for detecting IgE sensitisation in children at 2 years of age. Allergy 61: 337–343.
33. Wickman M, Ahlstedt S, Lilja G, van Hage HM (2003) Quantification of IgE antibodies simplifies the classification of allergic diseases in 4-year-old children. A report from the prospective birth cohort study—BAMSE. Pediatr Allergy Immunol 14: 441–447.
34. Sorensen M, Bisgaard H, Stage M, Loft S (2007) Biomarkers of exposure to environmental tobacco smoke in infants. Biomarkers 12: 38–46.
35. Sichert-Hellert W, Wenz G, Kersting M (2006) Vitamin intakes from supplements and fortified food in German children and adolescents: results from the DONALD study. J Nutr 136: 1329–1333.
36. Miyake Y, Sasaki S, Tanaka K, Hirota Y (2010) Dairy food, calcium and vitamin D intake in pregnancy, and wheeze and eczema in infants. Eur Respir J 35: 1228–1234.
37. Wjst M (2006) The vitamin D slant on allergy. Pediatr Allergy Immunol 17: 477–483.
38. Litonjua AA (2009) Childhood asthma may be a consequence of vitamin D deficiency. Curr Opin Allergy Clin Immunol 9: 202–207.
39. Yim S, Dhawan P, Ragunath C, Christakos S, Diamond G (2007) Induction of cathelicidin in normal and CF bronchial epithelial cells by 1,25-dihydroxyvitamin D(3). J Cyst Fibros 6: 403–410.

Vitamin D Deficiency Causes Defective Resistance to *Aspergillus fumigatus* in Mice via Aggravated and Sustained Inflammation

Pei Li[1], Xiaoyong Xu[1], Ehong Cao[1], Bo Yu[2], Wanchun Li[2], Ming Fan[3], Mei Huang[3], Lining Shi[4], Rong Zeng[4], Xin Su[1]*, Yi Shi[1]*

1 Department of Respiratory and Critical Care Medicine, Jinling Hospital, Nanjing University School of Medicine, Nanjing Jiangsu Province, People's Republic of China, **2** Department of Pathology, Jinling Hospital, Nanjing University School of Medicine, Nanjing Jiangsu Province, People's Republic of China, **3** Department of Clinical Microbiology, Jinling Hospital, Nanjing University School of Medicine, Nanjing Jiangsu Province, People's Republic of China, **4** Department of Clinical Laboratory, Jinling Hospital, Nanjing University School of Medicine, Nanjing Jiangsu Province, People's Republic of China

Abstract

Background: Vitamin D plays an important role in pulmonary resistance and immunity, and its deficiency has been linked to various respiratory infections. Little is known about the effect of vitamin D deficiency on host pulmonary defense to *Aspergillus fumigatus* (*A. fumigatus*).

Methods: Mice raised on vitamin D sufficient or deficient diets were infected intratracheally with *A. fumigatus* conidia. Mortality, fungal growth, weight loss and lung histology were monitored. Alveolar macrophages (AMs) were stimulated with *A. fumigatus* conidia *in vitro*. The kinetics of pro-inflammatory cytokines (TNF-α, IL-1β and IL-6), chemokines (CXCL1, CCL3), and pattern recognition receptors (Toll-like receptor [TLR] 2, TLR 4 and dectin-1) expression in the lungs and AMs were measured.

Results: Upon *A. fumigatus* infection, vitamin D deficient mice showed higher mortality, greater fungal load, and more weight loss than its sufficient counterparts. Vitamin D deficient mice demonstrated aggravated and prolonged histological evidence of lung inflammation as well as enhanced BAL cell counts, dominated by neutrophils after *A. fumigatus* inoculation. Increased basal levels of pro-inflammatory cytokines in the lungs and AMs from naïve vitamin D deficient mice were observed. Upon *A. fumigatus* exposure, vitamin D deficiency led to enhanced and sustained expression of TNF-α, IL-1β, IL-6, CXCL1 and CCL3 both *in vivo* and *in vitro*. Up-regulation of TLR2, TLR4 and dectin-1was observed in the lungs and AMs from vitamin D deficient mice both at baseline and after *A. fumigatus* exposure.

Conclusions: Vitamin D deficiency causes defective pulmonary resistance to *A. fumigatus* in mice, possibly by the enhanced basal expression of pattern recognition receptors and pro-inflammatory cytokines, which induced excessive inflammatory response in response to *A. fumigatus* challenge.

Editor: Joy Sturtevant, Louisiana State University, United States of America

Funding: This work was supported by National Natural Science Foundation of China (NSFC 81270064). The funders had no role in study design, data collection and analysis, decision to publish, or preparation of the manuscript.

Competing Interests: The authors have declared that no competing interests exist.

* E-mail: suxinjs@hotmail.com (XS); shiyi56@126.com (YS)

These authors contributed equally to this work.

Introduction

It is increasingly recognized that vitamin D plays an important role in pulmonary defense, immunity, and inflammatory processes [1,2]. The active vitamin D generating enzyme, 1α-hydroxylase, is expressed by the airway epithelium[3], alveolar macrophages (AMs)[4] and dendritic cells[5], indicating that active vitamin D can be produced locally within the lungs, that it acts in an autocrine or paracrine fashion, and is responsible for many immunomodulatory actions. Immune effects of vitamin D include increased secretion of the antimicrobial peptide cathelicidin, decreased chemokine production, inhibition of dendritic cell activation, and alteration of T-cell activation [6]. These cellular effects are important for host responses against infection and impaired vitamin D status would compromise the immune activity of vitamin D.

Vitamin D deficiency and insufficiency is a global issue which has significant implications for health [7,8]. Multiple studies have identified a correlation between vitamin D deficiency and various respiratory infections, especially increased risk of tuberculosis, influenza and viral respiratory tract infections [9,10,11,12]. *A. fumigatus* remains the most common Aspergillus species that cause respiratory infections in humans, in particular in the immunocompromised patient population [13]. However, little has been done to assess the impact of impaired vitamin D status on the host control of pulmonary *A. fumigatus* infection. Vitamin D deficiency has been proposed as a risk factor for Allergic Bronchopulmonary Aspergillosis (ABPA) in cystic fibrosis (CF) patients[14]. Based on the fact that local synthesis of active vitamin D in lung can act to support immunomodulation at this barrier site, we hypothesized that vitamin D deficiency may compromise pulmonary resistance to *A. fumigatus*. In the current study, we sought to test this hypothesis by inducing pulmonary *A. fumigatus* infection in mice raised on vitamin D sufficient (VitD+) or vitamin D deficient (VitD-) diets.

Materials and Methods

Animals

This study was carried out in strict accordance with the recommendations in the Guide for the Care and Use of Laboratory Animals of the National Institutes of Health. All mouse experiments were approved by the Animal Care and Use Committee at Nanjing University and Jingling Hospital under university-approved standards. Three-week old female C57BL/6J mice (Institute of Laboratory Animal Sciences, the Chinese Academy of Medical Sciences) were housed in groups of five together on hardwood chip bedding in micro-isolator cages in specific pathogen-free enviroment within small animal care facilities, at a room temperature of 22.5±1°C, and a relative humidity of 52±5%. Mice were exposed to a 12 hr light/dark cycle and had ad libitum access to the assigned diet and tap water. Cage maintenance was performed twice weekly, and the animals were handled by the same individuals at all times. Mice were weighed weekly and monitored for changes in health status. After one week acclimatization, the mice were randomized to VitD- diet (AIN-93G/No vitamin D) or VitD+ diet (AIN-93G) for at least eight weeks. The vitamin D replete diet contained 1000 IU vitamin D3/kg of food. All diets were procured from Research Diets, Inc. (New Brunswick, NJ). Every two weeks, three mice from each group were bled from the retro-orbital venous plexus. The blood was centrifuged at 1,000–1,500 rpm for 10 min and the serum collected for 25-OH VitD3 (25-(OH)D3) analysis. Serum 25-(OH)D3 levels were measured by ELISA kit (IDS) to confirm vitamin D deficiency. Ketamine-xylazine anesthesia was used for retro-orbital venous plexus puncture. Under ketamine-xylazine anesthesia, animals were sacrificed by cervical dislocation for each experiment. All efforts were made to minimize animal suffering.

Preparation of *A. fumigatus*

The strain of *A. fumigatus* was obtained from a patient with a fatal case of pulmonary aspergillosis at the Department of Respiratory and Critical Care Medicine, Jinling Hospital, Nanjing University School of Medicine. Conidia were harvested by washing a 7 day-old slant culture on Sabouraud dextrose agar with PBS supplemented with 0.1% Tween 20. The suspension was filtered through a 40 μm cell strainer (Falcon) to separate conidia from the contaminating mycelium and the absence of mycelium in the filtrate was verified microscopically.

In vivo *A. fumigatus* infection, survival and tissue burden assessment, and histology

Mice were lightly anesthetized with ketamine-xylazine and administered intratracheally with 2–7×10^7 per 50 μl viable conidia while being held in a vertical position. Afterword, mice were placed on their backs during recovery from anesthesia. After inoculation, all animals fully recovered within 1–2 hrs and were normal in appearance until signs of disease became apparent 24–30 hrs after infection. Survival, clinical appearance and body weight were monitored daily for each group. For survival studies, mice were monitored every 6 hr post-*A. fumigatus* challenge. Mice were observed on a regular basis during the day and were weighed each morning. Body temperature was taken in the morning and evening with a digital thermometer inserted into the vagina. Time of death or premature euthanasia was recorded, and deaths that occurred at night were assigned a time of death midway between the last evening observation and the first morning observation. Criteria for premature euthanasia were labored breathing, a 25% weight loss, and severe hypothermia (body temperature <32°C). Fungal burden in lungs was determined by a quantitative colony forming units (CFUs) assay. At selected time points post infection (p.i.) lungs were aseptically removed and their wet masses determined using a precision balance (±0.01 g). Tissue specimens were homogenized using a mechanical homogenizer for 1 min at a 1:5 dilution (w/v) in sterile PBS. Primary homogenate dilutions were quantitatively cultured by serial dilution, plated in triplicate on SDA plates, incubated at 37°C for 24–48 hrs, and the number of CFUs per gram of tissue was enumerated. Results were expressed as $\log_{10}$CFU per lung. Sections of formalin fixed lung were stained with hematoxylin and eosin (HE) for histological analysis, with Grocott's methenamine silver (GMS) for the detection of conidia and hyphae. Histopathologic scoring (HPS) was performed by a pathologist in a blinded manner. This HPS system assigned values of 0–26 (the higher the score, the greater the inflammatory changes) as described by Cimolai et al.[15]. Lungs were evaluated for inflammatory infiltrates and assigned a cumulative score in the following five categories: (1) peribronchiolar and bronchial infiltrates, (2) bronchiolar and bronchial luminal exudates, (3) perivascular infiltrates, (4) the number of neutrophils, and (5) parenchymal pneumonia.

Bronchoalveolar lavage (BAL) for cell recovery

Airway contents were recovered by 4 rounds of filling the lungs with 0.8 ml PBS and withdrawing as much of the liquid as possible through a 20-gauge needle inserted into the trachea after cervical dissection. The bronchoalveolar lavage fluid (BALF) was centrifuged, the supernatant was removed and immediately frozen and stored at −80°C. The recovered BAL cells were resuspended in PBS and enumerated under a light microscope in the presence of trypan blue using a hemocytometer.

Morphological leukocyte differential analysis

Cells were visually counted by standard morphological criteria in Wright-Giemsa-stained samples of BAL cell suspensions cytospun onto glass slides. For Wright-Giemsa staining, the slides were fixed for 2 min with a one-step methanol-based Wright-Giemsa stain (Sigma) followed by steps 2 and 3 of the Diff-Quik whole blood stain kit (Baxter Scientific). A total of 200 to 300 cells were counted from randomly chosen high-power microscope fields for each sample.

Isolation and stimulation of AMs

AMs were harvested from mouse lungs with 0.8 ml ice-cold PBS (10 times) through a 20-gauge needle inserted into the trachea after cervical dissection. For stimulation assays, cells were separated from BALF by centrifugation at 300×g for 8 min at 4°C and suspended at a concentration of 2×10^6/ml of RPMI1640 supplemented with penicillin (100 U/ml), streptomycin (100 μg/ml), and 5% heat-inactivated FBS. Aliquots of 250 μl (5×10^5 cells) were added to 24-well plates, and allowed to adhere for 2 h at 37°C under a humidified atmosphere with 5% CO_2. All wells were then washed three times with RPMI1640. Fresh RPMI 1640 supplemented with 10% FBS was added prior to challenge with conidia. AMs were incubated in medium alone or in the presence of viable *A. fumigatus* conidia at a microbe to cell ratio of 1:10 (MOI = 0.1). After 6, 10, 14, and 18 hr of co-culture, total RNA from AMs was extracted, reverse-transcribed to cDNA, and stored at −20°C.

Flow cytometry analysis

Cellular population in BALF were washed and resuspended at a concentration of 0.5×10^6 to 1×10^6/50 µl FA buffer (Difco) plus 0.1% NaN_3, and Fc receptors were blocked by the addition of unlabeled anti-CD16/32(Fc blocking, eBioscience Inc.). After Fc receptor blocking, immunostaining for cell surface molecules was performed for 30 min at 4°C. Cells were washed twice with FA buffer, resuspended in 200 µl of 4% formalin (Sigma). A minimum of 10000 events were acquired on a FACSCanto flow cytometer (BD Pharmingen) using CellQuest software (BD Pharmingen). The data acquired were analyzed with FlowJo software (Tree Star, Stanford, CA). Fluorochrome-conjugated antibodies directed against the following antigens were obtained: CD45-PE, Gr-1-FITC, CD11c-APC, TLR2-FITC, TLR4-PE, (eBioscience Inc.), and Dectin-1-PE (R&D). Numbers of relevant cell types were determined by combining flow cytometry data (percentage of a given cell type).

Gene expression

Gene expression was assessed by quantitative real-time PCR with TaqMan probes specific for mouse GAPDH (GU214026.1), TNF-α (NM_013693.2), IL-1β (NM_008361.3), IL-6 (NM_031168.1), CXCL1 (NC_000004.12), CCL3 (NC_000017.11), TLR2 (NM_011905.3), TLR4 (NM_021297.2), and dectin-1 (NM_020008.2) obtained from Applied Biosystems. RNA was isolated from lung tissue or cultured cells, and cDNA synthesis was performed using the RevertAid First Strand cDNA Synthesis Kit (Thermo Scientific) according to manufacturer's instructions. Data were expressed using the delta-delta Ct method and normalized to the housekeeping gene GAPDH. Each PCR run included a no-template control.

Western blot analysis

Equal amounts of protein from tissue homogenates were electrophoresed through SDS-PAGE 8–18% gradient gels. The material in the gels was blotted onto a polyvinylidene difluoride (PVDF) membrane (Bio-Rad), and the membrane was blocked with 3% BSA in TBS buffer pH 7.5 for 2 hr. After washes (TBS pH 7.5, 0.02% Tween 20), immunolabeling was performed using the primary antibody at 4°C overnight. The following primary antibodies were used: anti-dectin-1 at 1:1000, anti-TLR2 at 1:1500, and anti-TLR4 at 1:500 (Abcam). Then membranes were incubated with the appropriate secondary antibodies (Cell Signaling, 1:2000) for 2 h at room temperature. Anti-GAPDH (1:1000 Santa Cruz Biotechnology) was used as loading control. After washing, protein bands were visualized with Chemiluminescent HRP Substrate (Millipore) for 5 min at room temperature and exposed to X-ray film (Fuji Hyperfilm). Relative changes in protein expression were estimated from the mean pixel density using Quantity One software 4.6.2 (Bio-Rad), normalized to GAPHD and presented as relative density units.

Cytokine assays

The protein levels of TNF-α, IL-1β, IL-6, CXCL1, and CCL3 in BALF were measured by commercially available cytokine-specific mouse ELISA kits (R&D) according to the manufacturers recommendations.

Statistical analyses

Statistical analysis was performed using the Graph Pad Prism 5.0 software. Differences of survival rates were analyzed using the Log-rank and Wilcoxon tests. Parametric data were expressed as mean±SE and analyzed by t-tests. Non-parametric data were presented as median and analyzed using the Mann-Whitney test. P-values <0.05 were considered significant. All experiments were performed in triplicate.

Results

Vitamin D deficiency defected host resistance to *A. fumigatus*

To investigate whether vitamin D deficiency alters host resistance to *A. fumigatus*, we generated C57BL/6J mice that were nutritionally deficient in vitamin D as previously described [16]. After 8 wk on the diet, VitD- mice had 25-(OH)D3 levels of 5.1±0.25 ng/mL compared to VitD+ mice with 25-(OH)D3 levels of 82.04±1.74 ng/mL (Table 1, $p<0.0001$). No significant changes were observed in serum calcium and phosphorus concentrations at 8 wk on the diet (data not show). Average weight was similar in mice on VitD- and VitD+ chow over the 8 wk period (Table 1). Then, mice were infected intratracheally with viable *A. fumigatus* conidia and parameters of resistance to infection in terms of mortality, fungal growth and weight loss were evaluated.

Infection with 5×10^7 conidia resulted in significantly higher mortality in VitD- mice than in VitD+ mice (45%; 9/20 mice versus 15%; 3/20 mice, respectively) (Fig. 1A). Increasing the inoculum to 7×10^7 resulted in 61% mortality in VitD- mice by 4 days (Fig. 1B). Although infection with 2×10^7 conidia resulted in no death in either group of mice in a 28-day mortality assay (data not show), vitamin D deficiency impaired pulmonary clearance of *A. fumigatus*, as determined by a significantly higher pulmonary fungal load in VitD- mice at 24, 48 and 72 hr after infection with 2×10^7 conidia (Fig. 1C). Upon challenge with 2×10^7 conidia, weight loss was more pronounced in VitD- mice, and weight gain in VitD- mice was far less than in VitD+ mice (Fig. 1D). All these date suggested that vitamin D deficiency resulted in a defective host pulmonary resistance to *A. fumigatus*.

Aggravated and sustained inflammatory response in *A. fumigatus*-challenged VitD- mice

Histological evidence of aggravated and sustained inflammatory response in *A. fumigatus*-challenged VitD- mice. HE staining of lung tissue sections revealed the presence of inflammatory cells, mainly neutrophils, centered on bronchi/bronchioles and blood vessels with signs of peribronchial necrosis in both groups of mice (Fig. 2A, upper, 72 hr after challenge with 5×10^7 *A. fumigatus* conidia). The inflammatory lesions in VitD- mice were more severe and diffused, with peribronchiolar edema, consolidation of the inflammatory response, and disappearance of alveolar structure (Fig. 2A). GMS staining of lung tissue sections revealed *A. fumigatus* germinating conidia and septate-branching hyphae in VitD- mice as opposed to the relatively fewer germinating conidia and no hyphae in VitD+ mice (Fig. 2A, below).

Infection with 2×10^7 conidia resulted in no death in either group of mice. So lung histopathology was analyzed sequentially (Fig. 2B) and lung inflammation was quantified by HPS (Fig. 2C) after challenge with this amount of inocula. By 6 hr, lung sections

Table 1. Serum concentrations of Vitamin D and weights of mice in the two dietary groups after dietary restriction.

weeks	two		four		six		eight	
	VitD+	VitD-	VitD+	VitD-	VitD+	VitD-	VitD+	VitD-
25-(OH)D3 (ng/ml)	43.4±0.67	22.3±0.89***	63.2±1.02	12.3±0.32***	75.6±1.21	8.56±0.21***	82.04±1.74	5.1±0.25***
Weight(g)	16.8±0.38	16.7±0.26	18.3±0.26	18.7±0.28	19.9±0.27	19.2±0.2	20.65±0.17	20.75±0.16

C57BL/6 mice were raised on VitD+ and VitD- diets from weaning. Every two weeks thereafter, three mice from each group were bled from the retro-orbital venous plexus and the serum concentrations of 25-(OH)D3(ng/ml) were analyzed. Values represent mean±SE (n = 3,repeated three times each). Statistical significance between the two groups of mice was evaluated using a Student's t-test $p<0.001$(***).

remained without significant histological changes. By 12 hr and 24 hr, early scattered areas of inflammation were observed, and were more apparent in VitD- mice. By 48 hr and 72 hr, differences were notable, with more profound and intense inflammatory response in VitD- mice. By 7 d, the inflammation in the VitD+ lung sections apparently subsided, while inflammatory cell infiltration and fibrinous exudation were still noted in VitD- mice. The HPS first increased at 12 hr, peaked at 48 hr, and declined thereafter, and it was significantly higher in VitD- mice than in VitD+ mice at 48 hr, 72 hr and 7 d p.i. (Fig. 2C). Thus, histopathologic analysis revealed more severe inflammation with delayed resolution in VitD- mice compared to their VitD-sufficient counterparts, although germinating conidia and hyphae could hardly be found in both groups of lungs at all the indicated times p.i. (no shown).

Increased infiltration of inflammatory cells in the lungs of *A. fumigatus*-challenged VitD- mice. We investigated cell numbers and composition in BALF after *A. fumigatus* challenge. Mice were challenged with 2×10^7 *A. fumigatus* conidia, and the amounts of cells in BALF were enumerated using a hemocytometer. BAL Cells were identified by morphology after staining with Wright-Giemsa stain, subsequently sorted by flow cytometry.

At baseline (no exposures), the BALF consisted predominantly of AMs (Fig. 3A). No differences were observed in the basal counts of BAL cells from VitD+ and VitD- mice (Fig. 3B). *A. fumigatus* challenge resulted in significant increase in the number of inflammatory cells in BALF (Fig. 3B), which was accounted for by an increase in neutrophils (Fig. 3A, arrow indicated). BAL cells were dominated by neutrophils from 12 hr to 72 hr p.i., eosinophils and lymphocytes could hardly be found in the BAL smears (Fig. 3A). The total number of inflammatory cells in BALF peaked at 48 hr p.i., and was greater in VitD- mice compared with VitD+ mice at all the indicated time points p.i., except 6 hr (Fig. 3B). We found no differences in the proportion of neutrophils in the BAL smears between VitD+ and VitD- mice at any of the indicated times p.i. (data not shown).

Based upon the morphological observation of BAL smears and the staining strategies previously reported [17,18], a panel of cell surface antibodies against CD45, CD11c, and Gr-1 was used for differential flow cytometry staining of cells obtained by BAL. $CD45^+$ BAL cells fell within one of four distinct populations on a Gr-1/CD11c plot. The $Gr\text{-}1^-CD11c^-$ population in the BALF consisted of lymphocytes, $Gr\text{-}1^+CD11c^-$ of neutrophils, $Gr\text{-}1^{lo/-}CD11c^{hi}$ and $Gr\text{-}1^+CD11c^{hi}$ of macrophages [17,19]. At baseline (no exposures), within the $CD45^+$ population of cells, the major cell types were macrophages ($Gr\text{-}1^{lo/-}CD11c^{hi}$ and $Gr\text{-}1^+CD11c^{hi}$), accounting for 95% of $CD45^+$ cells (Fig. 3D). Following inoculation with *A. fumigatus*, there was a rapid and substantial increase in the numbers of neutrophils ($Gr\text{-}1^+CD11c^-$), which were dramatically increased from <2% of total BAL leukocytes at baseline to 50% of total BAL leukocytes by 6 hr, accounted for >85% of total BAL leukocytes at 24 hr and 48 hr p.i. (Fig. 3D). No differences were observed in the percentage of neutrophils in BAL leukocytes from VitD+ and VitD- mice at any time point p.i. (Fig. 3C). We also did not observe any differences in the proportion of macrophages in BAL leukocytes (data not show). Lymphocytes ($Gr\text{-}1^-CD11c^-$) were no more than 5% of total BAL leukocytes at any of the indicated times. The numbers of cell populations returned to the baseline at 7 days p.i. (Fig. 3C, D).

Altogether, these data demonstrated that *A. fumigatus* challenge induced infiltration of inflammatory cells, dominated by neutrophils. Vitamin D deficiency did not affect the proportion of neutrophils in BAL leukocytes in response to *A. fumigatus* challenge.

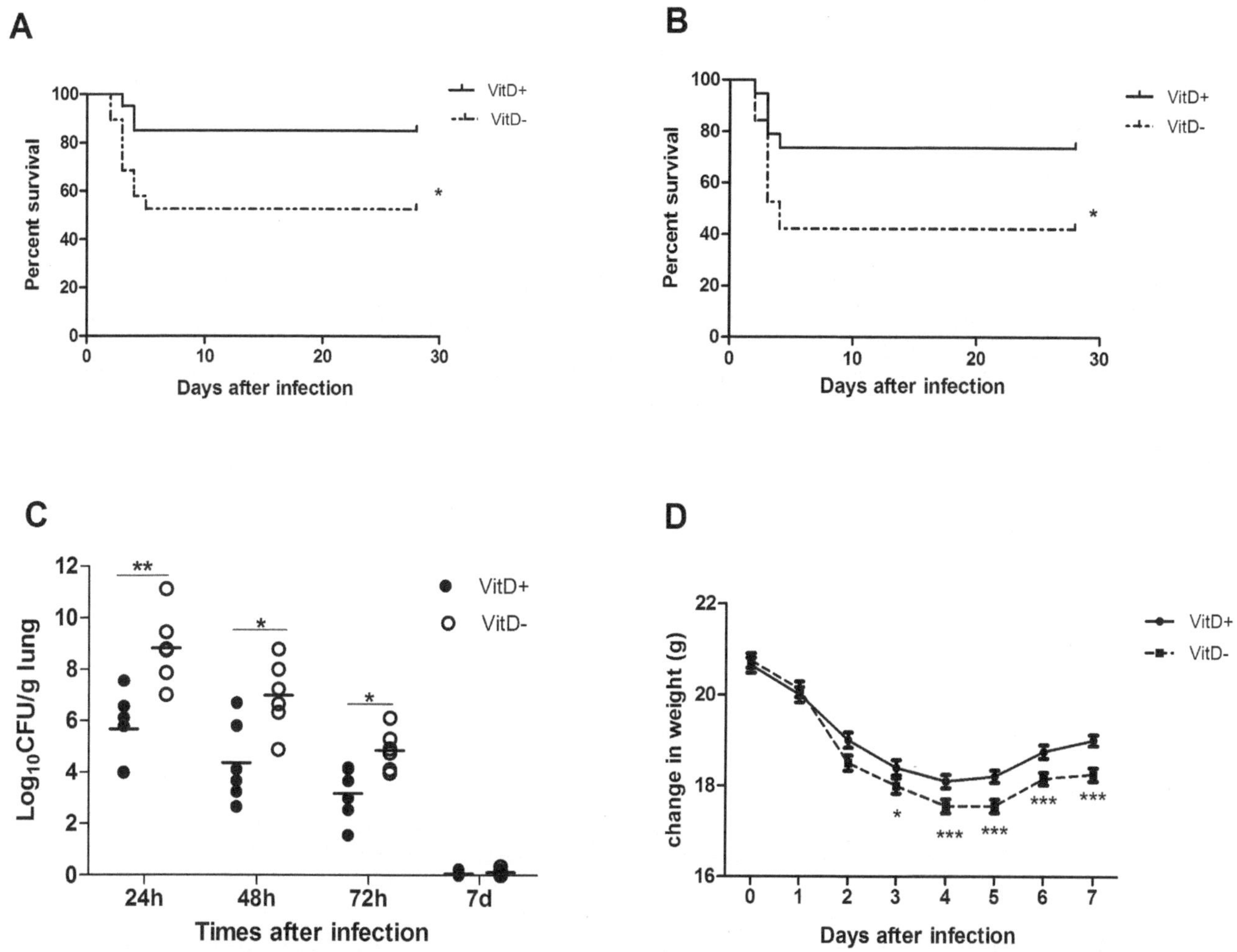

Figure 1. Enhanced susceptibility of VitD- mice after challenge with *A. fumigatus*. VitD+ and VitD- mice were challenged intratracheally with 5×10^7 (A), or 7×10^7 (B) *A. fumigatus* conidia in a volume of 50 µl. Survival was monitored for 28 days (n = 7 per group) and expressed as percentage of survival. This figure illustrates cumulative results from three independent studies per inoculum dose. The difference between survival rates was significant at $p<0.05$ (Log-rank test and Wilcoxon test). C. Fungal growth in the lungs of VitD+ and VitD- mice challenged intratracheally with 2×10^7 *A. fumigatus* conidia. Mice were sacrificed at the indicated times p.i., and serial dilutions of tissue homogenates were plated for CFU determination. Results are expressed as $\log_{10}$ of CFU average values determined in triplicate of three independent experiments (three for each dilution using two animals of each group). Each data point represents one mouse. Differences in CFU between VitD+ and VitD- mice were significant at $p<0.05$(*) and $p<0.01$(**) (Mann–Whitney U test). D. Infection-induced weight changes in mice were determined daily after intratracheal challenge with 2×10^7 *A. fumigatus* conidia. Values repersent means±SE (n = 12). $p<0.001$(***), $p<0.01$(**), $p<0.05$(*) (paired Student's t test).

Enhanced pro-inflammatory cytokine and chemokine production in the lungs of *A. fumigatus*-challenged VitD- mice. We next investigated the kinetic production of pro-inflammatory cytokine and chemokine in lung to better understand the inflammatory responses occurring after exposure. Vitamin D deficiency significantly enhanced the basal expression of IL-1β, IL-6, and TNF-α in the lungs of mice, while did not influence the basal expression of CXCL1 and CCL3 (Fig. 4A). *A. fumigatus* infection elicited a robust inflammatory response in lung, characterized by the increased production of IL-1β, IL-6, and TNF-α. This response was more profound in the lungs of VitD- mice at all the indicated times p.i. (Fig. 4A). Upon infection, the levels of these cytokines were elevated from 6 hr on; in VitD+ mice they peaked at 12 hr, returned to baseline at 7 d; in contrast in VitD- mice, they peaked at 48 hr, and were still significantly elevated over baseline levels at 7 d p.i. VitD- mice had significantly higher amounts of CXCL1 and CCL3 versus VitD+ mice at 12 to72 hr, and 7 d p.i. (Fig. 4A). In VitD+ mice they peaked at 48 hr, returned to baseline at 7 d p.i.; while in VitD- mice they peaked at 72 hr, and were still significantly higher than baseline at 7 d p.i.

Because AMs are a critical source for pro-inflammatory cytokine and chemokine production in response to *A. fumigatus* [20], we isolated AMs from naïve VitD+ and VitD-mice and assessed the kinetic pro-inflammatory cytokine and chemokine production in response to live *A. fumigatus* conidia *in vitro*. Results showed that compared with VitD+ AMs, VitD- AMs had significantly higher basal levels of IL-1β, IL-6, and TNF-α (Fig. 4B). In response to *A. fumigatus* conidia, VitD- AMs still had higher levels of them versus VitD+ AMs at all the indicated times. No differences in the basal levels of CXCL1 and CCL3 expression were observed between VitD+ and VitD- AMs (Fig. 4B). In response to *A. fumigatus* conidia, VitD- AMs had significantly higher amounts of CXCL1 and CCL3 versus VitD+ AMs at 10 hr, 14 hr and 18 hr. Furthermore, the up-regulation of cytokines and chemokines in VitD+ AMs peaked at 14 hr,

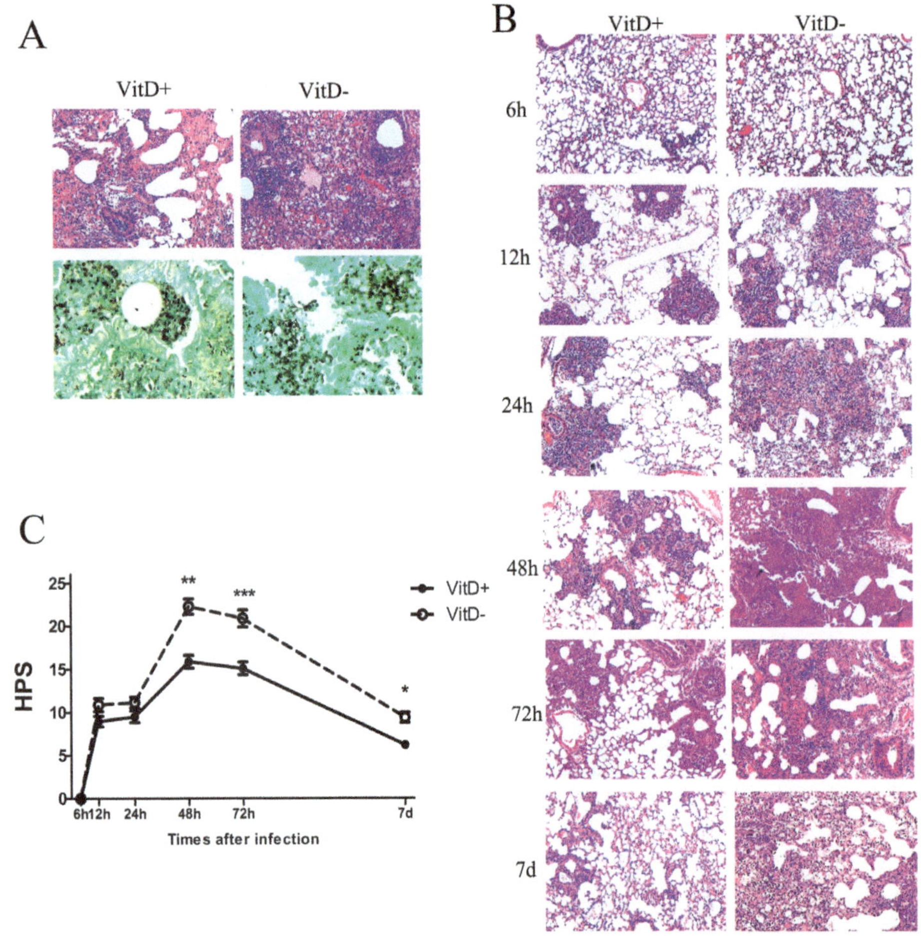

Figure 2. Histological evidence of aggravated and sustained inflammation in VitD- mice challenged with *A. fumigatus* conidia. A. Representative lung sections from VitD+ and VitD- mice three days post intratracheal challenge with 5×10^7 *A. fumigatus* conidia. Sections were stained with HE (upper, magnification 100x) for analysis of inflammation, and with GMS (lower, magnification 400x) for the detection of conidia and hyphae. B. Representative HE-stained lung sections (magnification 100x) from VitD- and VitD+ mice are shown at the indicated times after intratracheal challenge with 2×10^7 *A. fumigatus* conidia. C. HPS of serial HE-stained lung sections between 6 h and 7 d after intratracheal challenge with 2×10^7 *A. fumigatus* conidia. HPS is presented as mean±SE. Data are representative of three independent experiments (n = 3/group). Statistical analysis was performed by a Mann-Whitney rank sum test. $p<0.001$(***), $p<0.01$(**), $p<0.05$(*).

decreased rapidly thereafter; while in VitD- AMs their expression showed a continuously rising trend for 18 hr (Fig. 4B).

These results suggested that vitamin D deficiency enhanced the basal levels of pro-inflammatory cytokines in the lungs of mice. Upon *A. fumigatus* infection, vitamin D deficiency led to enhanced and sustained expression of pro-inflammatory cytokines and chemokines both *in vivo* and *in vitro*.

Enhanced up-regulation of pattern recognition receptors (PRRs) both at baseline and post A. fumigatus challeng in the lungs of VitD- mice. The initial sensing of fungal infection is mediated by PRRs, such as TLRs and lectin receptors, which trigger intracellular signaling cascades, leading to transcriptional expression of inflammatory mediators [21,22]. TLR2, TLR4 and _β-glucan receptor dectin-1 are key PRRs known to be involved in *A. fumigatus* recognition [21]. Hence, we investigated whether vitamin D deficiency modulates the expression of those PRRs in the lungs of mice (Fig. 5). Results showed that vitamin D deficiency increased pulmonary TLR2, TLR4 and dectin-1 expression at baseline both at mRNA and protein levels. Upon *A. fumigatus* challenge, these PRRs expression were up-regulated significantly, while VitD- mice still had higher mRNA and protein levels of these PRRs than VitD+ mice at all the indicated times. In VitD+ mice, these PRRs peaked at 12 hr, returned to baseline levels at 7 d p.i. While, in VitD- mice, they peaked at 48 hr, declined slowly thereafter, and were still much higher than basal levels at 7 d p.i.

Because AMs are of the main cells that express PRRs and recognize microorganism [20]. We investigated whether vitamin D deficiency affects the expression of TLR2, TLR4, and dectin-1 on AMs at baseline by flow cytometry. We found that the expression of these PRRs on AMs isolated from naïve VitD- mice was up-regulated significantly compared to AMs from naïve VitD+ mice (Fig. 6A). We further investigated the expression of these PRRs on AMs in response to *A. fumigatus in vitro*. AMs were isolated and co-cultured with viable *A. fumigatus* conidia. Gene expression of TLR2, TLR4, and dectin-1 was analyzed by q-PCR. Results showed that *A. fumigatus* challenge significantly increased the expression of these PRRs *in vitro* (Fig. 6B). Similar to what was found in vivo, increased expression of these PRRs was more pronounced in VitD- AMs compared with VitD+ AMs (Fig.6B). The up-regulation of PRR genes in VitD+ AMs peaked at 14 hr p.i. and decreased rapidly thereafter, while PRR gene expression

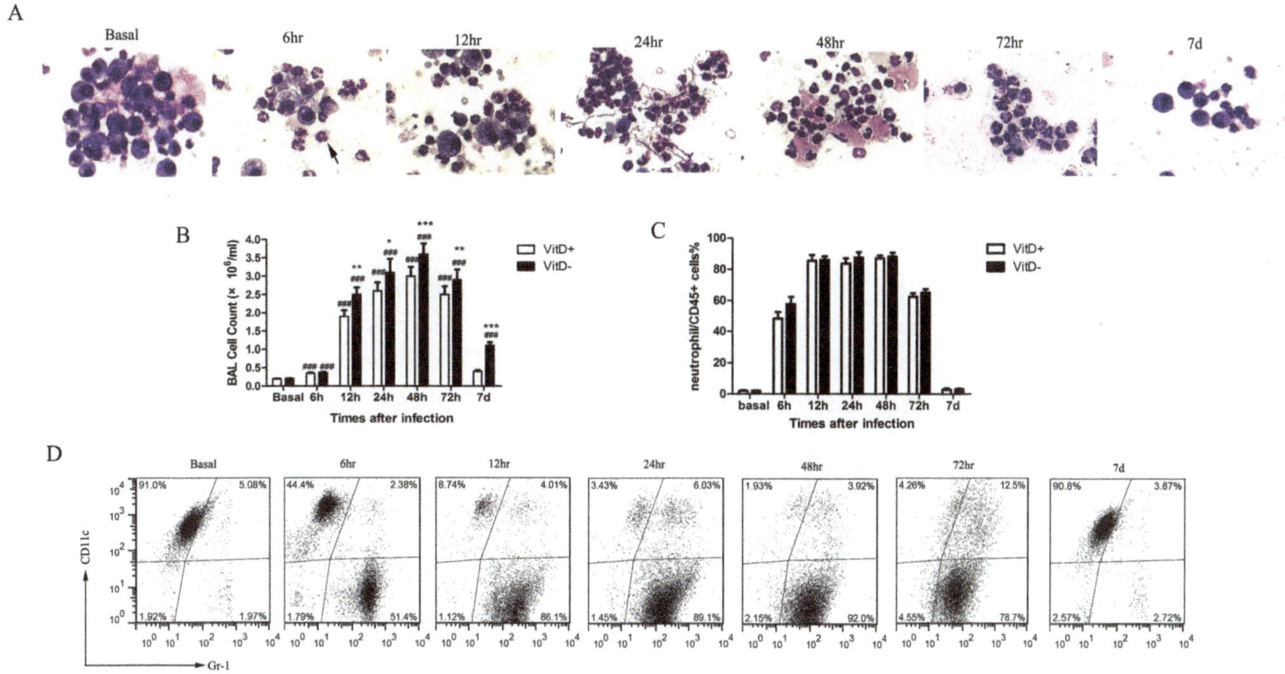

Figure 3. Increased infiltration of inflammatory cells in the lungs of *A. fumigatus*-challenged VitD- mice. A. BAL cells were stained with Wright-Giemsa stain and examined under a light microscope after intratracheal challenge with 2×10^7 *A. fumigatus* conidia (magnification 400x). B. Total cell counts in BALF were enumerated on a hemacytometer of individual mice after intratracheal challenge with 2×10^7 conidia. Data are representative of three independent experiments with n = 3 per group (mean±SE) and analyzed by paired Student's t test. p<0.001(###), for comparison of *A. fumigatus*-challenged VitD+/VitD- mice versus baseline levels; p<0.001(***), p<0.01(**), p<0.05(*), for comparison of VitD+ with VitD- mice. C. BAL cells were analyzed by flow cytometry after intratracheal challenge with 2×10^7 conidia. Lavage cells were gated by $CD45^+$; the resulting populations were further identified on the basis of CD11c and Gr-1expression and sorted as shown by the density plots. Within the $CD45^+$ population, the major cell types were macrophages ($CD11c^+Gr\text{-}1^{+/-}$) at baseline, neutrophils ($CD11c^-Gr\text{-}1^+$) became the major cell types 6–72 hr post infection. Flow cytometry was performed to quantify the percentage of cell types in $CD45^+$ cells. D. Flow cytometry was performed to quantify the percentage of neutrophils in $CD45^+$ cells in BALF after intratracheal challenge with 2×10^7 conidia. Neutrophils ($CD11c^-Gr\text{-}1^+$) were gated from the $CD45^+$ cells based on Gr-1 and CD11c expression profiles. Data are representative of three independent experiments with n = 3 per group (mean±SE), and analyzed by paired Student's t test.

showed a continuously rising trend for 18 hr in VitD- AMs (Fig. 6B).

Thus, vitamin D deficiency caused enhanced up-regulation of TLR2, TLR4 and dectin-1 in the lungs of mice both at baseline and post *A. fumigatus* challenge.

Discussion

Our results showed that VitD- mice demonstrated higher mortality after lung challenge with *A. fumigatus* coupled with impaired early clearance of the organism from the lungs. VitD- mice demonstrated aggravated and prolonged histological evidence of lung inflammation as well as enhanced BAL cell counts, dominated by neutrophils after *A. fumigatus* inoculation. Increased basal levels of pro-inflammatory cytokines in the lungs and AMs from naïve VitD- mice were observed. Upon *A. fumigatus* exposure, vitamin D deficiency led to enhanced and sustained expression of pro-inflammatory cytokines and chemokines both *in vivo* and *in vitro*. Up-regulation of key PRRs involved in *A. fumigatus* recognition was observed in the lungs and AMs from VitD- mice both at baseline and after *A. fumigatus* exposure.

Our survival experiments were performed with inocula of 5–7×10^7conidia, based on published reports using inocula at this level when assessing mortality and fungal clearance in animals that were not dually immunosuppressed with cyclophosphamide and cortisone [23,24]. Our experiments were not conducted in the presence of immunosuppressive drugs (cyclophosphamide, cortisone acetate, etc.) or during transient neutropenia (i.e., Ab-mediated depletion of neutrophils). Our position was that induction of immunosuppression before infection might exaggerate or underestimate the role of vitamin D whose importance in lung clearance of *A. fumigatus* in immunocompetent mice was clearly supported by the data of our experiments.

An important finding of this study was that the expression of pro-inflammatory cytokines (TNF-α, IL-1β and IL-6) and key PRRs involved in *A. fumigatus* recognition (TLR2, TLR4, and dectin-1) was significantly elevated in the lungs and AMs of VitD- mice versus VitD+ mice already at baseline. Microbial infection causes cytokine-associated inflammation to remove pathogens. The initial sensing of infection is mediated by innate PRRs. The intracellular signaling cascades triggered by PRRs recognition lead to transcriptional expression of inflammatory mediators that coordinate the elimination of pathogens and infected cells [22]. Studies have confirmed that naïve mice lacking dectin-1 or TLRs signaling were more sensitive to intratracheal challenge with *A. fumigatus* than control mice, and demonstrated impaired pro-inflammatory cytokines production and insufficient lung neutrophil recruitment [24,25]. Mice lacking TNF-α, or CCR1 (receptor for CCL3), were more susceptible to *A. fumigatus* lung infection, also through impaired neutrophil recruitment [26,27]. We thus expected that the increased basal levels of these PRRs and pro-inflammatory cytokines in the lungs of VitD- mice, which led to

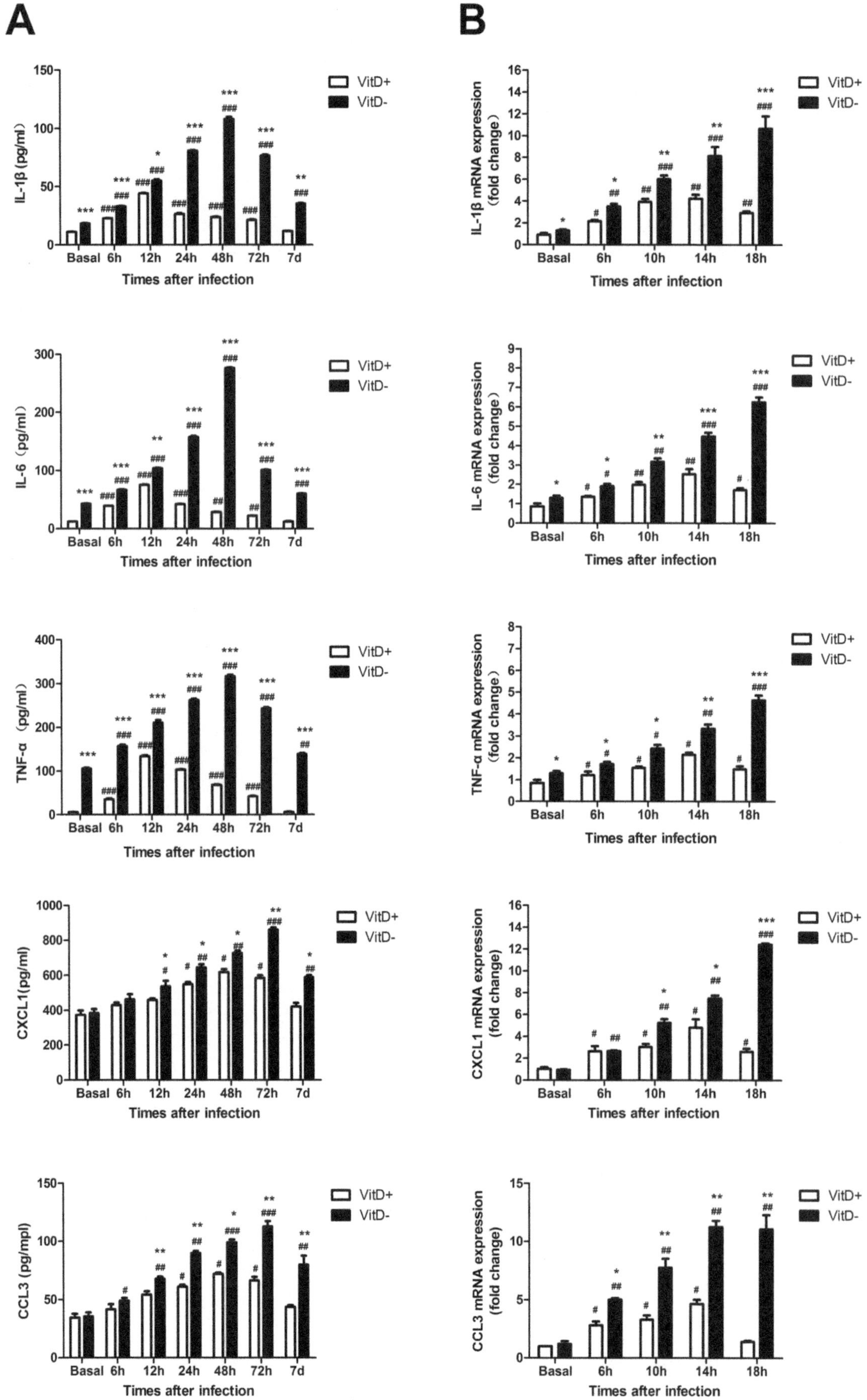
A
B
VitD+
VitD-
IL-1β (pg/ml)
IL-6 (pg/ml)
TNF-α (pg/ml)
CXCL1(pg/ml)
CCL3 (pg/mpl)
Basal 6h 12h 24h 48h 72h 7d
Times after infection
IL-1β mRNA expression (fold change)
IL-6 mRNA expression (fold change)
TNF-α mRNA expression (fold change)
CXCL1 mRNA expression (fold change)
CCL3 mRNA expression (fold change)
Basal 6h 10h 14h 18h
Times after infection

Figure 4. Enhanced pro-inflammatory cytokine and chemokine production in the lungs of *A. fumigatus*-challenged VitD- mice. A. Mice were infected intratracheally with 2×10^7*A. fumigatus* conidia. At specific times p.i. BALF collected from mice was analyzed for cytokine and chemokine content by ELISA. Data are representative of three independent experiments with n=5 per group (mean±SE). p<0.001(###), p<0.01(##), p<0.05(#), for comparison of *A. fumigatus*-challenged VitD+/VitD- mice versus baseline levels; p<0.001(***), p<0.01(**), p<0.05(*), for comparison of VitD+ with VitD- mice using paired Student's T-test. B. AMs isolated from naïve mouse lungs by BAL, were incubated in medium alone or in the presence of viable *A. fumigatus* conidia (MOI=0.1) *in vitro*. Total RNA from AMs was extracted at indicated times. Transcript abundance was measured by real-time RT-PCR. Representative data from three independent experiments with n=3 per group are shown. P<0.001(###), P<0.01(##), P<0.05(#), for comparison of *A. fumigatus*-challenged VitD+/VitD- AMs versus basal levels; P<0.001(***), P<0.01(**), P<0.05(*), for comparison of VitD+ and VitD- AMs using paired Student's T-test.

enhanced release of pro-inflammatory cytokines and chemokines after lung challenge with *A. fumigatus*, accompanied by more neutrophil infiltration in the lungs in our model, might increase host defense to *A. fumigatus*. However, the data in our study showed that up-regulation of them did not improve host resistance to *A. fumigatus*.

Excessive or uncontrolled release of pro-inflammatory cytokines can be fatal, which causes immunodeficiency, septic shock, or induction of autoimmunity, and may eventually impair disease eradication [22,28,29]. Influenza A virus and some Gram-negative bacteria trigger life-threatening "cytokine storms" in the host resulting in significant pathology and ultimately death [28,30]. It has been proposed that in invasive fungal infections, disease pathology may also be attributable to an aggravated or dysregulated host inflammatory response that results in extensive tissue damage [14,29,31]. In mice with chronic granulomatous disease, the intrinsic, genetically determined failure to control inflammation after exposure to sterile fungal components determines the animals' inability to resolve an infection with *A. fumigatus*[32]. Chronic disseminated candidiasis (CDC) is typically observed during neutrophil recovery in patients with acute leukemia, and the efficacy of corticosteroid therapy supports the pathophysiological hypothesis that CDC is a fungus-related immune reconstitution inflammatory syndrome [33]. The active form of vitamin D has been proved to inhibit *M. tuberculosis*, virus and bacteria through the induction of the cathelicidin antimicrobial peptide and β-defensins[34,35], or autophagy[36], while decreasing the inflammatory response to microbial infections[37,38,39,40,41]. Upon *in vitro* LPS, *C. albicans*, and *M. tuberculosis* stimulation, the active form of vitamin D has been observed to inhibit the production of TNF-α, IL-1β, and IL-6 by monocytes directly, or through down-regulating the expression of TLR2, TLR4 and dectin-1 on monocytes [39,40,41,42,43]. An increased serum vitamin D3 level in summer was associated with a significant drop in pro-inflammatory cytokines production by human monocytes *in vitro*, when compared to cytokine production in winter [44]. In addition, the reduced expression of TLR2 and TLR4 on human monocytes was associated with elevated vitamin D levels during summer, and the reduction of TLR2 expression during summer was accompanied by a corresponding drop in TNF-α production by human monocytes *in vitro* [44]. The active vitamin D can be produced locally within the lungs. Vitamin D deficiency resulted in decreased synthesis of active vitamin D in lung. Therefore, it is possible that lack of vitamin D increased the basal levels of pro-inflammatory cytokines and PRRs in the lungs

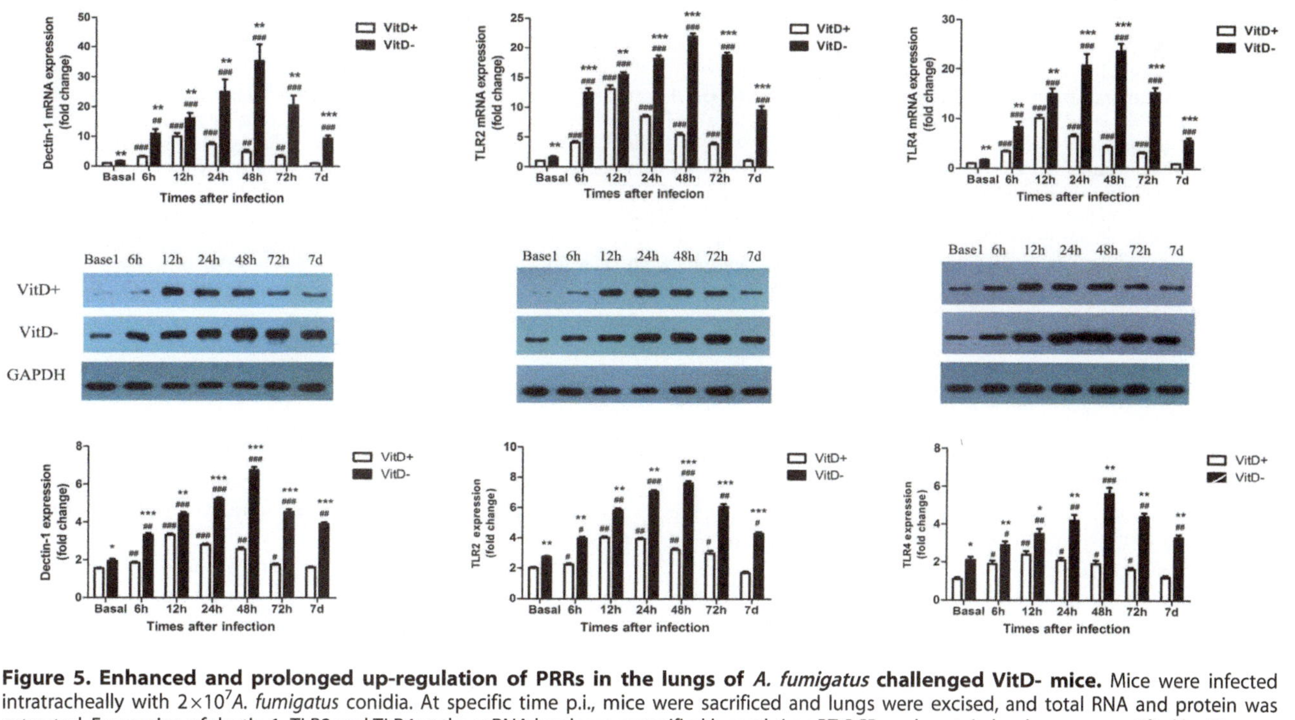

Figure 5. Enhanced and prolonged up-regulation of PRRs in the lungs of *A. fumigatus* challenged VitD- mice. Mice were infected intratracheally with 2×10^7*A. fumigatus* conidia. At specific time p.i., mice were sacrificed and lungs were excised, and total RNA and protein was extracted. Expression of dectin-1, TLR2 and TLR4 at the mRNA level was quantified by real-time RT-PCR, and protein levels were quantified by Western blotting (shown in middle panel). Representative data from three independent experiments are shown with n=3 per group (mean±SE). p<0.001(###), p<0.01(##), p<0.05(#), for comparison of *A. fumigatus*-challenged VitD+/VitD- versus baseline levels; p<0.001(***), p<0.01(**), p<0.05(*), for comparison of VitD+ and VitD- mice using paired Student's T-test.

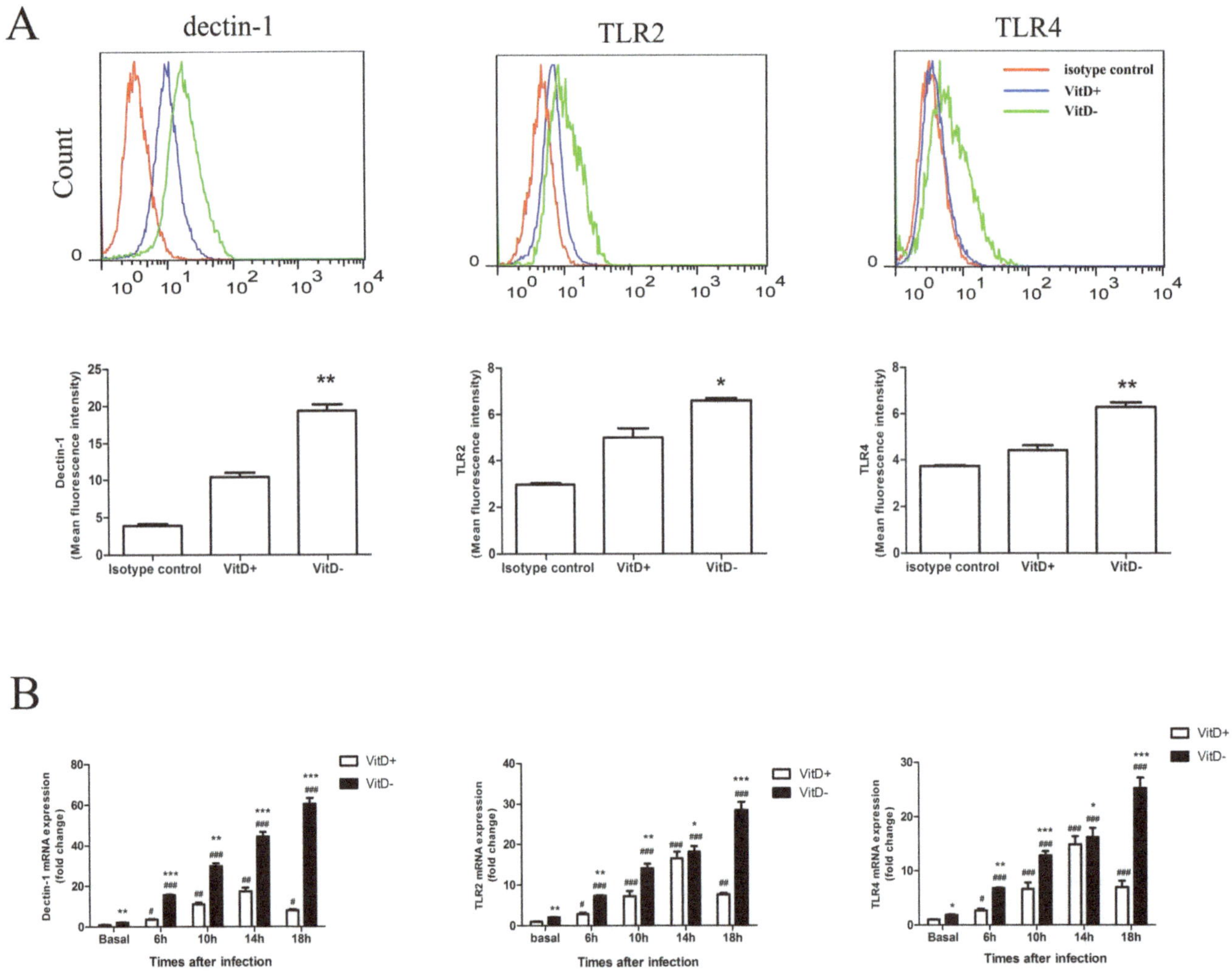

Figure 6. Enhanced and prolonged up-regulation of PRRs on *A. fumigatus*-stimulated VitD- AMs. A. Expression of surface TLR2, TLR4 and dectin-1 on AMs isolated from VitD- or VitD+ mice. AMs were isolated from mouse lungs by BAL, and stained for CD11c, dectin-1, TLR2 or TLR4 and then analyzed using flow cytometry. The data show the expression of dectin-1, TLR2 and TLR4 on CD11c-positive cells (red line, isotype control; blue line, VitD+ AMs; green line, VitD- AMs). The values shown in the flow cytometry profiles are the mean fluorescence intensity (MFI) indices. Data are representative of three independent experiments with $n=3$/group. $p<0.01$(**), $p<0.05$(*) using paired Student's T-test. B. mRNA expression of TLR2, TLR4 and dectin-1 in AMs after co-cultured with live *A. fumigatus* conidia *in vitro*. AMs were isolated from naïve mouse lungs by BAL, incubated in medium alone or in the presence of viable *A. fumigatus* conidia (MOI = 0.1). Total RNA from AMs was extracted at indicated times. Transcript abundance was measured by real-time RT-PCR. Representative data from three independent experiments with $n=3$ per group are shown. $P<0.001$(###), $P<0.01$(##), $P<0.05$(#), for comparison of A. f.-challenged VitD+/VitD- versus baseline levels; $P<0.001$(***), $P<0.01$(**), $P<0.05$(*), for comparison of VitD+ and VitD- using paired Student's T-test.

of mice, which subsequently led to a hyper-inflammatory response to *A. fumigatus* in lung and impaired host resistance to *A. fumigatus*.

Neutrophils are essential in initiation and execution of the acute inflammatory response in fungal infection [45]. 1 alpha, 25-Dihydroxyvitamin D3 was demonstrated to inhibit neutrophil motivation by decreasing ICAM-1 and ELAM-1 expressions on pulmonary microvascular endothelial cells [46], and inhibited neutrophil recruitment in lung in animal models of acute lung injury[47,48]. In addition, the active form of vitamin D was observed to suppress IL-8 production in Pseudomonas-stimulated neutrophils and have benefit for resisting persistent *P. aeruginosa* lower respiratory tract infection [49]. Thus, vitamin D deficiency might lead to more neutrophils infiltration in lung in response to *A. fumigatus* challenge, which aggravated pulmonary inflammatory response.

Moreover, our experiments were conducted in immunocompetent mice. In this case, the increased fungal burden in the lungs of VitD- mice might further enhance the PRRs signal, and exacerbated the values of inflammatory mediators, which aggravated the inflammation in the lungs, and eventually led to a poor prognosis.

Human diseases caused by *A. fumigatus* have been considered under three categories: invasive infections; infections caused by the colonization of mucosal surfaces without invasion into tissue; and hypersensitivity diseases. The key determinant of the pathogenicity of Aspergillus species, and the reason for the diversity of host outcomes, is hypothesized to be the nature of the immune response of the host [50], and the diseases may be conceptualized as points along a spectrum of abnormal immune responses of the host. Vitamin D may have a role in inhibiting *A. fumigatus* infections, while modulating and limiting any unnecessary inflammatory response generated by the host. In recent years, vitamin D deficiency in humans has received significant attention [7,51,52]. It has been shown to play a potent role in the susceptibility to respiratory infectious diseases [53,54]. A still unresolved question arising from ongoing laboratory and clinical research is the serum vitamin D concentrations needed to elicit an optimal immune response [55]. Our study indicates that vitamin D deficiency might lead to an aberrant immune response to *A. fumigatus*.

In conclusion, we have identified an important role of vitamin D for host defense against *A. fumigatus* in an immunocompetent host. By modifying the pro-inflammatory cytokine responses, and influencing on the major PRRs involved in *A. fumigatus* recognition, vitamin D deficiency causes an aggravated and prolonged inflammatory response in challenge with *A. fumigatus* infection. We therefore feel these studies lay the foundation for further examination of vitamin D status in individuals who are at risk for Invasive Pulmonary Aspergillosis (IPA), which may provide valuable insight into the role of vitamin D in susceptibility to IPA in immunosuppressed patients.

Acknowledgments

The authors would like to thank Ming Fan and Mei Huang for providing highly purified *Aspergillus fumigatus*. We also would like to thank Yongjun Jiang, Xiaoxiang Guan and Weiming Gan for his help in editing and submitting this manuscript.

Author Contributions

Conceived and designed the experiments: YS XS. Performed the experiments: PL XX EC BY WL RZ. Analyzed the data: PL XS. Contributed reagents/materials/analysis tools: WL MF MH LS RZ. Wrote the paper: PL.

References

1. Hughes DA, Norton R (2009) Vitamin D and respiratory health. Clin Exp Immunol 158: 20–25.
2. Hansdottir S, Monick MM (2011) Vitamin D effects on lung immunity and respiratory diseases. Vitam Horm 86: 217–237.
3. Hansdottir S, Monick MM, Hinde SL, Lovan N, Look DC, et al. (2008) Respiratory epithelial cells convert inactive vitamin D to its active form: potential effects on host defense. J Immunol 181: 7090–7099.
4. Adams JS, Gacad MA (1985) Characterization of 1 alpha-hydroxylation of vitamin D3 sterols by cultured alveolar macrophages from patients with sarcoidosis. J Exp Med 161: 755–765.
5. Sigmundsdottir H, Pan J, Debes GF, Alt C, Habtezion A, et al. (2007) DCs metabolize sunlight-induced vitamin D3 to 'program' T cell attraction to the epidermal chemokine CCL27. Nat Immunol 8: 285–293.
6. Baeke F, Takiishi T, Korf H, Gysemans C, Mathieu C (2010) Vitamin D: modulator of the immune system. Curr Opin Pharmacol 10: 482–496.
7. Thacher TD, Clarke BL (2011) Vitamin D insufficiency. Mayo Clin Proc 86: 50–60.
8. Holick MF, Chen TC (2008) Vitamin D deficiency: a worldwide problem with health consequences. Am J Clin Nutr 87: 1080S–6S.
9. Wilkinson RJ, Llewelyn M, Toossi Z, Patel P, Pasvol G, et al. (2000) Influence of vitamin D deficiency and vitamin D receptor polymorphisms on tuberculosis among Gujarati Asians in west London: a case-control study. Lancet 355: 618–621.
10. Wayse V, Yousafzai A, Mogale K, Filteau S (2004) Association of subclinical vitamin D deficiency with severe acute lower respiratory infection in Indian children under 5 y. Eur J Clin Nutr 58: 563–567.
11. Laaksi I, Ruohola JP, Tuohimaa P, Auvinen A, Haataja R, et al. (2007) An association of serum vitamin D concentrations <40 nmol/L with acute respiratory tract infection in young Finnish men. Am J Clin Nutr 86: 714–717.
12. Science M, Maguire JL, Russell ML, Smieja M, Walter SD, et al. (2013) Low Serum 25-Hydroxyvitamin D Level and Risk of Upper Respiratory Tract Infection in Children and Adolescents. Clin Infect Dis .
13. Dagenais TR, Keller NP (2009) Pathogenesis of Aspergillus fumigatus in Invasive Aspergillosis. Clin Microbiol Rev 22: 447–465.
14. Kreindler JL, Steele C, Nguyen N, Chan YR, Pilewski JM, et al. (2010) Vitamin D3 attenuates Th2 responses to Aspergillus fumigatus mounted by CD4+ T cells from cystic fibrosis patients with allergic bronchopulmonary aspergillosis. J Clin Invest 120: 3242–3254.
15. Cimolai N, Taylor GP, Mah D, Morrison BJ (1992) Definition and application of a histopathological scoring scheme for an animal model of acute Mycoplasma pneumoniae pulmonary infection. Microbiol Immunol 36: 465–478.
16. Lagishetty V, Misharin AV, Liu NQ, Lisse TS, Chun RF, et al. (2010) Vitamin D deficiency in mice impairs colonic antibacterial activity and predisposes to colitis. Endocrinology 151: 2423–2432.
17. Gonzalez-Juarrero M, Shim TS, Kipnis A, Junqueira-Kipnis AP, Orme IM (2003) Dynamics of macrophage cell populations during murine pulmonary tuberculosis. J Immunol 171: 3128–3135.
18. Shreiner AB, Murdock BJ, Sadighi AAA, Falkowski NR, Christensen PJ, et al. (2012) Repeated exposure to Aspergillus fumigatus conidia results in CD4+ T cell-dependent and -independent pulmonary arterial remodeling in a mixed Th1/Th2/Th17 microenvironment that requires interleukin-4 (IL-4) and IL-10. Infect Immun 80: 388–397.
19. Tighe RM, Li Z, Potts EN, Frush S, Liu N, et al. (2011) Ozone inhalation promotes CX3CR1-dependent maturation of resident lung macrophages that limit oxidative stress and inflammation. J Immunol 187: 4800–4808.
20. Segal BH (2007) Role of macrophages in host defense against aspergillosis and strategies for immune augmentation. Oncologist 12 Suppl 2: 7–13.
21. van de Veerdonk FL, Kullberg BJ, van der Meer JW, Gow NA, Netea MG (2008) Host-microbe interactions: innate pattern recognition of fungal pathogens. Curr Opin Microbiol 11: 305–312.
22. Takeuchi O, Akira S (2010) Pattern recognition receptors and inflammation. Cell 140: 805–820.
23. Bellocchio S, Montagnoli C, Bozza S, Gaziano R, Rossi G, et al. (2004) The contribution of the Toll-like/IL-1 receptor superfamily to innate and adaptive immunity to fungal pathogens in vivo. J Immunol 172: 3059–3069.
24. Werner JL, Metz AE, Horn D, Schoeb TR, Hewitt MM, et al. (2009) Requisite role for the dectin-1 beta-glucan receptor in pulmonary defense against Aspergillus fumigatus. J Immunol 182: 4938–4946.
25. Bretz C, Gersuk G, Knoblaugh S, Chaudhary N, Randolph-Habecker J, et al. (2008) MyD88 signaling contributes to early pulmonary responses to Aspergillus fumigatus. Infect Immun 76: 952–958.
26. Mehrad B, Strieter RM, Standiford TJ (1999) Role of TNF-alpha in pulmonary host defense in murine invasive aspergillosis. J Immunol 162: 1633–1640.
27. Gao JL, Wynn TA, Chang Y, Lee EJ, Broxmeyer HE, et al. (1997) Impaired host defense, hematopoiesis, granulomatous inflammation and type 1-type 2 cytokine balance in mice lacking CC chemokine receptor 1. J Exp Med 185: 1959–1968.
28. Tisoncik JR, Korth MJ, Simmons CP, Farrar J, Martin TR, et al. (2012) Into the eye of the cytokine storm. Microbiol Mol Biol Rev 76: 16–32.
29. Romani L (2011) Immunity to fungal infections. Nat Rev Immunol 11: 275–288.
30. Cheng XW, Lu J, Wu CL, Yi LN, Xie X, et al. (2011) Three fatal cases of pandemic 2009 influenza A virus infection in Shenzhen are associated with cytokine storm. Respir Physiol Neurobiol 175: 185–187.
31. Miceli MH, Maertens J, Buve K, Grazziutti M, Woods G, et al. (2007) Immune reconstitution inflammatory syndrome in cancer patients with pulmonary aspergillosis recovering from neutropenia: Proof of principle, description, and clinical and research implications. Cancer 110: 112–120.
32. Romani L, Fallarino F, De Luca A, Montagnoli C, D'Angelo C, et al. (2008) Defective tryptophan catabolism underlies inflammation in mouse chronic granulomatous disease. Nature 451: 211–215.
33. Legrand F, Lecuit M, Dupont B, Bellaton E, Huerre M, et al. (2008) Adjuvant corticosteroid therapy for chronic disseminated candidiasis. Clin Infect Dis 46: 696–702.
34. Gombart AF (2009) The vitamin D-antimicrobial peptide pathway and its role in protection against infection. Future Microbiol 4: 1151–1165.
35. White JH (2010) Vitamin D as an inducer of cathelicidin antimicrobial peptide expression: past, present and future. J Steroid Biochem Mol Biol 121: 234–238.
36. Campbell GR, Spector SA (2012) Vitamin D inhibits human immunodeficiency virus type 1 and Mycobacterium tuberculosis infection in macrophages through the induction of autophagy. PLoS Pathog 8: e1002689.
37. Hansdottir S, Monick MM, Lovan N, Powers L, Gerke A, et al. (2010) Vitamin D decreases respiratory syncytial virus induction of NF-kappaB-linked chemokines and cytokines in airway epithelium while maintaining the antiviral state. J Immunol 184: 965–974.
38. Xue ML, Zhu H, Thakur A, Willcox M (2002) 1 alpha,25-Dihydroxyvitamin D3 inhibits pro-inflammatory cytokine and chemokine expression in human corneal epithelial cells colonized with Pseudomonas aeruginosa. Immunol Cell Biol 80: 340–345.
39. Zhang Y, Leung DY, Richers BN, Liu Y, Remigio LK, et al. (2012) Vitamin D inhibits monocyte/macrophage proinflammatory cytokine production by targeting MAPK phosphatase-1. J Immunol 188: 2127–2135.
40. Khoo AL, Chai LY, Koenen HJ, Oosting M, Steinmeyer A, et al. (2011) Vitamin D(3) down-regulates proinflammatory cytokine response to Mycobacterium tuberculosis through pattern recognition receptors while inducing protective cathelicidin production. Cytokine 55: 294–300.

41. Khoo AL, Chai LY, Koenen HJ, Kullberg BJ, Joosten I, et al. (2011) 1,25-dihydroxyvitamin D3 modulates cytokine production induced by Candida albicans: impact of seasonal variation of immune responses. J Infect Dis 203: 122–130.
42. Sadeghi K, Wessner B, Laggner U, Ploder M, Tamandl D, et al. (2006) Vitamin D3 down-regulates monocyte TLR expression and triggers hyporesponsiveness to pathogen-associated molecular patterns. Eur J Immunol 36: 361–370.
43. Zarrabeitia MT, Riancho JA, Amado JA, Olmos JM, Gonzalez-Macias J (1992) Effect of calcitriol on the secretion of prostaglandin E2, interleukin 1, and tumor necrosis factor alpha by human monocytes. Bone 13: 185–189.
44. Khoo AL, Chai LY, Koenen HJ, Sweep FC, Joosten I, et al. (2011) Regulation of cytokine responses by seasonality of vitamin D status in healthy individuals. Clin Exp Immunol 164: 72–79.
45. Barnes PD, Marr KA (2007) Risks, diagnosis and outcomes of invasive fungal infections in haematopoietic stem cell transplant recipients. Br J Haematol 139: 519–531.
46. Chen SF (1995) 1 alpha, 25-Dihydroxyvitamin D3 decreased ICAM-1 and ELAM-1 expressions on pulmonary microvascular endothelial cells and neutrophil motivation. J Steroid Biochem Mol Biol 52: 67–70.
47. Takano Y, Mitsuhashi H, Ueno K (2011) 1alpha,25-Dihydroxyvitamin D(3) inhibits neutrophil recruitment in hamster model of acute lung injury. Steroids 76: 1305–1309.
48. Takano Y, Mitsuhashi H, Ishizuka S, Takahashi K, Chokki M, et al. (2012) TEI-A00114: a new vitamin D3 analogue that inhibits neutrophil recruitment in an acute lung injury hamster model while showing reduced hypercalcemic activity. Steroids 77: 1535–1542.
49. Matsumoto K (1995) New approaches to Pseudomonas aeruginosa lower respiratory tract infections. Verh K Acad Geneeskd Belg 57: 109–122.
50. Casadevall A, Pirofski LA (2003) The damage-response framework of microbial pathogenesis. Nat Rev Microbiol 1: 17–24.
51. van Schoor NM, Lips P (2011) Worldwide vitamin D status. Best Pract Res Clin Endocrinol Metab 25: 671–680.
52. Heaney RP (2012) Vitamin D—baseline status and effective dose. N Engl J Med 367: 77–78.
53. Dini C, Bianchi A (2012) The potential role of vitamin D for prevention and treatment of tuberculosis and infectious diseases. Ann Ist Super Sanita 48: 319–327.
54. Khoo AL, Chai L, Koenen H, Joosten I, Netea M, et al. (2012) Translating the role of vitamin D3 in infectious diseases. Crit Rev Microbiol 38: 122–135.
55. Vieth R (2006) What is the optimal vitamin D status for health. Prog Biophys Mol Biol 92: 26–32.

8

The Effects of Vitamin D Supplementation on Hepatic Dysfunction, Vitamin D Status, and Glycemic Control in Children and Adolescents with Vitamin D Deficiency and Either Type 1 or Type 2 Diabetes Mellitus

Benjamin Udoka Nwosu[1]*, Louise Maranda[2]

1 Division of Endocrinology, Department of Pediatrics, University of Massachusetts Medical School, Worcester, Massachusetts, United States of America, 2 Department of Quantitative Health Sciences, University of Massachusetts Medical School, Worcester, Massachusetts, United States of America

Abstract

Background: The effects of vitamin D supplementation on mild hepatic dysfunction and glycemic control are unclear in children and adolescents with either type 1 (T1D) or type 2 diabetes (T2D).

Hypothesis: Vitamin D supplementation will improve hepatic dysfunction and glycemic control.

Aim: To determine the effect of vitamin D supplementation on alanine transaminase (ALT), hemoglobin A1c (HbA1c), and serum 25-hydroxyvitamin D [25(OH)D] concentration.

Subjects and Methods: A retrospective study of 131 subjects with either T1D (n = 88:46 females, 42 males), or T2D (n = 43:26 females, 17 males) of ages 3–18 years between 2007–2013. All subjects had (1) a diagnosis of diabetes for >12 mo, (2) received vitamin D supplementation for the management of vitamin D deficiency (3) had baseline and subsequent simultaneous measurements of HbA1c, ALT, and 25(OH)D. Vitamin D deficiency was defined as 25(OH)D concentration of < 50 nmol/L (20 ng/mL).

Results: At baseline, vitamin D deficiency occurred in 72.1% of patients with T2D and in 37.5% of T1D patients ($p<0.001$). Patients with T2D had significantly higher values for BMI SDS ($p<0.001$), alanine transaminase (ALT) ($p = 0.001$), but lower 25(OH)D ($p<0.001$), and no difference in HbA1c ($p = 0.94$), and total daily dose (TDD) of insulin per kg body weight ($p = 0.48$) as compared to T1D patients. After 3 months of vitamin D supplementation, there was a significant increase in 25(OH)D in both T2D ($p = 0.015$), and T1D patients ($p<0.001$); significant reduction in BMI SDS ($p = 0.015$) and ALT ($p = 0.012$) in T2D, but not in T1D. There was a clinically-significant decrease in HbA1c in T2D from $8.5\pm2.9\%$ at baseline to 7.7 ± 2.5 at 3 mo, but not in T1D, 8.5 ± 1.2 to $8.53\pm1.1\%$.

Conclusions: Vitamin D supplementation in subjects with T2D was associated with statistically significant decreases in BMI SDS, ALT, and a clinically-significant decrease in HbA1c.

Editor: Marta Letizia Hribal, University of Catanzaro Magna Graecia, Italy

Funding: This study was funded in part by a grant to Benjamin U. Nwosu from the Department of Pediatrics, and the Faculty Diversity Scholars Program, University of Massachusetts Medical School, Worcester, MA. He is also a member of the UMass Diabetes and Endocrine Research Center (DK32520). The funders had no role in study design, data collection and analysis, decision to publish, or preparation of the manuscript.

Competing Interests: The authors have declared that no competing interests exist.

* E-mail: Benjamin.Nwosu@umassmemorial.org

Introduction

The management of diabetes mellitus remains an enigma even though its symptoms were described more than 2000 years ago. This is because the central therapeutic goal of diabetes management, euglycemia, is influenced by complex physiologic and pathologic processes, some of which are clearly understood, while others are less clear. Suboptimal glycemic control is a recognized risk factor for acute and chronic complications of diabetes including microvascular and macrovascular diseases [1–3]. However, the role of comorbid states such as nonalcoholic fatty liver disease (NAFLD) and vitamin D deficiency on glycemic control in children and adolescents has not been fully elucidated. Poor glycemic control remains a growing problem in patients with type 1 (T1D) or type 2 diabetes (T2D) [4] despite improvements in insulin formulation, delivery and adjunctive therapies [5]. A recent national study reported that a high proportion of youth with diabetes had elevated hemoglobin A1c (HbA1c) values, with 17% of patients with TIDM and 27% of those with T2DM showing significantly poor control, defined as HbA1c ≥9.5% [4].

NAFLD is the most common form of liver dysfunction in children [6], and the leading cause of elevated liver enzymes in obese youth [7]. Even though its prevalence is rising in parallel with the prevalence of childhood obesity [8], its role in poor glycemic control in diabetes is unknown. NAFLD represents a spectrum of conditions characterized by macrovesicular hepatic steatosis and little or no exposure to alcohol [8]. The hepatic pathology encompasses a range from isolated fatty infiltration to steatohepatitis, advanced fibrosis, and cirrhosis [6].

NAFLD has been strongly associated with vitamin D deficiency [9,10], IR [11], prediabetes [12], and T2D [10,13–17]. Several studies have reported associations between liver dysfunction and low vitamin D levels [9,10,18–20] on one hand, and liver dysfunction and poor glycemic control on the other [21]. Our group showed that hepatic dysfunction, characterized by elevated transaminases, was associated with vitamin D deficiency and poor glycemic control in children and adolescents with T2D, but not T1D [22]. This has led to the hypothesis that mild hepatic dysfunction could impair the conversion of vitamin D to 25-hydroxyvitamin D [25(OH)D], and consequently result in vitamin D deficiency. The resultant vitamin D deficiency is believed to impair insulin sensitivity [23].

Vitamin D deficiency is prevalent in children and adolescents with diabetes mellitus [22,24,25]. The etiology of this vitamin D deficiency is often attributed to the lack of sun exposure, poor intake of vitamin D-containing foods such as salmon, or due to either volumetric dilution [26], or sequestration of vitamin D in fat depots [27]. However, a crucial step in the metabolism of vitamin D, the hydroxylation of vitamin D at the 25 position, occurs in the liver. The role of NAFLD on this critical step in vitamin D metabolism in children and adolescents with diabetes has not been fully studied [22]. Equally, the effects of the resultant vitamin D deficiency on glycemic control in these patients are unclear. A study in healthy, non-diabetic adults with normal glucose tolerance using the hyperglycemic clamp technique showed a positive correlation of 25(OH)D level with insulin sensitivity [23]. Extrapolation of the data suggested that increasing the serum concentration of 25(OH)D from 25–80 nmol/L would increase insulin sensitivity by 60% [23], indicating that perhaps vitamin D supplementation offers promise as an adjunctive therapy for those with diabetes mellitus [28]. Recent studies in non-diabetic children and adolescents showed that low levels of 25(OH)D were associated with increasing insulin resistance in patients at risk for diabetes [29], while a 12-week study involving children, adolescents and young adults with T1D showed improved HbA1c level following a combined vitamin D and calcium supplementation protocol [30].

Therefore, to achieve the elusive goal of glycemic control in diabetes, euglycemia, it is necessary to evaluate the role of comorbid states such as hepatic dysfunction and vitamin D deficiency on glycemic control. Even though our group showed that hepatic dysfunction was associated with vitamin D deficiency and poor glycemic control in patients with T2D and not in those with T1D, the effects of vitamin D supplementation on the coexistence of hepatic dysfunction, vitamin D deficiency, and poor glycemic control have not been adequately studied in children and adolescents with either T1D or T2D. We hypothesize that vitamin D supplementation would improve vitamin D status, reduce hepatic dysfunction, and in turn lead to improved glycemic control in children and adolescents with diabetes mellitus. The study's aim was to determine the effect of vitamin D supplementation on ALT, HbA1c, and 25(OH)D in patients with vitamin D deficiency and either T1D or T2D.

Subjects and Methods

Ethics Statement

The study protocol was approved by the University of Massachusetts Institutional Review Board. All patient records and information were anonymized and de-identified prior to analysis.

Subjects

The clinical records of children and adolescents of ages 3–18 years who were treated for T1D and T2D at the Children's Medical Center of the University of Massachusetts between 2007 and 2013 were reviewed. Subjects were included if they had a diagnosis of diabetes for >12 mo, had HbA1c and 25(OH)D obtained simultaneously, and were on no vitamin D or calcium supplements. Subjects were excluded if they had vitamin D or calcium supplementation at baseline, or the disorders of calcium metabolism, hemoglobinopathies, or malabsorption syndrome such as celiac disease. Eighty-eight subjects with T1D (46 females, 42 males) and 43 subjects with T2D (26 females and 17 males) fulfilled these criteria (Table 1). The diagnosis of T2D was based on fasting blood glucose of ≥7 mmol/L (126 mg/dL), and/or 2-hour postprandial glucose of ≥11.1 mmol/L (200 mg/dL), and/or random blood glucose of ≥11.1 mmol/L (200 mg/dL) with symptoms of polyuria and/or polydipsia. All patients with T2D had negative results for T1D-associated antibodies (insulin, islet cell, glutamic acid decarboxylase, and insulinoma associated-2). Because 25(OH)D level could vary with sunlight exposure, we categorized each subject's visit according to the seasons as follows: fall (September 22–December 21), winter (December 22–March 21), spring (March 22–June 21), and summer (June 22-September 21) [31]. All subjects with T1D received insulin only. Of the 43 patients with T2D, 17 patients received a combination of insulin and metformin, 15 patients received metformin only, while 8 patients received insulin monotherapy.

The Procedure for Vitamin D Therapy

The rationale for the vitamin D supplementation in these patients was based on recent reports of high prevalence of vitamin D deficiency in children and adolescents with either T1D or T2D [22,24,25]. It is the standard practice at the Children's Medical Center to monitor the vitamin D status of children and adolescents with diabetes mellitus during patients' yearly blood draw for the evaluation of complications of diabetes mellitus, or at one of the patients' quarterly visits for routine diabetes care. Patients with serum 25(OH)D concentration of <50 nmol/L were started on vitamin D supplementation using either ergocalciferol or cholecalciferol with the aim of raising the 25(OH)D level to >75 nmol/L.

All participants received either ergocalciferol or cholecalciferol for a period ranging from 8 weeks for those receiving 7000 IU/day, through 12–16 weeks for subjects receiving 400–4000 IU/day as shown in Table 2. The dose of vitamin D was based on patient's age and weight according to reports showing that 25(OH)D response to vitamin D supplementation is directly related to dose and body size [32].

Anthropometry

Height was measured to the nearest 0.1 cm using a wall-mounted stadiometer (Holtain Ltd, Crymych, Dyfed, UK). Weight was measured to the nearest 0.1 kg using an upright scale. Body mass index (BMI) was derived using the formula weight/height^2 (kg/m^2), and expressed as SDS for age and gender based on National Center for Health Statistics (NCHS) data [33].

Table 1. Comparison of the characteristics of patients with type 1 diabetes vs. type 2 diabetes.

Parameters	Type 1 Diabetes (n = 88)	Type 2 Diabetes (n = 43)	*p*
Age (years)	12.6±3.6	16.2±2.2	**<0.001**
Sex: males (%)	42 (47.7%)	17 (39.5%)	0.38*
Race: white (Non-Hispanic) (%)	73 (83.0%)	23 (53.5%)	**0.001***
Height SDS (baseline)	0.04±1.1	0.2±1.2	0.57
Height SDS (3mo)	0.04±1.1	0.04±1.2	1.0
Weight SDS (baseline)	0.69±1.0	2.3±0.9	**<0.001**
Weight SDS (3mo)	0.71±1.0	2.3±1.0	**<0.001**
Body Mass Index SDS (baseline)	0.80±0.9	2.2±0.6	**<0.001**
Body Mass Index SDS (3mo)	0.81±0.8	2.14±0.7	**<0.001**
Alanine Transaminase (U/L)	19.2±6.2	48.3±47.4	**0.001**
25(OH)D level (nmol/L)	53.7±14.6	41.2±15.3	<0.001
25(OH)D level (nmol/L) in Whites	54.0±14.3	42.0±15.9	0.004
Percentage Vitamin D Deficiency [25(OH)D <50 nmol/L] (%)	33 (37.5%)	31 (72.1%)	**<0.001***
Hemoglobin A1c (%)	8.5±1.2	8.5±2.9	0.94
Seasons (Summer-Fall)	50/88 (56.8%)	17/43 (39.5%)	*0.063
Duration of Diabetes Mellitus	2.9±1.2	2.03±1.29	0.001

* = p values by Chi Square for proportions; SDS = standard deviation score; 25(OH)D = 25hydroxyvitamin D.

Biochemical Studies

Data were collected from quarterly HbA1c estimation during clinic visits. Data on serum concentrations of alanine transaminase (ALT) were obtained simultaneously with HbA1c during routine clinic visit before and after vitamin D supplementation in both T1D and T2D patients. Specifically, ALT, 25(OH)D and other laboratory studies were estimated annually or bi-annually, as part of a routine screening protocol for complications of diabetes mellitus. Patients with vitamin D deficiency were started on vitamin D supplementation, and had a follow up laboratory evaluation for 25(OH)D level at their follow up quarterly visit. Vitamin D supplementation was either discontinued if vitamin D levels became normal upon retesting, or supplementation was continued for another cycle of treatment to attain normal vitamin D status. Data were collected on HbA1c levels obtained 3 months prior to the date of vitamin D supplementation, at the time of the initiation of vitamin D supplementation, and at +3mo, +6mo, and +9mo for the evaluation of the temporal effect of vitamin D supplementation on HbA1c levels.

Assays

Hemoglobin A1c was measured by DCA 2000+ Analyzer (Bayer, Inc., Tarrytown, NY, USA) based on Diabetes Control and Complications Trial standards [34]. Serum levels of 25(OH)D were analyzed using 25-hydroxy chemiluminescent immunoassay (DiaSorin Liaison; Stillwater, Minnesota), which has a 100% cross-reactivity with both metabolites of 25(OH)D namely, 25(OH)D_2 and 25(OH)D_3 and thus measures total serum 25(OH)D content. Its functional sensitivity is 10 nmol/L (4 ng/mL), and its intra- and inter-assay coefficients of variation are 5% and 8.2% respectively.

Vitamin D Status

Vitamin D sufficiency was defined as a 25(OH)D concentration ≥30 ng/mL (75 nmol/L); vitamin D insufficiency as 25(OH)D of 20 to 29.9 ng/mL (50 to 75 nmol/L); and vitamin D deficiency as 25(OH)D level <20 ng/mL (50 nmol/L) according to the Endocrine Society criteria [35].

Statistical Analyses

Statistical analyses were performed using the Predictive Analytics SoftWare v.21 (IBM Corporation, Armonk, NY).

Table 2. Summary of Patients' Vitamin D Treatment Plan.

Treatment Plan	Number of Subjects	
Dose of Vitamin D (IU/day)	**Type 1 diabetes**	**Type 2 diabetes**
<1000	3	1
1000–2000	81	26
4000	4	6
7000	0	10

Means, standard deviations, and percentages were calculated for descriptive summary statistics. The values for ALT were log transformed before analysis to approximate normal distributions. Comparisons between independent means were made using two-tailed Student's t test and ANOVA. Non-independent measurements over time were compared using paired t test and repeated-measures ANOVA. Proportions were compared using Chi square test; Fisher's exact test was used where marginal totals were <5. Height, weight, and BMI were expressed as a standard deviation score (SDS).

Power analysis. The study's primary goal was to detect significant changes in HbA1c in subjects with either T1D or T2D during the 3 mo period of vitamin D supplementation, and secondarily to determine if there was a persistence of the changes in HbA1c over a 9 mo period. The small effect size of +0.03% change in HbA1c during the 3 mo of vitamin D supplementation in the 88 patients with T1D yielded a power of 7.5%, while the clinically-significant effect size of −0.6% in 37 subjects with T2D who had pre- and post-treatment values for HbA1c yielded a power of 60.4% at a *p* value of 0.024. Further extrapolation showed that 1,982 subjects with T1D would be needed to achieve a power of 60.4%; while 3,175 patients with T1D, and 58 patients with T2D would be needed to achieve a power of 80%.

Results

One hundred and thirty one subjects of ages 3–18 years (male 13.8±3.4 years, female 13.7±3.8, p = 0.80) were studied. This consisted of 88 subjects (42 males, 46 females) with T1D of mean age 12.6±3.6 years (males 13.1±3.5; females 12.1±3.6, p = 0.23); and 43 subjects (17 males, 26 females) with T2D of mean age 16.2±2.2 years (males 15.8±2.2; females 16.4±2.2, p = 0.36) (Table 1).

At baseline, 72.1% of patients with T2D had vitamin D deficiency compared to 37.5% of T1D patients (p<0.001). Patients with T2D had significantly higher values than those with T1D for BMI SDS (2.2±0.6 vs. 0.80±0.9, p<0.001), ALT (48.3±47.4 vs. 19.2±6.2, p = 0.001), but lower mean 25(OH)D level (41.2 nmol/L ±15.3 vs. 53.7±14.6, p<0.001), and no difference in HbA1c (8.5±2.9% vs. 8.5±1.2, p = 0.94) and total daily dose (TDD) of insulin per kg body weight (0.85 units/kg ±0.4 vs. 0.88±0.3, p = 0.48) (Table 3).

At 3 months, following vitamin D supplementation, 25(OH)D increased significantly in patients with T1D from a baseline of 53.3±14.6 nmol/L to a peak of 67.6±20.6 at 3 mo, and then decreased to 62.4±18.4 nmol/L (ANOVA p<0.001) (Figure 1). Similarly, in patients with T2D, 25(OH)D rose significantly from a baseline value of 41.8±15.0 nmol/L to a peak of 60.7±27.7 at 3 months and then subsequently decreased to 49.2±16.6 nmol/L (ANOVA p<0.011). There was neither a change in the TDD of insulin per kg body weight in either T1D or T2D, nor in the TDD of metformin per kg body weight in T2D patients (Table 3). Following vitamin D supplementation, there was a significant decrease in ALT in T2D (50.7±50.9 U/L to 35.0±31.0, p = 0.012), but not in T1D (18.0±6.0 U/L to 15.7±2.0 (p = 0.46) (Figure 2).

An analysis of the anthropometric changes in the subjects during the 3-month period of vitamin D supplementation showed no differences in weight SDS in either the T1D (0.70±1.0 to 0.71±1.0, p = 0.31) or T2D (2.31±0.96 to 2.26±0.96, p = 0.13) cohort. In contrast, there was a significant decrease in BMI SDS in patients with T2D (2.21±0.62 to 2.14±0.66, p = 0.015), but not in patients with T1D (0.80±0.88 to 0.81±0.84, p = 0.61).

A comparison of changes in HbA1c level over a period of 9 mo from the time of the initiation of vitamin D supplementation in subjects with either T1D or T2D showed a significant difference in HbA1c between the subjects with T1D and those with T2D (ANOVA p = 0.011). A focused analysis of the changes in HbA1c over the 9-month period showed a statistically significant, but clinically non-significant increase in HbA1c from baseline to 9 mo (p = 0.001) in the T1D cohort, while the patients with T2D had no change in A1c (p = 0.52). A closer examination of the HbA1c trends during the 9 mo showed that in patients with T1D, HbA1c levels increased consistently over time from 8.5±1.2 through 8.9±1.2% (ANOVA p = 0.001), while in patients with T2D, the HbA1c value decreased at the beginning of the supplementation (8.5±2.9% at baseline through 7.7±2.5% at 3 mo) but slowly returned toward the baseline value of 8.2±2.3% at the end of 9 months (Figure 3). To investigate whether pre-treatment excursions in HbA1c accounted for the changes in HbA1c described above for T1D and T2D, we compared the mean of the HbA1c levels drawn 3 mo before the start of vitamin D supplementation to the mean of the baseline HbA1c drawn just before the start of vitamin D therapy. There were no significant differences in HbA1c values in T1D (8.4±1.3% vs. 8.5±1.2, p = 0.57), and in T2D (8.9±3.3 vs. 8.5±2.9, p = 0.26).

Discussion

This study evaluated the effects of vitamin D supplementation on hepatic dysfunction and glycemic control in children and adolescents with vitamin D deficiency and either T1D or T2D. At baseline, a greater proportion of subjects with T2D were obese, and had both vitamin D deficiency and elevated ALT levels compared to those with T1D. The 3-mo period of vitamin D supplementation in subjects with T2D was associated with

Table 3. Comparison of the changes in the doses of insulin and metformin during the period of vitamin D supplementation.

Parameters	Type I Diabetes (n = 88)		*p*	Type 2 Diabetes (n = 43)		*p*
Time (months)	**0**	**3**		**0**	**3**	
TDD of insulin (units)	48.0±26.4	49.4±26.7	**0.008**	75.6±36.1	73.1±35.8	0.23
TDD of insulin per kg body weight (units/kg)	0.90±0.3	0.91±0.3	0.54	0.85±0.4	0.80±0.41	0.067
TDD of metformin (mg)	N/A	N/A	N/A	1105.0±687.4	122.3±670.0	0.052
TDD of metformin per kg body weight (mg/kg)	N/A	N/A	N/A	10.71±7.5	12.3±8.0	0.060

TDD = total daily dose.

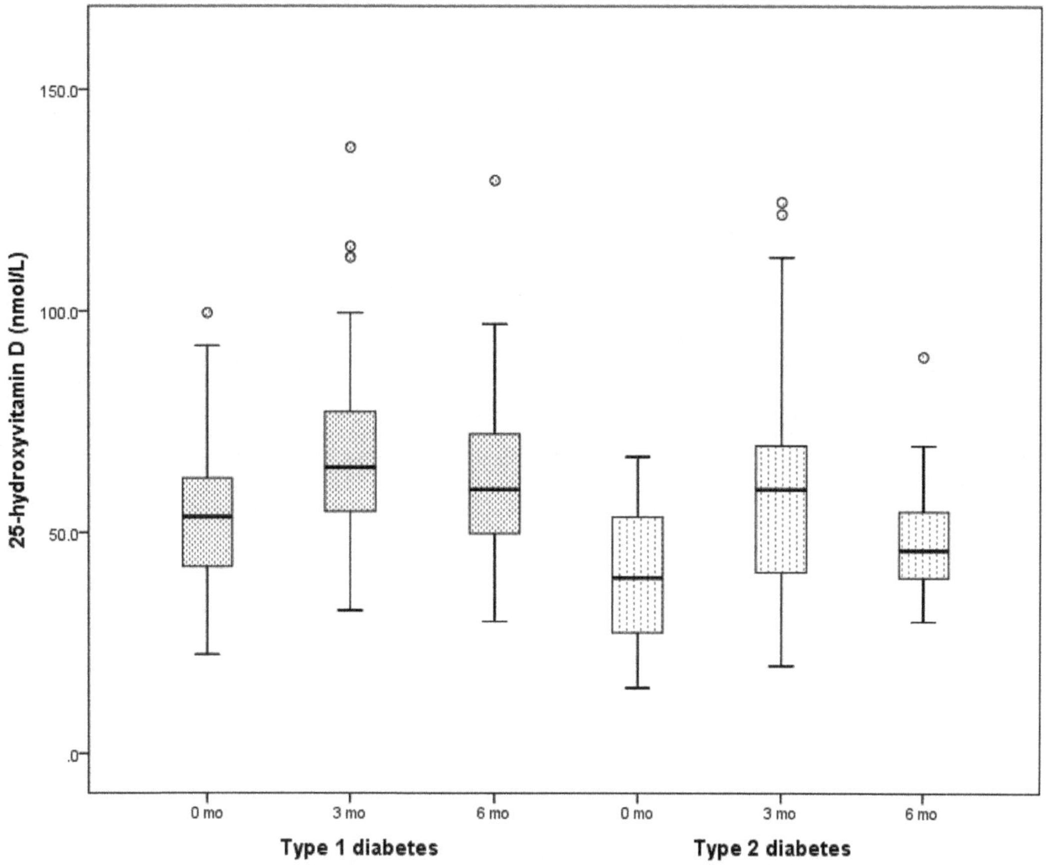

Figure 1. Graph showing a rise in the serum concentrations of 25-hydroxyvitamin D [25(OH)D] during vitamin D supplementation in patients with either type 1 diabetes or type 2 diabetes. In patients with type 1 diabetes, 25(OH)D rose from a baseline of 53.3±14.6 nmol/L to a peak of 67.6±20.6 at 3 mo, and then decreased to 62.4±18.4 (ANOVA $p<0.001$). In patients with type 2 diabetes 25(OH)D rose from a baseline value of 41.8±15.0 to a peak of 60.7±27.7 at 3 months and then decreased to 49.2±16.6 (ANOVA $p=0.011$).

significant reduction in BMI SDS, ALT, and a clinically-significant decrease in HbA1c which was followed by a gradual return toward pretreatment HbA1c values. These reductions in BMI SDS, ALT, and HbA1c [36] in T2D patients were not associated with significant changes in the doses of either insulin or metformin. These data and our earlier report [22] suggest that vitamin D deficiency may be associated with mild hepatic dysfunction which could in turn impair glycemic control in patients with T2D. The normalization of serum vitamin D concentration through vitamin D supplementation appeared to transiently improve glycemic control in patients with T2D.

Our data are in agreement with studies showing a higher prevalence of vitamin D deficiency in pediatric patients with T2D compared to those with T1D [37]. The clinically-significant reduction in HbA1c in our T2D cohort (Figure 2) is consistent with reports of significant associations between vitamin D and glycemic control in T2D [38], as well as earlier reports linking vitamin D deficiency with glucose intolerance [39], hyperinsulinemia [40], obesity [41], and T2D. This clinically-significant reduction in HbA1c in subjects with T2D is similar to the findings of a meta-analysis [36] on the effect of exercise on HbA1c in patients with T2D, which reported a decrease in HbA1c of 0.6%, with associated significant reductions in both visceral and subcutaneous adipose tissues in the study patients.

Vitamin D Deficiency and Type 1 Diabetes

Though vitamin D deficiency has been associated with increased risk of developing T1D [42,43], the relationship between 25(OH)D and glycemic control in patients with T1D is not fully understood. Our previous study [22] found no significant relationship between 25(OH)D and HbA1c in patients with T1D, while this study found a statistically significant, but clinically non-significant increase in HbA1c value following vitamin D supplementation. These results differ from the conclusions of a study in children, adolescents, and young adults with T1D which found a significant reduction in HbA1c level following a supplementation regimen consisting of both vitamin D and calcium [30]. It is possible that vitamin D alone has no significant role on improving glycemic control in patients with T1D.

Vitamin D Deficiency and Type 2 Diabetes

There is no consensus on the effect of vitamin D supplementation on HbA1c level in T2D. Even though previous studies [22,44,45] had reported strong inverse relationship between 25(OH)D and HbA1c, this association alone is not enough to demonstrate a cause and effect relationship. Evidence from two randomized controlled trials (RCT) suggests that vitamin D supplementation effectively reduces insulin resistance (IR) [46,47], but three smaller RCTs [48–50] of vitamin D supplementation in patients with T2D reported no change in HbA1c following vitamin D supplementation. A closer examination of these three

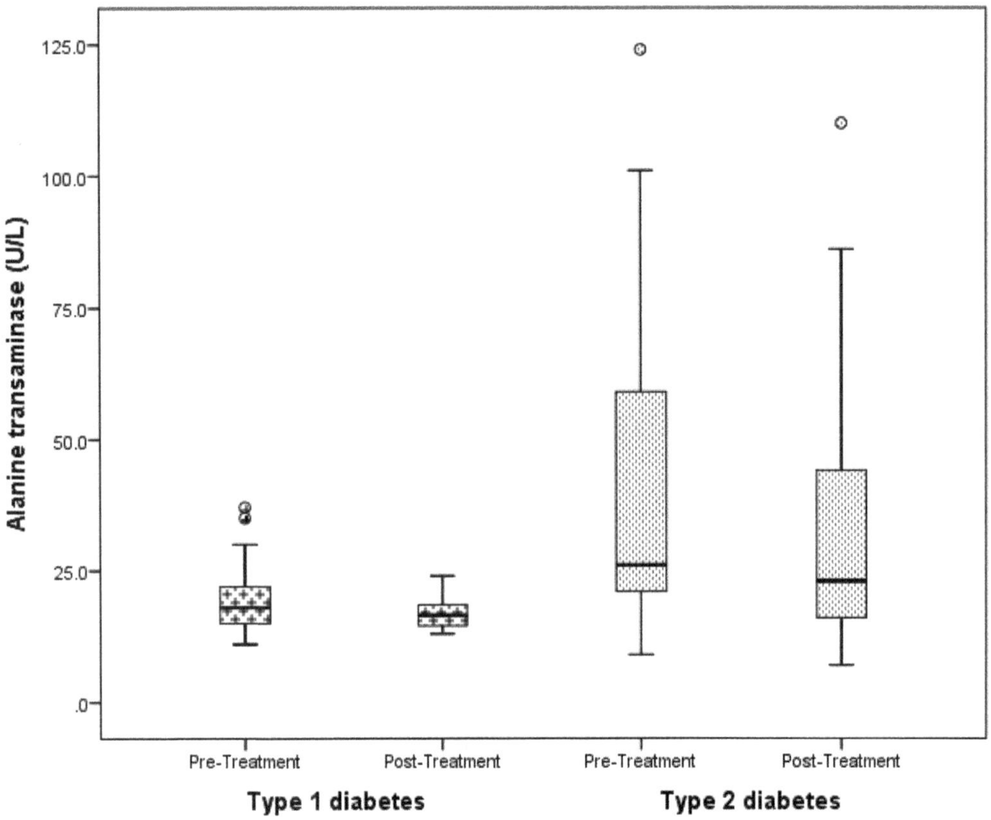

Figure 2. Bar graph showing the temporal change in the levels of alanine transaminases (ALT) following vitamin D supplementation. ALT decreased from 18.0±6.0 U/L to 15.7±2.0 (p = 0.46) in patients with type 1 diabetes; and from 50.7±50.9 to 35.0±31.0 (p = 0.012) in those with type 2 diabetes.

RCTs showed several limitations: (1) all three studies were underpowered (only 16–20 participants per arm), (2) only one study [50] was designed for glycemic outcomes, but it recruited only about half of the planned cohort, and studied patients with normal 25(OH)D levels; (3) only one study [48] reported baseline use of diabetes medications; however, in that study metformin use rate was much higher in the vitamin D arm; (4) changes in diabetes medications were not reported and were not taken into account in the analyses; and (5) all three trials used large infrequent doses of vitamin D. Two recent randomized studies reported improved glycemic control in patients with T2D who either received vitamin D alone [51] or vitamin D fortified yogurt drink [52] while another study reported decreased levels of inflammatory markers following vitamin D supplementation in patients with T2D [53]. However, a Japanese study reported no change in HbA1c following 2000 IU per day of vitamin D_3 with calcium for 24 weeks in patients with T2D [54]. Thus, the effects of vitamin D supplementation on glycemic control in patients with T2D are unclear in adults, and more so in children and adolescents where there are only a few published studies.

There was a significant decrease in BMI SDS in patients with T2D following vitamin D supplementation. The high prevalence of obesity and vitamin D deficiency at baseline in subjects with T2D is consistent with a report that characterized vitamin D deficiency as a risk factor for obesity and T2D [55]. The decrease in BMI SDS concurs with earlier studies indicating that vitamin D repletion could potentiate weight loss and improve metabolic markers [47,56,57]. Vitamin D is believed to regulate adipocyte apoptosis leading to decreased fat mass [58,59]. This vitamin D-associated weight loss may have contributed to the significant decrease in ALT concentrations in our T2D cohort.

Vitamin D Deficiency and Alanine Transaminase

There was a significant decrease in ALT following vitamin D supplementation in patients with T2D compared to those with T1D. Several studies have reported an association between liver enzymes or calculated surrogate measures of NAFLD, such as fatty liver index, and the incidence of diabetes mellitus [13–16]. Recent studies suggest that NAFLD predicts prediabetes [12], and that the resolution of fatty liver could reduce the risk of incident diabetes mellitus [18]. We previously showed a strong inverse relationship between ALT and 25(OH)D in children and adolescents with T2D [22], while this present study reports a significant decrease in ALT levels in patients with T2D who received vitamin D supplementation for the management of hypovitaminosis D.

The mechanism of the transient, clinically-significant improvement in glycemic control in patients with T2D during the period of vitamin D supplementation is not clear. Vitamin D supplementation has been shown to improve β-cell function [23] and the augmentation of insulin synthesis and secretion once it is activated to its active form, 1,25-dihydroxyvitamin D, by 1α-hydroxylase enzyme which is expressed in β cells [60] [61–63]. This study however, suggests that an improvement in hepatic dysfunction, as shown by reduced ALT, could also be associated with an improved glycemic control.

One of the limitations of our study is its retrospective nature which could have introduced selection bias as only patients who fulfilled the inclusion and exclusion criteria were studied. We also

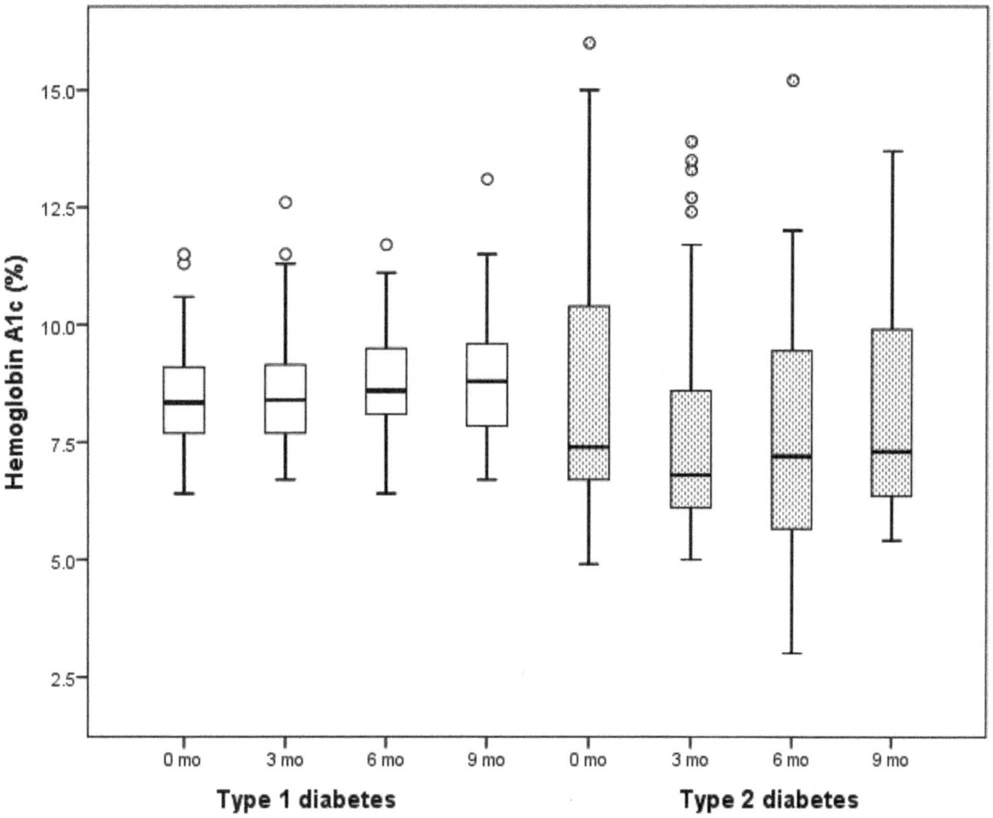

Figure 3. A 9-month analysis of the changes in hemoglobin A1c (HbA1c) level following a three-month vitamin D supplementation in patients with either type 1 diabetes or type 2 diabetes. There was a statistically-significant, but clinically non-significant rise in HbA1c level over 9 months in T1D (8.5±1.2 through 8.9±1.2%, ANOVA $p = 0.001$). In T2D, there was a clinically significant decrease in HbA1c [36] in the first 3 months (during the period of vitamin D supplementation) from 8.5±2.9% at baseline through 7.7±2.5% at 3 mo, followed by a slow return to pretreatment values of 8.2±2.3% at 9 mo. There was however, no statistical significant difference in HbA1c between the time points (ANOVA $p = 0.52$).

did not directly evaluate subjects' compliance with their vitamin D therapy. However, the post-treatment vitamin D levels were significantly elevated in patients with either T1D or T2D. Another limitation was that the vitamin D supplementation was not continued for longer than three months, and thus it was unclear whether the effect of vitamin D supplementation on glycemic control could have been sustained over a longer period of time. The lack of a relationship between ALT and 25(OH)D in T1D patients may be due to the fact that a fewer number of patients with T1D had ALT measured as compared to the larger proportion of patients with T2D who had ALT values. Specifically, forty two (47.7%) of the patients with T1D, and 36 (83.7%) of the subjects with T2D had ALT measured at baseline, while 12 (13.6%) of T1D and 29 (67.4%) of the T2D patients had ALT values following vitamin D supplementation. Another reason for a lack of an association between ALT and 25(OH)D could be due to the fact that subjects with T1D had normal mean serum ALT concentration at baseline compared to patients with T2D.

The strengths of this study stem from the fact that both the patients with either T1D or T2D received their care within the same clinical system, which is located in a similar geographical area around latitude 42° N, thus ensuring similar levels of insolation around the year. We had a relatively good sample size to enable us determine the differences in the various parameters studied. The availability of post-treatment 25(OH)D values confirmed that the subjects received the interventional therapy, while the availability of serial HbA1c values enabled us to establish a longitudinal model for the investigation of the duration of the glycemic effects of vitamin D supplementation on HbA1c and ALT in both T1D and T2D. Even though this is a retrospective study, it provides the much needed data on the effect of routine vitamin D supplementation on HbA1c, 25(OH)D, and ALT values in children and adolescents with either T1D or T2D. Such data will help establish the rationale for further investigation on the effects of vitamin D supplementation on these parameters in children and adolescents with diabetes mellitus.

Conclusions

This study demonstrates that routine vitamin D supplementation in patients with diabetes mellitus is associated with a significant reduction in BMI SDS, ALT, and an initial, clinically-significant reduction in HbA1c in patients with T2D, but not T1D. The changes in these parameters were not associated with significant changes in the doses of either insulin or metformin. Even though these findings suggest that vitamin D deficiency could impair hepatic processes that promote β-cell function and glycemic control in patients with T2D; and that this hepatic dysfunction could be ameliorated by vitamin D supplementation with resultant improvement in glycemic control, our data are not adequate to confirm these conclusions. Further randomized controlled trials are warranted to determine the effect of vitamin D supplementation on glycemic control in T2D, and the optimal dose of adjunctive vitamin D therapy for the maintenance of long-term glycemic control in children and adolescents with diabetes mellitus.

Acknowledgments

BUN is a member of the UMass Diabetes and Endocrine Research Center (DK32520). We thank Mr. Francis M. Wanjau for his help with data management, and Ms. Jessica L. Kowaleski for her clerical assistance.

Data Depository

Our study data files are publicly deposited in the University of Massachusetts Medical School's institutional repository, eScholarship@UMMS. The permanent link to the data is http://escholarship.umassmed.edu/datasets/2/.

Author Contributions

Conceived and designed the experiments: BUN. Performed the experiments: BUN LM. Analyzed the data: LM BUN. Contributed reagents/materials/analysis tools: LM. Wrote the paper: BUN.

References

1. (1995) Effect of intensive diabetes management on macrovascular events and risk factors in the Diabetes Control and Complications Trial. Am J Cardiol 75: 894–903.
2. de Boer IH, Sibley SD, Kestenbaum B, Sampson JN, Young B, et al. (2007) Central obesity, incident microalbuminuria, and change in creatinine clearance in the epidemiology of diabetes interventions and complications study. J Am Soc Nephrol 18: 235–243.
3. (1998) Intensive blood-glucose control with sulphonylureas or insulin compared with conventional treatment and risk of complications in patients with type 2 diabetes (UKPDS 33). UK Prospective Diabetes Study (UKPDS) Group. Lancet 352: 837–853.
4. Petitti DB, Klingensmith GJ, Bell RA, Andrews JS, Dabelea D, et al. (2009) Glycemic Control in Youth with Diabetes: The SEARCH for Diabetes in Youth Study. J Pediatr 155: 668–672.
5. Heinemann L (2010) New ways of insulin delivery. Int J Clin Pract Suppl: 29–40.
6. Schwimmer JB, Deutsch R, Kahen T, Lavine JE, Stanley C, et al. (2006) Prevalence of fatty liver in children and adolescents. Pediatrics 118: 1388–1393.
7. Burgert TS, Taksali SE, Dziura J, Goodman TR, Yeckel CW, et al. (2006) Alanine aminotransferase levels and fatty liver in childhood obesity: associations with insulin resistance, adiponectin, and visceral fat. J Clin Endocrinol Metab 91: 4287–4294.
8. Schwimmer JB, Deutsch R, Rauch JB, Behling C, Newbury R, et al. (2003) Obesity, insulin resistance, and other clinicopathological correlates of pediatric nonalcoholic fatty liver disease. J Pediatr 143: 500–505.
9. Barchetta I, Angelico F, Del Ben M, Baroni MG, Pozzilli P, et al. (2011) Strong association between non alcoholic fatty liver disease (NAFLD) and low 25(OH) vitamin D levels in an adult population with normal serum liver enzymes. BMC Med 9: 85.
10. Manco M, Ciampalini P, Nobili V (2010) Low levels of 25-hydroxyvitamin D(3) in children with biopsy-proven nonalcoholic fatty liver disease. Hepatology 51: 2229; author reply 2230.
11. Cusi K (2009) Nonalcoholic fatty liver disease in type 2 diabetes mellitus. Curr Opin Endocrinol Diabetes Obes 16: 141–149.
12. Zelber-Sagi S, Lotan R, Shibolet O, Webb M, Buch A, et al. (2013) Non-alcoholic fatty liver disease independently predicts prediabetes during a 7-year prospective follow-up. Liver Int 33: 1406–1412.
13. Fraser A, Harris R, Sattar N, Ebrahim S, Davey Smith G, et al. (2009) Alanine aminotransferase, gamma-glutamyltransferase, and incident diabetes: the British Women's Heart and Health Study and meta-analysis. Diabetes Care 32: 741–750.
14. Ford ES, Schulze MB, Bergmann MM, Thamer C, Joost HG, et al. (2008) Liver enzymes and incident diabetes: findings from the European Prospective Investigation into Cancer and Nutrition (EPIC)-Potsdam Study. Diabetes Care 31: 1138–1143.
15. Monami M, Bardini G, Lamanna C, Pala L, Cresci B, et al. (2008) Liver enzymes and risk of diabetes and cardiovascular disease: results of the Firenze Bagno a Ripoli (FIBAR) study. Metabolism 57: 387–392.
16. Balkau B, Lange C, Vol S, Fumeron F, Bonnet F, et al. (2010) Nine-year incident diabetes is predicted by fatty liver indices: the French D.E.S.I.R. study. BMC Gastroenterol 10: 56.
17. Ali R, Cusi K (2009) New diagnostic and treatment approaches in non-alcoholic fatty liver disease (NAFLD). Ann Med 41: 265–278.
18. Sung KC, Wild SH, Byrne CD (2013) Resolution of fatty liver and risk of incident diabetes. J Clin Endocrinol Metab 98: 3637–3643.
19. Liangpunsakul S, Chalasani N (2011) Serum vitamin D concentrations and unexplained elevation in ALT among US adults. Dig Dis Sci 56: 2124–2129.
20. Vozarova B, Stefan N, Lindsay RS, Saremi A, Pratley RE, et al. (2002) High alanine aminotransferase is associated with decreased hepatic insulin sensitivity and predicts the development of type 2 diabetes. Diabetes 51: 1889–1895.
21. Nadeau KJ, Klingensmith G, Zeitler P (2005) Type 2 diabetes in children is frequently associated with elevated alanine aminotransferase. J Pediatr Gastroenterol Nutr 41: 94–98.
22. Nwosu BU, Stavre ZG, Maranda L, Cullen K, Lee MM (2012) Hepatic dysfunction is associated with vitamin D deficiency and poor glycemic control in diabetes mellitus. J Pediatr Endocrinol Metab 25: 181–186.
23. Chiu KC, Chu A, Go VL, Saad MF (2004) Hypovitaminosis D is associated with insulin resistance and beta cell dysfunction. Am J Clin Nutr 79: 820–825.
24. Greer RM, Portelli SL, Hung BS, Cleghorn GJ, McMahon SK, et al. (2013) Serum vitamin D levels are lower in Australian children and adolescents with type 1 diabetes than in children without diabetes. Pediatr Diabetes 14: 31–41.
25. Svoren BM, Volkening LK, Wood JR, Laffel LM (2009) Significant vitamin D deficiency in youth with type 1 diabetes mellitus. J Pediatr 154: 132–134.
26. Drincic AT, Armas LA, Van Diest EE, Heaney RP (2012) Volumetric dilution, rather than sequestration best explains the low vitamin D status of obesity. Obesity (Silver Spring) 20: 1444–1448.
27. Liel Y, Ulmer E, Shary J, Hollis BW, Bell NH (1988) Low circulating vitamin D in obesity. Calcif Tissue Int 43: 199–201.
28. Inzucchi SE, Maggs DG, Spollett GR, Page SL, Rife FS, et al. (1998) Efficacy and metabolic effects of metformin and troglitazone in type II diabetes mellitus. N Engl J Med 338: 867–872.
29. Kelly A, Brooks LJ, Dougherty S, Carlow DC, Zemel BS (2011) A cross-sectional study of vitamin D and insulin resistance in children. Arch Dis Child 96: 447–452.
30. Aljabri KS, Bokhari SA, Khan MJ (2010) Glycemic changes after vitamin D supplementation in patients with type 1 diabetes mellitus and vitamin D deficiency. Ann Saudi Med 30: 454–458.
31. Ostergard M, Arnberg K, Michaelsen KF, Madsen AL, Krarup H, et al. (2011) Vitamin D status in infants: relation to nutrition and season. Eur J Clin Nutr 65: 657–660.
32. Drincic A, Fuller E, Heaney RP, Armas LA (2013) 25-hydroxyvitamin d response to graded vitamin d3 supplementation among obese adults. J Clin Endocrinol Metab 98: 4845–4851.
33. Kuczmarski RJ, Ogden CL, Grummer-Strawn LM, Flegal KM, Guo SS, et al. (2000) CDC growth charts: United States. Adv Data: 1–27.
34. Tamborlane WV, Kollman C, Steffes MW, Ruedy KJ, Dongyuan X, et al. (2005) Comparison of fingerstick hemoglobin A1c levels assayed by DCA 2000 with the DCCT/EDIC central laboratory assay: results of a Diabetes Research in Children Network (DirecNet) Study. Pediatr Diabetes 6: 13–16.
35. Holick MF, Binkley NC, Bischoff-Ferrari HA, Gordon CM, Hanley DA, et al. (2011) Evaluation, treatment, and prevention of vitamin D deficiency: an Endocrine Society clinical practice guideline. J Clin Endocrinol Metab 96: 1911–1930.
36. Thomas DE, Elliott EJ, Naughton GA (2006) Exercise for type 2 diabetes mellitus. Cochrane Database Syst Rev: CD002968.
37. Di Cesar DJ, Ploutz-Snyder R, Weinstock RS, Moses AM (2006) Vitamin D deficiency is more common in type 2 than in type 1 diabetes. Diabetes Care 29: 174.
38. Kostoglou-Athanassiou I, Athanassiou P, Gkountouvas A, Kaldrymides P (2013) Vitamin D and glycemic control in diabetes mellitus type 2. Ther Adv Endocrinol Metab 4: 122–128.
39. Hypponen E, Power C (2006) Vitamin D status and glucose homeostasis in the 1958 British birth cohort: the role of obesity. Diabetes Care 29: 2244–2246.
40. Baynes KC, Boucher BJ, Feskens EJ, Kromhout D (1997) Vitamin D, glucose tolerance and insulinaemia in elderly men. Diabetologia 40: 344–347.
41. Hahn S, Haselhorst U, Tan S, Quadbeck B, Schmidt M, et al. (2006) Low serum 25-hydroxyvitamin D concentrations are associated with insulin resistance and obesity in women with polycystic ovary syndrome. Exp Clin Endocrinol Diabetes 114: 577–583.
42. Hypponen E, Laara E, Reunanen A, Jarvelin MR, Virtanen SM (2001) Intake of vitamin D and risk of type 1 diabetes: a birth-cohort study. Lancet 358: 1500–1503.
43. (1999) Vitamin D supplement in early childhood and risk for Type I (insulin-dependent) diabetes mellitus. The EURODIAB Substudy 2 Study Group. Diabetologia 42: 51–54.
44. Kositsawat J, Freeman VL, Gerber BS, Geraci S (2010) Association of A1C levels with vitamin D status in U.S. adults: data from the National Health and Nutrition Examination Survey. Diabetes Care 33: 1236–1238.
45. Perez-Ferre N, Torrejon MJ, Fuentes M, Fernandez MD, Ramos A, et al. (2012) Association of low serum 25-hydroxyvitamin D levels in pregnancy with glucose homeostasis and obstetric and newborn outcomes. Endocr Pract 18: 676–684.
46. von Hurst PR, Stonehouse W, Coad J (2010) Vitamin D supplementation reduces insulin resistance in South Asian women living in New Zealand who are

insulin resistant and vitamin D deficient - a randomised, placebo-controlled trial. Br J Nutr 103: 549–555.

47. Nagpal J, Pande JN, Bhartia A (2009) A double-blind, randomized, placebo-controlled trial of the short-term effect of vitamin D3 supplementation on insulin sensitivity in apparently healthy, middle-aged, centrally obese men. Diabet Med 26: 19–27.
48. Sugden JA, Davies JI, Witham MD, Morris AD, Struthers AD (2008) Vitamin D improves endothelial function in patients with Type 2 diabetes mellitus and low vitamin D levels. Diabet Med 25: 320–325.
49. Witham MD, Dove FJ, Dryburgh M, Sugden JA, Morris AD, et al. (2010) The effect of different doses of vitamin D(3) on markers of vascular health in patients with type 2 diabetes: a randomised controlled trial. Diabetologia 53: 2112–2119.
50. Jorde R, Figenschau Y (2009) Supplementation with cholecalciferol does not improve glycaemic control in diabetic subjects with normal serum 25-hydroxyvitamin D levels. Eur J Nutr 48: 349–354.
51. Strobel F, Reusch J, Penna-Martinez M, Ramos-Lopez E, Klahold E, et al. (2013) Effect of a Randomised Controlled Vitamin D Trial on Insulin Resistance and Glucose Metabolism in Patients with Type 2 Diabetes Mellitus. Horm Metab Res.
52. Nikooyeh B, Neyestani TR, Farvid M, Alavi-Majd H, Houshiarrad A, et al. (2011) Daily consumption of vitamin D- or vitamin D+calcium-fortified yogurt drink improved glycemic control in patients with type 2 diabetes: a randomized clinical trial. Am J Clin Nutr 93: 764–771.
53. Shab-Bidar S, Neyestani TR, Djazayery A, Eshraghian MR, Houshiarrad A, et al. (2012) Improvement of vitamin D status resulted in amelioration of biomarkers of systemic inflammation in the subjects with type 2 diabetes. Diabetes Metab Res Rev 28: 424–430.
54. Ryu OH, Lee S, Yu J, Choi MG, Yoo HJ, et al. (2013) A prospective randomized controlled trial of the effects of vitamin D supplementation on long-term glycemic control in type 2 diabetes mellitus of Korea. Endocr J.
55. Grineva EN, Karonova T, Micheeva E, Belyaeva O, Nikitina IL (2013) Vitamin D deficiency is a risk factor for obesity and diabetes type 2 in women at late reproductive age. Aging (Albany NY) 5: 575–581.
56. Ortega RM, Lopez-Sobaler AM, Aparicio A, Bermejo LM, Rodriguez-Rodriguez E, et al. (2009) Vitamin D status modification by two slightly hypocaloric diets in young overweight/obese women. Int J Vitam Nutr Res 79: 71–78.
57. Zittermann A, Frisch S, Berthold HK, Gotting C, Kuhn J, et al. (2009) Vitamin D supplementation enhances the beneficial effects of weight loss on cardiovascular disease risk markers. Am J Clin Nutr 89: 1321–1327.
58. Sun X, Zemel MB (2008) 1Alpha, 25-dihydroxyvitamin D and corticosteroid regulate adipocyte nuclear vitamin D receptor. Int J Obes (Lond) 32: 1305–1311.
59. Zemel MB, Sun X (2008) Calcitriol and energy metabolism. Nutr Rev 66: S139–146.
60. Christakos S, Norman AW (1979) Studies on the mode of action of calciferol. XVIII. Evidence for a specific high affinity binding protein for 1,25 dihydroxyvitamin D3 in chick kidney and pancreas. Biochem Biophys Res Commun 89: 56–63.
61. Norman AW, Frankel JB, Heldt AM, Grodsky GM (1980) Vitamin D deficiency inhibits pancreatic secretion of insulin. Science 209: 823–825.
62. Ford ES, Ajani UA, McGuire LC, Liu S (2005) Concentrations of serum vitamin D and the metabolic syndrome among U.S. adults. Diabetes Care 28: 1228–1230.
63. Scragg R, Sowers M, Bell C (2004) Serum 25-hydroxyvitamin D, diabetes, and ethnicity in the Third National Health and Nutrition Examination Survey. Diabetes Care 27: 2813–2818.

9

Responses of a Triple Mutant Defective in Three Iron Deficiency-Induced *BASIC HELIX-LOOP-HELIX* Genes of the Subgroup Ib(2) to Iron Deficiency and Salicylic Acid

Felix Maurer[1¤], Maria Augusta Naranjo Arcos[1,2], Petra Bauer[1,2]*

1 Dept. Biosciences-Plant Biology, Saarland University, Saarbrücken, Germany, **2** Institute of Botany and Cluster of Excellence on Plant Sciences (CEPLAS), Heinrich Heine University, Düsseldorf, Germany

Abstract

Plants are sessile organisms that adapt to external stress by inducing molecular and physiological responses that serve to better cope with the adverse growth condition. Upon low supply of the micronutrient iron, plants actively increase the acquisition of soil iron into the root and its mobilization from internal stores. The subgroup Ib(2) *BHLH* genes function as regulators in this response, however their concrete functions are not fully understood. Here, we analyzed a triple loss of function mutant of *BHLH39*, *BHLH100* and *BHLH101* (*3xbhlh* mutant). We found that this mutant did not have any iron uptake phenotype if iron was provided. However, under iron deficiency the mutant displayed a more severe leaf chlorosis than the wild type. Microarray-based transcriptome analysis revealed that this mutant phenotype resulted in the mis-regulation of 198 genes, out of which only 15% were associated with iron deficiency regulation itself. A detailed analysis revealed potential targets of the bHLH transcription factors as well as genes reflecting an exaggerated iron deficiency response phenotype. Since the *BHLH* genes of this subgroup have been brought into the context of the plant hormone salicylic acid, we investigated whether the *3xbhlh* mutant might have been affected by this plant signaling molecule. Although a very high number of genes responded to SA, also in a differential manner between mutant and wild type, we did not find any indication for an association of the *BHLH* gene functions in SA responses upon iron deficiency. In summary, our study indicates that the bHLH subgroup Ib(2) transcription factors do not only act in iron acquisition into roots but in other aspects of the adaptation to iron deficiency in roots and leaves.

Editor: Abidur Rahman, Iwate University, Japan

Funding: This work has been partly funded by the University of Saarland and the Heinrich Heine University Düsseldorf. Funding by the Deutsche Forschungsgemeinschaft grant No. DFG-Ba1610/5-1to PB is was provided. The funders had no role in study design, data collection and analysis, decision to publish, or preparation of the manuscript.

Competing Interests: The authors have declared that no competing interests exist.

* E-mail: petra.bauer@hhu.de

¤ Current address: Department of Anaesthesiology, Intensive Care and Pain Therapy, Saarland University Medical Center and Saarland University Faculty of Medicine, Homburg, Germany

Introduction

Iron (Fe) deficiency is among the most prevalent micronutrient deficiencies in humans. Since plants constitute the primary source of nutrients for a large part of the world's population, the improvement of plants in terms of nutrient bioavailability is considered a priority [1]. Micronutrients like Fe are often present in an un-soluble form in the soil. Plants are able to mobilize such nutrients for uptake into the roots. Plants can also mobilize Fe from internal stores. Understanding the regulation of Fe acquisition and internal Fe utilization is of high importance for precision breeding of crops that are improved to either tolerate growth on alkaline and calcareous soils with poor Fe bio-availability or to accumulate a higher content of this micronutrient in bio-available form in the edible plant parts.

Genetic traits have been associated with micronutrient content and usage in plants, for example [2,3]. Another trait was found in soybean as being linked to transcription factor genes encoding the soybean homologs of *BHLH38* and *BHLH39* [4]. The potential importance of these two transcription factor genes for Fe mobilization had previously been uncovered in studies on the plant model *Arabidopsis thaliana*. *BHLH38* and *BHLH39* belong to the so-called subgroup Ib(2) *BHLH* genes [5] and they are functionally redundant [6–8]. In fact, *BHLH38* and *BHLH39* are tandem duplicates on the chromosome, and they share similarity with two other *BHLH* genes, namely *BHLH100* and *BHLH101* [6,9–11]. All these four subgroup Ib(2) *BHLH* genes are highly induced by low Fe supply in roots and leaves while they are not usually found expressed under sufficient Fe supply [6]. Expression of *BHLH39* and *BHLH101* in response to iron can be followed using the public microarray data in Arabidopsis [12–16] and it was found that they occur in a co-expression network along with several Fe homeostasis genes like *FERRIC REDUCTASE OXIDASE3* (*FRO3*), *NATURAL RESISTANCE-ASSOCIATED MACROPHAGE PROTEIN4* (*NRAMP4*) and *NICOTIANAMINE SYNTHASE4* (*NAS4*) [17]. From the co-expression with Fe homeostasis genes it can be concluded that the subgroup Ib(2) *BHLH* transcription factor genes likely perform regulatory functions in the context of Fe homeostasis and internal Fe mobilization. The bHLH protein POPEYE (PYE, belonging to another bHLH subgroup) is also induced by Fe deficiency within this co-expression network and it acts as a negative regulator of *FRO3*, *NRAMP4* and *NAS4*, presumably to avoid over-activation of Fe mobilization [18]. PYE is regulated by BRUTUS (BTS) that is also found in this co-expression network [17,18]. bHLH subgroup Ib(2) can physically interact with the bHLH FER-LIKE IRON DEFICIENCY-INDUCED TRANSCRIPTION FACTOR (FIT) [8,19]. FIT is expressed specifically in roots and has been shown to be essential for Fe uptake [20–23] by regulating the expression of the genes encoding ARABIDOPSIS H^+-ATPASE2 (AHA2) [17], Fe reductase FERRIC OXIDASE2 (FRO2) [22,24] and the IRON-REGULATED TRANSPORTER1 (IRT1) [22,25]. From ectopic FIT expression experiments along with yeast promoter activation assays and inducible FIT activation in plants, it can be concluded that FIT targets *FRO2* and *IRT1* gene promoters [22,23,26,27]. However, FIT induces *IRT1* and *FRO2* only upon Fe deficiency even when overexpressed [22,26]. The activation of FIT at low Fe can be explained with the presence of bHLH subgroup Ib(2) factors. Indeed, the double overexpression of FIT together with either bHLH subgroup Ib(2) protein leads to an increase of Fe acquisition responses under sufficient Fe supply conditions, and it was therefore proposed that the function of bHLH subgroup Ib(2) might be to induce Fe deficiency responses in conjunction with FIT [8,19]. However, the occurrence of *BHLH* subgroup Ib(2) genes in the *PYE* coexpression network, their non-expression upon sufficient Fe (where *FIT* and *IRT1* are active although at low level) and their high induction upon Fe deficiency not only in roots but also in leaves (in contrast to Fe acquisition genes) renders this hypothesis questionable. Moreover, contradictory results have been published with regard to the function of bHLH subgroup Ib(2) proteins. In one report, double *bhlh100 bhlh101* knockout mutants were demonstrated to develop a more severe leaf chlorosis than the wild type upon Fe deficiency, while no phenotype was apparent upon Fe sufficiency. Although some Fe homeostasis genes appeared mis-expressed, the gene knockouts did not affect the plants' abilities for Fe uptake and the regulation of *FRO2* and *IRT1* upon sufficient or deficient Fe supply [7]. In contrast to that, in another report, bHLH subgroup Ib(2) knockouts including *bhlh100 bhlh101* and a triple knockout *bhlh39 bhlh100 bhlh101* were demonstrated to affect Fe acquisition responses and to have low *FRO2* and *IRT1* expression upon sufficient or deficient Fe supply [28]. This latter finding was rather puzzling, and it was not further explained how this finding fits to the observation that the *BHLH* genes are not normally expressed upon sufficient Fe supply, when Fe also needs to be acquired via FRO2 and IRT1 [22,29]. Thus, the function of the bHLH subgroup Ib(2) transcription factors in Fe uptake is still open for debate.

Very interestingly, it has been shown that *BHLH38* and *BHLH39* were induced after application of salicylic acid (=SA) by the SA-inducible Dof (=DNA binding with one finger) transcription factor OBF BINDING PROTEIN3 (OBP3) [30]. Binding of OBP3 to promoter elements in *BHLH38* and *BHLH39* genes and their subsequent activation was demonstrated (in these studies *BHLH38* and *BHLH39* were named *OBP3 RESPONSIVE GENE2*, *ORG2*, and *OBP3 RESPONSIVE GENE3*, *ORG3*) [30]. Jasmonic acid negatively affects the onset of Fe mobilization and the induction of *FRO2* and *IRT1* [31], while ethylene enhances the responses [32–34]. Since SA, jasmonic acid and ethylene act in stress response networks, the possibility exists that perhaps, there is a link between SA and the up-regulation of Fe deficiency responses.

Here, we made use of the triple knockout mutant *bhlh39 bhlh100 bhlh101* (*3xbhlh*) that we constructed to investigate the functions of

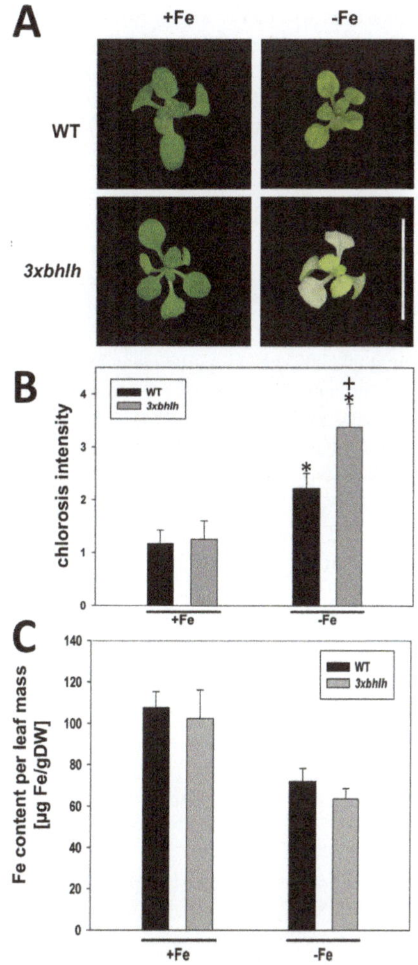

Figure 1. Leaf chlorosis phenotypes of the *3xbhlh* mutant. A, 10 d-old WT and *3xbhlh* plants grown at +Fe and −Fe; bar = 5 mm; B, Strength of leaf chlorosis; the leaf chlorosis scale used was 1 = green, 2 = green, partially yellow, 3 = yellow-green, 4 = yellow; 5 = white-yellow; n = 12; C, Fe content per leaf dry mass; n = 4; indicates a significant change ($p<0.05$) of −Fe versus +Fe; + indicates a significant change ($p<0.05$) of *3xbhlh* versus WT.

these *BHLH* genes in the Fe deficiency response and to further shed light on the question whether SA is involved in mediating the onset of Fe uptake via the induction of *BHLH* subgroup Ib(2) genes. We discuss that *BHLH39*, *BHLH100* and *BHLH101* are essential for a subset of Fe deficiency responses but not including up-regulation of *IRT1* and *FRO2*. We suggest that these transcription factors are involved in adapting stress responses and internal metabolic responses to Fe deficiency.

Materials and Methods

Plant Materials

Wild type was Col-0. The *3xbhlh* mutant line was generated from the single T-DNA insertion mutants *bhlh39-1* (SALK_025676), *bhlh100-1* (SALK_074568) and *bhlh101-1* (SALK_011245) [6]. A homozygous *bhlh39-1* plant was crossed with a *bhlh100-1 bhlh10-1* double mutant plant. In the F2 progeny a triple homozygous *bhlh39-1 bhlh100-1 bhlh101-1* plant was identified by genotyping and multiplied to obtain a triple homozygous line, hereafter named *3xbhlh*. The SA mutant line *npr1-1* (hereafter named *npr1*) with a defect in a central regulator component of SA signaling resulting in the failure of the expression of the *PR1* gene was obtained from the NASC stock center (N3726) [35]. The lines *NaHG* and *sid2-2* were provided by Fred Ausubel, Massachusetts General Hospital [36].

Plant Growth

Arabidopsis seeds were surface-sterilized with 6% NaOCl, 0.1% Triton-X for 10 minutes, and washed 5 times with distilled water. Seeds were stratified for 2 days in 0.1% plant agar in the dark at 4°C. For the 6-day growth assay seeds were placed on Hoagland agar medium containing 50 μM FeNaEDTA (sufficient Fe supply, hereafter termed +Fe) or 0 μM FeNaEDTA (deficient Fe supply, hereafter termed −Fe), germinated and grown for 6 d under long-day conditions with 8 h dark and 16 h light [34]. On day 6, seedlings were harvested for analysis.

For the 2-week growth assay, seeds were germinated and seedlings grown for 14 d on Hoagland agar medium as described above containing 50 μM FeNaEDTA, then transferred for 3 days to fresh medium containing either 0 μM FeNaEDTA (−Fe) or 50 μM FeNaEDTA (+Fe). Then, leaves and roots were harvested separately for RNA or protein analysis. If indicated in the text 100 μM methyl-salicylic acid (hereafter named SA, Sigma-Aldrich, USA) was added to the growth medium and plants exposed for the indicated time.

Physiological Analysis

The degree of leaf chlorosis was assessed according to a previously published procedure [37]. The leaf chlorosis scale is mentionned in the figure legend of Fig. 1.

For metal determination, plant parts exposed to plant medium were washed with 100 mM $Ca(NO_3)_2$ prior to harvest to eliminate metal residues from the growth medium. Plant material was dried overnight at room temperature, then for 1 d at 120°C and powdered with an achat mortar. Quantification of metal contents of the plant samples was performed using atomic absorption spectroscopy coupled with a graphite tube atomizer as described [34]. Four technical replicate measurements were carried out with weighted samples of 50–120 μg for every atomisation (2300°C) and mean mass per dry weight values were calculated for each biological sample. Four biological replicates were produced and mean values calculated.

Iron reductase activity assays were performed using a liquid ferrozine assay [38] and biological replicates were performed as described in the figure legends. Statistical analysis was performed using the t-test.

Gene Expression using Reverse Transcription-qPCR

Reverse transcription-quantitative real-time PCR was performed as previously described [39]. Briefly, DNase-treated RNA was used for cDNA synthesis. SYBR green I-based real-time PCR analysis was performed by using the TaKaRa Premix (TaKaRa, Japan) in the real-time ICycler (Bio-Rad, USA). For each gene, the absolute quantity of initial transcript was determined by standard curve analysis using mass standards. Absolute expression data was normalized against the averaged expression values of the internal control gene *EF1BALPHA2* [39]. Each biological cDNA sample was tested in two technical replicates and the values averaged. Statistical analysis was performed by ANOVA using the values of biological replicates. Information on oligonucleotide primer sequences is available in Table S1.

Gene Expression using Microarray Analysis

Wild type and *3xbhlh* seedlings were grown in the 6-day growth system at –Fe, treated for six hours with 100 μM SA or were mock-treated and harvested for RNA preparation. Three biological replicates were generated. RNA was purified using the Qiagen kit and checked for integrity. Microarray hybridization was performed using the Agilent one-color gene expression V4 chip

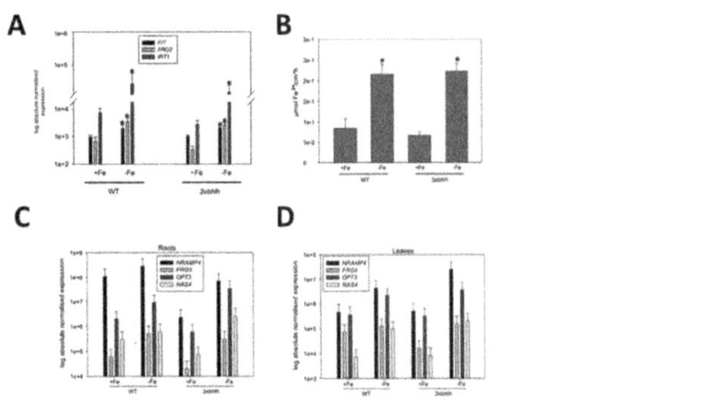

Figure 2. Molecular and physiological Fe acquisition responses of the *3xbhlh* mutant. A, Gene expression of *FIT, FRO2, IRT1* in roots; B, Fe reductase activity; C, *NRAMP4, FRO3, OPT3, NAS4*, gene expression in roots; D, *NRAMP4, FRO3, OPT3, NAS4*, gene expression in leaves; 14 d-old plants were transferred for three days to + and −Fe. Roots were harvested for analysis. n = 4; * indicates a significant change ($p<0.05$) of −Fe versus +Fe; + indicates a significant change ($p<0.05$) of *3xbhlh* versus WT. Gene expression was studied using reverse transcription-qPCR.

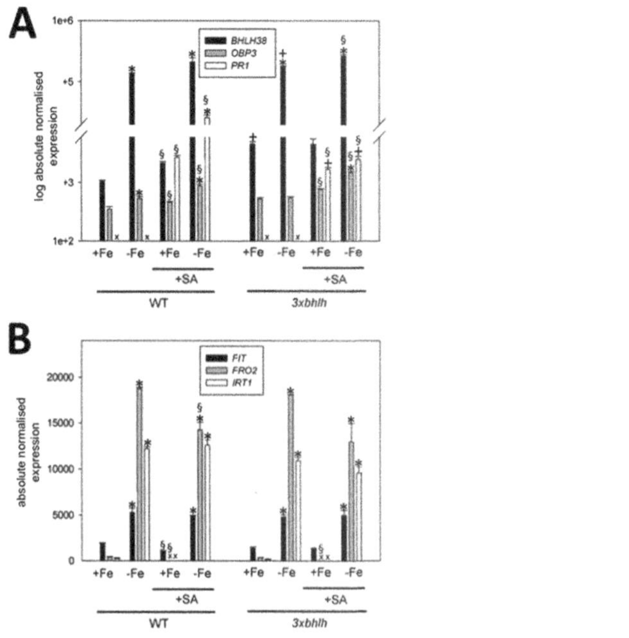

Figure 3. Gene expression of Fe deficiency and SA response genes in *3xbhlh* and wild type plants in response to SA and Fe. A, *BHLH38, OBP3, PR1*; B, *FIT, FRO2, IRT1*; *3xbhlh* and wild type seedlings were grown for 6 d at + and −Fe and exposed for 6 h to 100 μM SA (+SA) or were mock-treated (−SA). Whole seedlings were harvested for analysis. n = 2; * indicates a significant change ($p<0.05$) of −Fe versus +Fe; + indicates a significant change ($p<0.05$) of *3xbhlh* versus WT; § indicates a significant change ($p<0.05$) of +SA versus -SA. Gene expression was studied using reverse transcription-qPCR.

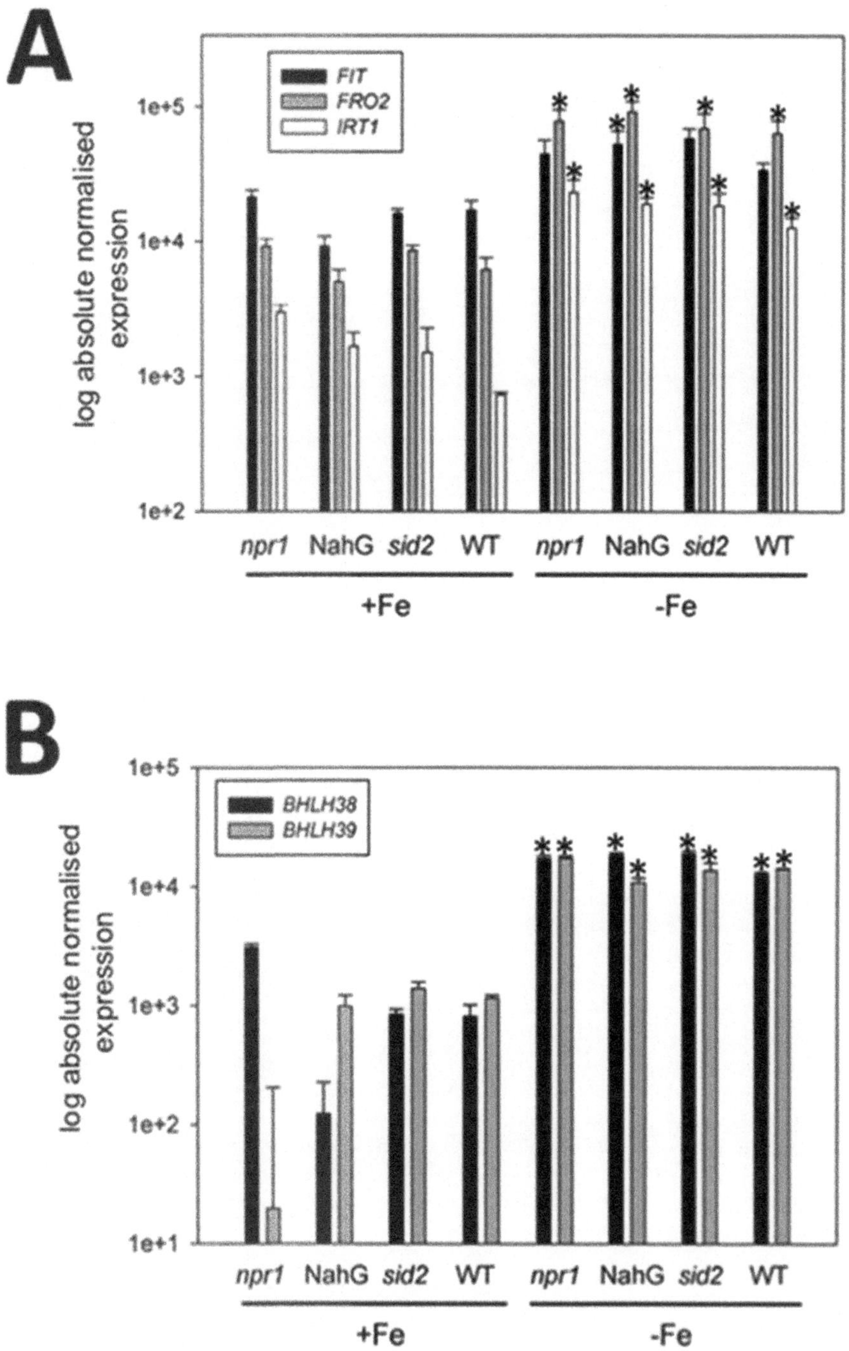

Figure 4. Gene expression of Fe deficiency response genes in various SA mutants and wild type plants. A, *FIT, FRO2, IRT1*; B, *BHLH38, BHLH39*; SA mutants and wild type seedlings were grown for 11 d at + and −Fe. Roots were harvested for analysis. n = 2; * indicates a significant change ($p<0.05$) of −Fe versus +Fe; + indicates a significant change ($p<0.05$) of SA mutant versus WT. Gene expression was studied using reverse transcription-qPCR.

(4×44 k) for *Arabidopsis thaliana*. Microarray chip hybridization and processing were done by ATLAS Biolabs GmbH, Berlin, Germany. The obtained data were further processed, checked for quality and filtered using the GeneSpring Software, Agilent Technologies, USA, according to the GeneSpring protocol. Full microarray data are available from the NCBI site of Gene Expression Omnibus under the series GSE41774. Interesting probes were identified based on fold change analysis with a fold change cut-off of 1.5 in four pairs of conditions which were *3xbhlh* versus wild type, *3xbhlh* + SA versus wild type + SA, wild type + SA versus wild type and *3xbhlh* + SA versus *3xbhlh*. Probes were retained if they passed the moderated t-test with $p<0.05$. The differentially regulated probes of the four pairs of conditions were then used to construct Venn diagrams to identify groups with unique and commonly regulated probes. Probe names of these groups were converted into Arabidopsis gene ID numbers. The groups of differentially expressed genes were then further analyzed using Venn diagrams, the ATTED co-expression tool [40], the

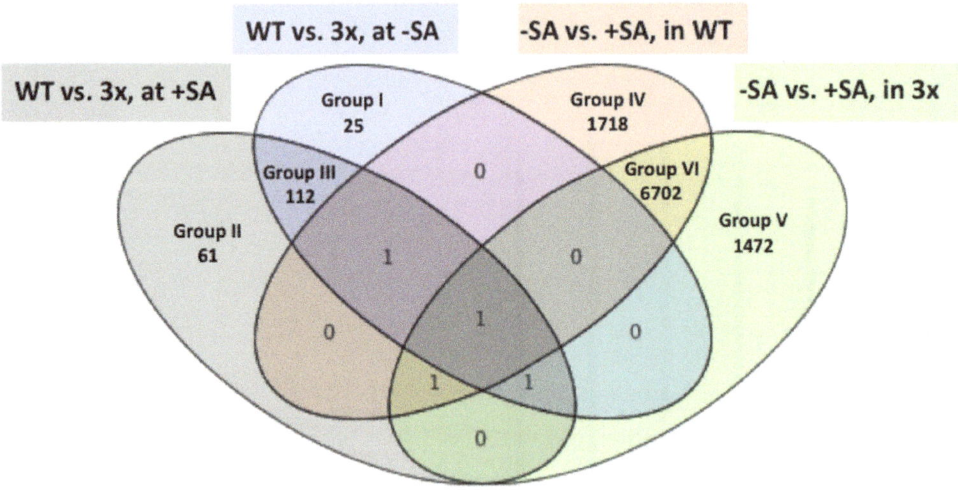

Figure 5. Venn diagram showing overlap of differentially regulated genes identified in microarray analysis. Four lists of genes that were differentially expressed at least 1.5-fold between the indicated conditions were used to construct the Venn diagram. The genes of groups I–V are listed in Tables S3, S4. Groups I to III contain genes differentially expressed between *3xbhlh* and wild type. Groups IV and V contain genes that show differential regulation between + and -SA treatment but not between wild type and mutant.

GOrilla GO annotation tool [41] and the Genevestigator tool [42].

Results

The *3xbhlh* Mutant was Sensitive to Fe Deficiency but not Affected in Fe Acquisition and Fe Transport to Shoots

To analyze the functions of *BHLH* subgroup Ib(2) genes, we generated a multiple loss of function mutant. The triple homozygous *bhlh39-1 bhlh100-1 bhlh101-1* knockout mutant, hereafter named *3xbhlh*, was fully fertile and did not express any full-length *BHLH39*, *BHLH100* and *BHLH101* transcripts while it expressed *BHLH38* at a higher level at Fe deficiency (hereafter termed −Fe) in roots and leaves. *BHLH38* was also found induced in the *3xbhlh* mutant roots at sufficient Fe (hereafter termed +Fe) compared to wild-type roots (Fig. S1A, B). In the same experiment, all four *BHLH* genes were highly expressed at –Fe in wild type plants, while they were not expressed or expressed at low level at +Fe (Fig. S1A, B), as expected [6]. The increased *BHLH38* expression in the *3xbhlh* mutant especially at –Fe might be due to a feedback control conferred by the triple loss of function phenotype.

To determine whether the triple *3xbhlh* mutant had any Fe deficiency phenotype at + or –Fe, we grew *3xbhlh* and wild type plants at +Fe and –Fe. Morphological alterations in root and shoot growth were not apparent at +Fe. However, at –Fe, the *3xbhlh* mutant plants had a stronger leaf chlorosis than wild type, while root growth was normal (Fig. 1A, B). This observation suggested that *3xbhlh* mutants might be perhaps Fe deficient. This assumption was tested and could be rejected after the determination of shoot Fe contents. Neither under + nor –Fe, we could detect any differences in Fe content in the mutant versus the wild type (Fig. 1C), suggesting that the mutant was not Fe deficient. After retransfer of *3xbhlh* mutants from –Fe to +Fe the leaf chlorosis phenotype disappeared within 1–2 days (data not shown). This observation confirmed that indeed the triple *3xbhlh* mutant was able to acquire Fe. We verified this point by analyzing gene expression of Fe acquisition genes. We observed that *IRT1*, *FRO2* and *FIT* were significantly up-regulated at –Fe in wild type and *3xbhlh* plants, and that no significant difference in the expression levels between wild type and mutant was detected (Fig. 2A). A reduced expression of these Fe acquisition genes is typical for mutants affected in the regulation of Fe deficiency responses, such as the chlorotic *fit* mutant [22]. Fe reductase activity was also detected at comparable levels in mutant and wild type (Fig. 2B). An increase of Fe reductase activity was noted at –Fe but due to high standard deviations it was not found significant, but clearly was not lower than in the wild type (Fig. 2B; [22]).

In addition, we tested whether two of the PYE-regulated Fe homeostasis genes of the *PYE/BHLH39/BHLH101* co-expression network that function in internal Fe mobilization were affected in the mutant. No differences in gene expression were noted for *NRAMP4* and *FRO3* in roots and leaves (Fig. 2C, D).

Taken together, *3xbhlh* mutant plants were fully capable of regulating internal and external Fe mobilization, Fe acquisition and Fe transport genes despite of the lack of the three transcription factors. The *3xbhlh* mutant was also able to mobilize Fe from roots into the shoots. Thus, the strong leaf chlorosis of the triple mutant at –Fe cannot be the consequence of a defect in Fe acquisition and mobilization responses.

SA and SA Signaling do not Affect Fe Deficiency Responses

Since the *BHLH39*, *BHLH100* and *BHLH101* genes were dispensable for Fe uptake, but yet the plants showed a chlorosis phenotype at –Fe, we reasoned that the chlorosis phenotype could be the result of an altered adaptation to Fe deficiency stress. Since previous reports established a connection between the *BHLH* subgroup Ib(2) genes and SA signaling [30] we hypothesized that perhaps SA responses interfered with Fe deficiency regulation via the bHLH subgroup Ib(2) proteins in the process of adaptation to –Fe. To test this hypothesis, we analyzed available gene expression data of *OBP3* (At3g55370), the regulator of *BHLH38* and *BHLH39* [30]. *OBP3* is not in a co-expression network with any known Fe-regulated metal homeostasis genes. However, its expression was reported to occur in the root stele where the subgroup Ib(2) gene promoters are also active [6,43]. SA plays a role throughout plant development and hence this could require an adaptation to Fe homeostasis [44]. To test a possible interference of SA and Fe signaling, we first tested using the seedling growth assay whether

A

WT - Fe vs + Fe	*3xbhlh* vs WT at - Fe	AGI number	encoding
	only at - SA		
up	up	AT3G01600	ANAC044
	at + SA and - SA		
up	down	AT1G53310	PPC1
up	down	AT3G07720	kelch-repeat
up	down	AT3G12900	oxidoreductase
up	down	AT4G31940	CYP82C4
up	up	AT1G01060	LHY
up	up	AT1G10370	ERD9
up	up	AT1G32900	starch synthase
up	up	AT2G15020	unknown
up	up	AT2G46830	CCA1
up	up	AT4G00050	UNE10
up	up	AT4G31870	ATGPX7
up	up	AT5G13170	SAG29
down	down	AT1G07050	CONSTANS-like
down	down	AT1G29395	COR414-TM1
down	down	AT1G31330	PSAF
down	down	AT1G34440	unknown
down	down	AT2G26500	petM
down	down	AT2G39920	acid phosphatase
down	down	AT3G47860	CHL
down	down	AT3G61870	unknown
down	down	AT4G13250	short-chain dehydrogenase
down	down	AT5G61410	RPE
	only at + SA		
up	down	AT3G58810	MTPA2
down	down	AT2G21130	CYP2
down	down	AT1G60950	FED A
down	down	AT5G23240	DNAJ heat shock
down	down	AT2G21650	MEE3
down	down	AT1G56300	DNAJ heat shock

B

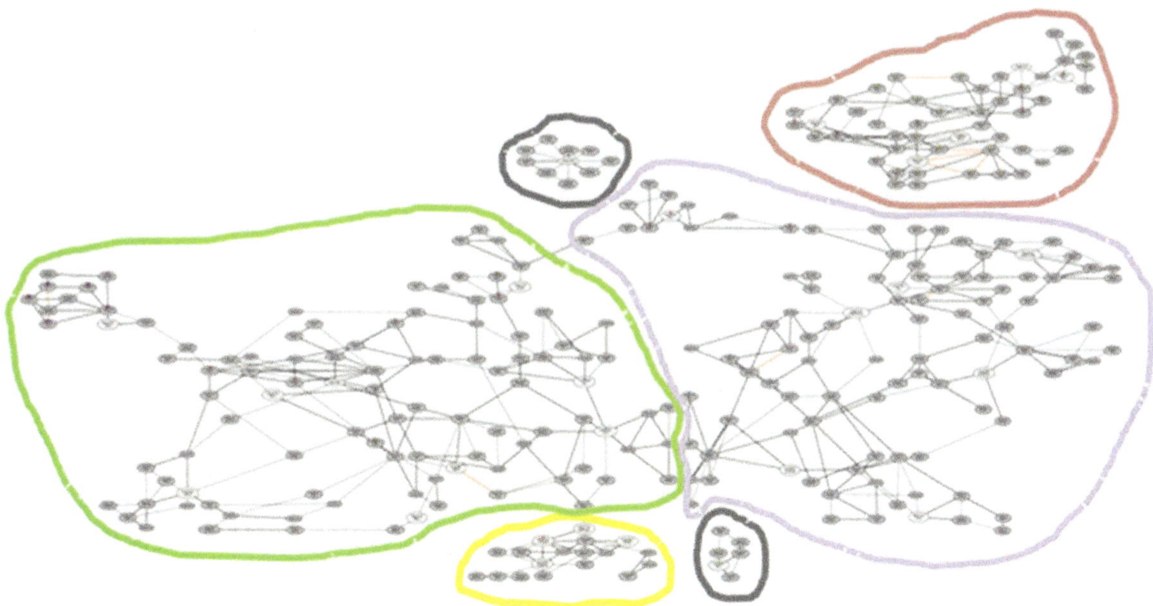

Figure 6. Regulation of the subset of 29 Fe-regulated genes out of groups I, II and III identified in microarray analysis. The list of Fe-regulated genes in wild type seedlings that we had published earlier [12] was used to compare with the list obtained in this work for the groups I–III.

29 genes of the groups I–III were found Fe-regulated in [12]. A, Regulation patterns, annotation and co-expression of the subset of 29 genes; the regulation at +Fe versus –Fe in the wild type is represented in the left-most column (in dark green up = up-regulated, in red down = down-regulated); the regulation in the *3xbhlh* mutant versus WT is shown in the middle column (in light green up = up-regulated and in yellow or violet down = down-regulated; note that the yellow color indicates that these genes do not follow in the *3xbhlh* mutant the regulation expected from –Fe versus +Fe in the left column and hence could be direct targets of bHLH39, bHLH100 and bHLH101). The Arabidopsis gene identification (AGI) numbers and annotations are shown on the right side, whereby the color code indicates the belonging to different co-expression networks as determined using the ATTED tool (ref), represented in B; B, Co-expression network analysis of the 29 genes; the ATTED tool was utilized for construction; the different networks are highlighted in color and the AGI numbers belonging to those networks are highlighted by the same color in A. The grey color indicates genes that are part of isolated co-expression networks. A high-resolution image of the co-expression networks is shown in Fig. S3.

the SA response gene *PATHOGENESIS RELATED1* (*PR1*) as a marker for SA responses [35], *OBP3* and *BHLH38* were regulated by SA and Fe deficiency treatments in wild type and *3xbhlh* mutant plants. As expected, *PR1* was induced by 100 μM SA in the wild type, while *BHLH38* was induced by –Fe (Fig. 3A). These two marker genes were not per se induced by the respective other treatment, and in two out of three experiments, the expression levels were not affected in the *3xbhlh* mutant (Fig. 3A). *OBP3* was hardly induced by SA treatment and did not show any regulation by Fe or in response to the *3xbhlh* mutant. We did also not detect any differences in gene expression levels of *IRT1*, *FRO2* and *FIT* at + versus –SA treatment (Fig. 3B). Therefore, we conclude that a clear SA response did not take place upon –Fe and that the *3xbhlh* mutant did not show an altered SA response upon SA application.

Since it is possible, that SA might have a more subtle effect in the regulation of Fe deficiency responses, we also tested Fe deficiency gene regulation in various SA mutants grown under + and −Fe supply. The *non-repressor of pr1* (*npr1*) mutant is defective in SA signaling [35]. *sid2* mutant plants are defective in SA production due to lack of isochorismate synthesis, and *NahG* plants overexpress a bacterial SA hydroxylase so that SA is rapidly transformed into catechol and consequently does not accumulate [36]. We found that in these mutants Fe acquisition genes *IRT1*, *FRO2* and *FIT* were up-regulated by –Fe as in the wild type (Fig. 4A). *IRT1* was slightly up-regulated at +Fe in *npr1* compared to the wild type in one experiment. *BHLH38* and *BHLH39* expression was not affected in the mutants (Fig. 4B).

Hence, we exclude an apparent effect of SA treatment or SA signaling on Fe deficiency regulation. The up-regulation of *BHLH* subgroup Ib(2) genes under –Fe was not likely the consequence of a SA signal.

Wild Type and *3xbhlh* Mutants Differ in Gene Expression Patterns at –Fe and in the Presence of SA

To get further hints on the Fe deficiency phenotype we performed a transcriptome comparison between *3xbhlh* and wild type seedlings (Fig. S2). This analysis was conducted under –Fe conditions since we expected most of the differential gene expression to occur at –Fe as deduced from the *3xbhlh* leaf chlorosis phenotype at –Fe. SA was included as a treatment to search for changes in gene expression in response to SA. 6-day old seedlings were grown on –Fe, transferred for 6 h to + or − 100 μM SA containing –Fe medium and harvested. Microarray analysis was performed using the Agilent V4 gene chip (26.283 Arabidopsis genes). In parallel, we used the same RNA samples to perform real time quantitative reverse transcription-PCR to assess the technical quality of the method and the biological quality of the samples in this experiment (Fig. S2).

At first, we identified from the microarray data those genes that showed differential regulation at least 1.5-fold between wild type and the *3xbhlh* mutant in the absence and presence of SA in a statistically significant manner. The differentially regulated genes were grouped according to expression patterns using Venn diagrams (Fig. 5). 198 genes were identified as being regulated between mutant and wild type (Table S2; Fig. 5). 25 of these genes were only found deregulated in the mutant in the absence of SA (group I) and 61 genes only in the presence of SA (group II). 112 genes were regulated between mutant and wild type in the presence and absence of SA (group III). An important control for the quality of our microarray hybridization experiment was represented by the *BHLH39*, *BHLH100* and *BHLH101* genes which we found down-regulated in the *3xbhlh* mutant compared to the wild type in the group III, as was expected (Table S2). On the other hand, 9892 genes were differentially regulated between + and − SA in the wild type or in the *3xbhlh* mutant (Fig. 5). Among these latter genes 1718 were only differentially expressed in response to SA in the wild type (group IV), while 1472 other genes were specifically affected by SA in the mutant (group V) (Table S3; Fig. 5). 6702 genes were regulated by SA in wild type and in the *3xbhlh* mutant (group VI) and were not further investigated as they reflected purely SA-dependent genes. (Fig. 5). The high numbers of SA-regulated genes might indicate that the SA treatment affected the transcriptomes in a strong manner than did the *3xbhlh* mutations. However, we found that genes of groups IV and V were only mis-regulated by a maximum level of 5-fold (Table S3). On the other hand, among the small number of genes mis-regulated between mutant and wild type (groups I–III) some genes reached differential expression up to 60-fold (Table S2).

Analysis of Functional Categories Differentially Regulated between *3xbhlh* and Wild Type Plants (Groups I to III)

Next, we assessed whether any specific functional pathways were affected in the *3xbhlh* mutant. At first, we analyzed the functions of the genes of groups I, II and III by analyzing whether specific gene ontology categories were hit among them using the GOrilla tool [41]. Among the DOWN-regulated genes of group I we found weak enrichment of categories related to lactate metabolism and cell wall, and among the UP-regulated genes of group I of categories RNA metabolism and transcription (Table S4-1, S4-2). In group II we found an enrichment for the categories flavonoid biosynthesis, UV responses, inositol metabolism and transpiration among the UP-regulated genes (Table S4-1, S4-2). In group III the categories metal response and copper binding were among the DOWN-regulated genes and again inositol metabolism among the UP-regulated genes (Table S4-1, 4-2). This analysis indicates that loss of the BHLH subgroup Ib(2) functions in the *3xbhlh* mutant at –Fe resulted in altered stress regulation and adaptation to stress.

Then, we checked whether the three groups I–III contained known Fe-regulated genes. In a previous work, we have grown six day-old Arabidopsis seedlings in + and −Fe conditions in the same system as utilized here. From these previous experiments we have obtained a list of iron-regulated genes in the seedlings [12,15,17]. The list of Fe-regulated genes in wild type seedlings published in [12] was used to compare with the list of genes in groups I–III. To our surprise we could only find 29 Fe-regulated genes among the 197 genes of the groups I–III, which corresponded to only 15% of these genes (Fig. 6A). Interestingly, these 15% of the *3xbhlh*-

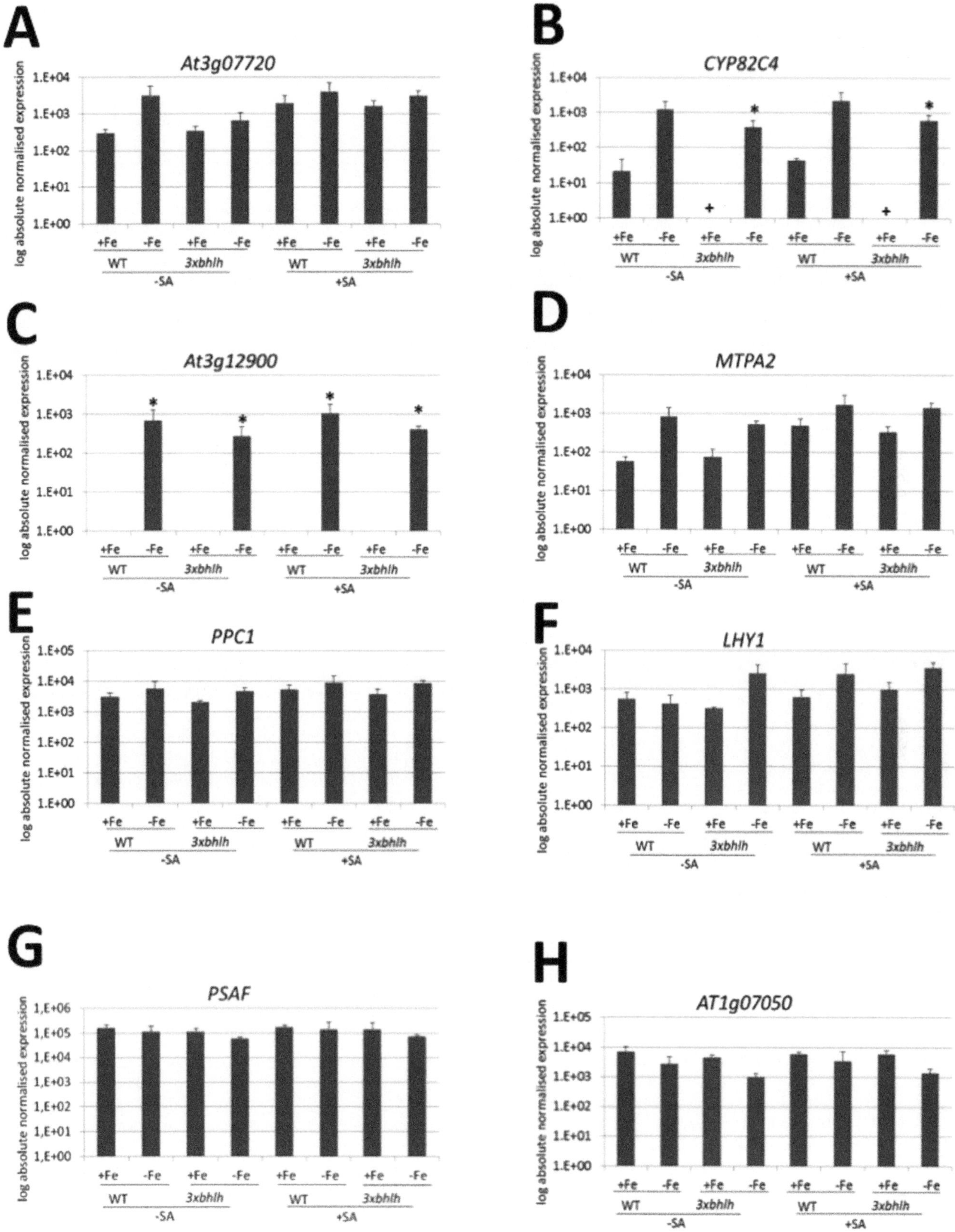

Figure 7. Gene expression of Fe and *3xbhlh*-regulated genes (groups I–III), identified from microarray analysis. A, At3g07720; B, *CYP82C4*; C, At3g12900; D, *MTPA2*; E, *PPC1*; F, *LHY1*; G, At1g07050; H, *PSAF*; The genes in A–E were identified as potential downstream targets of bHLH subgroup Ib(2) factors, while the genes in F–H indicated a more intense response to –Fe in the mutant (compare to Fig. 6). *3xbhlh* and wild type seedlings were grown for 6 d at + and −Fe and exposed for 6 h to 100 μM SA (+SA) or were mock-treated (−SA). Whole seedlings were harvested for analysis. n = 3; the –Fe cDNA samples were derived from the RNAs used in the microarray (Fig. S2); * indicates a significant change ($p<0.05$) of −Fe

versus +Fe; + indicates a significant change ($p<0.05$) of *3xbhlh* versus WT; § indicates a significant change ($p<0.05$) of +SA versus –SA. Gene expression was studied using reverse transcription-qPCR.

regulated genes could be further subdivided into 9 genes that were up-regulated by –Fe in the wild type and up-regulated in the mutant versus the wild type at –Fe as well as 15 genes that were down-regulated by –Fe in the wild type and down-regulated in the mutant versus the wild type at –Fe. Hence, the expression patterns of these 24 genes reflected the situation that the *3xbhlh* mutant was more sensitive to Fe deficiency than the wild type and that the Fe deficiency leaf chlorosis response was enhanced. Very interestingly, five genes showed an opposite expression pattern of being highly expressed at –Fe in the wild type, but expressed at low level in the *3xbhlh* mutant versus the wild type. These five genes were At1g53310 encoding PPC1, At3g07720, encoding a putative Kelch-repeat protein, At3g12900, an oxidoreductase gene, At4g31940 encoding CYP82C4 and At3g58810 encoding the metal transporter MTPA2. Therefore, it can be assumed that these five genes could represent specific target genes of the transcription factors bHLH39, bHLH100 and bHLH101. We also noted that the genes encoding the Fe acquisition machinery in Arabidopsis like *IRT1* and *FRO2* were not found among the differentially expressed genes which confirms above expression studies. We used the 29 genes to build co-expression networks using the ATTED tool [40], and in total we could identify four co-expression networks (Fig. 6B, Fig. S3). One network contained four out of the five putative bHLH targets. As mentioned above, this co-expression network was previously identified as the FIT target network [17]. Another network contained six genes up-regulated at –Fe and in the chlorotic triple mutant and one gene down-regulated in these respective conditions. This network was enriched with gene functions in flavonoid synthesis, secondary metabolism and circadian rhythm. A third network contained seven genes being down-regulated by –Fe and in the triple mutant, and this network was enriched for circadian rhythm functions. The fourth co-expression network comprised another five genes that were down-regulated at –Fe and in the *3xbhlh* mutant, and enrichment was found for photosynthetic functions and secondary metabolism. Similar functional categories were also evident for the 29 genes when using GOrilla as a GO annotation tool, namely metal response, inositol metabolism, protein folding, photosystem II and other chloroplast functions and circadian clock (Table S4-3, S4-4). In summary, co-expression analysis, functional annotation and enrichment analysis indicated that the expression of the 24 Fe-regulated genes was different in *3xbhlh* as a consequence of the increased leaf chlorosis of the triple mutant at –Fe, while the expression of five co-expressed genes indicates that they might be targets of the transcription factors in roots.

On the other hand, 85% of the genes of group I–III were not regulated by Fe deficiency. It was then interesting to determine whether these genes represented specific pathways. The functional categories were again related to inositol metabolism, circadian rhythm and UV response (Table S4-3, S4-4).

Hence, the Fe-regulated and non-Fe-regulated genes of groups I to III play functions in regulating adaptive stress processes suggesting that these functions are central for the bHLH proteins.

Validation of Differential Gene Expression in Groups I to III by Reverse Transcription-qPCR

To verify the regulatory expression patterns identified in the microarray experiments, we verified some of the gene expression results by reverse transcription-qPCR studies, especially by studying the Fe-regulated genes. Reverse transcription-qPCR was performed on the same biological samples as used for the microarray (Fig. S2). We also used the samples derived from plants grown at +Fe that we had raised in parallel. Three biological replicates have been analyzed. Due to the low number of three samples the differences were not found to be significant with $p< 0.05$ in all expected cases, which we designated then as "tendency". We found a tendency for up-regulation of *IRT1*, *FRO2* and *BHLH038* at –Fe versus +Fe irrespective of genotype and SA treatment which was significant for *IRT1* at −Fe versus +Fe in the *3xbhlh* mutant (Fig. S4A, B, C). *PR1* expression was significantly increased in all +SA versus –SA samples, as expected (Fig. S4D). Hence, these control gene expression results confirm that the plants had reacted as expected to Fe and salicylic acid supply in the experiment. Then, we studied gene expression of the Fe-regulated targets of the bHLH factors from groups I–III, namely of the four coexpressed genes At3g07720, *CYP82C4*, At3g12900 and *MTPA2* as well as of *PPC1*. All five genes showed a tendency to be up-regulated by –Fe in the wild type and in the *3xbhlh* mutant compared to +Fe, which was significant with $p< 0.05$ for *CYP82C4* in *3xbhlh* and for At3g12900 (Fig. 7A–E; compare to Fig. 6, yellow co-expression network and *PPC1*). The expression of these five genes had a tendency to be lower in the mutant than in the wild type at –Fe. In the presence of SA the five genes were similarly regulated than in the absence of SA, whereby the basal expression levels at +Fe in the wild type were found higher in tendency at +SA than at −SA for At3g07720 and *MTPA2*.

Next, we verified gene expression of the Fe-regulated group III genes, namely *LHY1*, *PSAF* and At1g07050 (Fig. 7F–H; compare to Fig. 6, green, violet and pink coexpression networks, respectively). We found that *LHY1* followed a tendency to be more expressed at –Fe versus +Fe in the mutant and in the presence of SA. At1g07050 and *PSAF* followed a tendency to be expressed at lower level at –Fe versus +Fe, especially in the *3xbhlh* mutant.

Taken together, the reverse transcription-qPCR data confirmed in their tendency the gene regulation changes detected in the comparative transcriptome analysis. This result underlined the technical and biological reproducibility, however the number of only three biological replicates did not allow obtention of $p<0.05$ statistical values in each comparison.

Analysis of Functional Categories Differentially Regulated between + and −SA (Groups IV and V)

Different genes were regulated by SA in the wild type (group IV) and *3xbhlh* plants (group V). We used again the GOrilla tool [41] to analyze whether specific categories were hit in the two cases. In group IV we identified the categories RNA and post-transcriptional genes silencing, organelle organization, GTP activity and chloroplast functions among the DOWN-regulated genes in the wild type, while the categories lipid metabolism, cellular starvation response and transition metal transport were hit among the UP-regulated genes (Table S4-1, 4-2). In group V the categories DNA replication, transmembrane receptor signaling, cell division, histone modification, protein binding and chloroplast thylakoid were hit among the DOWN-regulated genes and defense and heat response, signaling, kinase activity and ADP binding were identified as pathways among the UP-regulated genes (Table S4-1, 4-2).

Hence from the high number of regulated genes and the categories we deduce that SA affects stress responses and cell division in a different manner in the wild type and the *3xbhlh* mutant upon SA treatment. Thus, the *3xbhlh* mutant is in a different manner sensitive to SA than the wild type.

Discussion

In this report we show that *BHLH* subgroup Ib(2) genes *BHLH39*, *BHLH100* and *BHLH101* acted in the adaptation to the stress caused by the Fe deficiency but not for Fe acquisition itself. Although *BHLH38* and *BHLH39* may act in the SA pathway we did not find any evidence that SA responses interfered with Fe deficiency regulation via the *BHLH* genes.

Contradictory reports in the literature rendered it difficult to establish a clear function for *BHLH* subgroup Ib(2) genes in the regulation of Fe deficiency responses in Arabidopsis. On one side, it was shown that a triple mutant *bhlh39 bhlh100 bhlh101* was affected in the ability to up-regulate Fe reductase activity upon –Fe [28], while a double mutant *bhlh100 bhlh101* was not [7]. However, in both these studies the mutants were described to display a leaf chlorosis at –Fe but not at +Fe. Here we demonstrate that the *3xbhlh* triple mutant *bhlh39 bhlh100 bhlh101* developed a leaf chlorosis only at –Fe but not at +Fe. We found and confirmed that this phenotype was clearly not associated with a reduced uptake of Fe.

When we analyzed the triple *3xbhlh* mutant we observed that this mutant was able to mobilize and acquire Fe, in contrast to the report mentioned above [28]. The first evidence came from the fact that the leaf chlorosis was restrained to –Fe, while no such phenotype was observed at +Fe. The *3xbhlh* mutants had similar Fe levels as the wild type, and hence, these plants were able to utilize Fe at +Fe like the wild type. In addition, the *3xbhlh* mutants were able to induce *FIT*, *IRT1* and *FRO2* at –Fe versus +Fe. The three Fe uptake genes did also not occur among the groups I–III that comprised the genes differentially expressed between mutant and wild type. Fe reductase activity was clearly inducible in the triple mutant at least to the same extent as in the wild type. An alternative possibility to explain the increased leaf chlorosis of *3xbhlh* mutant compared to wild type plants at –Fe could be linked with a reduced ability of the mutant to utilise internal iron. However, we did not find evidence that typical genes for internal Fe utilization were changed in their expression, like *NRAMP4* [45], *FRO3* [46], *OPT3* [47] and *NAS4* [48,49]. Taken together, we can say that the leaf chlorosis of *3xbhlh* plants was not the consequence of impaired Fe uptake and utilisation. Since *BHLH38* was still expressed in the *3xbhlh* mutant, even to a higher level than in the wild type, we cannot conclude that none of the subgroup Ib(2) *BHLH* genes are required for Fe uptake or Fe mislocalization. Since *BHLH38* is hardly expressed at +Fe (when Fe is available for uptake), it is not likely required for Fe uptake, either. Due to the tandem location of *BHLH38* and *BHLH39* in the genome, a quadruple insertion mutant with a full knockout of all *BHLH* functions cannot be readily generated to confirm this. We predict that a quadruple mutant would have more severe leaf chlorosis symptoms than the wild type at –Fe.

The question remains what is the cause of the increased leaf chlorosis of *3xbhlh* mutants at –Fe. One clue to that question could come from the functions of the genes that we found differentially expressed in the mutant versus the wild type.

Five genes were regulated in an opposite manner in the *3xbhlh* mutant than in the wild type in response to iron. These genes might be targets for bHLH39, bHLH100 and bHLH101, namely *PPC1*, At3g07720, the oxidoreductase At3g12900, *CYP82C4* and *MTPA2*. The latter four are coexpressed with target genes of the transcription factor FIT, such as *IRT1*. However, some of the FIT targets of the co-expression network were found here not be mis-regulated in the *3xbhlh* mutant. This result can be explained. We suggest that the four bHLH transcription factors of the subgroup Ib(2) show functional divergence. bHLH38 in conjunction with FIT namely acts on the induction of the targets *IRT1* and *FRO2*, while bHLH39, bHLH100 and bHLH101 presumably together with FIT more specifically target the other genes in this co-expression network that we have found here.

Another set of Fe-regulated genes of groups I–III, which are differentially expressed in the mutant versus the wild type, indicated that the Fe deficiency responses were augmented in the mutant. For example, genes which are up-regulated at –Fe versus +Fe in the wild type showed an exaggerated up-regulation response in the comparison of mutant versus wild type at –Fe. Or, genes which are down-regulated at –Fe versus +Fe in the wild type showed a stronger down-regulation response in the mutant versus wild type at –Fe. From these expression patterns it is unlikely that these genes are regulated directly by the bHLH subgroup Ib proteins since otherwise we would have expected opposite trends of regulation between +/−Fe and mutant/wild type. The differential regulation of these genes is rather a pleiotropic effect due to the *3xbHLH* mutations. Since the most obvious phenotype was the increased leaf chlorosis, the differential regulation of these genes was likely an effect of the severe leaf chlorosis. Indeed, several of these genes have functions in the leaves related to the clock and in chloroplasts. Previous reports have established an effect of iron deficiency on the biological clock [50–52].

On the other hand, 170 genes were differentially expressed between mutant and wild type without that any differential expression of these genes had been noted in response to Fe supply in previous experiments [12]. Therefore, we deduce that the three *BHLH* genes regulate an adaptation response to the stress caused by the Fe deficiency. This would also explain why these *BHLH* genes are only activated at –Fe, but not at +Fe, and why they are induced in leaves and in roots. And in addition, it explains that in the absence of the genes in the *3xbhlh* mutant such a high number of genes are differentially expressed whereby in the wild type the expression appears unchanged. A further question is what could be the function of the 170 genes not regulated by Fe supply. One possibility could have been that these 170 genes are regulated by salicylic acid, a stress hormone. *BHLH38* and *BHLH39* have been brought into the context of SA regulation [30], and as a stress hormone SA signaling could be effective upon Fe deficiency stress. However, we exclude that the 170 genes are SA-regulated since none of them was in the intersections with the 50 times higher number of SA-regulated genes in the Venn diagrams, as revealed in our microarray experiments. The main functional categories that these 170 genes belong to are inositol metabolism, circadian rhythm again and UV responses. Hence, it can be concluded that the bhlh functions are important for adapting leaf responses to Fe deficiency stress. The absence of proper regulation would thus result in a more increased leaf chlorosis due to improper adaptation. Since the bHLH genes of the subgroup Ib(2) are expressed in leaves and there induced by Fe deficiency, it is plausible to predict that the leaf regulation is the main function of the bHLH genes which takes place independent of FIT.

In conclusion, it will be very interesting in the future to study the connection between leaf responses as an adaptation to Fe deficiency conferred by bHLH subgroup Ib(2) proteins.

Supporting Information

Figure S1 Gene expression of *BHLH* subgroup Ib genes in *3xbhlh* and wild type plants in response to Fe. A, in roots; B, in leaves; *3xbhlh* and wild type seedlings were grown for 14 d at +Fe and exposed for 3 d to + or −Fe. Roots and leaves were harvested for analysis. n = 4; * indicates a significant change ($p<0.05$) of −Fe versus +Fe; + indicates a significant change ($p<0.05$) of *3xbhlh* versus WT. Gene expression was studied by reverse transcription-qPCR.

Figure S2 Overview of one biological replicate set of microarray and reverse transcription-qPCR experiments; *3xbhlh* and wild type seedlings were grown for 6 d at + and −Fe and exposed for 6 h to 100 µM SA (+SA) or were mock-treated (−SA). RNA and cDNA was prepared from all samples for use in reverse transcription-qPCR analysis (see Fig. 7). Microarray analysis was only conducted with -Fe samples (see Fig. 5, 6). For reverse transcription-PCR and microarray analysis a total of three biological replicates was performed.

Figure S3 High-resolution image of the co-expression network analysis of the 29 Fe-regulated genes out of groups I, II and III. The ATTED tool was utilized for construction. Further analysis and additional information are provided in Fig. 6.

Figure S4 Gene expression of Fe deficiency and SA marker genes in the samples used for microarray analysis. A, *FIT*; B, *IRT1*; C, *FRO2*; D, *PR1*; *3xbhlh* and wild type seedlings were grown for 6 d at + and −Fe and exposed for 6 h to 100 µM SA (+SA) or were mock-treated (−SA). Whole seedlings were harvested for analysis. n = 3; the -Fe cDNA samples were derived from the RNAs used in the microarray (Fig. S2); * indicates a significant change ($p<0.05$) of −Fe versus +Fe; + indicates a significant change ($p<0.05$) of *3xbhlh* versus WT; § indicates a significant change ($p<0.05$) of +SA versus -SA. Gene expression was studied using reverse transcription-qPCR.

Table S1 Primer sequences.

Table S2 List of genes of the groups I, II and III with differential expression between *3xbhlh* and wild type at -Fe in the presence and absence of 100 µM SA.

Table S3 List of genes of the groups IV and V with differential expression of either *3xbhlh* or wild type at -Fe in the presence and absence of 100 µM SA.

Table S4 GO annotation of the differentially regulated genes of groups I to V.

Acknowledgments

This work has been funded by the Saarland University and the Heinrich Heine University Düsseldorf. Funding by the Deutsche Forschungsgemeinschaft grant No. DFG-Ba1610/5-1 to PB is kindly acknowledged. The authors thank Dr. Claudia Fink-Straube, Saarbrücken, for iron content determination. We thank Angelika Anna for excellent technical assistance regarding plant growth.

Author Contributions

Conceived and designed the experiments: PB. Performed the experiments: FM MN. Analyzed the data: FM MN PB. Wrote the paper: PB.

References

1. de Benoist B, McLean E, Egli I, Cogswell M (2008) Worldwide prevalence of anaemia 1993–2005. ISBN: 978 92 4 159665 7.
2. Uauy C, Distelfeld A, Fahima T, Blechl A, Dubcovsky J (2006) A *NAC* gene regulating senescence improves grain protein, zinc, and iron content in wheat. Science 314: 1298–1301.
3. Baxter IR, Vitek O, Lahner B, Muthukumar B, Borghi M, et al. (2008) The leaf ionome as a multivariable system to detect a plant's physiological status. Proc Natl Acad Sci U S A 105: 12081–12086.
4. Peiffer GA, King KE, Severin AJ, May GD, Cianzio SR, et al. (2012) Identification of candidate genes underlying an iron efficiency quantitative trait locus in soybean. Plant Physiol 158: 1745–1754.
5. Pires N, Dolan L (2010) Origin and diversification of basic-helix-loop-helix proteins in plants. Mol Biol Evol 27: 862–874.
6. Wang HY, Klatte M, Jakoby M, Baumlein H, Weisshaar B, et al. (2007) Iron deficiency-mediated stress regulation of four subgroup Ib *BHLH* genes in *Arabidopsis thaliana*. Planta 226: 897–908.
7. Sivitz AB, Hermand V, Curie C, Vert G (2012) Arabidopsis bHLH100 and bHLH101 control iron homeostasis via a FIT-independent pathway. PLoS One 7: e44843.
8. Wang N, Cui Y, Liu Y, Fan H, Du J, et al. (2012) Requirement and functional redundancy of Ib subgroup bHLH proteins for iron deficiency responses and uptake in *Arabidopsis thaliana*. Mol Plant 6: doi:10.1093/mp/sss1089.
9. Heim MA, Jakoby M, Werber M, Martin C, Weisshaar B, et al. (2003) The basic helix-loop-helix transcription factor family in plants: a genome-wide study of protein structure and functional diversity. Mol Biol Evol 20: 735–747.
10. Li X, Duan X, Jiang H, Sun Y, Tang Y, et al. (2006) Genome-wide analysis of basic/helix-loop-helix transcription factor family in rice and Arabidopsis. Plant Physiol 141: 1167–1184.
11. Toledo-Ortiz G, Huq E, Quail PH (2003) The Arabidopsis basic/helix-loop-helix transcription factor family. Plant Cell 15: 1749–1770.
12. Bauer P, Blondet E (2011) Transcriptome analysis of *ein3 eil1* mutants in response to iron deficiency. Plant Signal Behav 6.
13. Buckhout TJ, Yang TJ, Schmidt W (2009) Early iron-deficiency-induced transcriptional changes in Arabidopsis roots as revealed by microarray analyses. BMC Genomics 10: 147.
14. Dinneny JR, Long TA, Wang JY, Jung JW, Mace D, et al. (2008) Cell identity mediates the response of Arabidopsis roots to abiotic stress. Science 320: 942–945.
15. Schuler M, Keller A, Backes C, Phillipar K, Lenhof HP, et al. (2011) Transcriptome analysis by GeneTrail revealed regulation of functional categories in response to alterations of iron homeostasis in *Arabidopsis thaliana*. BMC Plant Biol 11: 87.
16. Yang TJ, Lin WD, Schmidt W (2010) Transcriptional profiling of the Arabidopsis iron deficiency response reveals conserved transition metal homeostasis networks. Plant Physiol 152: 2130–2141.
17. Ivanov R, Brumbarova T, Bauer P (2011) Fitting into the harsh reality: Regulation of iron deficiency responses in dicotyledonous plants. Mol Plant 5: 27–42.
18. Long TA, Tsukagoshi H, Busch W, Lahner B, Salt DE, et al. (2010) The bHLH transcription factor POPEYE regulates response to iron deficiency in Arabidopsis roots. Plant Cell 22: 2219–2236.
19. Yuan Y, Wu H, Wang N, Li J, Zhao W, et al. (2008) FIT interacts with AtbHLH38 and AtbHLH39 in regulating iron uptake gene expression for iron homeostasis in Arabidopsis. Cell Res 18: 385–397.
20. Bauer P, Ling HQ, Guerinot ML (2007) FIT, the FER-LIKE IRON DEFICIENCY INDUCED TRANSCRIPTION FACTOR in Arabidopsis. Plant Physiol Biochem 45: 260–261.
21. Colangelo EP, Guerinot ML (2004) The essential basic helix-loop-helix protein FIT1 is required for the iron deficiency response. Plant Cell 16: 3400–3412.
22. Jakoby M, Wang HY, Reidt W, Weisshaar B, Bauer P (2004) *FRU* (*BHLH029*) is required for induction of iron mobilization genes in *Arabidopsis thaliana*. FEBS Lett 577: 528–534.
23. Yuan YX, Zhang J, Wang DW, Ling HQ (2005) AtbHLH29 of Arabidopsis thaliana is a functional ortholog of tomato FER involved in controlling iron acquisition in strategy I plants. Cell Res 15: 613–621.
24. Robinson NJ, Procter CM, Connolly EL, Guerinot ML (1999) A ferric-chelate reductase for iron uptake from soils. Nature 397: 694–697.
25. Eide D, Broderius M, Fett J, Guerinot ML (1996) A novel iron-regulated metal transporter from plants identified by functional expression in yeast. Proc Natl Acad Sci USA 93: 5624–5628.

26. Meiser J, Lingam S, Bauer P (2011) Post-translational regulation of the Fe deficiency bHLH transcription factor FIT is affected by iron and nitric oxide. Plant Physiol 157: 2154–2166.
27. Sivitz A, Grinvalds C, Barberon M, Curie C, Vert G (2011) Proteasome-mediated turnover of the transcriptional activator FIT is required for plant iron-deficiency responses. Plant J doi:10.1111/j.1365-313X.2011.04565.x.
28. Wang N, Cui Y, Liu Y, Fan H, Du J, et al. (2013) Requirement and functional redundancy of Ib subgroup bHLH proteins for iron deficiency responses and uptake in Arabidopsis thaliana. Mol Plant 6: 503–513.
29. Vert G, Grotz N, Dedaldechamp F, Gaymard F, Guerinot ML, et al. (2002) IRT1, an Arabidopsis transporter essential for iron uptake from the soil and for plant growth. Plant Cell 14: 1223–1233.
30. Kang HG, Foley RC, Oñate-Sánchez L, Lin C, Singh KB (2003) Target genes for OBP3, a Dof transcription factor, include novel basic helix-loop-helix domain proteins inducible by salicylic acid. Plant J 35: 362–372.
31. Maurer F, Müller S, Bauer P (2011) Suppression of Fe deficiency gene expression by jasmonate. Plant Physiol Biochem 49: 530–536.
32. García MJ, Lucena C, Romera FJ, Alcántara E, Pérez-Vicente R (2010) Ethylene and nitric oxide involvement in the up-regulation of key genes related to iron acquisition and homeostasis in Arabidopsis. J Exp Bot 61: 3885–3899.
33. García MJ, Suárez V, Romera FJ, Alcántara E, Pérez-Vicente R (2011) A new model involving ethylene, nitric oxide and Fe to explain the regulation of Fe-acquisition genes in Strategy I plants. Plant Physiol Biochem 49: 537–544.
34. Lingam S, Mohrbacher J, Brumbarova T, Potuschak T, Fink-Straube C, et al. (2011) Interaction between the bHLH transcription factor FIT and ETHYLENE INSENSITIVE3/ETHYLENE INSENSITIVE3-LIKE1 reveals molecular linkage between the regulation of iron acquisition and ethylene signaling in *Arabidopsis*. Plant Cell 23: 1815–1929.
35. Cao H, Glazebrook J, Clarke JD, Volko S, Dong X (1997) The Arabidopsis *NPR1* gene that controls systemic acquired resistance encodes a novel protein containing ankyrin repeats. Cell Res 88: 57–63.
36. Ferrari S, Plotnikova JM, De Lorenzo G, Ausubel FM (2003) Arabidopsis local resistance to *Botrytis cinerea* involves salicylic acid and camalexin and requires *EDS4* and *PAD2*, but not *SID2*, *EDS5* or *PAD4*. Plant J 35: 193–205.
37. Schuler M, Rellán-Álvarez R, Fink-Straube C, Abadía J, Bauer P (2012) Nicotianamine functions in the Phloem-based transport of iron to sink organs, in pollen development and pollen tube growth in Arabidopsis. Plant Cell 24: 2380–23400.
38. Klatte M, Schuler M, Wirtz M, Fink-Straube C, Hell R, et al. (2009) The analysis of Arabidopsis nicotianamine synthase mutants reveals functions for nicotianamine in seed iron loading and iron deficiency responses. Plant Physiol 150: 257–271.
39. Klatte M, Bauer P (2009) Accurate real-time reverse transcription quantitative PCR. Meth Mol Biol 479: 61–77.
40. Obayashi T, Kinoshita K, Nakai K, Shibaoka M, Hayashi S, et al. (2007) ATTED-II: a database of co-expressed genes and cis elements for identifying co-regulated gene groups in Arabidopsis. Nucl Acids Res 35: D863–869.
41. Eden E, Navon R, Steinfeld I, Lipson D, Yakhini Z (2009) GOrilla: a tool for discovery and visualization of enriched GO terms in ranked gene lists. BMC Bioinformatics 10: doi:10.1186/1471-2105-1110-1148.
42. Zimmermann P, Hirsch-Hoffmann M, Hennig L, Gruissem W (2004) GENEVESTIGATOR. Arabidopsis microarray database and analysis toolbox. Plant Physiol 136: 2621–2632.
43. Brady SM, Orlando DA, Lee JY, Wang JY, Koch J, et al. (2007) A high-resolution root spatiotemporal map reveals dominant expression patterns. Science 318: 801–806.
44. Rivas-San Vicente M, Plasencia J (2011) Salicylic acid beyond defence: its role in plant growth and development. J Exp Bot 62: 3321–3338.
45. Lanquar V, Lelievre F, Bolte S, Hames C, Alcon C, et al. (2005) Mobilization of vacuolar iron by AtNRAMP3 and AtNRAMP4 is essential for seed germination on low iron. EMBO J 24: 4041–4051.
46. Mukherjee I, Campbell NH, Ash JS, Connolly EL (2006) Expression profiling of the Arabidopsis ferric chelate reductase (FRO) gene family reveals differential regulation by iron and copper. Planta 223: 1178–1190.
47. Stacey MG, Patel A, McClain WE, Mathieu M, Remley M, et al. (2008) The Arabidopsis AtOPT3 protein functions in metal homeostasis and movement of iron to developing seeds. Plant Physiol 146: 589–601.
48. Koen E, Besson-Bard A, Duc C, Astier J, Gravot A, et al. (2013) Arabidopsis thaliana nicotianamine synthase 4 is required for proper response to iron deficiency and to cadmium exposure. Plant Science 209: 1–11.
49. Palmer CM, Hindt MN, Schmidt H, Clemens S, Guerinot ML (2013) MYB10 and MYB72 Are Required for Growth under Iron-Limiting Conditions. Plos Genetics 9.
50. Chen YY, Wang Y, Shin LJ, Wu JF, Shanmugam V, et al. (2013) Iron is involved in the maintenance of circadian period length in Arabidopsis. Plant Physiol 161: 1409–1420.
51. Hong S, Kim SA, Guerinot ML, McClung CR (2013) Reciprocal interaction of the circadian clock with the iron homeostasis network in Arabidopsis. Plant Physiol 161: 893–903.
52. Salome PA, Oliva M, Weigel D, Kramer U (2013) Circadian clock adjustment to plant iron status depends on chloroplast and phytochrome function. EMBO J 32: 511–523.

Association of Serum 25-Hydroxyvitamin D with Lifestyle Factors and Metabolic and Cardiovascular Disease Markers: Population-Based Cross-Sectional Study (FIN-D2D)

Maija E. Miettinen[1]*, Leena Kinnunen[1], Jaana Leiviskä[2], Sirkka Keinänen-Kiukaanniemi[3,4], Eeva Korpi-Hyövälti[5], Leo Niskanen[6,7], Heikki Oksa[8], Timo Saaristo[9,10], Jaakko Tuomilehto[1,5,11,12], Mauno Vanhala[7,13], Matti Uusitupa[14,15], Markku Peltonen[16]

1 Diabetes Prevention Unit, National Institute for Health and Welfare, Helsinki, Finland, **2** Disease Risk Unit, National Institute for Health and Welfare, Helsinki, Finland, **3** Institute of Health Sciences, University of Oulu, Oulu, Finland, **4** Unit of Primary Health Care, Oulu University Hospital, Oulu, Finland, **5** Department of Internal Medicine, South Ostrobothnia Central Hospital, Seinäjoki, Finland, **6** Finnish Medicines Agency, Helsinki, Finland, **7** Faculty of Health Sciences, University of Eastern Finland, Kuopio, Finland, **8** Tampere University Hospital, Tampere, Finland, **9** Pirkanmaa Hospital District, Tampere, Finland, **10** Finnish Diabetes Association, Tampere, Finland, **11** Center for Vascular Prevention, Danube-University Krems, Krems, Austria, **12** King Abdulaziz University, Jeddah, Saudi Arabia, **13** Primary Health Care Unit, Central Finland Central Hospital, Jyväskylä, Finland, **14** Institute of Public Health and Clinical Nutrition, University of Eastern Finland, Kuopio, Finland, **15** Research Unit, Kuopio University Hospital, Kuopio, Finland, **16** Department of Chronic Disease Prevention, National Institute for Health and Welfare, Helsinki, Finland

Abstract

Objectives: Low serum 25-hydroxyvitamin D (25OHD) level has been associated with an increased risk of several chronic diseases. Our aim was to determine lifestyle and clinical factors that are associated with 25OHD level and to investigate connection of 25OHD level with metabolic and cardiovascular disease markers.

Design: In total, 2868 Finnish men and women aged 45–74 years participated in FIN-D2D population-based health survey in 2007. Participants that had a serum sample available (98.4%; n = 2822) were included in this study. 25OHD was measured with chemiluminescent microparticle immunoassay method.

Results: The mean 25OHD level was 58.2 nmol/l in men (n = 1348) and 57.1 nmol/l in women (n = 1474). Mean 25OHD level was lower in the younger age groups than in the older ones ($p<0.0001$ both in men and women). This study confirmed that low physical activity ($p<0.0001$ both in men and women), smoking ($p = 0.0002$ in men and $p = 0.03$ in women) and high BMI ($p<0.0001$ in women) are factors that independently associate with low 25OHD level. Of the metabolic and cardiovascular disease markers high triglyceride concentration ($p = 0.02$ in men and $p = 0.001$ in women) and high apolipoprotein B/ apolipoprotein A1 ratio ($p = 0.04$ in men and $p = 0.03$ in women) were independently associated with low 25OHD level.

Conclusions: Higher age did not predict lower 25OHD level in this study population of aged 45–74 years which may derive from a healthy life-style of "active pensioners". Low physical activity and smoking came up as independent lifestyle factors associated with low 25OHD level. Defining the molecular mechanisms behind the associations of 25OHD with low physical activity and smoking are important objective in future studies. The association of 25OHD with BMI, high triglyceride concentration and apolipoprotein B/apolipoprotein A1 ratio may be related to the role of vitamin D in inflammation, but more detailed studies are needed.

Editor: Sreeram V. Ramagopalan, University of Oxford, United Kingdom

Funding: The study was funded by Finnish Foundation for Cardiovascular Research (www.sydantutkimussaatio.fi). The funders had no role in study design, data collection and analysis, decision to publish, or preparation of the manuscript.

Competing Interests: The authors have declared that no competing interests exist.

* Email: maija.miettinen@thl.fi

Introduction

Low serum 25-hydroxyvitamin D [25OHD] level has been associated with several diseases including cancer, type 2 diabetes, osteoporosis, autoimmune diseases, cardiovascular diseases and schizophrenia [1].

Vitamin D is naturally synthesized from 7-dehydrocholesterol by the skin's exposure to ultraviolet B radiation. The best estimate of an individual's vitamin D status is the measurement of circulating vitamin D, 25OHD [1], which provides an indication of vitamin D stores obtained from both UV-light and dietary intake. Dietary sources of Vitamin D include fatty fish and fortified foods like milk and margarine. At the time of sample collection of the present study (year 2007) fish was the most important dietary source of vitamin D for both sexes among Finns aged 25–64 years [2]. Vitamin D is first hydroxylated in the liver to 25OHD and again in the kidney to form the biologically active 1,25-dihydroxyvitamin D. Low 25OHD level may be a result of inadequate sun exposure, deficient consumption of vitamin D-rich products or malabsorption of vitamin D [3].

25OHD concentration of 25 nmol/l has traditionally been considered as a boundary for vitamin D deficiency [4,5]. However, in recent years several experts have suggested a cut-off level of 50 nmol/l for vitamin D deficiency [1,6]. Concentration of 75 nmol/l or higher has been suggested as an optimal 25OHD level [6]. However, a reverse J-shaped association between 25OHD level and all-cause mortality has been suggested in the NHANES study [7]. The nadir of risk was shown to be 81 nmol/l [7]. In traditionally living indigenous populations in East Africa the mean 25OHD level in adult population has been shown to be 115 nmol/l [8]. There is no consensus about the toxic 25OHD concentration, but 375–500 nmol/l and higher than 600 nmol/l have been suggested [9,10].

A combination of increased triglyceride-rich very low-density lipoproteins and small, dense low-density lipoproteins (LDL) and decreased high-density lipoproteins (HDL) is a common feature in metabolic syndrome (MetS) [11,12]. Apolipoprotein A1 (apoA1) is the main protein in HDL particles and apolipoprotein B (apoB) in all the other lipoproteins [13,14]. ApoB/apoA1 ratio combines the atherogenic and antiatherogenic lipoproteins and an elevated apoB/apoA1 ratio has been connected to MetS [15]. ApoB/apoA1 ratio has also been shown to be a good predictor of cardiovascular disease and atherosclerosis [15–19], and it has been suggested that ApoB/apoA1 ratio should be used instead of cholesterol concentrations as a risk marker of myocardial infarction [17]. Several studies have found an association between low 25OHD level and MetS [20,21], but little is known of the link between 25OHD level and different components of the lipid disorders related to MetS, like elevated triglyceride and apoB concentrations and an increased apoB/apoA1 ratio.

Our aim was to determine the lifestyle and clinical factors that are associated with 25OHD level and to investigate connection of 25OHD level with metabolic and cardiovascular disease markers. We found several factors associated with 25OHD level that should be considered when investigating the role of vitamin D in different diseases.

Materials and Methods

Subjects

This study is a part of the FIN-D2D health survey 2007, which is a joint project within the Finnish National Diabetes Prevention program FIN-D2D [22,23]. Initially, a random sample of 4500 people aged 45–74 years, stratified according to gender, 10-year age groups (45–54, 55–64, and 65–74 years), and geographical areas (Hospital Districts of Pirkanmaa, Central Finland and South Ostrobothnia), was selected from the National Population Register in August 2007. Sample size of the population where this cohort was extracted in 2007 was 349326. The study participants were invited by mail to a health examination. The participants attended a health examination carried out by a trained nurse according to the multinational monitoring of trends and determinants in cardiovascular disease (MONICA) protocol. A total of 2868 persons (64%) participated in the health examination during October, November and December in 2007. Of these persons those that had a serum sample available were included in the present study (98.4%; n = 2822). All participants signed an informed consent form. Ethical committee of the Hospital District of Helsinki and the Uusimaa approved the study.

Waist circumference, triglycerides, HDL cholesterol, blood pressure and fasting plasma glucose were used to define the presence of metabolic syndrome according to the International Diabetes Federation 2009 criteria [24]. Information on glucose tolerance status during 2 hour oral glucose tolerance test together with reported drug-treated type 2 diabetes was used to indicate presence of normal glucose regulation (NGR), impaired glucose tolerance (IGT), impaired fasting glucose (IFG), screen-detected type 2 diabetes (SDM) or type 2 diabetes according to the WHO 1999 diagnostic criteria [25]. Participant's cardiovascular risk was estimated with the Framingham [26] risk score, and with the apoB/apoA1 ratio.

Methods

Height was measured to the nearest 0.1 cm. Weight was measured in light clothing. Body mass index (BMI) was calculated as weight (kg) divided by the square of height (m). Waist circumference was measured midway between the lower rib margin and the iliac crest. Serum triglycerides, HDL cholesterol, and plasma glucose were measured by enzymatic methods with Abbott Architect analyzer (Abbott Laboratories, Abbott Park, IL, USA). ApoA1 and apoB were measured with immunoturbidimetric methods and high sensitivity C-reactive protein (hs-CRP) was measured with ultrasensitive immunoturbidimetric method using Abbott Architect reagents. The inter-assay coefficients of variation (CV) for triglycerides, HDL cholesterol, and glucose were 1.2%, 2.5%, and 1.4%, respectively. CVs for apoA1, apoB, and hs-CRP were 1.3%, 2.5% and 2.9%, respectively.

Data of education and total household income were used as indicators of the socio-economic status. Educational level was divided into groups according to years of completed education: low (0–9 years), medium (10–12 years) and high education (13 years or more). Total household income per year was reported in three categories: low (<30 000 €/year), medium (30 001–60 000 €/year) and high (60 001–80 000 or more €/year).

Vitamin D analyses

The serum samples were collected during the end of year 2007 within three months (October–December). The samples were stored frozen in −20°C until analysis (4 years). 25OHD was determined by chemiluminescent microparticle immunoassay by Architect *i* system (Abbott Laboratories, Abbott Park, IL, USA). The interassay CVs of 25OHD were 6.7% and 3.8% at the levels of 34 nmol/l and 102 nmol/l, respectively. The bias compared to all-laboratory trimmed mean in the Vitamin D International External Quality Assessment Scheme (DEQAS) was −6.4%±7.1 (mean ± SD). 25OHD concentration lower than50 nmol/l was considered as vitamin D deficiency, between 50 nmol/l and 75 nmol/l as vitamin D sufficiency and higher than 75 nmol/l as an optimal 25OHD level.

Statistical analyses

Descriptive statistics (means, standard deviations and proportions) were used to describe the study population. Age- and gender-specific 25OHD levels were calculated among the participants by lifestyle factors and cardiovascular disease markers. In these analyses, continuous variables were categorized in order to evaluate linearity in associations. Univariate comparisons between groups were evaluated by the chi-square test or logistic regression models. Analysis of covariance (ANCOVA) and logistic regression models were further used to evaluate the associations between

25OHD concentrations and lifestyle factors and metabolic disease markers adjusting for possible confounding factors. The possible confounding factors were pre-determined and included age, gender, BMI, month of sample collection, physical activity and smoking. Assumptions of the ANCOVA models were evaluated by graphical methods. The goodness of fit in logistic regression models was assessed with the Hosmer-Lemeshow test. No interaction terms were included in the models. Statistical analyses were carried out using the Stata statistical package 10.1 (StataCorp. 2007. Stata Statistical Software: Release 10.1. College Station, TX; StataCorp LP).

Results

Characteristics of the study subjects are shown in table 1. Information on age, month of sample collection, use of vitamin D supplements, HDL concentration, triglyceride concentration, fasting glucose, hs-CRP and apoB/apoA1 ratio (men) was available from 100% of the participants. Information on physical activity, smoking, education, waist circumference, blood pressure, Framingham score, and apoB/apoA1 ratio (women) was available from >95% of the participants. Information on household income and on use of hormone replacement therapy was available from > 90% of the participants. The main reason for the missing information was that the participants did not answer all questions in the questionnaire included in the study.

25OHD level and its relation to lifestyle and related factors

The results of the univariate analysis of the 25OHD level in men and women are presented in Table 2. Higher 25OHD level was associated with higher age (men $p<0.0001$; women $p<0.0001$). Month of sample collection was associated with 25OHD, the mean level being approximately 8% higher in samples collected during October than during November and December (men $p<0.0001$; women $p=0.001$). Higher BMI was associated with lower 25OHD level (men $p=0.04$; women $p<0.0001$). Only 1.5% (n = 20) of the men and 3.1% (n = 46) of the women had BMI lower than 20 and thus a meaningful analysis of this group separately was not possible. Low physical activity was associated with lower 25OHD level (men $p<0.0001$; women $p<0.0001$). Participants that did not use vitamin containing supplements had lower 25OHD level than those using supplements (men $p<0.0001$; women $p<0.0001$). Smokers had lower 25OHD level than the non-smokers (men $p<0.0001$; women $p=0.002$). Use of hormone replacement therapy and absence of menstruation was associated with higher 25OHD level ($p=0.02$ and 0.002, respectively). No association was seen between educational level and total household income with 25OHD level.

Statistically significant association of 25OHD level with age (in men and women $p<0.0001$), month of sample collection (in men $p<0.000$; in women $p=0.002$), physical activity (in men and in women $p<0.0001$), use of vitamin D supplements (in men and in women $p<0.0001$) and smoking (in men $p=0.0002$; in women $p=0.03$) remained in the multivariate model when adjusted for age, gender, BMI, month of sample collection, physical activity and smoking (table 2). The association of 25OHD with BMI remained significant only in women ($p<0.0001$). Use of hormone replacement therapy and presence of menstruation were not associated with 25OHD level in the multivariate model.

The proportion of men and women with 25OHD deficiency (< 50 nmol/l), sufficiency (50–75 nmol/l) and with an optimal 25OHD level (>75 nmol/l) was calculated. Of men 30.6% had vitamin D deficiency, 54.0% a sufficient and 15.4% an optimal 25OHD level. Of women 36.0% had vitamin D deficiency, 49.5% a sufficient and 14.5% an optimal 25OHD level. Vitamin D deficiency was more common among women than men ($p=0.01$). Only 1% (n = 13) of the men and 0.7% (n = 10) of the women had severe vitamin D deficiency (25OHD <25 nmol/l). Prevalence of vitamin D deficiency (25OHD <50 nmol/l) in different age and BMI groups is shown in figure 1 and 2.

Table 1. Characteristics of the study subjects of the FIN-D2D study (n = 2822).

	Men		Women		p
	Mean	SD	Mean	SD	
n (%)	1348 (47.8)		1474 (52.2)		
Age (years)	60.2	8.5	59.4	8.3	0.005
BMI (kg/m^2)	27.5	4.2	27.5	5.3	0.61
Use of vitamin D supplements (%)	18.0		37.0		<0.001
Smokers (%)	19.6		11.7		<0.001
Use of hormone replacement therapy (%)			24.8		
Menstruation			21.4		
Metabolic syndrome (%)	59.8		54.0		0.002
Waist circumference (cm)	100.0	11.8	90.4	13.3	<0.001
HDL cholesterol concentration (mmol/l)	1.32	0.32	1.55	0.34	<0.001
Triglyceride concentration (mmol/l)	1.49	0.99	1.28	0.61	<0.001
Diastolic blood pressure	83.0	9.9	80.4	9.0	<0.001
Systolic blood pressure	138.4	18.7	135.4	18.8	<0.001
Fasting glucose (mmol/l)	6.4	1.3	6.0	1.1	<0.001
Type 2 diabetes (%)	20.8		13.3		<0.001
hs-CRP	2.6	8.0	2.9	7.6	0.32

Table 2. 25OHD concentrations in the Finnish population aged 45–74 years.

	Men			Women		
Variable	**Mean 25OHD (nmol/l) ± SD (n)**	**p-value**	**p-value (adjusted*)**	**Mean 25OHD (nmol/l) ± SD (n)**	**p-value**	**p-value (adjusted*)**
All	58.2±16.9 (1348)			57.1±17.3 (1474)		
Age						
45–49 years	54.0±15.3 (193)	<0.0001	<0.0001	52.3±16.4 (221)	<0.0001	<0.0001
50–54 years	55.3±15.2 (198)			55.1±15.5 (261)		
55–59 years	58.5±17.8 (234)			58.2±18.7 (257)		
60–64 years	58.0±18.6 (215)			58.9±18.6 (247)		
65–69 years	61.7±16.9 (275)			58.3±16.4 (282)		
70–74 years	60.0±15.9 (233)			59.4±17.4 (206)		
Month of sample collection						
October	61.0±16.9 (559)	<0.0001	<0.0001	58.9±17.3 (687)	0.001	0.002
November	56.4±16.1 (532)			55.5±17.2 (543)		
December	56.0±17.7 (257)			55.6±17.2 (244)		
BMI						
<25 kg/m^2	59.7±18.5 (389)	0.04	0.12	60.0±17.0 (518)	<0.0001	<0.0001
25–29.9	58.0±15.9 (664)			58.4±18.7 (553)		
30–34.9	57.6±17.4 (224)			52.8±14.8 (278)		
>35	53.9±14.4 (70)			48.7±13.1 (124)		
Physical activity						
Low	53.9±17.8 (267)	<0.0001	<0.0001	51.8±17.5 (270)	<0.0001	<0.0001
Moderate	58.3±15.9 (760)			57.5±16.9 (872)		
High	62.1±17.4 (295)			60.6±17.6 (307)		
Use of vitamin D containing supplements						
No	57.0±16.8 (1105)	<0.0001	<0.0001	53.9±16.7 (929)	<0.0001	<0.0001
Yes	63.9±16.1 (243)			62.5±17.1 (545)		
Smoking						
No	59.6±16.3 (1069)	<0.0001	0.0002	57.6±17.3 (1308)	0.002	0.03
Yes	53.2±18.3 (261)			52.9±17.8 (153)		
Use of hormone replacement therapy						
No	-	-	-	56.4±17.4 (1016)	0.02	0.48
Yes	-	-	-	58.9±17.2 (335)		
Menstruation						
No	-	-	-	58.0±17.7 (1118)	0.002	0.27
Yes	-	-	-	54.4±16.0 (304)		
Educational level						
0–9 years	58.2±16.8 (557)	0.32	0.93	57.0±16.6 (507)	0.97	0.63
10–12 years	57.4±17.3 (381)			57.2±16.8 (434)		
>13 years	59.2±16.5 (393)			57.2±18.6 (506)		
Total household income						
<30 000 €/year	57.3±16.5 (529)	0.16	0.28	57.5±17.5 (640)	0.34	0.51
30 001–60 000 €/year	59.3±16.9 (534)			56.5±17.0 (513)		
60 001–80 000 or more €/year	58.6±15.3 (211)			58.5±18.3 (204)		

*adjusted for age, gender, BMI, month of sample collection, physical activity and smoking.

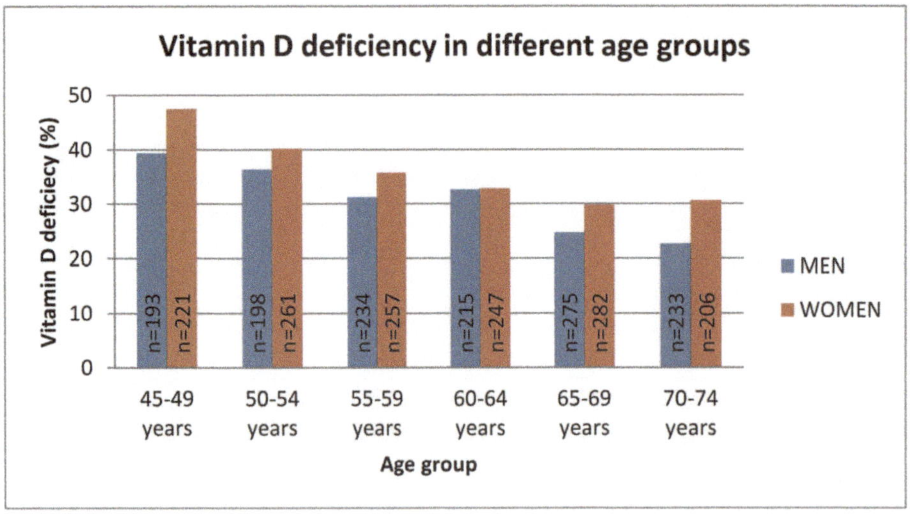

Figure 1. Prevalence of vitamin D deficiency (25OHD<50 nmol/l) in different age groups. P = 0.007 in men and p<0.0001 in women (adjusted for gender, BMI, month of sample collection, physical activity and smoking).

25OHD level in relation to features of MetS and glucose regulation

The association of 25OHD level with MetS, components of MetS and with glucose regulation is presented in table 3. In the univariate analysis the presence of MetS was associated with lower 25OHD level in women ($p = 0.0001$). Higher waist circumference in women ($p = 0.001$) and higher triglyceride concentration both in men ($p = 0.0007$) and in women ($p < 0.0001$) associated with low 25OHD level. 25OHD level was lower in those women that had hs-CRP concentration higher than 10 mg/l than those that had lower than 10 mg/l ($p = 0.04$).

In the multivariate model (adjusted for age, gender, BMI, month of sample collection, physical activity, smoking and waist circumference) association of 25OHD level with triglyceride concentration remained statistically significant both in men ($p = 0.02$) and women ($p = 0.001$), whereas association with presence of MetS, waist circumference and hs-CRP in women did not. No association between 25OHD and HDL concentration, blood pressure, fasting glucose, type 2 diabetes or glucose regulation was seen in this study.

25OHD level in relation to CVD markers

The association of 25OHD level with CVD markers is shown in figure 3 and 4. No association was found between 25OHD and Framingham score in the univariate analysis ($p = 0.67$ in men and $p = 0.44$ in women) or when adjusted for age, gender, BMI, month of sample collection, physical activity and smoking ($p = 0.47$ in men and $p = 0.44$ in women). Higher apoB/apoA1 ratio associated with lower 25OHD level in the univariate analysis both in men ($p = 0.0005$) and in women ($p < 0.0001$). Association remained statistically significant ($p = 0.04$ in men and $p = 0.03$ in women) when adjusted for age, gender, BMI, month of sample collection, physical activity, smoking and waist circumference.

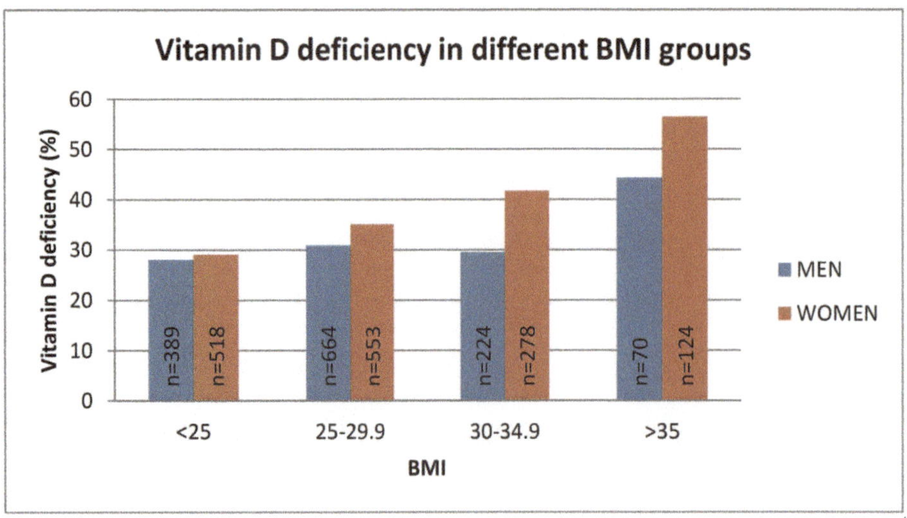

Figure 2. Prevalence of vitamin D deficiency (25OHD<50 nmol/l) in different BMI groups. P = 0.10 in men and p<0.0001 in women (adjusted for age, gender, month of sample collection and smoking).

Table 3. Association of 25OHD level with metabolic syndrome, type 2 diabetes and estimated cardiovascular disease risk (Framingham score) in the Finnish population aged 45–74 years.

	Men			Women		
	Mean 25OHD (nmol/l) (n)	**p-value**	**p-value (adjusted*)**	**Mean 25OHD (nmol/l) (n)**	**p-value**	**p-value (adjusted*)**
Metabolic syndrome (ref. 17)						
No	58.9±17.6 (540)	0.24	0.72	59.0±17.7 (675)	0.0001	0.15
Yes	57.8±16.4 (804)			55.4±16.9 (793)		
Metabolic syndrome components						
Waist circumference						
<94 cm (men); <80 cm (women);	59.0±18.6 (403)	0.34	0.59	59.9±16.8 (314)	0.001	0.82
>94 cm (men); >80 cm (women)	58.0±16.1 (942)			56.3±17.4 (1155)		
HDL						
>1.0 mmol/l (men); >1.3 mmol/l (women)	58.2±17.1 (1181)	0.86	0.44	57.5±17.7 (1130)	0.10	0.51
<1.0 mmol/l (men); <1.3 mmol/l (women)	58.4±15.4 (167)			55.7±16.1 (344)		
Triglycerides						
<1.7 mmol/l	59.1±16.9 (999)	0.0007	0.02**	58.2±17.6 (1203)	<0.0001	0.001**
>1.7 mmol/l	55.6±16.7 (349)			52.2±15.1 (271)		
Blood pressure						
Systolic<130 and/or diastolic<85 mm Hg	58.8±16.2 (341)	0.48	0.17	58.0±17.6 (458)	0.15	0.06
Systolic>130 and/or diastolic>85 mm Hg	58.1±17.1 (1006)			56.6±17.2 (1014)		
Fasting glucose						
<5.6 mmol/l	58.6±17.6 (164)	0.79	0.81	58.3±17.9 (451)	0.08	0.67
>5.6 mmol/l	58.2±16.8 (1184)			56.6±17.1 (1023)		
Glucose regulation						
Normal glucose regulation (NGR)	58.6±16.9 (479)	0.97	0.96	58.3±17.8 (813)	0.07	0.22
Type 2 diabetes (known and screen-detected together)	58.0±14.0 (104)			56.6±18.3 (71)		
Screen-detected diabetes mellitus (SDM)	57.5±18.4 (173)			55.8±16.2 (123)		
Impaired glucose tolerance (IGT)	58.5±16.2 (241)			55.2±16.1 (260)		
Impaired fasting glucose (IFG)	58.4±17.5 (337)			55.7±17.5 (188)		
hs-CRP						
<10 mg/l	58.3±16.8 (1314)	0.75	0.82	57.3±17.4 (1417)	0.04	0.93
>10 mg/l	57.3±20.2 (34)			52.5±15.9 (57)		

*adjusted for age, gender, BMI, month of sample collection, physical activity and smoking.
**adjusted for age, gender, BMI, month of sample collection, physical activity, smoking and waist circumference.

Discussion

In this population-based study representing a relatively large cohort, we analyzed association of 25OHD with several life-style factors and metabolic and cardiovascular disease markers. Our results are mainly consistent with a previous large (n = 5714) Finnish population-based study [27], where samples were collected during year 2000 (during year 2007 in the present study). The mean 25OHD level was higher in our study (58.2 nmol/l in men and 57.1 nmol/l in women) than in the previous study (45.5 nmol/l in men and 45.2 nmol/l in women). The difference may be explained by fortification of liquid dairy products with vitamin D since 2003 in Finland. Furthermore, better awareness of vitamin D deficiency has led to an increase in the use of vitamin D supplements; 10.2% of the participants used vitamin D supplements during year 2000, whereas in the present study 18% of men and 37% of women used vitamin D supplements. Methodological differences in 25OHD analysis in these two studies, however, may complicate reliable comparison of the mean 25OHD level between these two time points.

We found a positive association between 25OHD level and age in our study population aged 45–74 years. The result is somewhat unexpected since an inverse association between 25OHD and age has been shown in several previous large population-based studies [28–30], and since the elderly are thought to be at a special risk of vitamin D deficiency due to diminished outdoor activity, one-sided diet and a decline in the ability of the skin to synthesize vitamin D [28,31]. However, our results are consistent with a study of

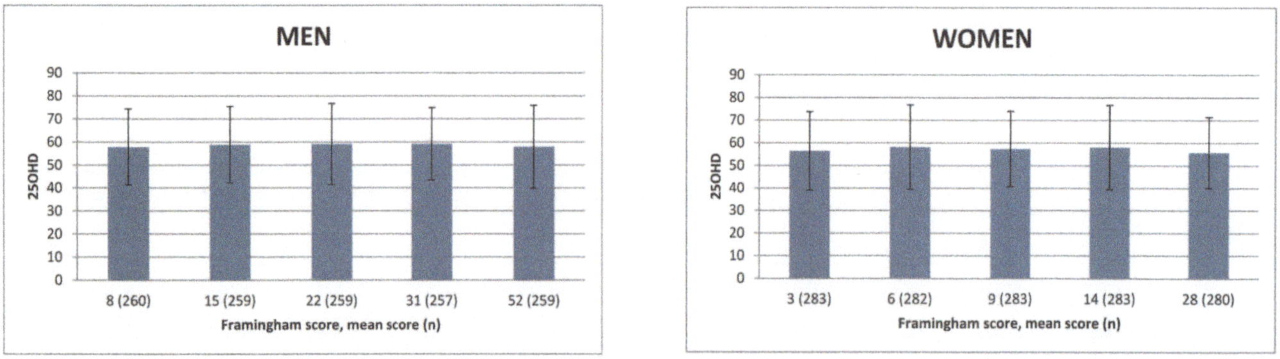

Figure 3. Association of 25OHD (nmol/l) with Framingham score. Mean Framingham risk score means the average risk score in each quintile of the study population. Higher score represents higher risk for CVD. P = 0.47 in men and p = 0.44 in women (adjusted for age, gender, BMI, month of sample collection, physical activity and smoking).

Jääskeläinen et al. [27], where a positive association between 25OHD and age was seen in Finnish population aged 30–79 years. Among Finnish people, the average retirement age was 60 years when the study was done. People aged 60–74 years could thus be regarded as "active pensioners", still quite healthy and spending time travelling abroad and in the home country. It is typical for Finnish pensioners to spend time at the summer cottages were outdoor living is usual. Eating fish is also more common among older than younger Finns [2]. It is thus possible that older Finns get more vitamin D from the diet and also from the sun by spending more time outdoors and by travelling, which is mirrored by higher 25OHD level of the older Finns all year round. However, since this study was restricted to people aged 74 years or less, and the study of Jääskeläinen et al. [27] to people aged 79 years or less, it cannot be determined if the positive association of 25OHD with age remains in the elderly aged 80 years or more.

In this study we found an inverse association between 25OHD level and BMI. Association of low 25OHD level and obesity has been seen in several studies [32–34]. It is likely that higher BMI leads to lower 25OHD level, whereas lower 25OHD is unlikely to have an effect on BMI [35]. It is not known whether low 25OHD level is due to for example changes in vitamin D metabolism in obese individuals or life style factors associated with obesity, for example low sun light exposure. It is known that 25OHD is stored in adipose tissue and muscle [36]. It is possible that bioavailability of 25OHD or its precursors stored in adipose tissue is poor [36]. Recently it has been suggested that muscle provides an extravascular pool through which 25OHD circulates [37,38]. This could explain the positive association between physical activity and 25OHD level found in this study. Also previously, high 25OHD level have been positively associated with outdoor activity [27,39,40] and indoor exercise [41]. 25OHD level is known to associate with muscle strength and function [42,43]. Low vitamin D status associates with poorer physical performance and a greater decline in physical performance and increases the risk of falls at least in the elderly [44,45].

The present study confirms that smoking is an independent lifestyle factor associated with low 25OHD level both in men and women. Also previously it has been shown that low 25OHD level is associated with smoking [27,46,47] and smoking related cancers [48]. It is not known whether the inverse association between 25OHD level and smoking is due to life-style factors not accessed in this study (for example diet). It has been suggested though that chemicals in tobacco smoke may have a direct effect on vitamin D metabolism and function [46]. There is evidence that smoking alters expression of several genes, among which are some genes acting in the metabolic pathway of vitamin D [46,49]. Low-grade chronic inflammation has been associated with low 25OHD level [50] and smoking increases inflammation [51]. There may be a benefit in increasing vitamin D supplementation among smokers,

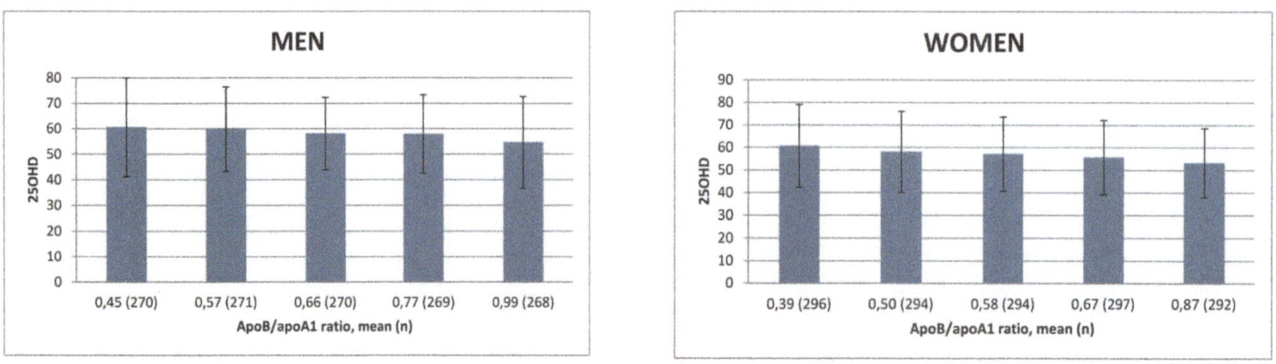

Figure 4. Association of 25OHD (nmol/l) with apoB/apoA1 ratio. Mean apoB/apoA1 ratio means the average ratio in each quintile of the study population. Higher ratio represents higher risk for CVD. P = 0.04 in men and p = 0.0002 in women (adjusted for age, gender, BMI, month of sample collection, physical activity, smoking and waist circumference).

since the biologically active form of vitamin D controls inflammation by for example inhibiting the differentiation and maturation of dendritic cells to antigen presenting cells, and by down-regulating Th1 cell associated cytokine production [52–54].

Vitamin D status of Finnish adult population seems to have improved since the last population-based study from year 2000 [27], although still approximately one third of the participants were found vitamin D deficient. Especially women that have high BMI, low physical activity and that do not use vitamin D supplements are at increased risk of vitamin D deficiency. There has been an increase in recommended vitamin D supplementation for people aged 60 years or more in Finland after the sample collection of the present study, and thus it is likely that mean 25OHD level is higher at the moment.

Association of 25OHD with glucose regulation and type 2 diabetes has been shown in several studies [55] including studies done in Finland [56]. 25OHD level has been associated with insulin sensitivity indices [57], and low 25OHD has been shown to predict later development of type 2 diabetes [58]. In this study, however, no association between 25OHD and type 2 diabetes or glucose regulation was found. The inverse association between 25OHD and triglycerides found in the present study has consistently been shown in previous studies as well [59]. However, intervention studies have for the most part failed to show improvement in triglyceride level after vitamin D supplementation [60,61] and thus a causal relationship has not been shown. In this study, 25OHD level was independently associated with apoB/apoA1-ratio. A positive association between apoA1 concentration and 25OHD level has been previously shown [62,63]. Obesity associates with both high triglyceride concentration and high apoB/apoA1 ratio. Low grade inflammation is associated with obesity as well as with CVD [64] and thus it is possible that associations of 25OHD with triglyceride concentration and apoB/apoA ratio relate to the known connection of vitamin D with inflammation [50]. However, in this study 25OHD level was not associated with hs-CRP, which was the only inflammation marker analyzed in this population.

Non-participation is a source for possible biases in this study since in population-based studies typically participants are healthier than the non-participants [65]. However, this would mean that the associations found between 25OHD and disease markers as well as between 25OHD and lifestyle factors representing unhealthy lifestyle can be assumed to be stronger rather than weaker in the whole population and thus does not explain the associations found in the present study. Also, it should be noted that in international comparison there are not many surveys which include a personal health examination with 2-hour glucose tolerance test with participation rate as high as in this survey (65%).

In conclusion, several lifestyle and clinical factors are associated with 25OHD level. These confounding factors should be taken into account when analysing the association of 25OHD with the risk for different diseases. The findings of the study indicate that in the future molecular mechanisms behind the associations of 25OHD e.g. with physical activity and smoking should be examined. Also, potential benefit of increased vitamin D supplementation for smokers should be evaluated. The association of 25OHD with BMI, high triglyceride concentration and apoB/apoA1 ratio may be related to the role of vitamin D in inflammation, but more detailed studies are needed.

Note: A part of the results of this study have been previously published in Finnish: Miettinen M, Kinnunen L, Keinänen-Kiukaanniemi S, Korpi-Hyövälti E, Niskanen L, Oksa H, Saaristo T, Sundvall J, Tuomilehto J, Vanhala M, Uusitupa M, Peltonen M. Prevalence of vitamin D insufficiency in Finnish adult population. Suom Lääkäril. 2013;4:29–33. [in Finnish].

Author Contributions

Conceived and designed the experiments: MM LK JL SK-K EK-H LN HO TS JT MV MU MP. Performed the experiments: JL. Analyzed the data: MM LK MP. Wrote the paper: MM LK JL SK-K EK-H LN HO TS JT MV MU MP.

References

1. Holick MF (2007) Vitamin D deficiency. N engl J Med 357(3):266–81.
2. The National Findiet 2007 Survey. Kansanterveyslaitoksen julkaisuja B 23/2008.
3. Sathe MN, Patel AS (2010) Update in pediatrics: focus on fat-soluble vitamins. Nutr Clin Pract 25(4):340–6.
4. Nordic Council of Ministers (2004) Nordic nutrition recommendations 2004. Integrating nutrition and physical activity. Århus, Denmark: Nordic Council of Ministers
5. UK Department of Health (1998) Nutrition and bone health: with particular reference to calcium and vitamin D. Report on health and social subjects (49). London, United Kingdom: The Stationary Office
6. Bischoff-Ferrari HA, Giovannucci E, Willett WC, Dietrich T, Dawson-Hughes B (2006) Estimation of optimal serum concentrations of 25-hydroxyvitamin D for multiple health outcomes. Am J Clin Nutr 84(1):18–28
7. Sempos CT, Durazo-Arvizu RA, Dawson-Hughes B, Yetley EA, Looker AC, et al. (2013) Is there a reverse J-shaped association between 25-hydroxyvitamin D and all-cause mortality? Results from the U.S. nationally representative NHANES. J Clin Endocrinol Metab 98(7):3001–9.
8. Luxwolda MF, Kuipers RS, Kema IP, Dijck-Brouwer DA, Muskiet FA (2012) Traditionally living populations in East Africa have a mean serum 25-hydroxyvitamin D concentration of 115 nmol/l. Br J Nutr 108(9):1557–61.
9. Jones G (2008) Pharmacokinetics of vitamin D toxicity. Am J Clin Nutr 88(2):582S–586S.
10. Hathcock JN, Shao A, Vieth R, Heaney R (2007) Risk assessment for vitamin D. Am J Clin Nutr 85(1):6–18.
11. Austin MA, King MC, Vranizan KM, Krauss RM (1990) Atherogenic lipoprotein phenotype. A proposed genetic marker for coronary heart disease risk. Circulation 82(2):495–506.
12. Rizzo M, Pernice V, Frasheri A, Di Lorenzo G, Rini GB, et al. (2009) Small, dense low-density lipoproteins (LDL) are predictors of cardio- and cerebro-vascular events in subjects with the metabolic syndrome. Clin Endocrinol (Oxf) 70(6):870–5.
13. Scanu AM, Edelstein C (2008) HDL: bridging past and present with a look at the future. FASEB J 22(12):4044–54
14. Prassl R, Laggner P (2009) Molecular structure of low density lipoprotein: current status and future challenges. Eur Biophys J 2009 38(2):145–58
15. Wallenfeldt K, Bokemark L, Wikstrand J, Hulthe J, Fagerberg B (2004) Apolipoprotein B/apolipoprotein A-I in relation to the metabolic syndrome and change in carotid artery intima-media thickness during 3 years in middle-aged men. Stroke 35(10):2248–52.
16. Raitakari OT, Mäkinen VP, McQueen MJ, Niemi J, Juonala M, et al. (2013) Computationally estimated apolipoproteins B and A1 in predicting cardiovascular risk. Atherosclerosis 226(1):245–51.
17. McQueen MJ, Hawken S, Wang X, Ounpuu S, Sniderman A, et al. (2008) Lipids, lipoproteins, and apolipoproteins as risk markers of myocardial infarction in 52 countries (the INTERHEART study): a case-control study. Lancet 372(9634):224–33.
18. Sierra-Johnson J, Fisher RM, Romero-Corral A, Somers VK, Lopez-Jimenez F, et al. (2009) Concentration of apolipoprotein B is comparable with the apolipoprotein B/apolipoprotein A-I ratio and better than routine clinical lipid measurements in predicting coronary heart disease mortality: findings from a multi-ethnic US population. Eur Heart J 30(6):710–7.
19. Juonala M, Viikari JS, Kähönen M, Solakivi T, Helenius H, et al. (2008) Childhood levels of serum apolipoproteins B and A-I predict carotid intima-media thickness and brachial endothelial function in adulthood: the cardiovascular risk in young Finns study. J Am Coll Cardiol 52(4):293–9.
20. Hyppönen E, Boucher BJ, Berry DJ, Power C (2008) 25-hydroxyvitamin D, IGF-1, and metabolic syndrome at 45 years of age: a cross-sectional study in the 1958 British Birth Cohort. Diabetes 57(2):298–305.
21. Kayaniyil S, Harris SB, Retnakaran R, Vieth R, Knight JA, et al. (2013) Prospective association of 25(OH)D with metabolic syndrome. Clin Endocrinol (Oxf) 80(4):502–7.

22. Saaristo T, Peltonen M, Keinänen-Kiukaanniemi S, Vanhala M, Saltevo J, et al. (2007) National type 2 diabetes prevention programme in Finland: FIN-D2D. Int J Circumpolar Health 66(2):101–12.
23. Saaristo T, Moilanen L, Korpi-Hyövälti E, Vanhala M, Saltevo J, et al. (2010) Lifestyle intervention for prevention of type 2 diabetes in primary health care: one-year follow-up of the Finnish National Diabetes Prevention Program (FIN-D2D). Diabetes Care 33(10):2146–51.
24. Alberti KG, Eckel RH, Grundy SM, Zimmet PZ, Cleeman JI, et al. (2009) Harmonizing the metabolic syndrome: a joint interim statement of the International Diabetes Federation Task Force on Epidemiology and Prevention; National Heart, Lung, and Blood Institute; American Heart Association; World Heart Federation; International Atherosclerosis society; and International Association for the Study of Obesity. Circulation 120(16):1640–5.
25. World Health Organization (1999) Definition, diagnosis and classification of diabetes mellitus and its complications: Report of a WHO Consultation. Part 1. Diagnosis and classification of diabetes mellitus. Geneva, World Health Organization.
26. Anderson KM, Wilson PWF, Odell PM, Kannel WB (1991) An updated coronary risk profile: a statement for health professionals. Circulation 83:357–363.
27. Jääskeläinen T, Knekt P, Marniemi J, Sares-Jäske L, Männistö S, et al. (2013) Vitamin D status is associated with sociodemographic factors, lifestyle and metabolic health. Eur J Nutr 52(2):513–25.
28. Jorde R, Sneve M, Emaus N, Figenschau Y, Grimnes G (2010) Cross-sectional and longitudinal relation between serum 25-hydroxyvitamin D and body mass index: the Tromsø study. Eur J Nutr 49(7):401–7.
29. Melamed ML, Michos ED, Post W, Astor B (2008) 25-hydroxyvitamin D levels and the risk of mortality in the general population. Arch Intern Med 168(15):1629–37.
30. Zittermann A, Ernst JB, Gummert JF, Börgermann J (2014) Vitamin D supplementation, body weight and human serum 25-hydroxyvitamin D response: a systematic review. Eur J Nutr 2014 Mar;53(2):367–74.
31. MacLaughlin J, Holick MF (1985) Aging decreases the capacity of human skin to produce vitamin D3. J Clin Invest 76(4):1536–8.
32. Liel Y, Ulmer E, Shary J, Hollis BW, Bell NH (1988) Low circulating vitamin D in obesity. Calcif Tissue Int 43:199–201.
33. McGill AT, Stewart JM, Lithander FE, Strik CM, Poppitt SD (2008) Relationships of low serum vitamin D3 with anthropometry and markers of the metabolic syndrome and diabetes in overweight and obesity. Nutr J 7:4–8.
34. Wortsman J, Matsuoka LY, Chen TC, Lu Z, Holick MF (2000) Decreased bioavailability of vitamin D in obesity. Am J Clin Nutr 72:690–3.
35. Vimeswaran K, Berry D, Lu C, Pilz S, Hiraki L, et al. (2013) Causal relationship between obesity and vitamin D status: Bi-directional mendelian randomization analysis of multiple cohorts. PLoS Med 10:1549–1676.
36. Heaney RP, Horst RL, Cullen DM (2009) Armas LA. Vitamin D3 distribution and status in the body,J Am Coll Nutr (3):252–6.
37. Abboud M, Puglisi DA, Davies BN, Rybchyn M, Whitehead NP, et al. (2013) Evidence for a specific uptake and retention mechanism for 25-hydroxyvitamin D (25OHD) in skeletal muscle cells. Endocrinology 154(9):3022–30.
38. Abboud M, Gordon-Thomson C, Hoy AJ, Balaban S, Rybchyn MS, et al. (2013) Uptake of 25-hydroxyvitamin D by muscle and fat cells. J Steroid Biochem Mol Biol pii: S0960-0760(13)00213-6. doi: 10.1016/j.jsbmb.2013.10.020. [Epub ahead of print]
39. Foo LH, Zhang Q, Zhu K, Ma G, Trube A, et al. (2009) Relationship between vitamin D status, body composition and physical exercise of adolescent girls in Beijing. Osteoporosis International 20:417–425.
40. Brock K, Cant R, Clemson L, Mason RS, Fraser DR (2007) Effects of diet and exercise on plasma vitamin D (25(OH)D) levels in Vietnamese immigrant elderly in Sydney, Australia. J Steroid Biochem Mol Biol 103:786–792.
41. Scragg R, Holdaway I, Jackson R, Lim T (1992) Plasma 25-hydroxyvitamin D3 and its relation to physical activity and other heart disease risk factors in the general population Ann Epidemiol 2(5):697–703.
42. Inderjeeth CA, Glennon D, Petta A, Soderstrom J, Boyatzis I, et al. (2007) Vitamin D and muscle strength in patients with previous fractures. N Z Med J 120(1262):U2730.
43. Mastaglia SR, Seijo M, Muzio D, Somoza J, Nuñez M, et al. (2011) Effect of vitamin D nutritional status on muscle function and strength in healthy women aged over sixty-five years. J Nutr Health Aging 15(5):349–354.
44. Murad MH, Elamin KB, Abu Elnour NO, Elamin MB, Alkatib AA, et al. (2011) Clinical review: The effect of vitamin D on falls: a systematic review and meta-analysis. J Clin Endocrinol Metab 96(10):2997–3006.
45. Wicherts IS, van Schoor NM, Boeke AJ, Visser M, Deeg DJ, et al. (2007) Vitamin D status predicts physical performance and its decline in older persons. J Clin Endocrinol Metab 92(6):2058–65.
46. Brot C, Jorgensen NR, Sorensen OH (1999) The influence of smoking on vitamin D status and calcium metabolism. Eur J Clin Nutr 53(12):920–6.
47. Laaksi I, Ruohola JP, Tuohimaa P, Auvinen A, Haataja R, et al. (2007) An association of serum vitamin D concentrations <40 nmol/L with acute respiratory tract infection in young Finnish men. Am J Clin Nutr 86(3):714–7.
48. Afzal S, Bojesen SE, Nordestgaard BG (2013) Low Plasma 25-Hydroxyvitamin D and Risk of Tobacco-Related Cancer. Clin Chem 59(5):771–80.
49. O'Shaughnessy PJ, Monteiro A, Bhattacharya S, Fowler PA (2011) Maternal smoking and fetal sex significantly affect metabolic enzyme expression in the human fetal liver. J Clin Endocrinol Metab 96(9):2851–60.
50. Hyppönen E, Berry D, Cortina-Borja M, Power C (2010) 25-Hydroxyvitamin D and pre-clinical alterations in inflammatory and hemostatic markers: a cross sectional analysis in the 1958 British Birth Cohort. PLoS One 24;5(5):e10801.
51. Brody JS (2012) Transcriptome alterations induced by cigarette smoke. Int J Cancer 15;131(12):2754–62.
52. Baeke F, Takiishi T, Korf H, Gysemans C, Mathieu C (2010) Vitamin D: modulator of the immune system. Curr Opin Pharmacol 10(4):482–96.
53. Guillot X, Semerano L, Saidenberg-Kermanac'h N, Falgarone G, Boissier MC (2010) Vitamin D and inflammation. Joint Bone Spine 77(6):552–7.
54. Penna G, Adorini L (2000) 1 Alpha,24-dihydroxyvitamin D3 inhibits differentiation, maturation, activation, and survival of dendritic cells leading to impaired alloreactive T cell activation. J Immunol 164(5):2405–11.
55. Forouhi NG, Ye Z, Rickard AP, Khaw KT, Luben R, et al. (2012) Circulating 25-hydroxyvitamin D concentration and the risk of type 2 diabetes: results from the European Prospective Investigation into Cancer (EPIC)-Norfolk cohort and updated meta-analysis of prospective studies. Diabetologia 2012 55(8):2173–82.
56. Hurskainen AR, Virtanen JK, Tuomainen TP, Nurmi T, Voutilainen S (2012) Association of serum 25-hydroxyvitamin D with type 2 diabetes and markers of insulin resistance in a general older population in Finland. Diabetes Metab Res Rev 28(5):418–23.
57. Chiu KC, Chu A, Go VL, Saad MF (2004) Hypovitaminosis D is associated with insulin resistance and beta cell dysfunction. Am J Clin Nutr 79(5):820–5.
58. Pittas AG, Sun Q, Manson JE, Dawson-Hughes B, Hu FB (2010) Plasma 25-hydroxyvitamin D concentration and risk of incident type 2 diabetes in women. Diabetes Care 33(9):2021–3.
59. Jorde R, Grimnes G (2011) Vitamin D and metabolic health with special reference to the effect of vitamin D on serum lipids. Prog Lipid Res 50(4):303–12.
60. Jorde R, Sneve M, Torjesen P, Figenschau Y (2010) No improvement in cardiovascular risk factors in overweight and obese subjects after supplementation with vitamin D for 1 year. J Intern Med 267:462–472.
61. Heikkinen AM, Tuppurainen MT, Niskanen L, Komulainen M, Penttilä I, et al. (1997) Long-term vitamin D3 supplementation may have adverse effects on serum lipids during postmenopausal hormone replacement therapy. Eur J Endocrinol 137:495–502.
62. Delvin EE, Lambert M, Levy E, O'Loughlin J, Mark S, et al. (2010) Vitamin D status is modestly associated with glycemia and indicators of lipid metabolism in French-Canadian children and adolescents. J Nutr 140(5):987–91.
63. John WG, Noonan K, Mannan N, Boucher BJ (2005) Hypovitaminosis D is associated with reductions in serum apolipoprotein A-I but not with fasting lipids in British Bangladeshis. Am J Clin Nutr 82(3):517–22.
64. Querfeld U (2012) Vitamin D and inflammation. Pediatr Nephrol 28(4):605–10.
65. Harald K, Salomaa V, Jousilahti P, Koskinen S, Vartiainen E (2007) Non-participation and mortality in different socioeconomic groups: the FINRISK population surveys in 1972–92. J Epidemiol Community Health 61(5):449–54.

11

Gene Expression Profiling in *Entamoeba histolytica* Identifies Key Components in Iron Uptake and Metabolism

Nora Adriana Hernández-Cuevas[1,2]*, Christian Weber[1,2], Chung-Chau Hon[1,2], Nancy Guillen[1,2]

1 Institut Pasteur, Unité Biologie Cellulaire du Parasitisme, Paris, France, 2 INSERM U786, Paris, France

Abstract

Entamoeba histolytica is an ameboid parasite that causes colonic dysentery and liver abscesses in humans. The parasite encounters dramatic changes in iron concentration during its invasion of the host, with relatively low levels in the intestinal lumen and then relatively high levels in the blood and liver. The liver notably contains sources of iron; therefore, the parasite's ability to use these sources might be relevant to its survival in the liver and thus the pathogenesis of liver abscesses. The objective of the present study was to identify factors involved in iron uptake, use and storage in *E. histolytica.* We compared the respective transcriptomes of *E. histolytica* trophozoites grown in normal medium (containing around 169 μM iron), low-iron medium (around 123 μM iron), iron-deficient medium (around 91 μM iron), and iron-deficient medium replenished with hemoglobin. The differentially expressed genes included those coding for the ATP-binding cassette transporters and major facilitator transporters (which share homology with bacterial siderophores and heme transporters) and genes involved in heme biosynthesis and degradation. Iron deficiency was associated with increased transcription of genes encoding a subset of cell signaling molecules, some of which have previously been linked to adaptation to the intestinal environment and virulence. The present study is the first to have assessed the transcriptome of *E. histolytica* grown under various iron concentrations. Our results provide insights into the pathways involved in iron uptake and metabolism in this parasite.

Editor: Pedro Lagerblad Oliveira, Universidade Federal do Rio de Janeiro, Brazil

Funding: The work was funded by the French National Research Agency through grants to NG (ANR-MIE-08 Intestinalamibe. The funders had no role in study design, data collection and analysis, decision to publish, or preparation of the manuscript.

Competing Interests: The authors have declared that no competing interests exist.

* Email: noraahc@gmail.com

Introduction

Entamoeba histolytica is a unicellular eukaryote that causes amebiasis in humans after the ingestion of contaminated water or food-containing cysts. Trophozoites (the vegetative form of *E. histolytica*) released into the intestinal lumen by excystation may then penetrate the intestinal mucosal layer and cause colitis and bloody diarrhea [1]. In some cases, virulent trophozoites may also invade the liver and cause liver abscesses. Given that the host environments of the intestinal lumen and the liver are dramatically different, the parasite's abilities to adapt to these environments are considered to be crucial for its parasitic lifestyle [2]. *Entamoeba histolytica*'s ability to efficiently use iron sources in the liver might be relevant to the parasite's survival and the pathogenesis of liver abscesses. In fact, amebic proteins such as ferredoxin, alcohol dehydrogenase 2 [3] and superoxide dismutase [4] require iron in order to function. Moreover, the fact that trophozoites grown under low-iron concentration *in vitro* show low cell adherence and cytotoxic activities suggests that iron metabolism has a role in the pathogenesis of amebiasis [3,5]. Despite iron's seemingly important roles in parasite survival and pathogenesis, the mechanisms underlying iron uptake, use and storage in *E. histolytica* have yet to be characterized.

Iron can enter eukaryotic cells by three major pathways: (i) uptake of ferrous iron (i.e., Fe^{2+}); (ii) endocytosis of iron-binding proteins; and (iii) acquisition of heme. In the first pathway, ferric iron (i.e., Fe^{3+}, the predominant form in the diet) is reduced to ferrous iron (Fe^{2+}) by intestinal ferric reductase (for a review, see [6,7]). Next, Fe^{2+} can be transported into enterocytes by the divalent metal transporter 1 (DMT1). In the second pathway, certain cell types acquire iron via transferrin receptor (TfR1)-mediated endocytosis of holotransferrin (transferrin (Tf) is the main iron carrier in plasma) [8]. Iron is transported into the cytoplasm by DMT1 after internalization of the transferrin-TfR1 complex. In the third pathway, iron is obtained from hemoglobin (Hb) or heme upon erythrocyte lysis. Heme and Hb are scavenged by hemopexin and haptoglobin, respectively. Hemoglobin's functions include oxygen transport from the lungs to the tissues, the removal of carbon dioxide and carbon monoxide from the body and the regulation of vascular tone through nitric oxide binding [7]. Heme is a prosthetic group in hemoproteins such as hemoglobin, myoglobin, cytochromes, catalases, and peroxidases. Enterocytes can internalize heme via the heme carrier protein 1 (HCP-1) transporter. Heme oxygenase-1 (HO-1) then cleaves the tetrapyrrole ring to yield α-biliverdin, carbon monoxide, and iron

[6,9]. Iron participates readily in redox reactions and produces reactive oxygen species (ROS) [10]. Since free iron is toxic to the cell, it is rapidly bound to ferritin and/or released into the circulation via the ferrous iron transporter ferroportin [11]. In the mitochondria, iron is used to synthesize heme and iron-sulfur (Fe-S) clusters. In microbial pathogens, heme acquisition and the endocytosis of iron-binding proteins are the main routes for iron uptake in host environments. Mechanisms of iron uptake have been best studied in bacteria and include (i) receptor-mediated binding of transferrin, lactoferrin and Hb, (ii) secretion of Fe^{3+}-chelating siderophores and (iii) hemophores (heme-chelating proteins that remove heme from diverse sources). The iron-siderophore and heme-hemophore complexes enter the cell via specialized receptors (for a review, see [12]).

It has been reported that *E. histolytica* is able to obtain iron from the bacterial flora and the host's iron-binding proteins (e.g., transferrin, hemoglobin, ferritin, and lactoferrin). These proteins are usually released when the amoeba lyses and phagocytes cells [13]. However, the fact that hemolytic activities have been detected in *E. histolytica* trophozoites [13] suggests that the parasites might be able to lyse red blood cells (RBCs) and liberate the host's heme via an non-phagocytic route. Furthermore, it has been suggested that two heme-binding proteins secreted by *E. histolytica* facilitate the scavenging of host heme [14]. Little is known about iron uptake, utilization and storage pathways in *E. histolytica*, with the exception of a few enzymes (i.e., NifS, NifU and rubrerythrin) involved in Fe-S cluster pathways [15,16].

The objective of the present study was to identify candidate factors involved in iron uptake, use and storage mechanisms in *E. histolytica*. We compared the transcriptome of *E. histolytica* trophozoites grown *in vitro* under four conditions: (i) normal iron concentrations (around 169 μM iron); (ii) low iron concentrations (around 123 μM); (iii) iron deficiency (91 μM) and (iv) iron deficiency with Hb replenishment. Considering the parasite's hemolytic activities and its phagocytosis of RBCs, Hb replenishment was used to mimic the transition from low iron levels in the intestine to high (Hb-derived) iron levels in the blood and liver. The differentially expressed candidate genes coded for proteins with a function in iron uptake (i.e., major facilitator transporters (MFTs) and ATP-binding cassette (ABC) transporters, which share homology with bacterial siderophores or heme transporters) or were homologous to important genes involved in heme biosynthesis and degradation in bacteria, plants, and humans (e.g., S-adenosylmethionine synthetase, glutamyl-tRNA synthetase, and monooxygenases). This study is the first to have assessed the transcriptome of *E. histolytica* grown with various iron concentrations and enabled us to identify candidates involved in iron uptake and metabolism in the parasite.

Methods

Entamoeba histolytica culture

The axenic, virulent *E. histolytica* strain HM1:IMSS was cultured in the TYI-S-33 medium at 37°C [17]. The TYI-S-33 medium contains 15% serum, 78 μM ammonium ferric citrate (AFC) and vitamins (Table S1 in File S1). The serum and peptone contribute 90.7 μM iron, meaning that the "normal iron" condition corresponds to ≈169 μM iron. In the "low iron" condition, 2×10^3 amoebae mL^{-1} grown in normal iron medium were grown for 6 days in modified TYI-S-33 medium (Table S1 in File S1) supplemented with just 32 μM AFC (yielding a final iron concentration of around 123 μM). The medium was changed at 72 and 96 hrs post-inoculation. The trophozoites were grown for 3 days in low iron and then were supplemented with 52 μM Hb (Sigma, H7379, France) for three days to determine the expression level of modulated genes by qRT-PCR assay. To obtain trophozoites adapted to "iron deficiency", trophozoites were grown for one month in TYI-S-33 medium in which the AFC supplementation was reduced in a step-wise manner every three days (from 80 μM AFC to 40 μM, 30 μM, 20 μM, 10 μM and 0 μM AFC). Hence, the "iron deficiency" condition corresponds to TYI-S-33ΔFe medium that contained only the iron contributed by serum and peptone (90.7 μM) (Table S1 in File S1). Trophozoites were growth for an additional seven weeks in iron-deficient medium prior to the extraction of RNA of transcriptomic analysis. Lastly, the iron-deficiency–adapted strain grown in TYI-S-33ΔFe was then supplemented with 84 μM Hb for 2 hours at 37°C (i.e. the "iron deficiency + Hb" condition). The number of amoebae was counted every day for five days using a hemocytometer (Neubauer, Germany). Reported values correspond to the mean of experiments performed in triplicate.

Quantification of iron in the culture medium

The ferrozine method [18] was used to quantify iron in the TYI-S-33 and TYI-S-33ΔFe media. Briefly, 100 μl of TYI-S-33 or TYI-S-33ΔFe medium were mixed with 100 μl of 10 mM HCl (the solvent of the iron standard $FeCl_3$) and 100 μl of the iron-releasing reagent (a freshly prepared solution containing equal volumes of 1.4 M HCl and 4.5% (w/v) $KMnO_4$) and were incubated for 2 hrs at 60°C. Next, 30 μl of the iron-detection reagent (6.5 mM ferrozine, 6.5 mM neocuproine, 2.5 M ammonium acetate, and 1 M ascorbic acid) were added to the samples. After a 30 min incubation, 280 μl aliquots of the sample solutions were transferred into the wells of a 96-well plate. Absorbance at 550 nm was measured in a microplate reader. Each sample's iron content was calculated with respect to a standard curve established with 0 to 300 μM $FeCl_3$ in the same reaction mixture. Reported values correspond to the mean of experiments performed in triplicate.

RNA preparation and microarray experiments

RNA prepared from trophozoites grown in the reference condition (normal iron) and the query conditions (i.e., iron deficiency, iron deficiency + Hb and low iron) was used for microarray analyses. RNA was obtained from three independent cultures grown with at least a one-week interval (i.e. three biological replicates). The differentially expressed genes mentioned below refer to genes expressed at significantly different levels in one or more of the three query conditions, relative to the reference condition. RNA was purified from 4×10^6 trophozoites using Trizol reagent (Invitrogen by LifeTechnologies Corp., USA), according to the manufacturer's protocol. The quality and integrity of the purified RNA was checked with spectrophotometry, electrophoresis on 0.8% agarose gels, and capillary electrophoresis in a Bioanalyser 2100 (Agilent Technologies, Les Ulis, France). The RNA was reverse-transcribed using Superscript III Reverse Transcriptase (45-0039, Invitrogen by LifeTechnologies Corp.) [19], according to the manufacturer's protocol. Cy3- or Cy5-labeled cDNA obtained from amoeba grown under each of the query conditions was cohybridized with Cy3- or Cy5-labeled cDNA from amoebae grown in the reference condition on EH2008 oligomicroarrays [19,20]. Standard dye-swap hybridizations were carried out. The EH2008 microarray is a custom-designed microarray developed by our group. It contains oligonucleotides covering the open reading frames from *E. histolytica* genome [21]. After pooling data from technical and biological replicates, differential expression analysis was carried out using both a paired Student's *t*-test and the variance estimating method in the VarMixt software package [22]. The raw *P*-values were adjusted using the Benjamini and Yekutieli method [23], which monitors the false discovery rate. Differentially expressed genes were considered to be those with a Benjamini and Yekutieli *P*-value <0.05 and a ≥2-fold change in expression level. Complete experimental details and data sets are available in the "ArrayExpress" MIAME-based database (www.ebi.ac.uk/arrayexpress/) with the accession number E-MTAB-1158.

Quantitative real-time PCR

RNA was reverse-transcribed with Superscript III Reverse Transcriptase (45-0039, Invitrogen by LifeTechnologies Corp., USA), according to the manufacturer's protocol and using the qRT-PCR primers listed in Table S7 in File S1. qRT-PCRs were performed on the RNA samples used in the microarray assay. After reverse transcription, qRT-PCRs were carried out using an ABI Prism 7900HT system (Applied BioSystems by LifeTechnologies Corp.). Reactions were performed in a 15 µl volume containing 667 nM of each primer, 1× PCR SYBR Green Master Mix (4309155, Applied Biosystems by LifeTechnologies Corp., USA) and 1 µg of template cDNA. A control curve (with 10-fold serial dilutions of cDNA) was used to check the amplification efficiency. The α-tubulin transcript was used to normalize cycle threshold (Ct) values because its expression levels were stable throughout all our microarray experiments. For each biological triplicate, the mean relative concentration was divided by the mean of the values obtained for the normal iron condition. This ratio represents the change in the tested gene's mRNA abundance under the different iron concentrations, relative to the normal iron condition.

Identification of iron-responsive-element-like structures in *Entamoeba histolytica*

The Searching for Iron-Responsive Elements (SIREs) web server (http://ccbg.imppc.org/sires/index.html) was used to identify iron-responsive-element (IRE)-like sequences in the set of *E. histolytica* mRNAs. The server's predictions have high, medium, and low levels of stringency. High- and medium-stringency predictions are mainly based on IREs that have been well characterized *in vivo* and/or *in vitro*, whereas low-level stringency predictions are based on mRNAs that interacted with novel iron-regulatory proteins (IRPs) in a recent genome-wide study. Some of these predictions have been validated *in vitro* but not *in vivo* [24]. The SIREs program also considers other criteria, including the motif type, apical loop, the nucleotide at position 25, the number of UG pairs, and the free energy of the stem-loop structures. The putative 5′- and 3′-UTRs (defined as the 100 nucleotides on each side of the coding sequences) and coding sequences (n = 8306, based on AmoebaDB version 1.3) were submitted for analysis using default parameters. The mouse ferredoxin sequence (NM_010239, which contains an IRE sequence) was included as a positive control in each submitted group.

Results

The growth conditions and their effects on trophozoites

The ferrozine method was used to quantify the iron levels in the TYI-S-33 and TYI-S-33ΔFe media (Table S1 in File S1). We measured the iron concentration in TYI-S-33 medium to be 168.9 µM±5.5 with 78 µM AFC supplementation and 90.7 µM±6.1 in the absence of supplementation (Table S1 in File S1). Serum and peptone contribute ≈55 µM and ≈40 µM, respectively (Table S1 in File S1). The iron concentration in low-iron medium is approximately 123 µM (Table S1 in File S1). Under low-iron conditions, the initial mortality rate was ≈30%. However, four days later, the surviving trophozoites grew at much the same rate as in normal TYI-S-33 medium. The iron concentration in the TYI-S-33ΔFe medium (90.7 µM) was supplemented with 84 µM Hb (Table S1 in File S1). In the iron deficiency condition, trophozoites showed a longer lag growth phase but achieved a normal growth rate after one day (Figure S1 in File S1).

To identify changes in gene expression in trophozoites grown with different iron concentrations, total RNA was purified and analyzed with microarrays. We analyzed the gene expression profiles of trophozoites grown with different iron concentrations in order to mimic the scenarios probably faced by *E. histolytica* during infection: adaptation to the low iron concentration in the intestine (mimicked by TYI-S-33 medium supplemented with only 32 µM AFC). We selected 32 µM AFC (Table S1 in File S1) because this was the threshold concentration for a subnormal growth rate (since trophozoites grew as well in TYI-S-33 medium supplemented with 40 µM AFC as they do in TYI-S-33 medium supplemented with around 78 µM AFC). Trophozoites initially grow in normal TYI-S-33 medium were able to adapt to and grow in iron-deficient medium (via stepwise reductions in the magnitude of AFC supplementation, see the Methods). These adapted trophozoites were then supplemented with Hb as an iron source for 2 hours, in order to mimic the higher iron concentrations encountered in the blood and liver blood. *E. histolytica* is known to use Hb as an iron source *in vitro* [13].

Genes differentially expressed under different iron conditions

The transcriptomes of trophozoites exposed to different iron concentrations were evaluated using our previously designed genome-wide microarray [21]. Differentially expressed genes refer to genes expressed at significantly different levels under low-iron, iron deficiency and/or iron deficiency + Hb conditions when compared with normal iron conditions. The gene expression profile of trophozoites in the iron deficiency condition revealed transcripts modulated upon adaptation to iron deficiency, whereas the gene expression of trophozoites in the iron deficiency + Hb condition revealed transcripts modulated upon uptake and further degradation of Hb (which is expected to rapidly increase intracellular iron levels). A comparison of the gene expression profiles under low-iron, iron deficiency and iron deficiency + Hb conditions with the profile in the normal iron condition revealed a total of 224 transcripts with significantly modulated ($P<0.05$ and at least a two-fold change) expression levels. The distribution and overlap of these transcripts under the various conditions is represented as a Venn diagram (Figure S2 in File S1). In iron deficiency, the transcriptome did not differ greatly from that seen with normal iron levels. Only a few genes were modulated (9 upregulated transcripts and 11 downregulated transcripts; Table S2 and Figure S2 in File S1), suggesting that the trophozoites were able to adapt to iron deficiency. Addition of Hb revealed 107 upregulated transcripts and 50 downregulated transcripts (Table S3 and Figure S2 in File S1). In cells grown under low-iron conditions, 34 transcripts were upregulated and 46 were down-regulated (Table S4 and Figure S2 in File S1). Of the 42 genes extracted from AmoebaDB using the keyword "iron", 2 (5%) were downregulated in iron deficiency and 10 (24%) were upregulated however after Hb supplementation.

The microarray results were validated by quantitative real-time PCR assays (Table 1). We selected 6 transcripts that were downregulated under low-iron conditions and 5 that were

Table 1. Fold-changes for genes differentially expressed in low iron as detected by microarray and quantitative real-time PCR.

Gene description	AmoebaDB ID	Genbank ID	Microarray	qRT-PCR
Cell division control protein 42	EHI_154270	XM_645351	4.5	3.9±1.1
Glutamyl-tRNA synthetase	EHI_155570	XM_650693	3.1	3.3±1.4
Regulator of nonsense transcripts	EHI_110840	XM_649191	3.0	36±19.4
S-adenosylmethionine synthetase	EHI_195110	XM_001913755	2.9	3.3±2.0
Hypothetical protein	EHI_023330	XM_650547	2.6	5.1±1.5
Fe-hydrogenase	EHI_005060	XM_647747	−2.9	−3.1±0.1
Grainin 2	EHI_167310	XM_645265	−3.1	−1.7±0.6
Actobindin	EHI_039020	XM_651745	−3.3	−1.7±0.1
Grainin 2	EHI_111720	XM_001913814	−3.3	−1.8±0.1
Actobindin	EHI_158570	XM_644616	−4.0	−3.2±0.1
Monooxygenase	EHI_009840	XM_652013	−4.4	−2.6±0.3

AmoebaDB ID and Genbank ID refers to the accession number of the gene in AmoebaDB and NCBI GenBank, respectively; Microarray and qRT-PCR refers to fold-change in the low iron condition as compared with the normal iron condition as detected using microarray.

upregulated. The qRT-PCR data agreed with the microarray results in all cases. Putative functions for the proteins encoded by the identified genes were annotated and browsed using tools that we had previously implemented for *E. histolytica* gene discovery [21]. These data are summarized in the following sections.

Genes that are differentially expressed in iron deficiency

Genes that are differentially expressed in iron deficiency might be important for the parasite's adaptation to long-term iron deficiency (Table 2 and Table S2 in File S1). Upregulated transcripts included genes coding for acyl-CoA synthetase, ComEC competence proteins, androgen-inducible gene 1 (AIG1) and NADPH-dependent oxidoreductase (EhNO$_2$). Acyl-CoA synthetase (coded for by EHI_153060) is essential enzyme for *de novo* lipid synthesis, fatty acid catabolism, vesicular trafficking, membrane remodeling. It is also involved in the post-translational modification of proteins and the regulation of gene expression [25]. The ComEC competence proteins are putative channels for DNA uptake in bacteria [26]. They contain seven transmembrane domains, a competence (COM) domain and a metallo-β-lactamase domain. The EHI_169340 and EHI_156240 proteins (annotated as "amebic ComEC") are smaller than the bacterial homologs and do not appear to contain a COM domain (Figure S3 in File S1). Functional activity has not yet been described for amebic ComEC proteins. The ComEC EHI_169340 and EHI_156240 transcripts were upregulated in iron deficiency. After Hb supplementation, the ComEC EHI_169340 transcript declined to normal levels but the ComEC EHI_156240 was still upregulated (Table 2). AIG1 is a member of the GTPase immunity-associated protein family [27,28]. Three AIG1 transcripts (EHI_115160, EHI_022500, and EHI_195260) were upregulated in iron deficiency (Table 2). These three genes are also upregulated in an *E. histolytica* cell line that produce large liver abscesses in a gerbil model but are not modified in an *E. histolytica* cell line that does not produce abscesses. Hence, Biller et coworkers have suggested that the AIG1 gene is a pathogenicity factor in *E. histolytica* [29]. The EHI_195260 transcript is downregulated in trifluoromethionine-resistant trophozoites [30]. Other members of the AIG gene family (such as EHI_144280 and EHI_144390) are known to be overexpressed in trophozoites during mouse intestinal colonization [31]. EhNO$_2$ is involved in redox homeostasis through L-cysteine and iron reduction [32] and was also upregulated in iron deficiency (Table 2).

We observed that a number of transcripts were modulated upon Hb supplementation after iron deficiency (Table 2). However, most of these encoded proteins of unknown function. The genes for alcohol dehydrogenase 3 (EHI_160670), acyl-CoA synthetase (EH_131880), kinase (EHI_140330), serine/threonine-protein kinase RIO1 (EHI_170330) and serine/threonine rich protein (STIRP, EHI_004340) were also upregulated (Table 2). The kinase RIO1 is involved in ribosome biogenesis, whereas STIRP is associated with pathogenicity.

Genes that are potentially responsible for iron uptake and heme/iron metabolism

Comparison of gene expression in the three different conditions enabled us to highlight factors that are likely to be important for iron or heme uptake and trafficking (Table 2). Six putative transmembrane transporters were upregulated in the iron deficiency + Hb condition; (i) three P-glycoprotein-5 transporters (PgP5, EHI_175450, EHI_125030, EHI_075410) and (ii) three ABC transporters (EHI_095820, EHI_178050, EHI_178580). Furthermore, an MFT family member (EHI_173950) (Table 2) also showed increased transcript levels in the iron deficiency + Hb condition. Transcript levels for EHI_178580, EHI_175450 and EHI_125030 were also upregulated under low-iron conditions (Table 2). The ABC transporter (EHI_095820) had already been identified in a proteomic analysis of mitosomes [33]. P-glycoprotein-5 (EHI_175450 and EHI_125030) shows 45% homology with the ATP-binding cassette LABCG5 protein that is involved in intracellular heme trafficking in the parasite *Leishmania* [34]. Furthermore, P-glycoprotein-5 (EHI_175450) and ABC transporters (EHI_095820, EHI_178580, and EHI_178050) show similarities with the domain architecture of the iroC siderophore exporter in *Salmonella typhi* (Figure S3 in File S1) [35]. P-glycoprotein-5 (EHI_125030) shows homology with the PvdE siderophore pyoverdin exporter in *Pseudomonas aeruginosa* [36] (Figure S3 in File S1). Moreover, MFT (EHI_173950) shows similarities with both MFS1 (the azotochelin siderophore exporter in *Azotobacter vineldii* [37]) and FLVCR1 (a human cytoplasmic heme exporter) [38,39]. Furthermore, MFT is overexpressed in response to L-cysteine deprivation, which suggests that it is involved in metabolite intake or efflux in *E. histolytica* [40].

Table 2. Differentially expressed genes relevant to the iron uptake, utilization and storage.

Gene description	AmoebaDB ID	Genebank ID	Iron deficiency	Iron def + Hb	Low iron
Genes that are preferentially upregulated in iron deficiency					
Acyl-CoA synthetase	EHI_153060	XM_651318	5.7	5.4	NM
AIG1 family protein	EHI_195260	XM_643194	2.6	NM	NM
AIG1 family protein	EHI_022500	XM_642923	2.3	NM	NM
AIG1 family protein	EHI_115160	XM_644114	2.2	NM	NM
Competence protein ComEC	EHI_156240	XM_647820	6.5	4.1	NM
Competence protein ComEC	EHI_169340	XM_650745	2.4	NM	NM
EhNO2	EHI_045340	XM_648481	2.2	NM	NM
Genes that are preferentially upregulated after Hb supplementation					
Acyl-CoA synthetase	EHI_131880	XM_647524	NM	2.2	NM
Alcohol dehydrogenase 3	EHI_160670	XM_001914165	NM	3.7	NM
Hypothetical protein	EHI_058920	XM_646161	2.4	4.2	NM
Hypothetical protein	EHI_009990	XM_651985	NM	4.1	NM
Hypothetical protein	EHI_187790	XM_643995	NM	3.7	NM
Hypothetical protein	EHI_174580	XM_648227	NM	3.7	NM
Hypothetical protein	EHI_075990	XM_649526	NM	3.7	NM
Hypothetical protein	EHI_159670	XM_645153	NM	3.2	NM
Hypothetical protein	EHI_148870	XM_652487	NM	2.6	NM
Hypothetical protein	EHI_112830	XM_651012	NM	2.6	NM
Hypothetical protein	EHI_031640	XM_648447	NM	2.1	NM
Hypothetical protein	EHI_151930	XM_652295	NM	4.5	NM
Hypothetical protein	EHI_169830	XM_650917	NM	3.6	NM
Hypothetical protein	EHI_087110	XM_651036	NM	2.5	NM
Hypothetical protein	EHI_050590	XM_651508	NM	2.4	NM
Protein kinase	EHI_140330	XM_646643	NM	3.7	NM
RIO1 family protein	EHI_170330	XM_645949	NM	4.5	NM
STIRP	EHI_004340	XM_001913561	NM	2.2	NM
ABC and Major Facilitator Transporters					
ATP binding cassette	EHI_095820	XM_649804	NM	2.9	NM
ATP binding cassette	EHI_178050	XM_646404	NM	2.0	NM
ATP binding cassette	EHI_178580	XM_001913406	NM	2.2	2.2
P-glycoprotein 5	EHI_175450	XM_644247	NM	3.2	2.4
P-glycoprotein 5	EHI_125030	XM_644884	NM	4.8	2.1
P-glycoprotein 5	EHI_075410	XM_001914252	NM	2.1	NM
Transporter major facilitator	EHI_173950	XM_647419	NM	2.5	NM
GluRS, SAMS and Monooxygenase					
Glutamyl-tRNA synthetase	EHI_155570	XM_650693	NM	3.4	3.1
Monooxygenase	EHI_009840	XM_652013	−3.7	−20.6	−4.4
S-adenosylmethionine synthetase	EHI_004920	XM_001913609	−2.3	NM	2.9
S-adenosylmethionine synthetase	EHI_174250	XM_647762	−3.5	NM	2.7
S-adenosylmethionine synthetase	EHI_195110	XM_001913755	−2.9	NM	2.5

AmoebaDB ID and Genbank ID refers to the accession number of the gene in AmoebaDB (http://amoebadb.org/amoeba/) and NCBI GenBank (http://www.ncbi.nlm.nih.gov/genbank/), respectively; iron deficiency refers to the fold changes of expression level in the iron deficiency condition as compared with the normal condition; Iron def + Hb refers to the fold-change of the expression level in iron deficiency following by hemoglobin supplementation as compared with the normal condition; low iron refers to the fold-change of expression level in low iron as compared with the normal condition; Please see methods for definition of iron deficiency, low iron, and normal iron condition. NM: non-modulated.

Further experiments are necessary to clarify the role of ABC transporters and MFTs in siderophore/hemophore transport in *E. histolytica*.

It is noteworthy that genes relevant for heme metabolism in bacteria were modulated in trophozoites grown under both iron deficiency and low-iron conditions. These include genes coding for three S-adenosylmethionine synthetases (SAMS; EHI_174250,

EHI_004920, and EHI_195110), a monooxygenase (EHI_009840) and glutamyl-tRNA synthetase (GluRS, EHI_155570) (Table 2). The SAMS transcripts were downregulated in iron deficiency but normal levels were restored after Hb supplementation (Table 2). S-adenosylmethionine synthetase is responsible for the biosynthesis of S-adenosylmethione (SAM); the latter is necessary in many biosynthetic pathways, including methionine-cysteine conversion [40] and heme biosynthesis [41,42]. S-adenosylmethionine synthetase is also involved in iron acquisition in plants and it is necessary for the synthesis of mugineic acid (MA) phytosiderophores through a well described pathway [43].

The monooxygenase-encoding transcript was downregulated moderately under low-iron and iron deficiency conditions and dramatically (20-fold) in the iron deficiency + Hb condition (Table 2). The monooxygenase (EHI_009840) presents significant homology (Figure in File S1) with bacterial monooxygenases (such as the heme-degrading monooxygenase (isdG) from *Staphylococcus aureus*). The *E. histolytica* gene coding for glutamyl-tRNA synthetase (EHI_155570) was upregulated under iron deficiency + Hb and low-iron conditions (Table 2). Expression of the amebic GluRS encoding gene did not change during iron starvation but was upregulated by a factor of 3.4 in the iron deficiency + Hb condition. Glutamyl-tRNA synthetase is involved in heme/tetrapyrrole biosynthesis in bacteria and plants.

We used qRT-PCR to further examine expression levels of SAMS, monooxygenase and GluRS transcripts by (Tables 3, S5 and S6 in File S1). The SAMS transcript (EHI_195110) was upregulated under low-iron conditions and was downregulated in iron deficiency. However, Hb supplementation was associated with a return to normal expression levels of SAMS (Tables 3). Glutamyl-tRNA synthetase gene expression was not modulated in the iron-deficient environment but was upregulated under both low-iron and iron deficiency + Hb environments. Moreover, we confirmed that SAMS and GluRS transcripts were modulated only in trophozoites having been exposed to below-normal iron concentrations, since the transcript levels did not vary significantly in trophozoites grown in normal iron medium supplemented with Hb for 2 hrs (qRT-PCR, Table S5 in File S1). Levels of monooxygenase transcript increased by a factor of 1.8 in normal iron medium supplemented with Hb for 2 hours (Table S5 in File S1) and decreased by a factor of 20 in the iron deficiency + Hb condition (Table 2), as observed with transcriptome analyses.

To confirm that SAMS, GluRS, and monooxygenase transcript levels were regulated by iron deficiency and that iron from Hb and/or AFC supplementation reestablished their expression, transcript amounts were determined in trophozoites grown in iron-deficient medium for only 24 hrs. In this condition, expression was similar to that observed under low-iron conditions; SAMS and GluRS expression levels were upregulated 2.9- and 2.5-fold, respectively (Table 2 and Table S6 in File S1). However, levels of the monooxygenase transcript were 6.3-fold lower. Transcript expression returned to baseline levels when the iron-deficient medium was replaced by normal medium for 24 hours (Table S6 in File S1). Overall, we confirmed the modulation of SAMS, GluRS, and monooxygenase transcripts by iron deficiency and thus validated the microarray data.

The differential regulation of the genes coding for GluRS and SAMS in *E. histolytica* grown in various iron concentrations may indicate a potential role in heme biosynthesis, given the enzymes' reported role in bacteria, plants, and humans. However, a heme biosynthesis pathway has not yet been described in *E. histolytica*. In a BLAST search for orthologous genes encoding enzymes responsible for the production of components within the heme biosynthesis pathway (from aminolevulinic acid to heme production), we observed that only two genes in *E. histolytica* (the hypothetical proteins EHI_138420 and EHI_095090) present homology with intermediate enzymes. The hypothetical protein EHI_138420 shows homology with uroporphyrin-III C-methyltransferase from *Actinobacillus pleuropneumoniae* (32% similarity), whereas the hypothetical protein EHI_095090 presents homology with ferrochelatase from *Nitrosomonas sp* (27.4% similarity) (Figure S3 in File S1). Ferrochelatase is an enzyme that catalyzes the terminal step in heme biosynthesis (conversion of protoporphyrin IX (PIX) into heme). Thus, further experiments are necessary to characterize the role of the hypothetical protein EHI_138420 and the ferrochelatase-like protein (EHI_095090) in *E. histolytica*.

Molecular functions that are potentially regulated by changes in iron levels

When considering the functional category, we found that differentially expressed genes belonged to groups related to oxidoreductase activity, sulfur-containing amino acid metabolism, general stress responses, DNA repair, RNA synthesis, cysteine proteinases (CP), and actin cytoskeleton rearrangements. The genes regulated within each of these categories are described below.

Oxidoreductase activity. Nineteen genes encoding proteins with oxidoreductase activity were upregulated in the iron deficiency + Hb condition (Table 4). *Entamoeba histolytica* lacks the components for MA siderophore biosynthesis. However, we found that *E. histolytica* aldose reductase shows homology with the deoxymugineic acid synthases from *Zea mays* (maize) and *Oryza sativa* (rice). Furthermore, an aldo-keto reductase from the green algae *Chlorella vulgaris* with aldehyde reductase activity is capable of functioning as a ferric reductase and driving the Fenton reaction. In the presence of Fe^{2+} as an electron donor, hydrogen peroxide is univalently reduced to produce the hydroxyl radical, which can then produce toxic ROS [44]. Three aldose reductase transcripts (EHI_157010, EHI_039190, and EHI_107560) were upregulated 5.0- to 5.6-fold under the iron deficiency + Hb condition only (Table 4). Hence, further work will have to clarify the function of aldose reductase in the siderophores biosynthesis and/or ROS formation in *E. histolytica*.

Table 3. Fold-changes for genes differentially expressed in low iron condition detected by quantitative real-time PCR.

Gene description	AmoebaDB ID	Genbank ID	Low iron	Low iron + Hb
S-adenosylmethionine synthetase	EHI_195110	XM_001913755	3.3±2.0	1.1±0.1
Glutamyl-tRNA synthetase	EHI_155570	XM_650693	3.3±1.4	1.2±0.5

AmoebaDB ID and Genbank ID refers to the accession number of the gene in AmoebaDB and NCBI GenBank, respectively; low iron refers to the to fold-change in low iron condition compared with normal iron condition detected by quantitative real-time PCR; Low iron + Hb refers to the to fold-change in low iron condition with hemoglobin supplementation compared with normal iron condition detected by quantitative real-time PCR.

Table 4. Differentially expressed genes relevant to oxidoreductase activity and sulfur-containing amino acid metabolism.

Gene description	AmoebaDB ID	Genbank ID	Iron deficiency	Iron def + Hb	Low iron
Oxidation-reduction					
Alcohol dehydrogenase	EHI_125950	XM_645327	NM	−3.9	−3.6
Alcohol dehydrogenase ADH3	EHI_160670	XM_001914165	NM	3.7	NM
Alcohol dehydrogenase ADH2	EHI_150490	XM_647208	NM	2.5	NM
Alcohol dehydrogenase ADH3	EHI_088020	XM_643978	NM	4.2	2.8
Aldehyde-alcohol dehydrogenase ADH2	EHI_160940	XM_650725	NM	2.2	NM
Aldehyde-alcohol dehydrogenase ADH2	EHI_024240	XM_001913618	NM	2.3	NM
Aldose reductase NADPH-dependent oxidoreductase	EHI_157010	XM_001914421	NM	5.6	NM
Aldose reductase NADPH-dependent oxidoreductase	EHI_039190	XM_648674	NM	5.1	NM
Aldose reductase NADPH-dependent oxidoreductase	EHI_107560	XM_001914234	NM	5.0	NM
Fe-hydrogenase	EHI_005060	XM_647747	NM	2.0	−2.9
Fe-S cluster assembly NifU	EHI_049620	XM_650796	NM	2.7	NM
Hydroxylamine reductase	EHI_004600	XM_644914	NM	2.5	NM
Iron sulfur flavoprotein	EHI_022600	XM_643169	−2.9	2.2	NM
Iron sulfur flavoprotein	EHI_067720	XM_643101	−2.6	2.0	NM
Iron sulfur flavoprotein	EHI_022270	XM_644774	−2.3	2.0	NM
Iron sulfur flavoprotein	EHI_103260	XM_001913434	−2.3	NM	NM
Iron sulfur flavoprotein, FprB2	EHI_138480	XM_650038	NM	3.3	2.8
Iron-containing superoxide dismutase (Fe-SOD)	EHI_159160	XM_643735	NM	2.5	NM
Malate dehydrogenase	EHI_014410	XM_001913511	NM	2.4	NM
Malate dehydrogenase	EHI_165350	XM_644664	NM	2.1	NM
NADP-dependent alcohol dehydrogenase	EHI_023110	XM_648415	NM	−2.4	−2.7
Sulfotransferase	EHI_197340	XM_646583	NM	2.0	2.8
Sulfur-containing amino acid metabolism					
Cysteine desulfurase NifS	EHI_136380	XM_650165	NM	3.2	NM
Cysteine synthase CS1	EHI_171750	XM_648014	NM	3.8	NM
Cysteine synthase CS2	EHI_160930	XM_643199	NM	3.9	2.5
D 3 phosphoglycerate dehydrogenase PGDH	EHI_060860	XM_647048	−2.0	−2.1	NM
Methionine gamma lyase	EHI_057550	XM_001913898	NM	−2.6	NM
Methionine gamma lyase MGL1	EHI_144610	XM_647004	NM	−2.1	NM
Phosphoglycerate dehydrogenase PSAT	EHI_026360	XM_650291	−2.0	−2.2	NM

For definition of columns please refer to footnote of Table 2.

An iron-containing superoxide dismutase transcript was also identified. Levels of this transcript were not altered in trophozoites grown under iron deficiency or low-iron conditions. Iron-containing superoxide dismutase has been identified as a dimeric enzyme responsible for superoxide radical ($O2\bullet^{-}$) detoxification in *E. histolytica* [45]. The downregulated genes in the iron deficiency condition included four iron sulfur flavoproteins (ISFs) (EHI_022600, EHI_022270, EHI_067720, and EHI_103260; Tables 4 and S2 in File S1). Expression of the ISF EHI_138480 gene expression was not altered by iron deficiency but was upregulated upon Hb supplementation and under low-iron conditions. The ISFs constitute a novel family of proteins that are broadly distributed across distantly related anaerobes. *Trichomonas vaginalis* and *E. histolytica* are the only eukaryotes to possess ISFs [40,46]. The ISF EHI_067720, EHI_103260, and EHI_138480 transcripts were upregulated during L-cysteine deprivation [40], and the ISF EHI_067720 was downregulated in a mouse model of intestinal amebiasis [31].

Alcohol dehydrogenase transcripts were upregulated in the iron deficiency + Hb condition; they included aldehyde-alcohol dehydrogenase 2 (EHI_024240; a 2.3-fold increase), which known to be involved in the internalization of human transferrin [47] and is regulated by iron [3]. Alcohol dehydrogenase (EHI_125950) and NADP-dependent alcohol dehydrogenase (EHI_023110) transcripts were downregulated in trophozoites grown under low iron concentrations and upon Hb supplementation. The Fe-hydrogenase (EHI_005060) transcript was downregulated 2.9-fold under low iron conditions (Table 4) and upregulated 2-fold after supplementation with Hb. Transcripts such as alcohol dehydrogenase (EHI_088020) and sulfotransferase (EHI_197340) were also differentially expressed in trophozoites cultured under low iron conditions (Table 4).

Sulfur-containing amino acid metabolism. Cysteine synthase CS1 (EHI_171750) and CS2 (EHI_190630) transcripts and cysteine desulfurase NifS (EHI_136380) transcripts were upregulated in the iron deficiency + Hb condition (Table 4). Together with the changes observed for SAMS (Table 2), this upregulation

Table 5. Differentially expressed genes relevant to heat shock stress, DNA repair, and RNA synthesis.

Gene description	AmoebaDB ID	Genbank ID	Iron deficiency	Iron def + Hb	Low iron
Stress response					
Chaperone clpB	EHI_090840	XM_001914528	NM	2.9	3.9
Chaperone clpB	EHI_155060	XM_001914269	NM	2.1	3.5
Chaperone clpB	EHI_094680	XM_001914511	NM	NM	2.7
Heat shock protein 101	EHI_076480	XM_001914516	NM	NM	3.3
Heat shock protein 101	EHI_013550	XM_001914488	NM	NM	2.8
Heat shock protein 101	EHI_156560	XM_001914239	NM	2.2	4.1
Heat shock protein 101	EHI_183680	XM_001914603	NM	2.1	3.9
Heat shock protein 101	EHI_178230	XM_001914365	NM	NM	3.8
Heat shock protein 101	EHI_094470	XM_001914472	NM	NM	2.5
Heat shock protein 90	EHI_196940	XM_648040	NM	2.0	NM
Heat shock protein Hsp20	EHI_125830	XM_651403	NM	−2.1	NM
Heat shock protein70 (hsp70A2)	EHI_015390	XM_001913629	NM	2.1	NM
DNA repair					
DNA directed RNA polymerase II subunit	EHI_056690	XM_643999	NM	2.1	NM
DNA directed RNA polymerase III subunit	EHI_050830	XM_651537	NM	2.0	NM
Double strand break repair protein MRE11	EHI_125910	XM_651393	NM	3.9	NM
RNA synthesis					
DEAD box ATP dependent RNA helicase 42	EHI_197990	XM_001914267	NM	2.0	NM
DEAD/DEAH box helicase	EHI_131080	XM_650428	NM	3.7	NM
Regulator of nonsense transcripts	EHI_070810	XM_649317	NM	3.7	3.8
Regulator of nonsense transcripts	EHI_110840	XM_649191	NM	2.7	3.0
Regulator of nonsense transcripts	EHI_035550	XM_651038	NM	2.0	NM
Regulator of nonsense transcripts	EHI_193520	XM_646961	NM	NM	2.2
RNA binding protein	EHI_151990	XM_652289	NM	2.2	NM

For definition of columns please refer to footnote of Table 2.

suggests that cysteine metabolism is activated and forms a key part of the metabolism of sulfur-containing amino acids in *E. histolytica* [48,49]. Upregulation of the NifS transcript also suggests that Fe-S cluster synthesis is activated in the presence of Hb as an iron source (Table 4). In contrast, serine metabolism appears to be downregulated, since transcripts of genes coding for D-3-phosphoglycerate dehydrogenase (PGDH, EHI_060860), methionine γ-lyase 1 (MGL1, EHI_144610), and phosphoserine aminotransferase (PSAT, EHI_026360) were downregulated in iron deficiency. The PGDH and PSAT transcripts were still downregulated after Hb supplementation.

Stress responses, DNA repair and RNA synthesis. A number of transcripts involved in stress responses were upregulated upon Hb replenishment, including heat shock proteins (HSPs) such as Hsp101 and ClpB (Table 5) and the chaperone Hsp90. Hsp101 and ClpB transcripts were also upregulated in the low-iron condition but not in the iron deficiency condition. Upon Hb replenishment, Hsp20 was downregulated and Hsp70A2 was upregulated. Thus, in an iron-deficient environment, the sudden supply of heme might induce a stress response in *E. histolytica*. Gene transcripts involved in DNA/RNA synthesis and DNA repair (such as the double strand break repair protein MRE11, DEAD/DEAH box helicase and the regulators of nonsense transcripts) were modulated by Hb supplementation (Table 5). Expression of three regulators of nonsense transcripts was observed in amoebae grown in the low-iron condition (Table 5) and upon supplementation with Hb. The regulators of nonsense transcripts present homology with the product of the human *Upf1* gene (regulator of nonsense transcripts 1, a RNA helicase that detects mRNA containing premature stop codons).

Cysteine proteinases and actin-related cytoskeleton. It has already been suggested that iron-limited conditions regulate cysteine proteinase levels in *E. histolytica* [50]. In the present analysis, we identified three annotated cysteine proteinases (CP-A4, CP-A5, and CP-A7) and the putative cysteine proteinase EHI_010850 (XP_001914429). Upon Hb supplementation, expression of CP-A5, CP-A7, and EHI_010850 was upregulated 2.4-, 4.5-, and 4.5-fold, respectively. Furthermore, CP-A4 was upregulated 3.0-fold in iron-starved trophozoites (Table 6). Transcripts encoding proteins involved in actin cytoskeleton organization (such as actobindin (EHI_158570, EHI_039020), cofilin (EHI_186840), and ARP 2/3 complex subunits (EHI_199690, EHI _045000)) (Table 6) were downregulated only in low-iron conditions. Reorganization of the actin cytoskeleton may thus be correlated with the previously reported loss of parasite adherence under low-iron conditions [5].

Overall, the results of our microarray analysis provide a new vision of iron-related functions in *E. histolytica*. There are clear similarities with bacterial iron-related pathways. Furthermore, our work is the first to highlight candidates for iron uptake and utilization studies *in E. histolytica*.

Table 6. Differentially expressed genes relevant to other notable molecular functions.

Gene description	AmoebaDB ID	Genbank ID	Iron deficiency	Iron def + Hb	Low iron
Cysteine Proteinases					
Cysteine proteinase	EHI_010850	XM_001914394	NM	4.5	NM
Cysteine proteinase (CP-A7)	EHI_039610	XM_643904	NM	4.5	NM
Cysteine proteinase (CP-A4)	EHI_050570	XM_651510	3.0	NM	NM
Cysteine proteinase (CP-A5)	EHI_168240	XM_645845	NM	2.4	NM
Actin cytoskeleton organization					
Actobindin	EHI_158570	XM_644616	NM	NM	−4.0
Actin binding protein cofilin/tropomyosin	EHI_186840	XM_651345	NM	NM	−2.4
Actin related protein 2/3 complex subunit 1A	EHI_045000	XM_652168	NM	NM	−2.0
Actobindin	EHI_039020	XM_651745	NM	NM	−3.3
ARP2/3 complex 34 kDa subunit	EHI_199690	XM_645477	NM	NM	−2.0
Other amoebic transcripts					
Acetyltransferase	EHI_039180	XM_001913968	NM	2.0	NM
Acetyltransferase	EHI_167080	XM_649690	NM	−2.1	NM
Aspartate ammonia lyase	EHI_082270	XM_001913840	NM	−2.3	−2.3
Aspartate ammonia lyase	EHI_150390	XM_650734	NM	−2.5	−2.0
Calmodulin	EHI_010020	XM_651988	NM	−2.0	−3.0
Grainin 1	EHI_167300	XM_645280	NM	NM	−2.8
Grainin 2	EHI_111720	XM_001913814	NM	NM	−3.3
Grainin 2	EHI_167310	XM_645265	NM	NM	−3.1
Molybdenum cofactor sulfurase	EHI_194600	XM_649637	NM	−2.1	NM
N system amino acid transporter 1	EHI_050900	XM_649086	NM	2.4	NM
WD domain containing protein	EHI_126260	XM_647361	NM	−2.0	NM

For definition of columns please refer to footnote of Table 2.

Identification of IRE-like sequences

By taking advantage of existing bioinformatics approaches, we screened *E. histolytica*'s entire genome for post-transcriptional regulatory elements controlling cellular iron homeostasis. In eukaryotes, key proteins involved in iron transport and storage (e.g., TfR1 and ferroportin) are regulated post-transcriptionally by *cis* elements present in their mRNA. These IREs are stem-loop structures containing the canonical sequences required to bind IRPs. Iron-responsive elements have been found in both the 5′ and 3′ untranslated regions (UTRs) of mRNAs and also in regions coding for proteins involved in iron transport and storage [51–53]. We used the SIREs web server to identify potential IRE structures in the *E. histolytica* transcripts identified by the microarray analysis [24]. We analyzed the 5′-UTR, 3′-UTR and coding mRNA sequences extracted from the *E. histolytica* genome. The results were then categorized into SIREs' three stringency levels and the presence of putative IRE-like stem-loop structures was determined by inspection of the SIREs output files. In the whole-genome analysis, we identified 550 transcripts containing IRE structures. Of these transcripts, 173 had high- or medium-stringency IREs, which were more present in coding regions than in 5′- and 3′-UTRs. Eighteen transcripts with putative IREs appeared to be significantly regulated in our microarray analyses (Table 7). Five of the latter had IRE-like structures with high and medium stringency levels. The proportion of differentially expressed genes with IRE-containing transcripts is similar to that in the genome as a whole. Furthermore, stem-loop IRE-like structures were identified in transcripts that were upregulated in iron-starved parasites or upon Hb replenishment (e.g., MFT, DEAD/DEAH helicase, AIP family members, and acyl-CoA synthetase) (Table 7). Stem-loop folds were also identified in transcripts that were not modulated (according to the microarray analysis) by iron starvation or Hb replenishment (e.g. thioredoxin and CP-A8). Thus, the presence of IRE-like structures in these mRNAs may control translation during changes in intracellular iron levels.

Discussion

Entamoeba histolytica must adapt its metabolism as a function of the changing iron concentrations encountered during host infection. It also needs to acquire iron from host sources. In the present study, we searched for genes whose *in vitro* expression level was modulated by differing iron conditions (i.e. cues for iron uptake, utilization and storage in *E. histolytica*). *Entamoeba histolytica* has hemophore-like proteins [14] and receptors for transferrin and lactoferrin [13]. The mechanisms of heme-hemophore and iron-siderophore uptake and the subsequent iron utilization and storage have not been described. In our transcriptome analysis, we identified several genes that encode factors with transporter functions (such as ABC proteins, P-glycoprotein 5 transporters and MFTs). Since homologs of these transporter families are involved in siderophore export/import in bacteria and heme export in humans [35–38], they are likely to have a role in siderophore or hemophore export in *E. histolytica* (although this remains to be explored).

Table 7. IRE-like sequences in differentially expressed genes.

Gene description	AmoebaDB ID	Genbank ID	Iron deficiency	Iron def + Hb	Low iron	RNA	IRE quality	Stem-loop
DEAD/DEAH box helicase	EHI_131080	XM_650428	NM	3.7	NM	CD	H	-
STIR	EHI_025700	XM_644280	NM	2.3	NM	CD	H	-
Hypothetical protein	EHI_092110	XM_649471	NM	NM	−2.4	5′ UTR	H	-
Transporter major facilitator	EHI_173950	XM_647419	NM	2.5	1.6	CD	M	YES
Calmodulin	EHI_023500	XM_650529	NM	−1.4	−2.0	5′ UTR	M	-
Proliferating cell nuclear antigen	EHI_128450	XM_646418	NM	4.2	NM	CD	L	YES
Leucine rich repeat / protein phosphatase 2C	EHI_137760	XM_648955	NM	3.9	NM	CD	L	-
Cysteine synthase A	EHI_160930	XM_643199	NM	3.9	2.5	CD	L	YES
Hypothetical protein	EHI_197520	XM_646601	NM	2.8	NM	CD	L	YES
DEAD/DEAH box helicase	EHI_119920	XM_644837	NM	2.0	NM	CD	L	YES
AIG1 family protein	EHI_022500	XM_642923	2.5	NM	NM	5′ UTR	L	YES
AIG1 family protein	EHI_195260	XM_643194	2.3	NM	NM	5′ UTR	L	YES
AIG1 family protein	EHI_115160	XM_644114	2.2	NM	NM	5′ UTR	L	YES
Acyl-CoA synthetase	EHI_131880	XM_647524	NM	2.2	NM	5′ UTR	L	YES
ARP2/3 complex 20 kDa subunit	EHI_152660	XM_643475	NM	−1.5	−1.8	CD	L	-
Threonine dehydratase	EHI_049910	XM_652079	NM	−1.7	−1.9	CD	L	YES
Hypothetical protein	EHI_053140	XM_001913728	NM	NM	−2.2	CD	L	-
Amino acid transporter	EHI_072120	XM_648362	NM	−2.0	NM	CD	L	-

NM: non-modulated; CD: coding region; 5′UTR: 5′ untranslated region; H: high stringency; M: medium stringency, and L: low stringency.

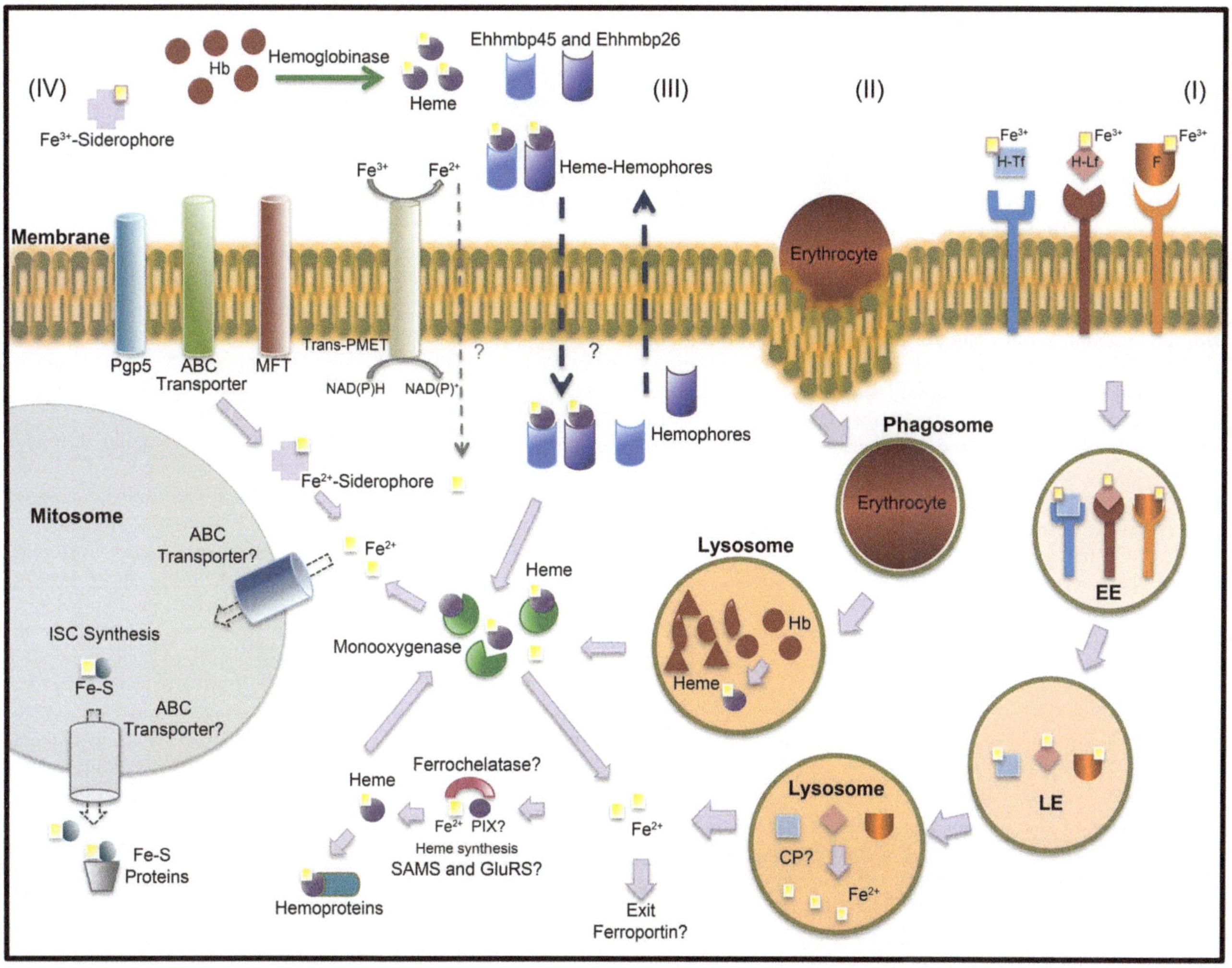

Figure 1. A model summarizing our hypothesis for iron uptake and metabolism in *Entamoeba histolytica*. The pathways described in (I), (II), (III), and (IV) refer to potential routes for iron entry into cells. (I) Trophozoites are able to obtain iron from host proteins such as holotransferrin (H-Tf), hololactoferrin (H-Lf), ferritin (F), and Hb that bind to cell surface proteins. The complexes are internalized in clathrin-coated vesicles (for ferritin and holotransferrin) or caveolin-like coated vesicles (for hololactoferrin). The ligand-receptor complexes dissociate in the endosomes (early endosome; EE and late endosome; LE) and the iron bound to proteins is released in the lysosomes. It is not clear whether iron transporter proteins are degraded by cysteine proteinases (as has been suggested by López-Soto et al [13]) or whether these transporters and cognate receptors are shuttled to the plasma membrane for reuse. (II) *E. histolytica* also acquires iron from Hb via heme internalization during the phagocytosis of human erythrocytes, which are degraded by hemolysin and phospholipases. It has been proposed that hemoglobinases and cysteine proteinases degrade Hb [13]. The monooxygenase heme oxygenase degrades heme and releases iron; we suggest that a monooxygenase (EHI_009840) could be responsible for heme degradation in *E. histolytica*. (III) Heme can also be scavenged by secreted hemophores such as hemoglobin-binding proteins 45 and 26 (Ehhmbp 45 and Ehhmbp 26), which are able to bind Hb and heme [14]. However, the mechanisms of hemophore export and heme-hemophore complex uptake are unknown (blue dashed arrows). An MFT (EHI_173950) and an ABC transporter (EHI_178050) may be involved in heme-hemophore uptake in *E. histolytica*. Once heme has entered the cell, it can be degraded by monooxygenase. (IV) Iron may be taken up by siderophores, since the ABC transporters, P-glycoprotein 5 transporters and the MFT family share homology with bacteria siderophore export systems. Lastly, a trans-plasma membrane electron transport (trans-PMET) system capable of transferring electrons from cytosolic electron donors to non-permeable electron acceptors may have an important role in iron reduction and acquisition (gray dashed arrow) [61]. The above-listed mechanisms deliver iron to cells. The iron could then be used (for example) in iron-sulfur cluster (ISC) biosynthesis in the mitosomes [16]. Heme synthesis has not been described in *E. histolytica*. Both GluRS and SAMS may be key sensors of iron status in this pathway. Ferroportin has not yet been identified in *E. histolytica*.

In eukaryotes, iron can be recovered from heme via the action of the endoplasmic reticulum heme oxygenase-1 (HO-1) [54]. A gene encoding a monooxygenase was strongly downregulated (20-fold) in iron-deficient trophozoites supplemented with Hb. In bacteria and human cells, monooxygenase is responsible for heme-degradation. Hence, the repression of monooxygenase in the iron deficiency + Hb condition may be required to avoid the production of ROS and Fe^{2+} via heme catabolism [55]. The identification of a monooxygenase protein in *E. histolytica* is noteworthy because the parasite may be able to recover iron from heme that is directly internalized or degraded after erythrophagocytosis.

We found that GluRS and SAMS transcripts were modulated by changes in the iron concentration. These enzymes are involved in several metabolic pathways, including heme biosynthesis [41,42]. The first step in heme biosynthesis is the production of

5-aminolevulinic acid (ALA) via two unrelated pathways: the C_5-pathway and the Shemin pathway. In the C_5-pathway, glutamate is metabolized to glutamyl-t-RNA, L-glutamate-1-semialdehyde and then ALA through the action of GluRS, glutamyl t-RNA reductase and glutamate-1-semialdehyde aminotransferase, respectively. In the Shemin pathway, ALA is produced from the condensation of glycine and succinyl co-enzyme A [56,57]. The condensation of eight molecules of ALA is necessary to form uroporphyrinogen III, which is then converted to protoporphyrin IX. In a reaction catalyzed by ferrochelatase, protoporphyrin IX can incorporate Fe^{2+} to produce heme [57]. S-adenosylmethionine synthetases are involved in this complex pathway by producing SAM (an essential cosubstrate for many enzymatic reactions, including the final steps of heme synthesis) [42]. For instance, a mutation in SAMS in *Rhodobacter sphaeroides* leads to the accumulation of the intermediate coproporphyrin III [42]. In parasites such as *Leishmania* and *Crithidia*, some (but not all) of the enzymatic machinery required for *de novo* heme synthesis is present [58]; genes in the genomes of symbiotic bacteria complement the absence of full heme synthesis in these parasites. Although the heme biosynthesis pathways in *E. histolytica* have not yet been characterized, the presence of SAMS, GluRS, and a hypothetical (EHI_095090) non-conserved ferrochelatase homolog suggests that iron-related biosynthetic pathways merit further exploration. In higher eukaryotes, heme and Fe-S cluster biosynthesis occurs in the mitochondria. However, heme biosynthesis also occurs in bacteria, which lack mitochondria. *E. histolytica* lacks mitochondria but does have mitosomes. Nevertheless, there is currently no evidence to suggest that amebic mitosomes are involved in heme biosynthesis.

On the basis of our current knowledge of iron uptake and metabolism in *E. histolytica*, we propose the following hypotheses: (i) *E. histolytica* is able to obtain iron and heme via phagocytosis and directly from host proteins through import mediated by hemophores [14] and siderophores; (ii) transporter and trafficking proteins (e.g., P-glycoprotein 5 proteins, ABC transporters and MFTs) are involved in the internalization and salvaging of iron/heme, as observed for *Leishmania* [34,58]; (iii) within the cell, iron ions may be released from these complexes through the action of monooxygenase and cysteine proteinases; and (iv) *E. histolytica* maintains a balance between free and protein-bound iron ions using Fe-S clusters. Experimental validation of these hypotheses is now required to confirm the roles of these factors in iron uptake and metabolism in *E. histolytica*. Our working hypothesis is summarized in Figure 1.

Putative IREs are present in prokaryotes and protozoans (e.g., *Plasmodium falciparum* [59] and *Trichomonas vaginalis*). For example, IRE-like structures are present in the mRNA for TVCP4 cysteine proteinase in *Trichomonas vaginalis* [53]. Furthermore, the α-actinin 3 protein (TvACTN3) is able to bind to this IRE-like structure and may be involved in the post-translational mechanism for iron regulation [60]. The amebic cysteine proteinases CP-A7, CP-A5, and CP-A4 were modulated in iron-starved amoebae supplemented with Hb. However, we did not identify IRE-like structures in these mRNAs in a SIREs screen. In contrast, we identified IRE-like structures in amebic STIRP, helicase, MFT, AIG1 and acyl-CoA synthetase mRNAs. Interesting, it has been suggested that the AIG1 genes are *E. histolytica* pathogenicity factors [29]. Iron-regulatory protein homologs that work with IRE elements have yet to be identified in *E. histolytica*. Thus, active IRE-like structures and α-actinin's role in iron regulation in *E. histolytica* have yet to be functionally confirmed.

In summary, we identified candidates for subsequent functional studies of iron/heme uptake, trafficking, and utilization in *E. histolytica*. These included ABC transporters, MFTs, GluRS, SAMS, a monooxygenase, and a ferrochelatase homolog. The regulation of these proteins in presence of ferritin (which is highly abundant in the liver) remains to be investigated.

Supporting Information

File S1 Supporting information. Figure S1, Growth of *Entamoeba histolytica* trophozoites under normal iron conditions (▲) and in iron-deficient medium (■). Trophozoites were counted in a Neubauer chamber every 24 hrs for 5 days. The cell count corresponds to the mean of three observations. Figure S2, A Venn diagram of genes differentially expressed in three conditions. Upper panel: upregulated genes. Lower panel: downregulated genes. A total of 224 transcripts were significantly modulated in one or more of the three conditions. In iron deficiency, 9 transcripts were upregulated and 11 were downregulated. In iron deficiency + Hb, 107 transcripts were upregulated and 50 were downregulated. Under low-iron conditions, 34 transcripts were upregulated and 46 were downregulated. Figure S3, Alignments of selected *E. histolytica* genes. A) amoebic ComEC orthologs (EHI_169340 and EHI_156240) and ComEC from *Bacillus licheniformis* (WP_003183688.1, 20% similarity), B) amebic P-glycoprotein-5 (EHI_125030) and PvdE from *Pseudomonas aeruginosa* (YP_002440490.1, 33% similarity), C) amoebic MFT (EHI_173950) and MFS1 exporter from *Azotobacter vineldii* (YP_002797373.1, 33% similarity), D) amoebic MFT (EHI_173950) and human FLVCR1 (NP_054772.1), E) amoebic hypothetical protein (EHI_009840) and heme-degrading monooxygenase (isdG) from *Staphylococcus aureus* (NP_645835.1, 38% similarity), F) amoebic hypothetical protein (EHI_095090) and ferrochelatase from *Nitrosomonas sp.* (YP_004294842.1, 27% similarity), and G) amoebic hypothetical protein (EHI_138420) and uroporphyrin-III C-methyltransferase from *Actinobacillus pleuropneumoniae* (WP_005597783.1, 32% similarity). Residues with 100% and 80% homology are highlight in gray and black, respectively. The comparisons were performed using the CLUSTALW alignment tool from the WebExPASy Molecular Biology Server (http://ca.expasy.org). Table S1, Quantification of iron in the TYI-S-33 and TYI-S-33ΔFe medium. *Footnote*: The ferrozine method described in the Material and Methods section was used to quantify iron in the TYI-S-33 medium, incomplete TYI-S-33ΔFe medium (no supplementation with AFC, vitamins and serum) and TYI-S-33ΔFe complete (no supplementation with AFC but supplemented with vitamins and serum) medium. Serum accounts for 55.5 μM iron, i.e. the difference between complete and incomplete media. Peptone accounts for 39.7 μM iron, i.e. the level determined in the incomplete TYI-S-33ΔFe medium. AFC accounts for 78 μM iron, i.e. the difference between the complete TYI-S-33 and complete TYI-S-33ΔFe media. AFC: ammonium ferric citrate; Hb: hemoglobin. Values correspond to the mean of experiments performed in triplicate. Table S2, Differentially expressed genes in iron deficiency. *Footnote*: FC: fold-change; BY: the false discovery rate according to Benjamini and Yekutieli multiple testing; rawp: the unadjusted *P*-value. Table S3, Differentially expressed genes in iron deficiency with Hb supplementation. *Footnote*: FC: fold-change; BY: the false discovery rate according to Benjamini and Yekutieli multiple testing; rawp: the unadjusted *P*-value. Table S4, Differentially expressed genes under low-iron conditions. *Footnote*: FC: fold-change; BY: the false discovery rate according to Benjamini and Yekutieli multiple testing; rawp: the unadjusted *P*-value. Table S5, Fold-changes for genes differentially expressed in normal medium + Hb for 2 hours. *Footnote*: The AmoebaDB ID and GenBank ID numbers refer to the gene's accession number in AmoebaDB and NCBI GenBank, respectively; "Normal iron + Hb for 2 h" refers to the fold-change in expression in TYI-S-33 medium supplemented with Hb for 2 hours, compared with the normal iron condition (as detected by quantitative real-time PCRs). Table S6, Fold-changes for genes differentially expressed in iron deficiency for 24 hours. *Footnote*: The AmoebaDB ID and GenBank ID numbers refer to the gene's accession number in AmoebaDB and NCBI GenBank, respectively; "Normal iron to iron deficiency for 24 h" refers to the fold-change in expression in TYI-S-33 medium without AFC supplementation for 24 hours, when compared with the normal iron condition (as detected by quantitative real-time PCRs). The trophozoites incubated in iron-deficient medium for 24 hours were recovered and incubated for an additional 24 hours in normal iron medium ("iron deficiency 24 h to normal iron 24 h"). Gene expression was detected using quantitative real-time PCRs. Table S7, List of primers used for real time-PCRs. *Footnote*: Position: the relative nucleotide position of the primer's 5′ end, where 0 refers to the first nucleotide of the start codon; Sequence: sequence of the primer from 5′ to 3′. Note that the reverse primer's sequence is reversed and complemented.

Acknowledgments

The authors thank Jean-Yves Coppée, Marie-Agnes Dillies, and Caroline Proux for advice on the statistical analysis and for technical assistance during the microarray experiments. We acknowledge Sherri Smith and Daniela Faust for critical reading and correction of the manuscript.

Author Contributions

Conceived and designed the experiments: NAHC NG CW. Performed the experiments: NAHC CCH. Analyzed the data: NAHC NG CCH. Contributed reagents/materials/analysis tools: NAHC NG CW CCH. Contributed to the writing of the manuscript: NAHC NG CCH.

References

1. Ralston KS, Petri Jr WA (2011) Tissue destruction and invasion by *Entamoeba histolytica*. Trends in Parasitology 27: 254–263.
2. Olivos-García A, Saavedra E, Ramos-Martínez E, Nequiz M, Pérez-Tamayo R (2009) Molecular nature of virulence in *Entamoeba histolytica*. Infection, Genetics and Evolution 9: 1033–1037.
3. Espinosa A, Perdrizet G, Paz-y-Mino CG, Lanfranchi R, Phay M (2009) Effects of iron depletion on *Entamoeba histolytica* alcohol dehydrogenase 2 (EhADH2) and trophozoite growth: implications for antiamoebic therapy. J Antimicrob Chemother 63: 675–678.
4. Tannich E, Bruchhaus I, Walter RD, Horstmann RD (1991) Pathogenic and nonpathogenic *Entamoeba histolytica*: identification and molecular cloning of an iron-containing superoxide dismutase. Molecular and Biochemical Parasitology 49: 61–71.
5. Lee J, Park S-J, Yong T-S (2008) Effect of Iron on Adherence and Cytotoxicity of *Entamoeba histolytica* to CHO Cell Monolayers. Korean J Parasitol 46: 37–40.
6. Evstatiev R, Gasche C (2012) Iron sensing and signalling. Gut 61: 933–952.
7. Cassat JE, Skaar EP (2013) Iron in Infection and Immunity. Cell Host & Microbe 13: 509–519.
8. Dunn LL, Rahmanto YS, Richardson DR (2007) Iron uptake and metabolism in the new millennium. Trends in Cell Biology 17: 93–100.
9. Wilks A, Schmitt MP (1998) Expression and Characterization of a Heme Oxygenase (Hmu O) from *Corynebacterium diphtheriae*. Journal of Biological Chemistry 273: 837–841.
10. Puntarulo S (2005) Iron, oxidative stress and human health. Molecular Aspects of Medicine 26: 299–312.
11. Richardson D, Huang M, Whitnall M, Becker E, Ponka P, et al. (2010) The ins and outs of mitochondrial iron-loading: the metabolic defect in Friedreich's ataxia. Journal of Molecular Medicine 88: 323–329.
12. Wandersman Cc, Delepelaire P (2004) BACTERIAL IRON SOURCES: From Siderophores to Hemophores. Annual Review of Microbiology 58: 611–647.
13. López-Soto F, León-Sicairos N, Reyes-López M, Serrano-Luna J, Ordaz-Pichardo C, et al. (2009) Use and endocytosis of iron-containing proteins by *Entamoeba histolytica* trophozoites. Infection, Genetics and Evolution 9: 1038–1050.
14. Cruz-Castañeda A, López-Casamichana M, Olivares-Trejo JJ (2011) *Entamoeba histolytica* secretes two haem-binding proteins to scavenge haem. Biochemical Journal 434: 105–111.
15. Ali V, Shigeta Y, Tokumoto U, Takahashi Y, Nozaki T (2004) An Intestinal Parasitic Protist, Entamoeba histolytica, Possesses a Non-redundant Nitrogen Fixation-like System for Iron-Sulfur Cluster Assembly under Anaerobic Conditions. Journal of Biological Chemistry 279: 16863–16874.
16. Maralikova B, Ali V, Nakada-Tsukui K, Nozaki T, Van Der Giezen M, et al. (2010) Bacterial-type oxygen detoxification and iron-sulfur cluster assembly in amoebal relict mitochondria. Cellular Microbiology 12: 331–342.
17. Diamond LS (1961) Axenic cultivation of *Entamoeba hitolytica*. Science 4: 336–337.
18. Riemer J, Hoepken HH, Czerwinska H, Robinson SR, Dringen R (2004) Colorimetric ferrozine-based assay for the quantitation of iron in cultured cells. Analytical Biochemistry 331: 370–375.
19. Weber C, Guigon G, Bouchier C, Frangeul L, Moreira S, et al. (2006) Stress by Heat Shock Induces Massive Down Regulation of Genes and Allows Differential Allelic Expression of the Gal/GalNAc Lectin in *Entamoeba histolytica*. Eukaryotic Cell 5: 871–875.
20. Santi-Rocca J, Weber C, Guigon G, Sismeiro O, Coppée J-Y, et al. (2008) The lysine- and glutamic acid-rich protein KERP1 plays a role in *Entamoeba histolytica* liver abscess pathogenesis. Cellular Microbiology 10: 202–217.
21. Santi-Rocca J, Smith S, Weber C, Pineda E, Hon C-C, et al. (2012) Endoplasmic Reticulum Stress-Sensing Mechanism Is Activated in *Entamoeba histolytica* upon Treatment with Nitric Oxide. PLoS ONE 7: e31777.
22. Delmar P, Robin Sp, Daudin JJ (2005) VarMixt: efficient variance modelling for the differential analysis of replicated gene expression data. Bioinformatics 21: 502–508.
23. Reiner A, Yekutieli D, Benjamini Y (2003) Identifying differentially expressed genes using false discovery rate controlling procedures. Bioinformatics 19: 368–375.
24. Campillos M, Cases I, Hentze MW, Sanchez M (2010) SIREs: searching for iron-responsive elements. Nucleic Acids Research 38: W360–W367.
25. Black PN, DiRusso CC (2007) Yeast acyl-CoA synthetases at the crossroads of fatty acid metabolism and regulation. Biochimica et Biophysica Acta (BBA) - Molecular and Cell Biology of Lipids 1771: 286–298.
26. Draskovic I, Dubnau D (2005) Biogenesis of a putative channel protein, ComEC, required for DNA uptake: membrane topology, oligomerization and formation of disulphide bonds. Molecular Microbiology 55: 881–896.
27. Wang Z, Li X (2009) IAN/GIMAPs are conserved and novel regulators in vertebrates and angiosperm plants. Plant Signaling & Behavior 4: 165–167.
28. Krücken J, Schroetel RMU, Müller IU, Saïdani N, Marinovski P, et al. (2004) Comparative analysis of the human gimap gene cluster encoding a novel GTPase family. Gene 341: 291–304.
29. Biller L, Davis P, Tillack M, Matthiesen J, Lotter H, et al. (2010) Differences in the transcriptome signatures of two genetically related *Entamoeba histolytica* cell lines derived from the same isolate with different pathogenic properties. BMC Genomics 11: 63.
30. Penuliar GM, Furukawa A, Nakada-Tsukui K, Husain A, Sato D, et al. (2012) Transcriptional and functional analysis of trifluoromethionine resistance in Entamoeba histolytica. Journal of Antimicrobial Chemotherapy 67: 375–386.
31. Gilchrist CA, Houpt E, Trapaidze N, Fei Z, Crasta O, et al. (2006) Impact of intestinal colonization and invasion on the *Entamoeba histolytica* transcriptome. Molecular and Biochemical Parasitology 147: 163–176.
32. Jeelani G, Husain A, Sato D, Ali V, Suematsu M, et al. (2010) Two Atypical l-Cysteine-regulated NADPH-dependent Oxidoreductases Involved in Redox Maintenance, l-Cystine and Iron Reduction, and Metronidazole Activation in the Enteric Protozoan *Entamoeba histolytica*. Journal of Biological Chemistry 285: 26889–26899.
33. Mi-ichi F, Yousuf MA, Nakada-Tsukui K, Nozaki T (2009) Mitosomes in *Entamoeba histolytica* contain a sulfate activation pathway. Proceedings of the National Academy of Sciences 106: 21731–21736.
34. Flannery AR, Renberg RL, Andrews NW (2013) Pathways of iron acquisition and utilization in Leishmania. Current Opinion in Microbiology 16: 716–721.
35. Crouch M-LV, Castor M, Karlinsey JE, Kalhorn T, Fang FC (2008) Biosynthesis and IroC-dependent export of the siderophore salmochelin are essential for virulence of *Salmonella* enterica serovar *Typhimurium*. Molecular Microbiology 67: 971–983.
36. Reimmann C, Patel HM, Serino L, Barone M, Walsh CT, et al. (2001) Essential PchG-Dependent Reduction in Pyochelin Biosynthesis of *Pseudomonas aeruginosa*. J Bacteriol 183: 813–820.
37. Page W, Kwon E, Cornish A, Tindale A (2003) The csbX gene of *Azotobacter vinelandii* encodes an MFS efflux pump required for catecholate siderophore export. FEMS Microbiology Letters 228: 211–216.
38. Keel SB, Doty RT, Yang Z, Quigley JG, Chen J, et al. (2008) A Heme Export Protein Is Required for Red Blood Cell Differentiation and Iron Homeostasis. Science 319: 825–828.

39. Quigley JG, Yang Z, Worthington MT, Phillips JD, Sabo KM, et al. (2004) Identification of a Human Heme Exporter that Is Essential for Erythropoiesis. Cell 118: 757–766.
40. Husain A, Jeelani G, Sato D, Nozaki T (2011) Global analysis of gene expression in response to L-Cysteine deprivation in the anaerobic protozoan parasite Entamoeba histolytica. BMC Genomics 12: 275.
41. Levicán G, Katz A, de Armas M, Núñez H, Orellana O (2007) Regulation of a glutamyl-tRNA synthetase by the heme status. Proceedings of the National Academy of Sciences 104: 3135–3140.
42. Sabaty M, Adryanczyk G, Roustan C, Cuine S, Lamouroux C, et al. (2010) Coproporphyrin Excretion and Low Thiol Levels Caused by Point Mutation in the *Rhodobacter sphaeroides* S-Adenosylmethionine Synthetase Gene. J Bacteriol 192: 1238–1248.
43. Kobayashi T, Nishizawa NK (2012) Iron Uptake, Translocation, and Regulation in Higher Plants. Annual Review of Plant Biology 63: 131–152.
44. Sato J, Takeda K, Nishiyama R, Fusayama K, Arai T, et al. (2010) *Chlorella vulgaris* Aldehyde Reductase Is Capable of Functioning as Ferric Reductase and of Driving the Fenton Reaction in the Presence of Free Flavin. Bioscience, Biotechnology, and Biochemistry 74: 854–857.
45. Tannich E, Bruchhaus I, Walter RD, Horstmann RD (1991) Pathogenic and nonpathogenicEntamoeba histolytica: identification and molecular cloning of an iron-containing superoxide dismutase. Molecular and Biochemical Parasitology 49: 61–71.
46. Zhao T, Cruz F, Ferry JG (2001) Iron-Sulfur Flavoprotein (Isf) from *Methanosarcina thermophila* Is the Prototype of a Widely Distributed Family. Journal of Bacteriology 183: 6225–6233.
47. Reyes-López M, Bermúdez-Cruz RM, Avila EE, De la Garza M (2011) Acetaldehyde/alcohol dehydrogenase-2 (EhADH2) and clathrin are involved in internalization of human transferrin by *Entamoeba histolytica*. Microbiology 157: 209–219.
48. Ali V, Hashimoto T, Shigeta Y, Nozaki T (2004) Molecular and biochemical characterization of d-phosphoglycerate dehydrogenase from Entamoeba histolytica. European Journal of Biochemistry 271: 2670–2681.
49. Mishra V, Kumar A, Ali V, Nozaki T, Zhang KYJ, et al. (2012) Glu-108 is essential for subunit assembly and dimer stability of d-phosphoglycerate dehydrogenase from *Entamoeba histolytica*. Molecular and Biochemical Parasitology 181: 117–124.
50. Park S-J, Lee S-M, Lee J, Yong T-S (2001) Differential gene expression by iron-limitation in *Entamoeba histolytica*. Molecular and Biochemical Parasitology 114: 257–260.
51. Hentze MW, Muckenthaler MU, Galy B, Camaschella C (2010) Two to Tango: Regulation of Mammalian Iron Metabolism. Cell 142: 24–38.
52. Leipuviene R, Theil E (2007) The family of iron responsive RNA structures regulated by changes in cellular iron and oxygen. Cellular and Molecular Life Sciences 64: 2945–2955.
53. Solano-González E, Burrola-Barraza E, León-Sicairos C, Avila-González L, Gutiérrez-Escolano L, et al. (2007) The trichomonad cysteine proteinase TVCP4 transcript contains an iron-responsive element. FEBS Letters 581: 2919–2928.
54. Kim HP, Pae H-O, Back SH, Chung SW, Woo JM, et al. (2011) Heme oxygenase-1 comes back to endoplasmic reticulum. Biochemical and Biophysical Research Communications 404: 1–5.
55. Tronel C, Rochefort GY, Arlicot N, Bodarf S, Chalon S, et al. (2013) Oxidative Stress Is Related to the Deleterious Effects of Heme Oxygenase-1 in an In Vivo Neuroinflammatory Rat Model. Oxidative medicine and cellular longevity 2013: 1–10.
56. Frankenberg N, Moser J, Jahn D (2003) Bacterial heme biosynthesis and its biotechnological application. Applied Microbiology and Biotechnology 63: 115–127.
57. Heinemann IU, Jahn M, Jahn D (2008) The biochemistry of heme biosynthesis. Archives of Biochemistry and Biophysics 474: 238–251.
58. Saurin W, Hofnung M, Dassa E (1999) Getting In or Out: Early Segregation Between Importers and Exporters in the Evolution of ATP-Binding Cassette (ABC) Transporters. Journal of Molecular Evolution 48: 22–41.
59. Loyevsky M, Mompoint F, Yikilmaz E, Altschul SF, Madden T, et al. (2003) Expression of a recombinant IRP-like *Plasmodium falciparum* protein that specifically binds putative plasmodial IREs. Molecular and Biochemical Parasitology 126: 231–238.
60. Calla-Choque JS, Figueroa-Angulo EE, Ávila-González L, Arroyo R (2014) α-Actinin TvACTN3 of Trichomonas vaginalis Is an RNA-Binding Protein That Could Participate in Its Posttranscriptional Iron Regulatory Mechanism. BioMed Research International 2014: 20.
61. Bera T, Nandi N, Sudhahar D, Akbar M, Sen A, et al. (2006) Preliminary evidence on existence of transplasma membrane electron transport in Entamoeba histolytica trophozoites: a key mechanism for maintaining optimal redox balance. Journal of Bioenergetics and Biomembranes 38: 299–308.

Serum Iron Concentration, but Not Hemoglobin, Correlates with TIMI Risk Score and 6-Month Left Ventricular Performance after Primary Angioplasty for Acute Myocardial Infarction

Ching-Hui Huang[1,2], Chia-Chu Chang[3,4], Chen-Ling Kuo[5], Ching-Shan Huang[5], Tzai-Wen Chiu[2], Chih-Sheng Lin[2]*, Chin-San Liu[5,6,7]*

1 Division of Cardiology, Department of Internal Medicine, Changhua Christian Hospital, Changhua, Taiwan, **2** Department of Biological Science and Technology, National Chiao Tung University, Hsinchu, Taiwan, **3** Division of Nephrology, Department of Internal Medicine, Changhua Christian Hospital, Changhua, Taiwan, **4** School of Medicine, Chung Shan Medical University, Taichung, Taiwan, **5** Vascular and Genomic Research Center, Changhua Christian Hospital, Changhua, Taiwan, **6** Department of Neurology, Changhua Christian Hospital, Changhua, Taiwan, **7** Graduate Institute of Integrative Medicine, China Medical University, Taichung, Taiwan

Abstract

Objective: Anemia is associated with high mortality and poor prognosis after acute coronary syndrome (ACS). Increased red cell distribution width (RDW) is a strong independent predictor for adverse outcomes in ACS. The common underlying mechanism for anemia and increased RDW value is iron deficiency. It is not clear whether serum iron deficiency without anemia affects left ventricular (LV) performance after primary angioplasty for acute myocardial infarction (AMI). We investigated the prognostic value of serum iron concentration on LV ejection fraction (EF) at 6 months and its relationship to thrombolysis in myocardial infarction (TIMI) risk score in post MI patients.

Methods: We recruited 55 patients who were scheduled to undergo primary coronary balloon angioplasty after AMI and 54 age- and sex-matched volunteers. Serum iron concentration and interleukin-6 levels were measured before primary angioplasty. LVEF was measured by echocardiography at baseline and after 6 months. TIMI risk score was calculated for risk stratification.

Results: Serum iron concentration was significantly lower in those in whom LVEF had not improved ≥10% from baseline (52.7±24.1 *versus* 80.8±50.8 μg/dl, $P = 0.016$) regardless of hemoglobin level, and was significantly lower in the AMI group than in the control group (62.5±37.7 *versus* 103.0±38.1 μg/dl, $P < 0.001$). Trend analysis revealed that serum iron concentration decreased as TIMI risk score increased ($P = 0.002$). In addition, lower serum iron concentrations were associated with higher levels of inflammatory markers. Multiple linear regression showed that baseline serum iron concentration can predict LV systolic function 6 months after primary angioplasty for AMI even after adjusting for traditional prognostic factors.

Conclusion: Hypoferremia is not only a marker of inflammation but also a potential prognostic factor for LV systolic function after revascularization therapy for AMI, and may be a novel biomarker for therapeutic intervention.

Editor: Yiru Guo, University of Louisville, United States of America

Funding: The study was supported by a research grant of Changhua Christian hospital (100-CCH-IRP-08). The funders had no role in study design, data collection and analysis, decision to publish, or preparation of the manuscript.

Competing Interests: The authors have declared that no competing interests exist.

* Email: lincs@mail.nctu.edu.tw (C-S Lin); liu48111@gmail.com (C-S Liu)

These authors contributed equally to this work.

Introduction

Functional iron deficiency is associated with impaired left ventricular (LV) performance in patients with chronic heart failure (CHF) [1]. Treatment with intravenous iron can improve the symptoms of CHF in patients with reduced LV ejection fraction even in the absence of anemia [2]. In heart failure, systemic and myocardial iron stores are depleted [3], which raises the possibility that iron deficiency rather than lack of hemoglobin (Hb) might be of primary concern in heart failure [4]. Red cell distribution width (RDW) represents the variability in the size of circulating erythrocytes [5]. Most recently, increased RDW was shown to be a strong independent predictor of increased morbidity and mortality in patients with acute coronary syndrome even in nonanemic patients [6–8]. The common underlying mechanism for anemia and increased RDW value is iron deficiency. RDW values are increased in iron deficiency anemia. Iron deficiency is a common cause of anemia; nevertheless Hb concentration may be normal in the presence of iron deficiency. Iron is essential to many biological processes, particularly in mitochondria, where it catalyzes enzymatic reactions and is involved in the regulation of oxidative stress. Heart tissue is rich in mitochondria, making iron of particular importance to cardiac function [9]. Several strands of evidence have shown that anemic patients have a worse outcome after acute myocardial infarction (AMI) [10–12]. Few studies, however, have fully explored whether iron status changes during the course of AMI, and whether serum iron concentration affects LV performance after primary angioplasty.

Longitudinal studies have demonstrated that Interleukin 6 (IL-6) is a better predictor of CHF after acute coronary syndrome (ACS) than C-reactive protein (CRP) [13], and that it is also an independent predictor of cardiovascular mortality [14]. To the best of our knowledge, however, no studies have analyzed the relation between IL-6 concentration and serum iron concentration in patients with acute ST-segment elevation myocardial infarction (STEMI).

In this study, we examined whether baseline serum iron concentration measured at the time of primary angioplasty is predictive of LV function 6 months after STEMI. We also examined whether there were associations between serum iron concentration and factors traditionally associated with outcome after myocardial infarction, such as the concentrations of circulating inflammatory cytokines and the thrombolysis in myocardial infarction (TIMI) risk score, a validated clinical risk score that predicts short- and long-term mortality after STEMI [15,16].

Methods

Subjects and study protocol

In this prospective study we enrolled 55 consecutive patients with *de novo* acute STEMI who underwent primary PCI and thromboaspiration between January 2010 and January 2011. We also enrolled a control group of 54 healthy age- and sex-matched volunteers to compare changes in serum iron and inflammatory cytokine levels after STEMI.

Serum iron and IL-6 concentrations were measured from specimens of venous blood obtained prior to PCI. A second sample was taken after an 8-hour fast to evaluate the lipid profile and measure serum glucose. Diagnosis of STEMI was based on a universal definition of myocardial infarction [17]. Specifically, symptoms of ischemia, ST segment elevation >0.2 mV in ≥2 contiguous electrocardiogram (ECG) leads, and an increase in systemic cardiac biomarkers (for example, troponin I and creatinine kinase (CK) MB mass) with at least one value above the 99th percentile of the upper reference limit within 24 hours of the onset of pain were considered diagnostic of AMI. The culprit vessel was identified based on clinical, ECG and angiographic findings. All patients were administered aspirin and clopidogrel before PCI. Echocardiography was undertaken within the first 2 days after primary PCI and 6 months later. Change in heart function was calculated by subtracting the LV ejection fraction at baseline from ejection fraction at 6 months, divided by baseline ejection fraction. Improvement in heart function was defined as a change in LVEF ≥10%, according to the clinical study results by Ndrepepa et al [18]. Data collected from the subjects included age, sex, and the presence of risk factors (*e.g.*, cigarette smoking, diabetes mellitus, hypertension, and hypercholesterolemia), clinical signs and current medication history. TIMI risk score for STEMI was calculated for each patient based on the description by Morrow et al. [15]. The protocol was approved by the Institutional Review Board of the Changhua Christian Hospital, Taiwan, and all subjects gave written and informed consent to participate.

Measurement of serum iron and IL-6 concentrations

Serum iron concentration was measured by a timed-endpoint method using a commercially available kit (Synchron Systems FE/IBCT Calibrator Kit; Beckman Coulter, Fullerton, CA, USA), which measures iron bound to transferrin. Serum IL-6 concentration was determined by a commercially available ELISA kit (Human IL-6 ELISA Ready-SET-Go!; eBioscience, San Diego, CA, USA).

Angiographic assessments

Quantitative coronary angiographic measurements were taken by a cardiologist blinded to the results of other investigations. The TIMI flow [19] and myocardial blush [20] grades for assessing microvascular perfusion were also reviewed by the same cardiologist. Characteristic coronary lesions were classified according to the American College of Cardiologists/American Heart Association classification [21].

Echocardiographic assessments

We used a modified Simpson's method to calculate LV ejection fraction as described by the American Echocardiographic Society [22]. Diastolic function was evaluated using Pulsed-wave Doppler recordings. Pulsed wave Doppler measurements were obtained from the apical four-chamber view. Peak E and A wave velocities and E wave deceleration time (DT) were measured from the mitral leaflet tip according to American Society of Echocardiography guidelines [23]. Regional wall motion score index (WMSI) were calculated as the sum of wall motion scores divided by the number of visualized segments (from 17-segment model), where 1 indicates normal; 2, hypokinesis; 3, akinesis; and 4, dyskinesis [24]. After AMI extensive regional wall motion abnormalities may be present but when compensated by regional hyperkinesis of the normal segments, LVEF will be (almost) normal; in these patients, WMSI could more correctly reflect the magnitude of myocardial damage [25].

Statistical analysis

We performed a sample size calculation according to the results of our pilot study because no case-control trials using the same laboratory test method for serum iron have been reported. A sample size of 19 patients in each group was determined to be sufficient to detect differences in serum iron concentration between the STEMI group and control group, assuming a standard deviation of 37.3, using a two-sided test of the difference between means, a type I error of 5%, and a power of 90%. We expended the sample size to 55 patients in the STEMI group and 54 subjects in the control group to enhance the reliability of the study. Based on current sample size, we had a mean of 62.5 μg/dl of serum iron and a standard deviation of 37.7 μg/dl in the STEMI group, and a mean of 103.0 μg/dl of serum iron and a standard deviation of 38.1 μg/dl in the control group, and then we have a power of 99.99%. We calculated the power from a reliable, freely available website is: http://www.stat.uiowa.edu/~rlenth/Power/index.html [26].

The Mann–Whitney U test was used to examine differences in serum iron concentration between patients whose LV ejection fraction had improved ≥10% over 6 months and those in whom ejection fraction improved <10%. A Spearman's rho correlation was used to analyze the relationships between serum iron concentration and patient characteristics. A general linear model

Table 1. Characteristics of patients grouped by change in left ventricular ejection fraction 6 months after percutaneous coronary interventions for acute myocardial infarction.

	Improvement in ejection fraction ≥10% (n = 19)	No improvement in ejection fraction (n = 36)	*P* value
Sex (M/F)	14/5	33/3	0.853
Age, years	53.3±14.7	59.1±8.9	0.124
BMI, kg/m^2	26.2±3.7	25.3±3.6	0.441
CPK, μ/l (Maximal)	2101±1817	2410±2140	0.862
CKMB, ng/ml (Maximal)	190±173	249±192	0.353
Troponin I, ng/ml	4.08±10.58	6.18±18.56	0.928
Fasting glucose, mg/dl	146±74	159±93	0.600
HBA1C, %	6.0±1.0	6.6±1.8	0.246
Cholesterol, mg/dl	193±51	194±46	0.894
HDL-C, mg/dl	38.9±9.5	42.9±9.7	0.098
LDL-C, mg/dl	134.8±40.9	138.0±39.9	0.614
Creatinine, mg/dl	1.01±0.24	1.01±0.36	0.537
hsCRP, mg/l	0.56±0.62	0.42±0.73	0.578
IL-6, pg/ml	19.8±9.8	16.1±8.5	0.993
Fibrinogen, mg/dl	439±102	449±89	0.452
Serum iron, μg/dl	80.8±50.8	52.7±24.1	0.016*
Statin used, %	80	89	0.324
TIMI risk score	2.53±1.20	2.91±1.07	0.191
LVMI, g/m^2	113.3±26.9	109.0±23.9	0.839
LV EF at baseline, %	57.8±11.3	62.2±10.3	0.135
LVEF at 6 M, %	67.9±10.1	59.8±11.4	0.005*
E/A ratio at baseline	1.07±0.46	1.05±0.46	0.866
DT at baseline, ms	162.5±44.3	187.7±53.2	0.104
E/A ratio at 6 M	1.08±0.50	0.93±0.32	0.252
DT at 6 M, ms	199.9±66.7	201.6±52.5	0.422
EDV at baseline, ml	80.9±26.4	73.2±17.9	0.396
ESV at baseline, ml	35.1±17.4	27.7±11.7	0.222
WMSI	1.29±0.21	1.26±0.19	0.730
Hb, g/dl	14.7±1.5	14.4±1.5	0.449
Hb at 6 M, g/dl	13.9±2.0	13.8±1.5	0.602
Hematocrit, %	42.7±4.4	53.5±7.7	0.410
Hematocrit at 6 M, %	40.5±6.0	40.9±3.9	0.759
RDW, %	13.58±0.74	13.79±0.84	0.416
RDW at 6 M, %	13.56±0.74	14.20±1.17	0.102
Culprit lesion	LAD (10)	LAD (20)	0.992
	LCX (3)	LCX (3)	
	RCA (6)	RCA (13)	
D2B time, minutes	85.5±38.4	84.3±38.0	0.916
Myocardial brush grade	2.10±0.87	2.00±0.93	0.693
Lesion length (mm)	19.8±7.9	19.1±5.8	0.726
Pre-PCI TIMI flow grade	0.35±0.79	0.88±1.20	0.079
Post-PCI TIMI flow grade	2.97±0.18	3.00±0.00	0.384
Lesion calcification	0.26±0.57	0.13±0.44	0.355
Lesion complexity	1.03±0.40	0.88±6.12	0.284

*$P<0.05$, Mann–Whitney U test.

6 M, six months; BMI, body mass index; CPK, creatine- phosphor-kinase; CKMB, creatine phosphokinase-MB; HbA1C, glycohemoglobin; HDL-C, high density lipoprotein cholesterol; LDL-C, low density lipoprotein cholesterol; hsCRP, high sensitivity C reactive protein; IL-6, interleukin 6; WMSI, wall motion score index; TIMI, thrombolysis in myocardial infarction; LVMI, left ventricular mass index; LVEF, left ventricular ejection fraction; E/A ratio, the ratio of the peak velocities of early (E wave) and late (A wave) diastolic filling; DT, the deceleration time of the E wave; EDV, left ventricular end diastolic volume; ESV, left ventricular end systolic volume; Hb, hemoglobin; RDW, red blood cell distribution width; LAD, left anterior descending artery; RCA, right coronary artery; LCX, left circumflex artery; D2B, door to balloon; PCI, percutaneous coronary interventions; TIMI, thrombolysis in myocardial infarction.

technique and linear regression were used to evaluate independent associations between serum iron and IL-6 concentrations. The Jonckheere-Terpstra test was used to analyze the association between the serum iron concentration and TIMI risk scores. Trend analysis for IL-6 concentrations after they had been divided into tertile groups was undertaken using the Jonckheere-Terpstra test, which was also used to analyze the association between IL-6 concentrations and serum iron concentrations. The Jonckheere-Terpstra test is similar to the Kruskal-Wallis test but is applied to samples with *a priori* ordering, such as TIMI risk scores, when it has greater statistical power. Parameters showing significant correlations in the univariate analyses were then included in multiple linear regression model to test for significant predictors of improvement in LV ejection fraction 6 months after primary angioplasty. A P value<0.05 was considered statistically significant. All statistical analyses were performed on a personal computer with the statistical package SPSS for Windows (Version 15.0, SPSS, Chicago, IL, USA).

Results

Baseline serum iron concentration was significantly lower in patients who did not show improvement in LV performance at 6-month follow-up

At 6-month follow-up after PCI, all of 55 AMI patients were alive and there were no adverse cardiac events. We divided the patients into two groups according to the LV performance at 6-month follow-up after PCI. Biochemical and physiological examinations of the patients were summarized in **Table 1**. There were no significant differences between the improvement and non-improvement groups in infarct-related artery location, lesion calcification, lesion complexity, maximal cardiac muscle enzyme concentrations-CKMB, troponin I concentrations, baseline Hb concentrations and 6 month follow-up Hb concentrations, baseline RDW values and 6 month follow-up RDW values, baseline LV ejection fraction, reperfusion quality-post PCI TIMI flow grade, myocardial brush grade and inflammatory marker-IL6. However, serum iron concentration was significantly lower in the non-improvement subgroup (80.8±50.8 *versus* 52.7±24.1 µg/dl, P = 0.016).

Factors correlated with serum iron concentration after AMI

Hb concentration, hematocrit, lymphocyte counts, the proportion of patients taking statins, and LV ejection fraction at 6 months were positively correlated with serum iron concentration (**Table 2**); however, TIMI risk score was negatively correlated with serum iron concentration.

Serum iron concentration significantly decreased as TIMI risk score increased after primary angioplasty

We divided AMI patients into four subgroups according to TIMI risk score for STEMI: group 1, TIMI risk score 1 (n = 8); group 2, risk score 2 (n = 15); group 3, risk score 3 (n = 19); and group 4, risk score ≥4 (n = 13). Trend analysis found that serum iron concentration significantly decreased as TIMI risk score rose (**Figure 1**; Jonckheere-Terpstra test, P = 0.002).

The relationship between serum iron and interleukin-6 levels in all study subjects

Serum iron concentration in the AMI group was significantly lower than in the control group (62.5±37.7 *vs.* 103.0±38.1 µg/dl, P<0.001) and IL-6 concentration was significantly higher in the AMI group than in the control group (17.80±13.19 *vs.* 6.98±8.26 pg/ml, P<0.001). Linear regression model was used to evaluate the independent associations between serum iron and IL-6 concentrations in all enrolled subjects. We found that serum iron concentration was negatively correlated with circulating IL-6 concentration (**Figure 2**; Serum iron = 95.994 − 1.246 (IL-6), R^2 = 0.133, P<0.001). We found no correlation between IL-6 and Hb concentration in all study subjects. Furthermore, we found that serum iron concentration in the control group was, on average, 35.494 µg/dl higher than that in the AMI group. For every one unit increase in IL-6 concentration, there was a decrease of 0.625 units in serum iron concentration (**Table 3**).

Trend analysis showed serum iron concentration, not Hb, was inversely proportional to IL-6 concentration

We divided AMI patients into three subgroups according to circulating IL-6 concentration tertile: group 1, IL-6 concentration ≤10.48 pg/ml (n = 19); group 2, IL-6 concentration between 10.49–19.67 pg/ml (n = 20); group 3, IL-6 concentration ≥19.68 pg/ml (n = 16). Trend analysis found that serum iron concentration significantly decreased as serum IL-6 concentration rose (**Figure 3**; Jonckheere-Terpstra test, P = 0.043).

Table 2. Univariate correlation between serum iron concentration and patient characteristics after acute myocardial infarction.

Variable	*Rho* correlation coefficient	*P* value
Hemoglobin, g/dl	0.273	0.036*
Hematocrit, %	0.257	0.047*
Lymphocyte, %	0.276	0.035*
Statin used	0.273	0.028*
TIMI risk score	−0.346	0.009*
EF 6 M, %	0.301	0.025*

*P<0.05, Spearman's rho correlation.6 M, six months; TIMI, thrombolysis in myocardial infarction; EF 6 M, left ventricular ejection fraction at 6–month follow-up.

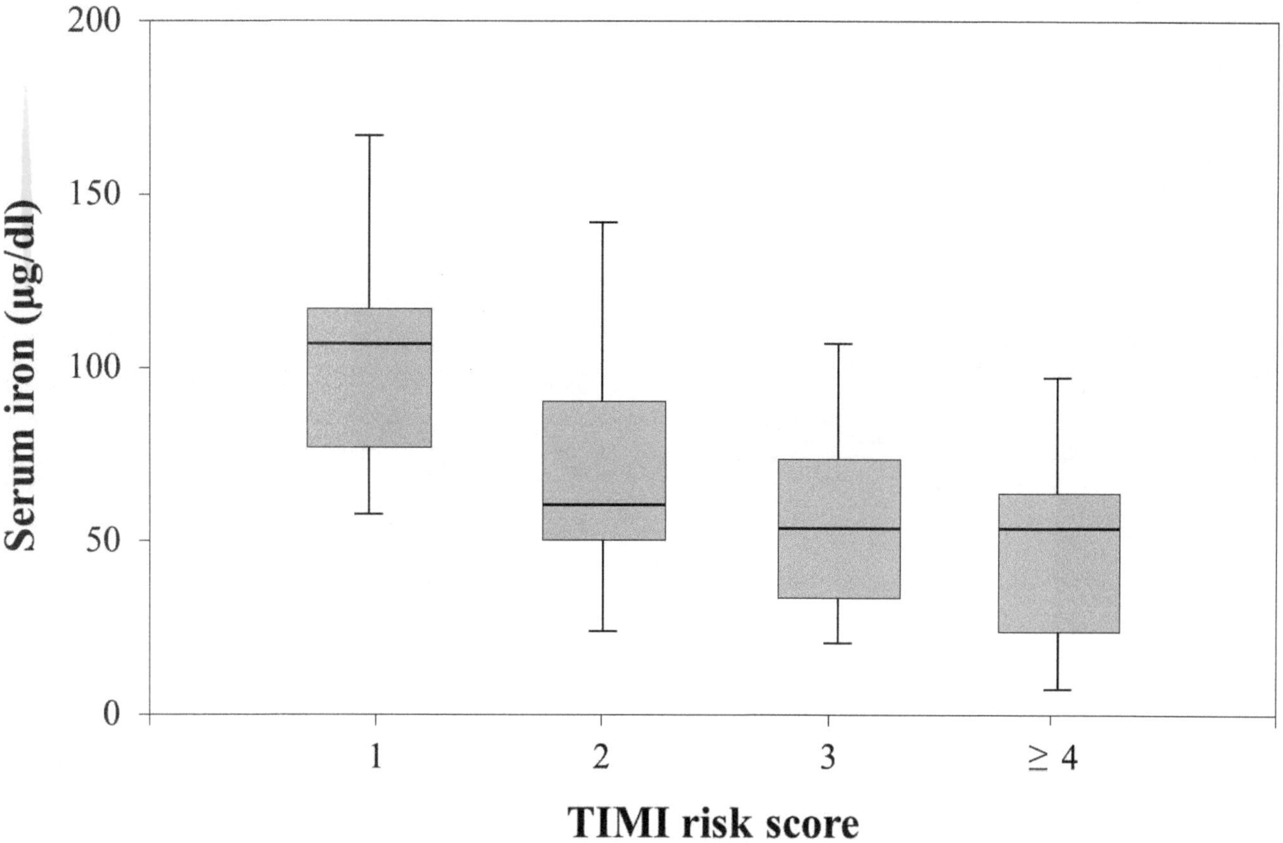

Figure 1. The relationships between serum iron concentration and TIMI risk scores after primary angioplasty for AMI. The AMI patients were divided into four subgroups according to TIMI risk score for STEMI: Group 1 (TIMI risk score 1, n = 8); Group 2 (TIMI risk score 2, n = 15); Group 3 (TIMI risk score 3, n = 19); and Group 4 (TIMI risk score ≥4, n = 13). Trend analysis with Jonckheere-Terpstra test found that serum iron concentration significantly decreased as TIMI risk score rose ($P = 0.002$).

Lower serum iron concentration is associated with higher TIMI risk score and has higher inflammatory markers after AMI

The patients in AMI group was divided into two subgroups, lower serum iron (<60 μg/dl) and higher serum iron (≥60 μg/dl), on the basis of the median serum iron concentration (**Table 4**). Patients in the lower serum iron subset had significantly higher concentrations of fibrinogen and IL-6 ($P<0.05$). Both fibrinogen and IL-6 are biomarkers of inflammation related with cardiovascular diseases. It is also noted that patients in the lower serum iron subset showed a higher TIMI risk score after AMI ($P<0.05$).

Baseline serum iron level predicts LV function 6 months after primary angioplasty for AMI

Multiple linear regression analysis of variables associated with LV performance 6 months after primary angioplasty was undertaken. The following variables were entered into the model: serum iron, IL-6, infarct related artery location, peak creatine kinase-MB and WMSI. It showed that serum iron concentration at the time of AMI could predict LV ejection fraction 6 months later, even when traditional prognostic factors such as LV wall motion score index, cardiac enzyme and IL-6 concentrations, and infarct locations were taken into account (**Table 5**). Baseline Hb concentrations, follow-up Hb concentrations, baseline RDW values and follow-up RDW values did not predict LV ejection fraction at 6 months when the same prognostic factors were considered.

Discussion

Our findings confirm the important role of serum iron in determining LV performance after STEMI. Furthermore, the recovery of LV function was impaired in those with lower serum iron concentration after revascularization. Anemia can be viewed as the net result of iron deficiency, but a normal Hb level does not necessarily mean that iron stores are adequate. An individual with normal body iron stores must lose a large portion of body iron before the Hb falls below the laboratory definition of anemia (generally, Hb<12 g/dl for women and Hb<13 g/dl for men). To investigate whether serum iron or Hb or RDW is the most important determinant of LV function after STEMI, multiple regression analyses were performed with serum iron or Hb concentration or RDW value as one of the covariates. In these analyses, serum iron concentrations were significantly predictive of LV systolic function after adjusting for possible confounding factors (such as infarct location, LV wall motion score index, and serum concentrations of cardiac enzymes and IL-6). Blood Hb concentrations and RDW values at baseline and at 6 months were found not to be significant predictors when the same prognostic factors were considered. These findings suggest that serum iron concentration is an independent predictor of LV systolic function after STEMI, rather than Hb level or RDW value. This conclusion is supported by a previous study that showed that the symptoms and signs of CHF can be ameliorated by the administration of intravenous iron regardless of whether the patient is anemic or not [2]. Furthermore, administration of an

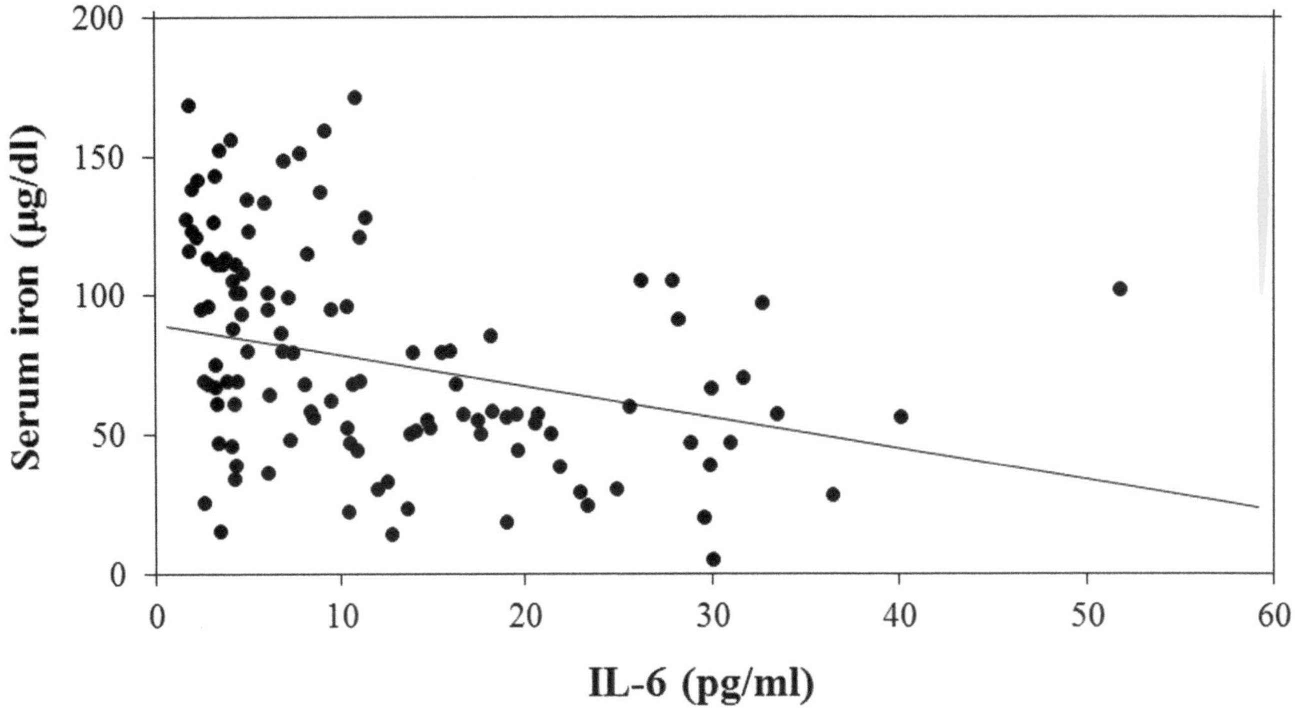

Figure 2. The relationship between serum iron concentration and IL-6 levels in all enrolled subjects. The result indicated that the serum iron concentration was negatively correlated with circulating IL-6 concentration in all study subjects. The linear relationship was well described by Serum iron = 95.994 − 1.246 (IL-6), $R^2 = 0.133$ and $P < 0.001$.

iron chelator after AMI but before PCI does not appear to get clinical benefit [27]. In addition, lower serum iron concentrations are associated with higher concentrations of proinflammatory markers and lower concentrations of the cardioprotectant insulin-like growth factor-1 in ischemic heart disease [28]. These data support the concept that serum ion is tightly regulated.

Iron is an essential micronutrient as it is required for satisfactory erythropoietic function, oxidative metabolism and cellular immune response. Functionally, iron exists in the body in two pools: utilized and stored [1]. Utilized iron consists of circulating and intracellular iron. Iron released into the circulation binds to transferrin and is transported to sites of use and storage [29]. The amount of transferrin-bound iron is around 4 mg, but this is the most important functional dynamic iron pool [29]. The vast majority of intracellular iron is in erythrocyte Hb and circulating reticulocytes. Iron pools interact with each other, and iron can be transferred between these compartments using tightly regulated mechanisms. A normal Hb level with a mean corpuscular Hb (MCH) in the lower limit of the normal range (28–35 pg) or an increased red cell distribution width (RDW, normal range 11–15%) indicates mild iron deficiency without anemia. Although a rising RDW may be an earliest indicator of iron deficiency, the main laboratory finding is a low serum ferritin concentration [1]. However, an RDW value within the reference interval can be used to exclude iron deficiency in those cases in which the serum ferritin concentration does not accurately reflect the iron stores owing to severe tissue damage, as in inflammation [30]. This is the reason why we did not check serum ferritin in STEMI. We also did not measure total iron-binding capacity (TIBC); hence, we were unable to determine participants' complete iron status. However, indirect data suggest that our subjects had normal iron stores, reflected in largely normal MCH and RDW values. Conceptually, a low serum iron concentration might be indicative of a diminished utilized iron pool. Cells with a high mitogenic potential (neoplastic, hematopoietic, immune) [31,32] and high-energy demand (hepatocytes, adipocytes, skeletal and cardiac myocytes, and renal cells) [33,34] are particularly sensitive to depleted iron supplies and/or abnormal iron utilization.

Table 3. The relationship between serum iron and interleukin-6 levels in all subjects.

Parameter	Estimate	SE	95% Confidence interval	*P* value
Intercept	71.872	6.984	58.040–85.704	<0.001**
Group (Control vs. AMI)	35.494	7.440	20.759–50.229	<0.001**
IL-6	−0.625	0.299	−1.218–−0.032	0.039*

(Dependent variable: serum iron concentration).
*$P<0.05$ and **$P<0.001$, general linear model. AMI, acute myocardial infarction; IL-6, interleukin 6; SE, standardized error. The intercept is the predicted value of serum iron concentration in AMI group. The predicted value is 71.872 µg/dl. The serum iron concentration in the control group was, on average, 35.494 µg/dl higher than that in the AMI group. For every one unit increase in IL-6 concentration, there was a decrease of 0.625 units in serum iron concentration.

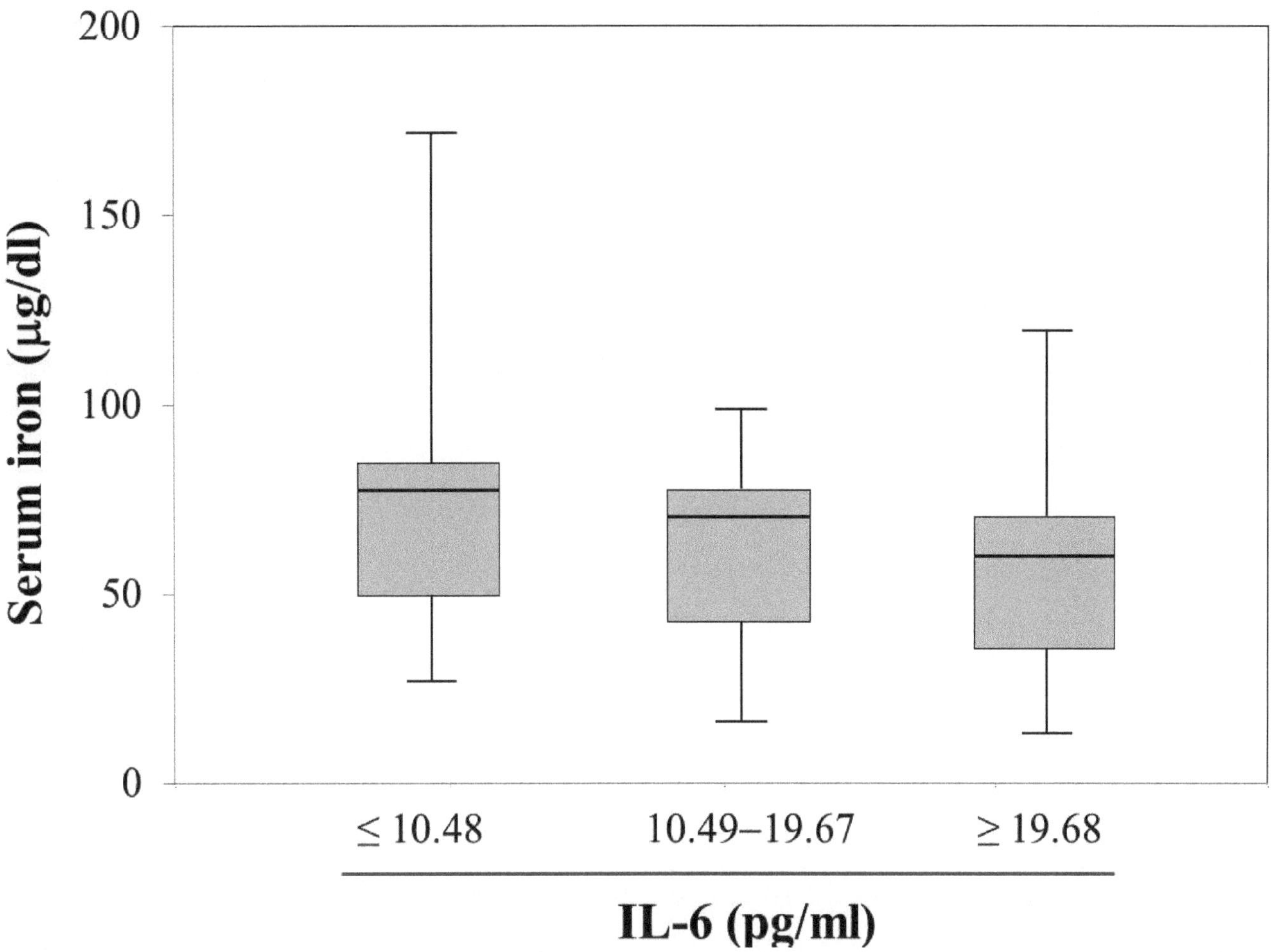

Figure 3. Trend analysis showed serum iron concentration was inversely proportional to IL-6 concentration in STEMI patients. AMI patients were divided into three subgroups according to circulating IL-6 concentration tertile: group 1, IL-6 concentration ≤10.48 pg/ml (n = 19); group 2, IL-6 concentration between 10.49–19.67 pg/ml (n = 20); group 3, IL-6 concentration ≥19.68 pg/ml (n = 16). Trend analysis showed serum iron concentration was inversely proportional to IL-6 concentration. (Jonckheere-Terpstra test, $P = 0.043$).

ACS is a disease characterized by inflammation-induced atherosclerotic plaque rupture, subsequent thrombus formation, coronary artery occlusion, and myocardial oxygen deficiency [35]. Hypoferremia is a common response to systemic infections or generalized inflammatory disorders. A recent longitudinal study demonstrated that IL-6 was a better predictor of CHF after ACS than CRP [13]. Our findings are in broad agreement with a previous report that elevated IL-6 concentrations immediately after AMI were negatively correlated with LV ejection fraction 6 months later [36]. We demonstrated clearly that serum iron concentration was inversely proportional to IL-6 concentration: For every one unit increase in IL-6 concentration, there was a decrease of 0.625 units in serum iron concentration. We also found that serum iron concentration in the control group was on average 35.494 μg/dl higher than that in the AMI group. However, there was no correlation between Hb concentrations and IL-6 concentration. One previous study conducted in human liver cell culture, mice and human volunteers reported that IL-6 was necessary and

Table 4. Lower serum iron concentration is associated with higher inflammatory markers and TIMI risk score after acute myocardial infarction.

	Lower serum iron (<60 μg/dl)	Higher serum iron (≥ 60 μg/dl)	*P* value
	n = 34	n = 21	
IL-6, pg/ml	19.8±14.6	14.2±9.4	0.042*
Fibrinogen, mg/dl	470±93	421±86	0.040*
TIMI risk score	3.10±1.00	2.43±1.27	0.025*

*$P<0.05$, Mann-Whitney U test. TIMI, thrombolysis in myocardial infarction; IL-6, interleukin 6.

Table 5. Multiple linear regression analysis of variables associated with ejection fraction 6 months after primary angioplasty for acute myocardial infarction.

Explanatory variable	Unstandardized Coefficients		Standardized Coefficients	t	*P* value
	B	Std. error	Beta		
(Constant)	106.249	7.684		13.833	0.000
Serum iron	0.069	0.029	0.227	2.415	0.020*
CPK MB	−0.012	0.006	−0.200	−1.965	0.055
IL-6	−0.006	0.082	−0.007	−0.068	0.946
WMSI	−36.606	6.510	−0.631	−5.723	<0.001**
IRA (LAD *vs.* RCA)	0.943	2.670	0.041	0.353	0.725
IRA (LCX *vs.* RCA)	9.890	3.825	0.269	2.585	0.013*

(Dependent variable: ejection fraction at 6 months).
$R^2 = 0.620$.
*$P<0.05$ and **$P<0.001$.
CPK MB, creatine phosphokinase-MB; IL-6, interleukin 6; WMSI, wall motion score index; IRA, infarct related artery; LAD, left anterior descending artery; RCA, right coronary artery; LCX, left circumflex artery.

sufficient for the induction of hepcidin during inflammation, and that the IL-6–hepcidin axis was responsible for inflammation-induced hypoferremia [37]. In rodents [38] and humans [39], AMI was accompanied by increased circulating hepcidin, which subsequently subsided during recovery. These findings led us to postulate that after AMI, circulating IL-6 level increases, followed by elevation in hepcidin and a decrease in serum iron concentrations. However, reduced serum iron concentration represents depletion of the main functional iron pool, which could modulate LV function. Our hypothesis is also supported by the finding that after AMI, increased circulating IL-6 concentrations at baseline and after hospital discharge were associated with heart failure and impaired LV ejection fraction [40]. Low serum iron concentration may explain why activation of proinflammatory factors is believed to enhance myocardial damage, leading to dysfunction and heart failure.

The novelty of our study is that we analyzed the relationship between serum iron concentration and TIMI risk score for STEMI. In patients with ACS, risk scores are useful short- and long-term predictors of death and cardiovascular complications [15,16]. The score is calculated from patients' age, body mass, blood pressure and heart rate on admission and the Killip class. It was significantly higher in patients with low baseline serum iron concentration and *vice versa*, suggesting that serum iron has a protective effect on myocardial function.

The major limitation of the study is that it does not provide mechanistic insight. Other limitations include the relatively small size of the cohort, and the fact that iron status markers were only measured at baseline. Therefore, larger studies of patients with STEMI that measure serum iron concentration, total iron binding capacity and ferritin are needed to further confirm our hypothesis. These might form the basis of intervention studies, to examine whether iron supplementation and/or control of serum IL-6 concentration might have a beneficial effect on the recovery of LV function after STEMI.

Conclusions

We found an association between lower serum iron concentration before PCI and impaired recovery of LV systolic function 6 months later. The circulating concentration of IL-6 was increased after STEMI and negatively correlated with serum iron concentration. Serum iron concentration was also negatively correlated with TIMI risk score. Our findings support the hypothesis that higher serum iron concentration is associated with a cardioprotective phenotype, and that it is a potential prognostic biomarker for complications after STEMI, and may be a novel biomarker that could therapeutic intervention.

Acknowledgments

We would like to thank Dr. Yu-Jun Chang for her contributions to the statistical analysis in the study.

Author Contributions

Conceived and designed the experiments: C-HH C-CC C-S Lin C-S Liu. Performed the experiments: C-LK C-SH. Analyzed the data: C-HH T-WC. Contributed reagents/materials/analysis tools: C-LK C-SH. Wrote the paper: C-HH C-CC. Performed the acquisition of data: C-HH. Contributed to the guidance of experiments: C-S Liu. Read the manuscript and revised it for important intellectual content: C-S Lin T-WC. Read and approved the final manuscript: C-S Lin C-HH C-CC C-LK C-SH T-WC C-S Liu.

References

1. Jankowska EA, von Haehling S, Anker SD, Macdougall IC, Ponikowski P (2013) Iron deficiency and heart failure: diagnostic dilemmas and therapeutic perspectives. European heart journal 34: 816–829.
2. Anker SD, Comin Colet J, Filippatos G, Willenheimer R, Dickstein K, et al. (2009) Ferric carboxymaltose in patients with heart failure and iron deficiency. New England Journal of Medicine 361: 2436–2448.
3. Maeder MT, Khammy O, dos Remedios C, Kaye DM (2011) Myocardial and Systemic Iron Depletion in Heart FailureImplications for Anemia Accompanying Heart Failure. Journal of the American College of Cardiology 58: 474–480.
4. McMurray J, Ponikowski P (2011) Heart FailureNot Enough Pump Iron? Journal of the American College of Cardiology 58: 481–482.
5. Simel DL, DeLong ER, Feussner JR, Weinberg JB, Crawford J (1988) Erythrocyte anisocytosis: visual inspection of blood films vs automated analysis of red blood cell distribution width. Archives of internal medicine 148: 822–824.
6. Uyarel H, Ergelen M, Cicek G, Kaya MG, Ayhan E, et al. (2011) Red cell distribution width as a novel prognostic marker in patients undergoing primary angioplasty for acute myocardial infarction. Coronary artery disease 22: 138–144.
7. Dabbah S, Hammerman H, Markiewicz W, Aronson D (2010) Relation between red cell distribution width and clinical outcomes after acute myocardial infarction. The American journal of cardiology 105: 312–317.

8. Ilhan E, Güvenç TS, Altay S, Çagdas M, Çalik AN, et al. (2012) Predictive value of red cell distribution width in intrahospital mortality and postintervention thrombolysis in myocardial infarction flow in patients with acute anterior myocardial infarction. Coronary artery disease 23: 450–454.
9. Rines AK, Ardehali H (2013) Transition metals and mitochondrial metabolism in the heart. Journal of molecular and cellular cardiology 55: 50–57.
10. Anker SD, Voors A, Okonko D, Clark AL, James MK, et al. (2009) Prevalence, incidence, and prognostic value of anaemia in patients after an acute myocardial infarction: data from the OPTIMAAL trial. European heart journal 30: 1331–1339.
11. Aronson D, Suleiman M, Agmon Y, Suleiman A, Blich M, et al. (2007) Changes in haemoglobin levels during hospital course and long-term outcome after acute myocardial infarction. European heart journal 28: 1289–1296.
12. Nikolsky E, Aymong ED, Halkin A, Grines CL, Cox DA, et al. (2004) Impact of anemia in patients with acute myocardial infarction undergoing primary percutaneous coronary interventionAnalysis from the controlled abciximab and device investigation to lower late angioplasty complications (cadillac) trial. Journal of the American College of Cardiology 44: 547–553.
13. Vasan RS, Sullivan LM, Roubenoff R, Dinarello CA, Harris T, et al. (2003) Inflammatory markers and risk of heart failure in elderly subjects without prior myocardial infarction the Framingham Heart Study. Circulation 107: 1486–1491.
14. Tan J, Hua Q, Li J, Fan Z (2009) Prognostic value of interleukin-6 during a 3-year follow-up in patients with acute ST-segment elevation myocardial infarction. Heart and vessels 24: 329–334.
15. Morrow DA, Antman EM, Charlesworth A, Cairns R, Murphy SA, et al. (2000) TIMI risk score for ST-elevation myocardial infarction: a convenient, bedside, clinical score for risk assessment at presentation an intravenous nPA for treatment of infarcting myocardium early II trial substudy. Circulation 102: 2031–2037.
16. Wiviott SD, Morrow DA, Frederick PD, Giugliano RP, Gibson CM, et al. (2004) Performance of the thrombolysis in myocardial infarction risk index in the National Registry of Myocardial Infarction-3 and-4A simple index that predicts mortality in ST-segment elevation myocardial infarction. Journal of the American College of Cardiology 44: 783–789.
17. Thygesen K, Alpert JS, White HD (2007) Universal definition of myocardial infarction. Journal of the American College of Cardiology 50: 2173–2195.
18. Ndrepepa G, Mehilli J, Martinoff S, Schwaiger M, Schömig A, et al. (2007) Evolution of left ventricular ejection fraction and its relationship to infarct size after acute myocardial infarction. Journal of the American College of Cardiology 50: 149–156.
19. Investigators GA (1993) The effects of tissue plasminogen activator, streptokinase, or both on coronary-artery patency, ventricular function, and survival after acute myocardial infarction. N Engl j Med 329: 1615–1622.
20. Gibson CM, Cannon CP, Murphy SA, Ryan KA, Mesley R, et al. (2000) Relationship of TIMI myocardial perfusion grade to mortality after administration of thrombolytic drugs. Circulation 101: 125–130.
21. Ellis SG, Vandormael MG, Cowley MJ, DiSciascio G, Deligonul U, et al. (1990) Coronary morphologic and clinical determinants of procedural outcome with angioplasty for multivessel coronary disease. Implications for patient selection. Multivessel Angioplasty Prognosis Study Group. Circulation 82: 1193–1202.
22. Schiller NB, Shah P, Crawford M, DeMaria A, Devereux R, et al. (1988) Recommendations for quantitation of the left ventricle by two-dimensional echocardiography. American Society of Echocardiography Committee on Standards, Subcommittee on Quantitation of Two-Dimensional Echocardiograms. Journal of the American Society of Echocardiography: official publication of the American Society of Echocardiography 2: 358–367.
23. Quiñones MA, Otto CM, Stoddard M, Waggoner A, Zoghbi WA (2002) Recommendations for quantification of Doppler echocardiography: a report from the Doppler Quantification Task Force of the Nomenclature and Standards Committee of the American Society of Echocardiography. Journal of the American Society of Echocardiography 15: 167–184.
24. Lang RM, Bierig M, Devereux RB, Flachskampf FA, Foster E, et al. (2005) Recommendations for chamber quantification: a report from the American Society of Echocardiography's Guidelines and Standards Committee and the Chamber Quantification Writing Group, developed in conjunction with the European Association of Echocardiography, a branch of the European Society of Cardiology. Journal of the American Society of Echocardiography 18: 1440–1463.
25. Feigenbaum H (1990) Role of echocardiography in acute myocardial infarction. The American journal of cardiology 66: H17–H22.
26. Lenth RV (2010) Java applets for power and sample size (computer software) 2006–9. Available: http://www.stat.uiowa.edu/~rlenth/Power. Accessed 2014 Jun 08.
27. Chan W, Taylor AJ, Ellims AH, Lefkovits L, Wong C, et al. (2012) Effect of Iron Chelation on Myocardial Infarct Size and Oxidative Stress in ST-Elevation–Myocardial Infarction. Circulation: Cardiovascular Interventions 5: 270–278.
28. Lee S-D, Huang C-Y, Shu W-T, Chen T-H, Lin JA, et al. (2006) Pro-inflammatory states and IGF-I level in ischemic heart disease with low or high serum iron. Clinica chimica acta 370: 50–56.
29. Muñoz M, García-Erce JA, Remacha ÁF (2011) Disorders of iron metabolism. Part 1: molecular basis of iron homoeostasis. Journal of clinical pathology 64: 281–286.
30. Zeben D, Bieger R, Wermeskerken RK, Castel A, Hermans J (1990) Evaluation of microcytosis using serum ferritin and red blood cell distribution width. European journal of haematology 44: 106–109.
31. Kell DB (2009) Iron behaving badly: inappropriate iron chelation as a major contributor to the aetiology of vascular and other progressive inflammatory and degenerative diseases. BMC medical genomics 2: 2.
32. Hower V, Mendes P, Torti FM, Laubenbacher R, Akman S, et al. (2009) A general map of iron metabolism and tissue-specific subnetworks. Molecular bioSystems 5: 422–443.
33. Cairo G, Bernuzzi F, Recalcati S (2006) A precious metal: Iron, an essential nutrient for all cells. Genes & nutrition 1: 25–39.
34. Beard JL (2001) Iron biology in immune function, muscle metabolism and neuronal functioning. The Journal of Nutrition 131: 568S–580S.
35. Libby P, Ridker PM, Maseri A (2002) Inflammation and atherosclerosis. Circulation 105: 1135–1143.
36. Karpiński L, Płaksej R, Kosmala W, Witkowska M (2008) Serum levels of interleukin-6, interleukin-10 and C-reactive protein in relation to left ventricular function in patients with myocardial infarction treated with primary angioplasty. Kardiologia polska 66: 1279–1285.
37. Nemeth E, Rivera S, Gabayan V, Keller C, Taudorf S, et al. (2004) IL-6 mediates hypoferremia of inflammation by inducing the synthesis of the iron regulatory hormone hepcidin. Journal of Clinical Investigation 113: 1271–1276.
38. Simonis G, Mueller K, Schwarz P, Wiedemann S, Adler G, et al. (2010) The iron-regulatory peptide hepcidin is upregulated in the ischemic and in the remote myocardium after myocardial infarction. Peptides 31: 1786–1790.
39. Suzuki H, Toba K, Kato K, Ozawa T, Tomosugi N, et al. (2009) Serum hepcidin-20 is elevated during the acute phase of myocardial infarction. Tohoku journal of experimental medicine 218.
40. Gabriel AS, Martinsson A, Wretlind B, Ahnve S (2004) IL-6 levels in acute and post myocardial infarction: their relation to CRP levels, infarction size, left ventricular systolic function, and heart failure. European Journal of Internal Medicine 15: 523–528.

13

Quercetin Inhibits Intestinal Iron Absorption and Ferroportin Transporter Expression *In Vivo* and *In Vitro*

Marija Lesjak[1,2]⁹, Rukshana Hoque[3]⁹, Sara Balesaria[1], Vernon Skinner[1], Edward S. Debnam[4], Surjit K. S. Srai[1]*, Paul A. Sharp[3]*

1 Research Department of Structural and Molecular Biology, Division of Biosciences, University College London, London, United Kingdom, **2** Department of Chemistry, Biochemistry and Environmental Protection, Faculty of Sciences University of Novi Sad, Novi Sad, Serbia, **3** Diabetes & Nutritional Sciences Division, King's College London, London, United Kingdom, **4** Research Department of Neuroscience, Physiology and Pharmacology, Division of Biosciences, University College London, Royal Free Campus, London, United Kingdom

Abstract

Balancing systemic iron levels within narrow limits is critical for maintaining human health. There are no known pathways to eliminate excess iron from the body and therefore iron homeostasis is maintained by modifying dietary absorption so that it matches daily obligatory losses. Several dietary factors can modify iron absorption. Polyphenols are plentiful in human diet and many compounds, including quercetin – the most abundant dietary polyphenol – are potent iron chelators. The aim of this study was to investigate the acute and longer-term effects of quercetin on intestinal iron metabolism. Acute exposure of rat duodenal mucosa to quercetin increased apical iron uptake but decreased subsequent basolateral iron efflux into the circulation. Quercetin binds iron between its 3-hydroxyl and 4-carbonyl groups and methylation of the 3-hydroxyl group negated both the increase in apical uptake and the inhibition of basolateral iron release, suggesting that the acute effects of quercetin on iron transport were due to iron chelation. In longer-term studies, rats were administered quercetin by a single gavage and iron transporter expression measured 18 h later. Duodenal FPN expression was decreased in quercetin-treated rats. This effect was recapitulated in Caco-2 cells exposed to quercetin for 18 h. Reporter assays in Caco-2 cells indicated that repression of FPN by quercetin was not a transcriptional event but might be mediated by miRNA interaction with the FPN 3′UTR. Our study highlights a novel mechanism for the regulation of iron bioavailability by dietary polyphenols. Potentially, diets rich in polyphenols might be beneficial for patients groups at risk of iron loading by limiting the rate of intestinal iron absorption.

Editor: James F. Collins, University of Florida, United States of America

Funding: This study was supported by a Biotechnology and Biological Sciences Research Council (BBSRC) project grant (BB/H003576/1) awarded to Kaila Srai. Marija Lesjak was supported by Dr. Willmar Schwabe Research Scholarship for Young Scientists awarded by Society for Medicinal Plant and Natural Product Research and Ministry of Education and Sciences Republic of Serbia (Grant No. 172058). Rukshana Hoque was supported by an MRC Doctoral Training Award. The funders had no role in study design, data collection and analysis, decision to publish, or preparation of the manuscript.

Competing Interests: The authors have declared that no competing interests exist.

* Email: k.srai@ucl.ac.uk (SKSS); paul.a.sharp@kcl.ac.uk (PAS)

⁹ These authors contributed equally to this work.

Introduction

Iron is an essential transition metal that plays an important role in all mammalian organisms. It is incorporated into a diverse array of proteins, including the oxygen carriers haemoglobin and myoglobin, cytochrome complexes involved in electron transfer in the mitochondria, and enzymes participating in nucleic acid processing such as ribonucleotide reductase [1,2]. Balancing systemic iron levels within narrow limits is critical for human health, as both iron deficiency and iron overload leads to serious haematological, metabolic and neurodegenerative disorders. In mammals there are no known pathways to eliminate excess iron from the body and therefore iron homeostasis is maintained by modifying dietary absorption so that it matches daily obligatory losses [1].

There are two forms of dietary iron, haem and non-haem iron. Non-haem iron is the major dietary form but its bioavailability depends on presence of other dietary factors which either enhance or inhibit absorption in the duodenum [3,4]. Non-haem iron is present almost entirely in the ferric (Fe^{3+}) form; however, to be bioavailable it must first be reduced to ferrous (Fe^{2+}). This is achieved by the combined action of duodenal cytochrome b (Dcytb), a ferri-reductase which resides on the apical membrane of duodenal enterocytes [5,6], or exogenous dietary reducing agents, such as ascorbic acid (reviewed in [4]). Reduced iron is then transported across the membrane into the enterocyte via the apical iron transporter, divalent metal transporter-1 (DMT1) [7]. Subsequently, ferrous iron is transferred across the basolateral membrane of the enterocyte via the iron exporter, ferroportin (FPN) [8–10] and re-oxidized by ferroxidase hephaestin [11] on the basolateral surface, prior to loading onto transferrin.

In addition to enhancers of iron bioavailability there are a number of dietary components that act as potent inhibitors of intestinal iron absorption, including phytic acid and polyphenolic compounds [4]. Polyphenols are natural products, which are abundant in food of plant origin, and are thus an integral part of our diet. Dietary polyphenols are receiving increasing attention due to their proven health benefits for a variety of disorders [12]. The inhibitory potential of flavonoid polyphenols on non-haem iron absorption in duodenum has been demonstrated both *in vivo* and *in vitro* [13–17]. These studies provide convincing evidence that polyphenols modify intestinal iron absorption in single meal studies in human volunteers and acute *in vitro* experiments; however, the longer-term effect of consuming elevated levels of polyphenolic compounds on iron status is less clear. It is possible that chronic consumption of diets poor in iron and rich in inhibitors of iron bioavailability could contribute to the burden of iron deficiency in certain population groups. However, there may be benefits of consuming a polyphenol-enriched diet for groups at risk of iron loading, for example patients with hereditary haemochromatosis.

The flavonol quercetin is the most abundant dietary flavonoid and is especially enriched in onions, tea and apples [18]. It is conservatively estimated that humans consume approximately 40 – 80 mg of flavonoids/day [19]; and that quercetin contributes approximately 25% of total flavonoid intake (i.e. 10–20 mg/day) [20]. In common with most polyphenols, quercetin is found almost exclusively in foods as glycoside conjugates but can be converted rapidly into the aglycone in the intestinal lumen via the actions of glycosidases [21,22]. In this study we have investigated the acute and longer-term effects of quercetin on iron metabolism *in vivo* (in rats) and *in vitro* (Caco-2 cells).

Material and Methods

Animals and treatments

Rats were supplied by the Comparative Biology Unit, Royal Free Campus, UCL Medical School, London, UK. All experimental procedures were approved by the University College London local animal ethics committee and were conducted in accordance with the UK Animals (Scientific Procedures) Act, 1986. After weaning (three weeks old) Sprague-Dawley male rats were placed on low iron (25 ppm) diet for two weeks and allowed free access to water throughout. At the end of the experimental procedure animals were killed by administering a terminal dose of pentobarbitone sodium (120 mg/Kg body weight).

Acute effects of quercetin on iron uptake

For acute studies, rats were anesthetized with 60 mg/Kg pentobarbitone sodium IP and 5 cm long segments of duodenum (starting 1 cm distal to the pylorus) were cannulated and rinsed free of their contents with warm saline (0.9% w/v of NaCl), followed by air. Uptake buffer (200 µL), containing Na-HEPES (14.6 mmol/L), NaCl (127.4 mmol/L), KCl (3.2 mmol/L), ascorbic acid (4.0 mmol/L), $^{59}FeCl_3$ (0.2 mmol/L) and 1 mmol/L of either quercetin (Sigma-Aldrich, UK) (Q) or 3-*O*-methylquercetin (Extrasynthese, France) (3MQ) or 4′-*O*-methylquercetin (Extrasynthese) (4′MQ) or quercetin 3,4′-dimethylquercetin (ABCR GmbH, Germany) (3,4′dMQ) or penta-methylquercetin (Extrasynthese) (PMQ) (Stock solutions prepared in DMSO:ethanol [1:1]) was instilled into the duodenal segment, which was then tied off. In control groups, DMSO:ethanol (1:1) was added to buffer instead of the polyphenols. Structures of polyphenolic compounds are shown in Figure S1. Rat body temperature was maintained at 37°C using a thermostatically controlled heating blanket. After 30 minutes, blood samples (≤2 mL) were collected via cardiac puncture and the segment of duodenum was removed and washed with approximately 40 mL of solution containing 154 mmol/L NaCl, 0.1 mmol/L ascorbic acid, 0.01 mmol/L $FeCl_3$ to displace any ^{59}Fe bound to the mucosal surface. Subsequently, the duodenal mucosa was scraped away, the blood and mucosa samples were weighed and gamma counted for determination of ^{59}Fe activity. Results were expressed as percentage of absorbed radioactive iron retained in duodenal mucosa or transferred to blood. The percentage of ^{59}Fe transferred to the entire blood volume of the animal was calculated using the equation: total blood volume = (body weight*0.06) +0.77 [23].

Effects of oral gavage of quercetin on iron metabolism

In order to investigate the longer-term effects of quercetin administration on non-haem iron absorption, animals were gavaged with a single dose of quercetin (50 mg/kg dissolved in 10% DMSO) or vehicle (control) eighteen hours before experiments. Animals were anesthetized with pentobarbitone sodium (60 mg/Kg body weight) injected IP. The duodenum and liver were collected, snap frozen in liquid N_2, and stored at −80°C for real-time PCR analysis and tissue non-haem iron determination.

RNA extraction and RT-PCR

Duodenal RNA was extracted with TRIzol (Invitrogen) according to the manufacturer's instructions. Total RNA (1 µg) was reverse transcribed using the Verso cDNA reverse transcription kit (Thermo-Fisher Scientific), according to the manufacturer's instructions. Real-time PCR reactions were performed using a Roche Lightcycler using GAPDH as internal standard. Each reaction was performed in duplicate and contained 10 pmol of specific primers (Table S1), 1× SYBR Green Mastermix (Qiagen), and 1 µL of cDNA in a 20 µL reaction. Samples without cDNA were included as negative controls. Cycle threshold (Ct) values were obtained for each gene of interest and the GAPDH internal standard. Gene expression was normalized to GAPDH and represented as ΔCt values. For each sample the mean of the ΔCt values was calculated. Relative gene expression was normalized to 1.0 (100%) of controls.

Levels of tissue non-haem iron

Quantitative measurement of non-haem iron was performed according to the modified method of Torrance and Bothwell [24]. Briefly, 20–50 mg of duodenum was dried at 55°C for 72 hours and subsequently weighed. Dried samples were digested in 1 mL acid mixture (30% (v/v) HCl and 10% (w/v) trichloroacetic acid) at 65°C for 20 hours. 1 mL of chromogen reagent (0.1% (w/v) bathophenanthrolinesulfonate; 1% (v/v) thioglycolic acid in 50% (w/v) sodium acetate solution) and samples were incubated at 37°C for 10 minutes, after which the absorbance of samples and iron standards was measured at 535 nm. Results were reported as µg iron/g tissue dry weight.

Serum biochemistry

Serum iron and transferrin saturation were measured using a commercial ferrozine-based colorimetric assay according to the manufacturer's instructions (Pointe Scientific, USA).

Cell culture

Caco-2 TC7 cells were originally obtained from Drs Monique Rousset and Edith Brot-Laroche (CRC, Jussieu, Paris) [25] and have been characterised for studies on iron transport [26]. Cells (passages 40-45) were seeded onto Transwell inserts in 6-well plates at a density of 40,000 cells per well and cultured for 19 d in DMEM containing 10% foetal bovine serum.

For acute uptake studies, cells were pre-treated with quercetin (10 or 100 µmol/L) for 15 min to permit equilibration in uptake buffer; quercetin remained present during the uptake assay. For chronic studies, cells were exposed for 18 h at their apical surface to quercetin. However, prior to uptake measurements, the incubation medium was discarded and cells were washed to remove quercetin.

In vitro iron transport

Iron uptake was measured as described previously [27]. Briefly, a transepithelial pH gradient was established by adding Mes-buffered saline (pH 5.5; 140 mmol/L NaCl, 5 mmol/L KCl, 1 mmol/L Na_2HPO_4, 1 mmol/L $CaCl_2$, 0.5 mmol/L $MgCl_2$, 5 mmol/L glucose, and 10 mmol/L Mes) and adding Hepes-buffered saline (pH 7.5; same ionic composition but containing 10 mmol/l Hepes in place of Mes and 0.2% bovine serum albumin) to the basolateral chamber. Studies were initiated by the addition of 10 µmol/L $^{55}FeCl_3$ complexed with 1 mmol/L ascorbic acid to the apical well of the Transwell plate. Uptake into the cells was measured over 20 min. To measure iron efflux, cells were incubated for 1 h in buffer containing $^{55}FeCl_3$, washed and placed in fresh medium, and incubated for a further 2 h at 37 C. At the end of the experiments cells were washed thoroughly in uptake buffer containing iron and solubilized in 0.2 mmol/L NaOH. Basolateral medium from efflux assays was collected and aliquots of the solubilized cell fraction and basolateral medium were subjected to liquid scintillation counting. Data were normalized to amounts of total protein/well.

PCR

Total RNA was isolated from cells cultured for 18 h in the presence of quercetin using TRIzol. Following first strand cDNA synthesis, expression levels of iron transporter mRNA and GAPDH mRNA (used as a housekeeping gene) were analysed by real-time quantitative PCR using an ABI Prism 7700HT Sequence Detection System and a Power SYBR Green PCR master mix kit (Applied Biosystems Cheshire, UK). The primer sequences used for each gene are given in Table S1. Quantitative measurements of iron transporter relative to GAPDH gene expression were derived using the ΔCt method. Data have been normalised to the untreated control group in each experiment and are presented as the mean ± S.E.M.

Western blotting

Caco-2 cells were harvested into ice-cold lysis buffer (PBS containing 1% sodium dodecyl sulphate and 10 mg/L protease inhibitor cocktail) and homogenized by repeated passing through at 25-gauge needle. Protein samples (40 µg) were solubilised in sample loading buffer and subjected to polyacrylamide gel electrophoresis. Following immobilization on nitrocellulose, the proteins were exposed to commercially available antibodies to either DMT1 (NRAMP24A; 1:1000 dilution, Alpha Diagnostics, TX, USA), FPN (MTP11A, 1:1000 dilution, Alpha Diagnostics) or β-actin (1:1000 dilution, Sigma-Aldrich). Cross-reactivity was observed using a horseradish peroxidase-linked secondary antibody (Dako) and ECL Plus (GE Healthcare).

Cell ferritin levels

Cells were incubated with 10 µmol/L $FeCl_3$ in the presence or absence of quercetin (0.1–10 µmol/L) for 18 h. Cells were washed with PBS before being lysed in ice-cold lysis buffer (10 mmol/L Tris-HCl, pH 7.5, 50 mmol/L NaCl, 1% Triton X-100, 10 mg/L protease inhibitor cocktail). 20 µg of cellular protein was used to measure cell ferritin using a commercially available ELISA kit (RAMCO Laboratories).

Reporter assays

FPN 5′-promoter-luciferase constructs were provided by Drs D-L Zhang and T. Rouault (National Institute of Child Health and Human Development, USA). MISSION FPN 3′-UTR-Renilla luciferase reporter construct was purchased from Sigma-Aldrich UK. Caco-2 cells were seeded in 24-well plates and grown to 60-80% confluence. Cells were transfected with reporter constructs and control plasmids using FuGENE HD transfection reagent (Promega UK). After 24 h, cells were treated with quercetin (10 µmol/L) for 18 h and luciferase activity measured (in duplicate, in 3 plates of cells, repeated in at least 2 individual passages; n = 6–9) using a Promega dual-luciferase reporter assay system.

Statistics

All data are expressed as means ± SEM. Statistical analysis was carried out using SigmaPlot (version 12, Systat Software Inc. IL, USA). Student's unpaired t-test or one-way ANOVA followed by Tukey's post-hoc test were used where appropriate to detect statistical differences ($P<0.05$) between control and test groups.

Results

Acute exposure to quercetin increases apical iron uptake but decreases basolateral iron efflux

To investigate the acute effects of quercetin on duodenal iron absorption, the *in situ* duodenal loop method was used [28] where either quercetin (aglycone) or methylated quercetin isoforms were introduced into rat duodenum together with radioactive iron. In the presence of quercetin, 3MQ, 4′MQ or 3,4′dMQ, but not PMQ, there was a significant increase in mucosal ^{59}Fe uptake compared with the untreated control group (Figure 1A). The increase in uptake was significantly higher in the presence of quercetin aglycone and 4′MQ compared with the other methylated forms. In contrast, ^{59}Fe release from the intestinal mucosa into the blood was significantly diminished in the presence of quercetin and 4′MQ compared with other methylated-quercetin compounds and the untreated controls (Figure 1B).

The acute stimulation of iron uptake as well as inhibition of iron efflux in the presence of quercetin aglycone was recapitulated in intestinal Caco-2 cell monolayers (Figure 1C,D).

Quercetin decreases intestinal FPN expression

18 hours after oral administration of a single dose of quercetin, quantitative RT-PCR analysis of rat duodenal iron transporters revealed significant down regulation of DMT1 and FPN mRNA levels (Figure 2A). In the same animals there was a significant increase in non-haem iron content of the duodenum, a significant decrease in serum iron and transferrin saturation and a decrease in liver hepcidin mRNA expression (60%) which did not reach statistical significance compared with control animals (Table 1).

To distinguish between the direct effects of quercetin on iron transporter expression, and possible indirect influences resulting from either increased duodenal iron content or changes in hepcidin levels, we employed Caco-2 cells as a model of human intestinal epithelial cells. In contrast to data from rat studies, there was no effect of quercetin on DMT1 mRNA or protein levels in Caco-2 cells (Figure 2B,D). However, FPN mRNA and protein expression were decreased significantly by exposure to quercetin in a dose-dependent manner (Figure 2C,E).

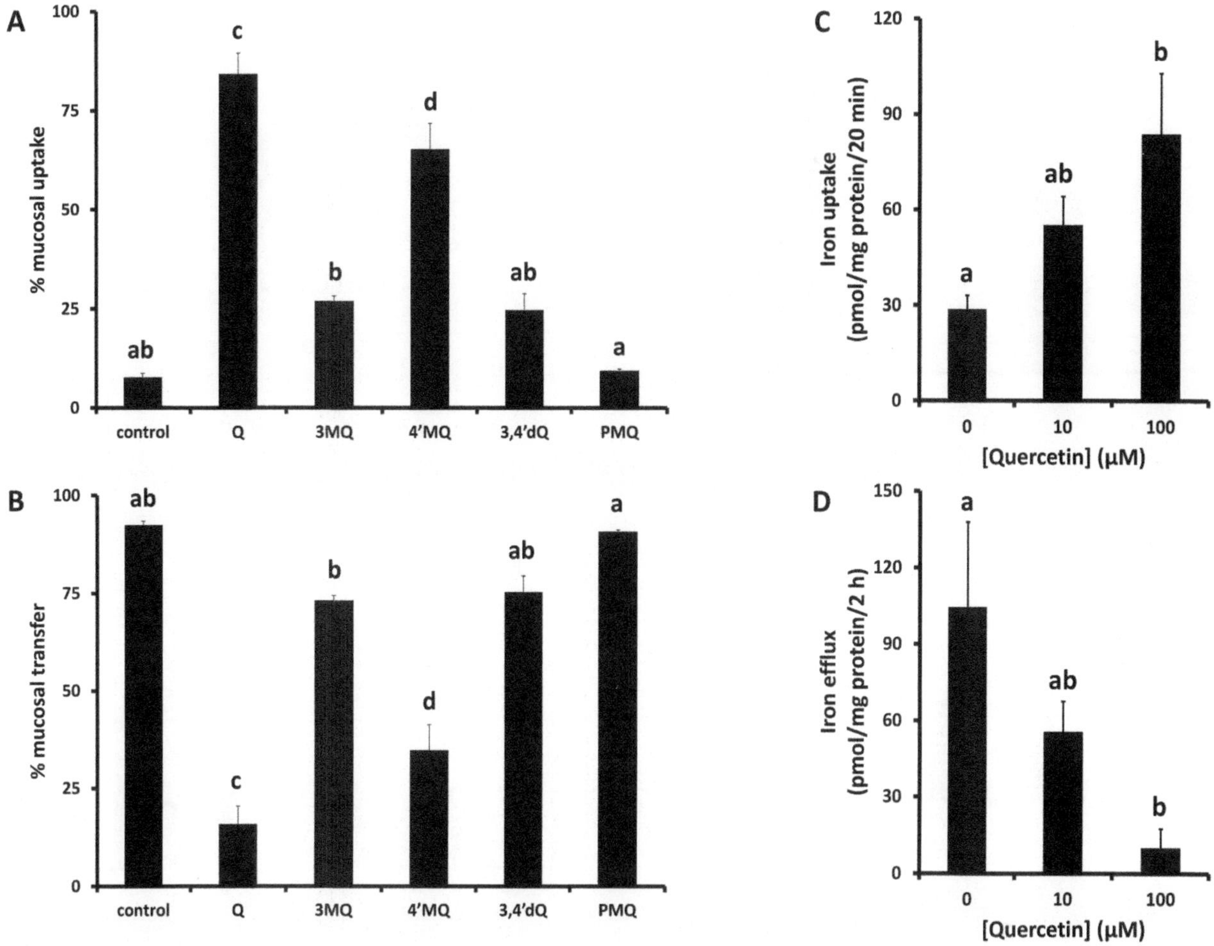

Figure 1. Acute effects of quercetin on intestinal iron transport. The acute effects of quercetin and its methylated analogues (3MQ, 4′MQ, 3,4′dMQ, PMQ) on iron transport *in vivo* were measured using the *in situ* duodenal loop method. ^{59}Fe (0.2 mmol/L) and polyphenol (1 mmol/L) were added to the lumenal uptake buffer and mucosal iron uptake (A) and mucosal transfer of iron into the circulation (B) measured. The effects of quercetin on iron uptake across the apical membrane (C) and iron efflux across the basolateral membrane (D) of human intestinal Caco-2 cells was also measured. Data are mean ± SEM of 4 (rat duodenum) or 4–5 (Caco-2 cells) observations in each group. Groups with no common letters are significantly different from each other (one-way ANOVA and Tukey's post hoc test; $P<0.05$).

To determine the cellular effects of quercetin on iron transport, Caco-2 cells were washed to remove any residual lumenal quercetin and placed in fresh quercetin-free uptake buffer prior to measurement of iron transport. The initial rate of iron uptake into cells was not significantly altered following quercetin treatment (Figure 3A). However, there was a significant decrease in iron efflux into the basolateral medium in cells exposed to quercetin (Figure 3B).

To investigate the cellular fate of cellular iron in quercetin-treated Caco-2 cells we measured cell ferritin content (the main cellular iron storage molecule). Following exposure to quercetin there was a significant decrease in ferritin protein levels (Figure 4).

Quercetin did not alter FPN 5′-promoter activity in Caco-2 cells

Next we investigated whether the inhibitory effects of quercetin on FPN protein and mRNA were mediate via altered gene transcription. Two FPN mRNA isoforms have been identified in Caco-2 cells; FPN1A and FPN1B, respectively [29]. Reporter assays with luciferase reporter constructs containing 1Kb of either the FPN1A or FPN1B 5′-promoter indicated that FPN1A is the dominant isoform in Caco-2 cells having 4-5 fold higher basal activity than the FPN1B promoter (Figure 5A). However, there was no effect of quercetin on the luciferase activity of either FPN promoter construct (Figure 5 B,C).

Quercetin decreases 3′-UTR reporter activity in Caco-2 cells

Polyphenols are known to be potent regulators of micro-RNA (miRNA) expression and activity. We therefore investigated whether quercetin might regulate FPN mRNA levels in Caco-2 cells via miRNA interaction with its 3′UTR. In reporter assays in Caco-2 cells transfected with a Renilla-luciferase reporter construct containing the 3′ UTR of human FPN, exposure to quercetin significantly decreased reporter activity (Figure 6A).

Next we attempted to identify potential miRNA species that might be involved in these regulatory events. First, we used arrays to identify miRNA species up-regulated by quercetin in Caco-2 cells. Expression of 33 miRNAs were increased >1.5-fold in quercetin-treated cells compared with untreated controls (Table S2). Next we used web-based bioinformatics packages (TargetScan www.targetscan.org; and miRBase www.mirbase.org) to determine

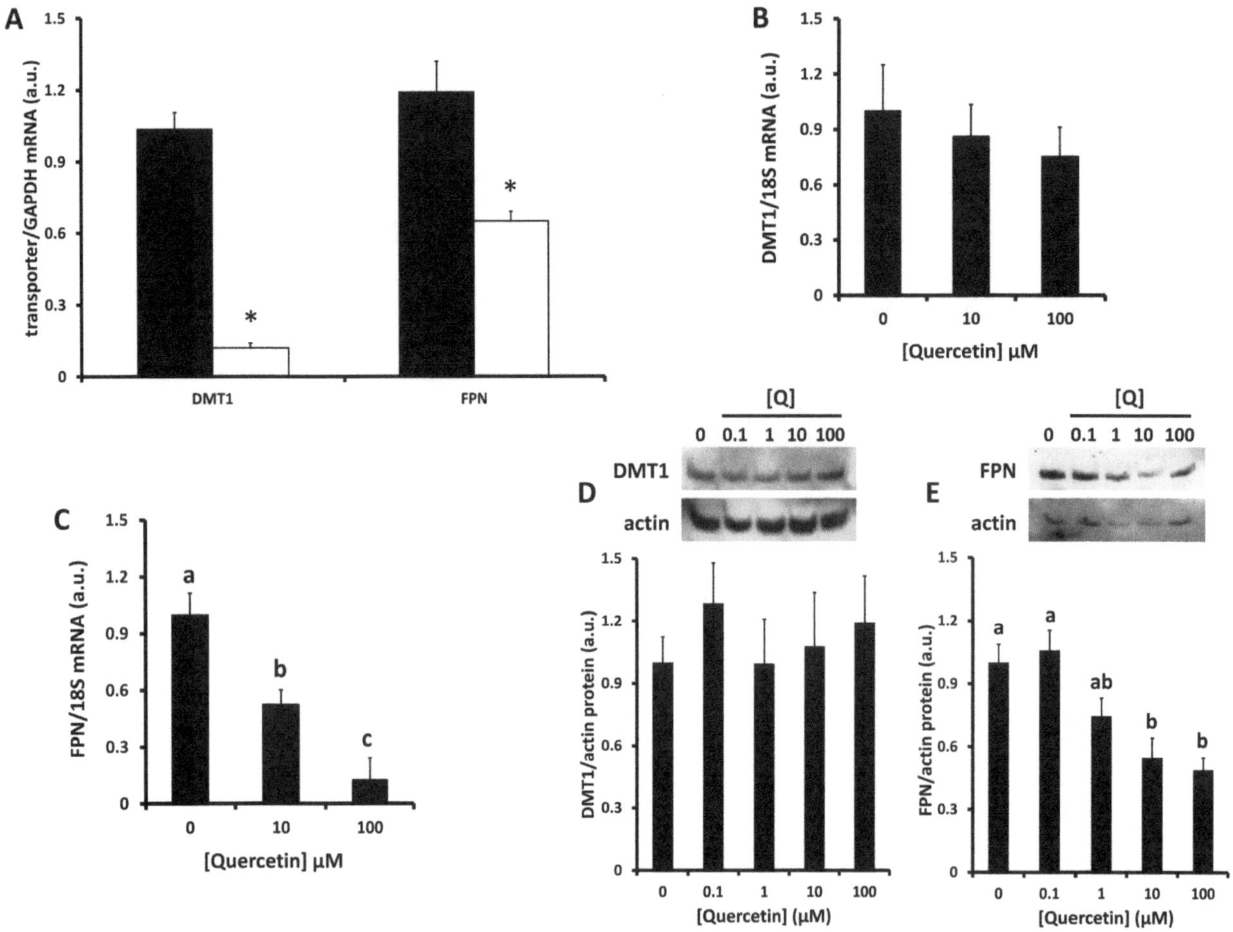

Figure 2. Effects of longer-term exposure to quercetin on intestinal iron transporter expression. Rats (A) were given a single gavage containing quercetin (50 mg/Kg body weight). Caco-2 cells (B & C) were exposed to quercetin (10 or 100 µM). After 18 h RNA was isolated from duodenal tissue (A) and Caco-2 cells (B,C) and used to measure changes in iron transporter mRNA expression. (D,E) Whole cell protein was isolated from Caco-2 cells and used for western blotting to measure DMT1 and FPN protein. Data are mean ± SEM of 4 (rat duodenum) or 7-18 (Caco-2 cells) observations in each group. (A) *P<0.05 compared with control group (Student's unpaired t-test). (B – E) Groups with no common letters are significantly different from each other (one-way ANOVA and Tukey's post hoc test; P<0.05). No letters indicates no significant difference between any of the groups.

if any up-regulated miRNAs had consensus binding sites in the human FPN 3′-UTR (Table S3). Binding sites for 2 members of the miR-17 family, miR-17-3p (bases 61-67 of the 3′UTR sequence) and miR-17-5p (2 sites at bases 1132-1138 and 1166-1172), respectively, were present in the FPN 3′UTR (Figure S2). Finally, we used qPCR to validate the array data to determine whether expression of the miR-17 species was altered following quercetin treatment. miR-17-3p was strongly up-regulated in quercetin-treated Caco-2 cells (Figure 6B). In contrast, there was no significant effect of quercetin on the expression of miR-17-5p (Figure 6C). Furthermore, expression levels of miR-485-3p, which has 2 consensus binding sites in the FPN 3′UTR (at bases 448-454 and 618–625, respectively) and has been shown to be involved in the inhibition of FPN expression by iron deficiency in HepG2 cells [30], were not altered in quercetin-treated Caco-2 cells (Figure 6D).

Table 1. Markers of iron status in control and quercetin-treated rats.

	Control	Quercetin-treated
Duodenal non-haem iron (µg/g dry weight)	22.9±1.2 (4)	32.5±1.5 (4)*
Serum iron (µg/dL)	140.9±15.1 (4)	90.7±3.9 (4)*
Transferrin saturation (%)	27.6±2.5 (4)	18.9±1.0 (4)*
Liver hepcidin mRNA (a.u.)	0.6±0.3 (4)	0.2±0.1 (4)[NS]

Data are means ± SEM (n). *P<0.05 compared with control group. [NS] Not significantly different from control group.

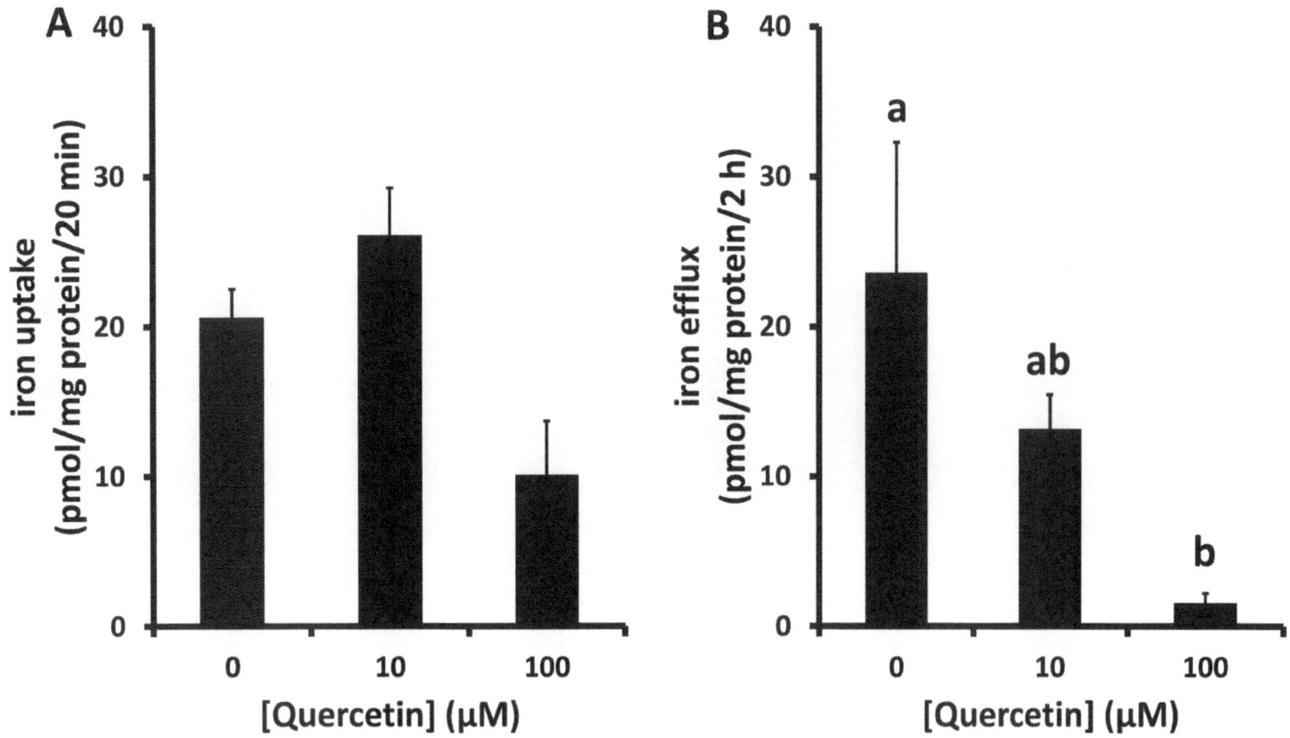

Figure 3. Effects of longer-term exposure to quercetin on iron transport in Caco-2 cells. Caco-2 cells were exposed to quercetin (10 or 100 µM) for 18 h. Quercetin was removed by washing and cells were incubated in quercetin-free uptake buffer containing ^{59}Fe. Uptake across the apical membrane (A) and efflux across the basolateral membrane (B) was determined. Data are mean ± SEM of 5-6 observations in each group. Groups with no common letters are significantly different from each other (one-way ANOVA and Tukey's post hoc test; $P<0.05$). No letters indicates no significant difference between any of the groups.

Discussion

Several independent studies have established that polyphenols significantly decrease non-haem iron absorption in duodenum [13–17]; however, the exact mechanism of action is unknown. Based on the data from our current study we discuss four possible mechanisms that might underlie the inhibitory effects of quercetin on intestinal iron transport: 1. Iron chelation; 2. Circulating iron and hepcidin levels; 3. Cellular iron levels; 4. Direct effects of quercetin on intestinal iron transporter expression.

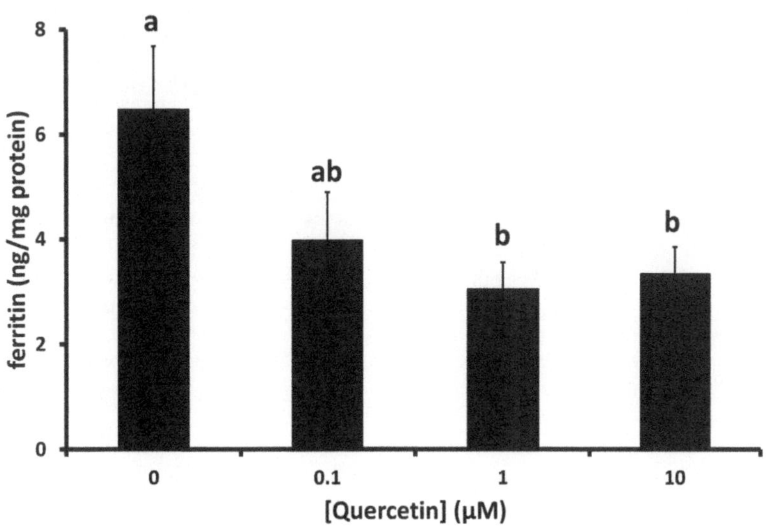

Figure 4. Effects of quercetin on ferritin protein levels in Caco-2 cells. Caco-2 cells were exposed to quercetin (10 or 100 µM) for 18 h. Cells were solubilised and aqueous extracts used to measured cell ferritin protein content using a commercially available ELISA. Data are mean ± SEM of 15 observations in each group. Groups with no common letters are significantly different from each other (one-way ANOVA and Tukey's post hoc test; $P<0.05$).

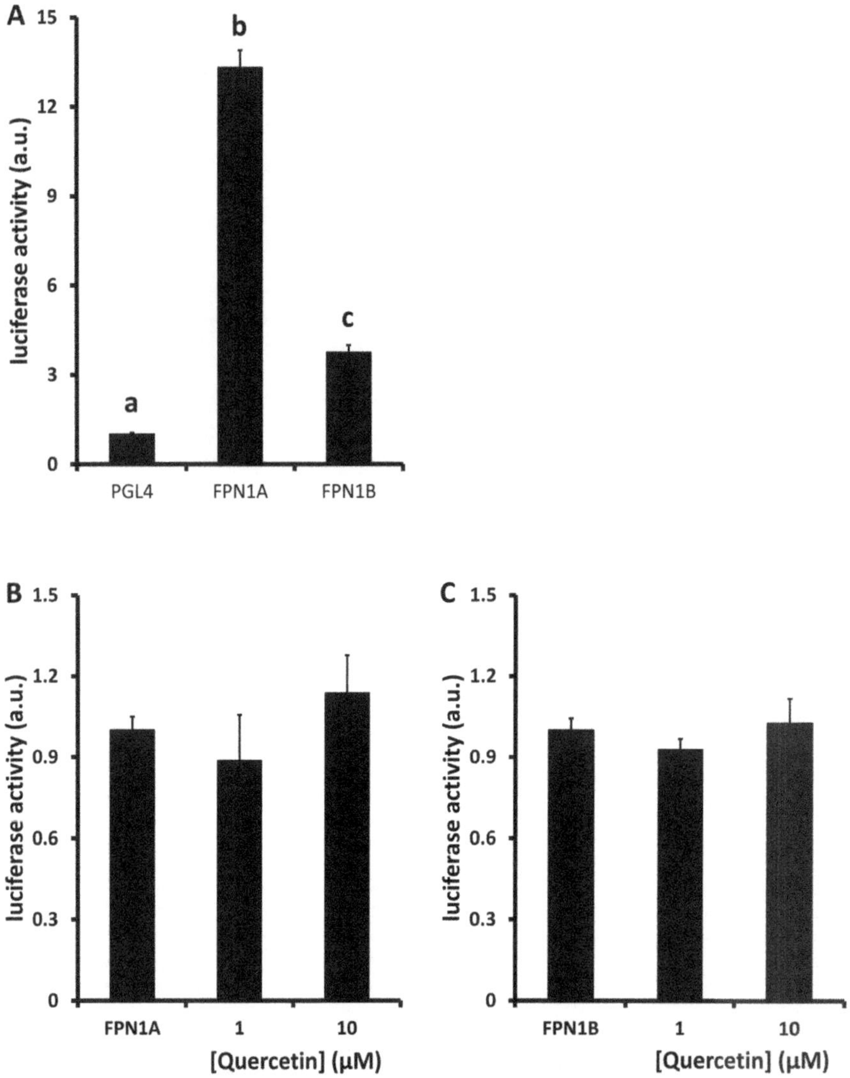

Figure 5. Effects of quercetin on FPN promoter activity. Caco-2 cells were transfected with luciferase reporter constructs containing 1Kb of either FPN1A or FPN1B 5′ promoter, or with the empty PGL4 plasmid. Luciferase activity (normalised to renilla) arising from basal activity of the promoters (A) and following exposure to quercetin (1 or 10 μM) for 18 h (B) was measured using the Dual Luciferase Reporter Assay (Promega). Data are mean ± SEM of 6-9 observations in each group. Groups with no common letters are significantly different from each other (one-way ANOVA and Tukey's post hoc test; $P<0.05$). No letters indicates no significant difference between any of the groups.

1. Iron chelation

Our acute *in vivo* iron transport data demonstrated that quercetin increases iron uptake and retention by the duodenal mucosa. We argued that iron chelation by quercetin could play important role in this phenomenon. It has previously been shown that the preferred site for iron chelation by quercetin is between the 3-hydroxyl and 4-carbonyl group; for complexes containing one iron and one quercetin molecule, binding strength has an order 3–4>4–5>3′–4′. Moreover, 3–4 chelation site is also preferred for complexes which are formed between one iron and two or three quercetin molecules [31]. We therefore performed uptake experiments with quercetin aglycone, and methylated forms of quercetin to determine whether replacing the putative iron binding groups would influence transepithelial iron transport. Our data clearly indicate that the greatest increase in transepithelial iron transport was observed with compounds where 3-hydroxyl groups were methylated (3MQ, 3,4′dMQ and PMQ). In contrast, when the 3-hydroxyl group was present, namely in quercetin and 4MQ, there was a decrease in transepithelial iron transport. These results demonstrate that chelation of iron by the 3-hydroxyl group of quercetin is an important determinate of iron uptake in duodenum. Potentially this mode of action could be ascribed to all dietary polyphenols that have demonstrable capacity to chelate iron, for example (-)-epigallocatechin-3-gallate, [16,32] and this information could be useful in the design of iron chelators based on the structure of these common dietary polyphenols.

The site of iron chelation by quercetin is unclear, i.e. whether binding takes place in the intestinal lumen or within the cytosol of the duodenal enterocytes. Quercetin aglycone can cross cell membranes via facilitated glucose (GLUT) transporters [33,34]. In addition, there is evidence from *in vitro* studies that quercetin-iron chelates may also be transported via GLUTs [35]. Thus there is scope for both lumenal and cytosolic iron chelation to lead to iron accumulation within enterocytes. The increase in duodenal iron content occurs largely as a consequence of a reduced rate of iron

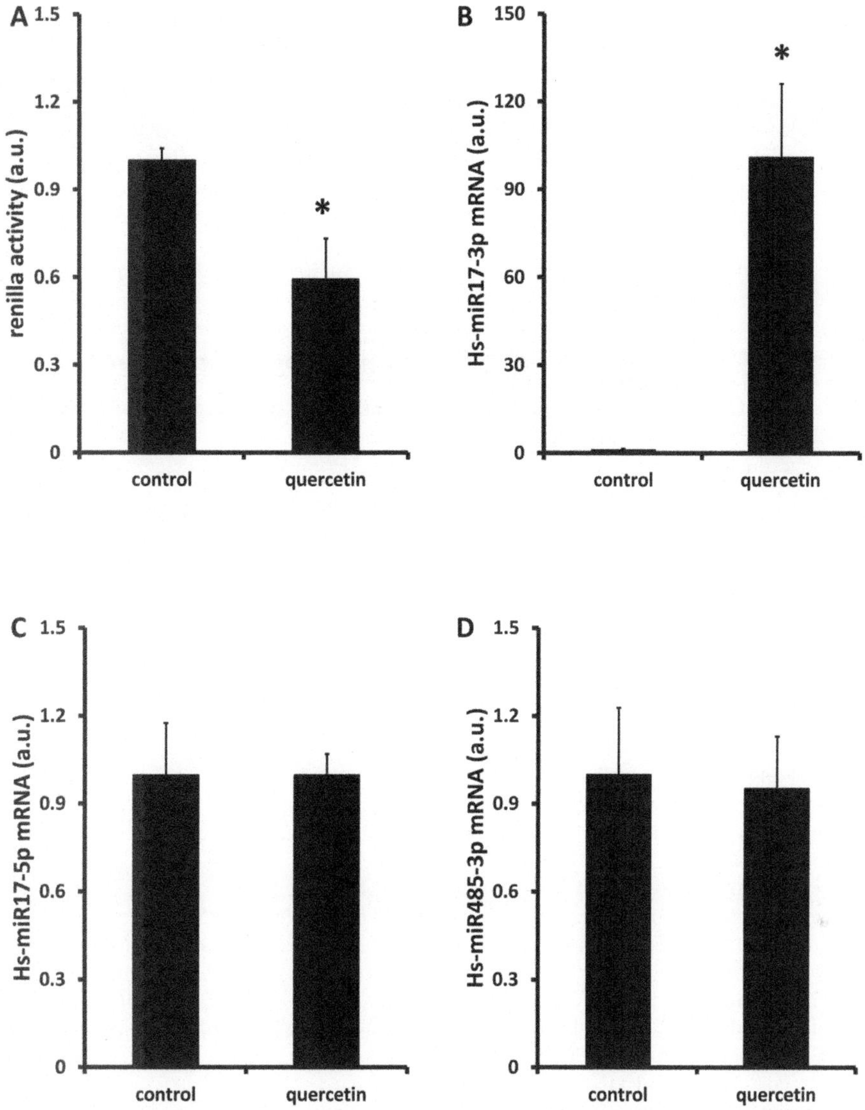

Figure 6. Effects of quercetin on the activity of FPN 3′ UTR. (A) Caco-2 cells were transfected with MISSION FPN 3′-UTR-Renilla luciferase reporter construct and exposed to quercetin (10 μM) for 18 h. (B-D) Quantitative PCR was used to determine the effects of quercetin on the expression of candidate microRNAs predicted to interact with the FPN 3′UTR. Data are mean ± SEM of 5-6 observations in each group. *$P<0.05$ compared with control group (Student's unpaired t-test).

efflux across the basolateral membrane into the blood. It is possible that intracellular quercetin-iron chelates might be too large to exit enterocytes via FPN, though some efflux through basolateral GLUTs remains a possibility. Furthermore, we cannot discount the possibility that quercetin or its metabolites have direct inhibitory effects on the function of FPN. Together these mechanisms could account for the increased mucosal iron retention observed in our studies.

2. Circulating iron and hepcidin levels

The longer term effects of quercetin on intestinal iron transport are less well studied. Here we have shown that oral administration of quercetin increased iron retention within the duodenum and resulted in a decrease in serum iron and transferrin saturation levels. In addition, there was a 60% decrease in liver hepcidin mRNA expression in quercetin-treated rats. These findings are consistent with previous data in rats fed an iron deficient diet [36]; however, crucially in this and previous studies iron deficiency was associated with a significant increase in both DMT1 [36,37] and FPN in the duodenum [10,36]. Furthermore, we and others have shown previously that intestinal FPN and DMT1 expression are down-regulated by prolonged exposure to elevated hepcidin levels [38–42]. Taken together these data suggest that low circulating iron and hepcidin levels do not mediate the inhibitory effects of quercetin on intestinal iron transport observed in the current study.

3. Cellular iron levels

The accumulation of iron in duodenal tissue observed in our *in vivo* experiments with quercetin-fed rats might also result in regulation of iron transporter expression. Previous studies in animals given a bolus of iron by gavage demonstrated a decrease in DMT1 expression [43–45]; however, iron efflux [43] and FPN expression [45] were largely unaffected. Therefore, the increase in duodenal iron accumulation in quercetin-fed rats is consistent with the decrease in DMT1 expression but does not explain the decrease in FPN.

The increase in duodenal iron content presents an apparent paradox since in quercetin-treated Caco-2 cells there was a significant decrease in levels of the iron storage protein ferritin, which is indicative of functional cellular iron deficiency rather than iron loading. In the cell culture model we envisage that cellular iron is sequestered by some other molecular entity, most likely quercetin. At this stage we do not know whether the iron retained within the rat duodenal mucosa in our *in vivo* model is also chelated by quercetin.

Even if we assume that quercetin treatment results in iron deficiency in Caco-2 cells this still cannot explain the effects of quercetin on transporter expression. We have shown that DMT1 expression in Caco-2 cells is decrease by iron [26;46] and increased following exposure to the iron chelator desferrioxamine (Figure S3). In contrast neither iron deficiency nor iron loading had a significant effect on FPN mRNA expression.

4. Direct effect of quercetin on intestinal FPN expression

Finally, we addressed the possibility that quercetin directly regulates FPN expression. In Caco-2 cells exposed to quercetin there was a significant dose-dependent decrease in FPN protein and mRNA and this was associated with a significant decrease in iron transport across Caco-2 cell monolayers. To elucidate the molecular mechanisms underlying these effects we employed luciferase-reporter assays containing either the FPN 5′-promoter or its 3′UTR. While there was no effect of quercetin on the activity of 5′-promoter, the activity of the 3′UTR construct was significantly decreased in the presence of quercetin. Regulation of the stability of the 3′UTR of mammalian mRNA has been shown to be controlled by a number of mechanisms including interactions with non-coding miRNA species. Interestingly, miRNAs have been shown to play a role in modulating the expression of a number of key players in iron homeostatic regulation, including hepcidin (miR-122; [47]), DMT1 (Let-7d; [48]) and FPN (miR-485-3p; [30]). While there was no significant effect of quercetin on miR-485-3p expression in Caco-2 cells, we identified miR-17-3p as a quercetin-induced candidate regulator of FPN mRNA expression. Expression of miR-17-3p was elevated significantly following exposure to quercetin, and bioinformatics identified a consensus binding site for miR-17-3p (bases 61-67 of the 3′UTR sequence) in the human FPN 3′UTR. The miR17 cluster is one of the most widely studied in microRNA biology and has been shown to play an important role in a number of biological processes in both health and disease [49]. Our data suggest a role for miR-17 and potentially other microRNAs in mediating diet-gene interactions that can influence nutrient bioavailability.

In summary, we have shown that quercetin can influence intestinal iron absorption acutely through chelation of iron within the intestinal lumen via its 3-hydroxyl group, and in the longer-term through direct regulation of FPN transporter expression, possibly through interactions between miRNA and 3′UTR of FPN mRNA. As potent inhibitors of iron bioavailability, diets rich in polyphenols might be beneficial for groups at risk of iron loading (e.g. patients with hereditary haemochromatosis), either by limiting the rate of intestinal iron absorption or by modifying tissue iron distribution. Further testing of quercetin and other phenolic compounds with iron chelating and cell signalling properties in animal models of iron overload could provide the basis for novel approaches for treating clinical iron overload in humans.

Supporting Information

Figure S1 Structures of quercetin and methylated-quercetin analogues.

Figure S2 Predicted binding sites for miR17-3p, miR17-5p and miR485-3p in human FPN 3′UTR.

Figure S3 Effects of desferrioxamine (DFO) and iron (FAC) on (A) DMT1 and (B) FPN mRNA expression in Caco-2 cells. Data are mean ± SEM of 5–6 observations in each group. Groups with no common letters are significantly different from each other (one-way ANOVA and Tukey's post hoc test; $P<0.05$). No letters indicates no significant difference between any of the groups.

Table S1 PCR primers used in the study.

Table S2 Fold changes (>1.5-fold) of human miRNA in Caco-2 cells exposed to 10 μM quercetin for 18 h. miRNA profiling was performed using the GeneChip miRNA array (Affymetrix, UK), which contains 847 specific probe sets for human miRNAs derived from the Sanger miRBase miRNA database v11. Results from the chip have been filtered to show human miRNA only and true significant changes ($p<0.05$) when compared to untreated controls.

Table S3 Predicted miRNAs interacting with FPN (SLC40A1); top 30 by rank. Data are from miRBase www.mirbase.org. Both miR17-3p (24th) and miR17-5p (12th) are among the top 30 miRNAs predicted to interact with the FPN 3′UTR.

Author Contributions

Conceived and designed the experiments: ESD SKSS PAS. Performed the experiments: ML RH SB VS ESD SKSS PAS. Analyzed the data: ML RH SB ESD SKSS PAS. Contributed to the writing of the manuscript: ML RH ESD SKSS PAS.

References

1. Sharp P, Srai SK (2007) Molecular mechanisms involved in intestinal iron absorption. World J Gastroenterol 13:4716–4724.
2. Evstatiev R, Gasche C (2011) Iron sensing and signalling. Gut. 61:933–952.
3. Hurrell R, Egli I (2010) Iron bioavailability and dietary reference values. Am J Clin Nutr 91:1461S–1467S.
4. Sharp P (2010) Intestinal iron absorption: regulation by dietary and systemic factors. Int J Vitamin Nutr Res 80:231–242.
5. McKie AT, Barrow D, Latunde-Dada GO, Rolfs A, Sager G, et al. (2001) An iron-regulated ferric reductase associated with the absorption of dietary iron. Science 291:1755–1759.
6. Wyman S, Simpson RJ, McKie AT, Sharp PA (2008) Dcytb (Cybrd1) acts as a ferric and cupric reductase and enhances cellular iron uptake. FEBS Lett 582:1901–1906.
7. Gunshin H, Mackenzie B, Berger UV, Gunshin Y, Romero M F, et al. (1997) Cloning and characterization of a mammalian proton-coupled metal-ion transporter. Nature 388:482–488.
8. Abboud S, Haile DJ (2000) A novel mammalian iron-regulated protein involved in intracellular iron metabolism. J Biol Chem 275:19906–19912.
9. Donovan A, Brownlie A, Zhou Y, Shepard J, Pratt S J, et al. (2000) Positional cloning of zebrafish ferroportin 1 identifies a conserved vertebrate iron exporter. Nature 403:776–781.

10. McKie AT, Marciani P, Rolfs A, Brennan K, Wehr K, et al. (2000) A novel duodenal iron-regulated transporter, IREG1, implicated in the basolateral transfer of iron to the circulation. Mol Cell 5:299–309.
11. Vulpe CD, Kuo Y M, Murphy TL, Cowley L, Askwith C, et al. (1999) Hephaestin, a ceruloplasmin homologue implicated in intestinal iron transport, is defective in the sla mouse. Nature Genet 21:195–199.
12. Havsteen BH (2002) The biochemistry and medical significance of the flavonoids. Pharmacol Ther 96:67–202.
13. Cook JD, Reddy MB, Hurrell RF (1995) The effect of red and white wine on non-heme iron absorption in humans. Am J Clin Nutr 61:800–804.
14. Hurrell RF, Reddy M, Cook JD (1999) Inhibition of non-haem iron absorption in man by polyphenolic-containing beverages. Br J Nutr 81:289–295
15. Samman S, Sandström B, Toft MB, Bukhave K, Jensen M, et al. (2001) Green tea or rosemary extract added to foods reduces nonheme-iron absorption. Am J Clin Nutr 73:607–612.
16. Kim E, Ham S, Shigenaga MK, Han O (2008) The inhibiting bioactive dietary polyphenolic compounds reduce nonheme iron transport across human intestinal cell monolayers. J Nutr 138:1647–1651.
17. Petry N, Egli I, Zeder C, Walczyk T, Hurrell R (2010) Polyphenols and phytic acid contribute to the low iron bioavailability from common beans in young women. J Nutr 140:1977–1982.
18. Kroon PA, Clifford MN, Crozier A, Day AJ, Donovan JL, et al. (2004) How should we assess the effects of exposure to dietary polyphenols in vitro? Am J Clin Nutr 80:15–21.
19. Aherne SA, O'Brien NM (2002) Dietary flavonols: chemistry, food content, and metabolism. Nutrition. 18:75–81.
20. Olthof MR, Hollman PCH, Vree T B, Katan MB (2000) Bioavailabilities of quercetin-3-glucoside and quercetin-4'-glucoside do not differ in humans. J Nutr 130:1200–1203.
21. Day AJ, Cañada FJ, Díaz JC, Kroon PA, Mclauchlan R, et al. (2000) Dietary flavonoid and isoflavone glycosides are hydrolysed by the lactase site of lactase phlorizin hydrolase. FEBS Lett 468:166–70
22. Day AJ, Gee JM, DuPont MS, Johnson IT, Williamson G (2003) Absorption of quercetin-3-glucoside and quercetin-4'-glucoside in the rat small intestine: the role of lactase phlorizin hydrolase and the sodium-dependent glucose transporter. Biochem Pharmacol 65:1199–206.
23. Lee HB, Blaufox MD (1985) Blood volume in the rat. J Nuclear Med 26:72–76.
24. Torrance JD, Bothwell T H (1980) Tissue iron stores, in Cook, J D (ed): Methods in Hematology. vol 1. 90–115, New York, NY, Churchill Livingstone.
25. Chantret I, Rodolosse A, Barbat A, Dussaulx E, Brot-Laroche E, et al. (1994) Differential expression of sucrase-isomaltase in clones isolated from early and late passages of the cell line Caco-2: evidence for glucose-dependent negative regulation. J Cell Sci 107:213–225.
26. Sharp PA, Tandy SR, Yamaji S, Tennant JP, Williams MR, et al. (2002) Rapid regulation of Divalent Metal Transporter (DMT1) protein but not mRNA expression by non-haem iron in human intestinal Caco-2 cells. FEBS Lett 510:71–76.
27. Tandy S, Williams M, Leggett A, Lopez-Jimenez M, Dedes M, et al. (2000) Nramp2 expression is associated with pH-dependent iron uptake across the apical membrane of human intestinal Caco-2 cells. J Biol Chem 275:1023–1029.
28. Johnston K, Johnson D, Marks J, Srai SK, Debnam ES, et al. (2006) Non-haem iron transport in the rat proximal colon. Eur J Clin Invest 36:35–40.
29. Zhang DL, Hughes RM, Ollivierre-Wilson H, Ghosh MC, Rouault TA (2009) A ferroportin transcript that lacks an iron-responsive element enables duodenal and erythroid precursor cells to evade translational repression. Cell Metab 9:461–473.
30. Sangokoya C, Doss JF, Chi JT. (2013) Iron-responsive miR-485-3p regulates cellular iron homeostasis by targeting ferroportin. PLoS Genet 9:e1003408.
31. Ren J, Meng S, Lekka ChE, Kaxiras E (2008) Complexation of flavonoids with iron: structure and optical signatures. J Phys Chem B 112:1845–1850.
32. Kim EY, Ham S, Bradke D, Ma Q, Han O (2011) Ascorbic acid offsets the inhibitory effect of bioactive dietary polyphenolic compounds on transepithelial iron transport in Caco-2 intestinal cells. J Nutr 141:828–834.
33. Strobel P, Allard C, Perez-Acle T, Calderon R, Aldunate R, et al. (2005) Myricetin, quercetin and catechin-gallate inhibit glucose uptake in isolated rat adipocytes. Biochem J 386:471–478.
34. Cunningham P, Afzal-Ahmed I, Naftalin RJ (2006) Docking studies show that D-glucose and quercetin slide through the transporter GLUT1. J Biol Chem 281:5797–5803.
35. Vlachodimitropolou E, Sharp PA, Naftalin RJ (2011) Quercetin-iron chelates are transported via glucose (GLUT) transporters. Free Radic Biol Med 50: 934–944.
36. Frazer DM, Wilkins SJ, Becker EM, Vulpe CD, McKie AT, et al. (2002) Hepcidin expression inversely correlates with the expression of duodenal iron transporters and iron absorption in rats. Gastroenterology 123:835–844.
37. Trinder D, Oates PS, Thomas C, Sadleir J, Morgan EH (2000) Localisation of divalent metal transporter 1 (DMT1) to the microvillus membrane of rat duodenal enterocytes in iron deficiency, but to hepatocytes in iron overload. Gut 46: 270–276.
38. Yamaji S, Sharp P, Ramesh B, Srai SK (2004) Inhibition of iron transport across human intestinal epithelial cells by hepcidin. Blood 104:2178–2180.
39. Chaston T, Chung B, Mascarenhas M, Marks J, Patel B, et al. (2008) Evidence for differential effects of hepcidin in macrophages and intestinal epithelial cells. Gut 57:374–382.
40. Mena NP, Esparza A, Tapia V, Valdés P, Núñez MT (2008) Hepcidin inhibits apical iron uptake in intestinal cells. Am J Physiol 294:G192–G198.
41. Chung B, Chaston TB, Marks J, Srai SKS, Sharp PA (2009) Hepcidin decreases iron transporter expression in vivo in mouse duodenum and spleen and in vitro in THP-1 macrophages and intestinal Caco-2 cells. J Nutr 139:1457–1462.
42. Brasse-Lagnel C, Karim Z, Letteron P, Bekri S, Bado A, et al. (2011) Intestinal DMT1 cotransporter is down-regulated by hepcidin via proteasome internalization and degradation. Gastroenterology 140: 1261–1271.
43. Oates PS, Trinder D, Morgan EH (2000) Gastrointestinal function, divalent metal transporter-1 expression and intestinal iron absorption. Pflügers Arch. 440:496–502.
44. Yeh KY, Yeh M, Watkins JA, Rodriguez-Paris J, Glass J (2000) Dietary iron induces rapid changes in rat intestinal divalent metal transporter expression. Am J Physiol 279:G1070–G1079.
45. Frazer DM, Wilkins SJ, Becker EM, Murphy TL, Vulpe CD, et al. (2003) A rapid decrease in the expression of DMT1 and Dcytb but not Ireg1 or hephaestin explains the mucosal block phenomenon of iron absorption. Gut 52: 340–346.
46. Johnson D, Yamaji S, Tennant JP, Srai SK, Sharp PA (2005) Regulation of divalent metal transporter (DMT1) expression in human intestinal epithelial cells following exposure to non-haem iron. FEBS Lett 579:1923–1929.
47. Castoldi M, Vujic Spasic M, Altamura S, Elmén J, Lindow M, et al. (2011) The liver-specific microRNA miR-122 controls systemic iron homeostasis in mice. J Clin Invest 121:1386–1396.
48. Andolfo I, De Falco L, Asci R, Russo R, Colucci S, et al. (2010) Regulation of divalent metal transporter 1 (DMT1) non-IRE isoform by the microRNA Let-7d in erythroid cells. Haematologica 95:1244–1252.
49. Mogilyansky E, Rigoutsos I (2013) The miR-17/92 cluster: a comprehensive update on its genomics, genetics, functions and increasingly important and numerous roles in health and disease. Cell Death Differ 20:1603–1614.

14

Metabolome Analysis of *Arabidopsis thaliana* Roots Identifies a Key Metabolic Pathway for Iron Acquisition

Holger Schmidt[1], Carmen Günther[1], Michael Weber[1], Cornelia Spörlein[2], Sebastian Loscher[2], Christoph Böttcher[3], Rainer Schobert[2,4], Stephan Clemens[1,4]*

1 Department of Plant Physiology, University of Bayreuth, Bayreuth, Germany, **2** Department of Organic Chemistry, University of Bayreuth, Bayreuth, Germany, **3** Department of Stress and Developmental Biology, Leibniz Institute of Plant Biochemistry, Halle/Saale, Germany, **4** Bayreuth Center for Molecular Biosciences, University of Bayreuth, Bayreuth, Germany

Abstract

Fe deficiency compromises both human health and plant productivity. Thus, it is important to understand plant Fe acquisition strategies for the development of crop plants which are more Fe-efficient under Fe-limited conditions, such as alkaline soils, and have higher Fe density in their edible tissues. Root secretion of phenolic compounds has long been hypothesized to be a component of the reduction strategy of Fe acquisition in non-graminaceous plants. We therefore subjected roots of *Arabidopsis thaliana* plants grown under Fe-replete and Fe-deplete conditions to comprehensive metabolome analysis by gas chromatography-mass spectrometry and ultra-pressure liquid chromatography electrospray ionization quadrupole time-of-flight mass spectrometry. Scopoletin and other coumarins were found among the metabolites showing the strongest response to two different Fe-limited conditions, the cultivation in Fe-free medium and in medium with an alkaline pH. A coumarin biosynthesis mutant defective in *ortho*-hydroxylation of cinnamic acids was unable to grow on alkaline soil in the absence of Fe fertilization. Co-cultivation with wild-type plants partially rescued the Fe deficiency phenotype indicating a contribution of extracellular coumarins to Fe solubilization. Indeed, coumarins were detected in root exudates of wild-type plants. Direct infusion mass spectrometry as well as UV/vis spectroscopy indicated that coumarins are acting both as reductants of Fe(III) and as ligands of Fe(II).

Editor: Gloria Muday, Wake Forest University, United States of America

Funding: The authors have no support or funding to report.

Competing Interests: The authors have declared that no competing interests exist.

* Email: stephan.clemens@uni-bayreuth.de

Introduction

Virtually all life forms depend on iron (Fe) for basic cell function, growth and development. The availability of its ferric (Fe^{3+}) and ferrous (Fe^{2+}) oxidation states under physiological conditions make the metal essential for a plethora of electron transfer reactions, e.g. in photosynthesis and respiration [1,2]. Consequently, Fe deficiency results in a number of adverse effects for organisms. In humans, undersupply with this micronutrient is the most widespread nutritional disorder in the world. Fe deficiency anemia is estimated to affect about 30% of the world's population. It substantially increases the risk of maternal and perinatal mortality and can be the cause of impaired mental development [3]. Since a large fraction of the human diet is plant-based, there is an urgent need for crops that more efficiently accumulate Fe in a bioavailable form in their edible parts. Prerequisite for this biofortification approach is the understanding of Fe uptake into and its distribution within plants for breeding or engineering new varieties [4,5].

Fe acquisition poses a major challenge. While the metal is one of the most prevalent elements in the Earth's crust and highly abundant in soils, it is not readily available for plant uptake in the presence of oxygen as it precipitates in the form of insoluble ferric oxides. This process is strongly enhanced at alkaline pH with dramatic consequences for plant productivity especially on calcareous soils. It is estimated that 30% of the world's arable land is too alkaline for optimal plant growth [6].

Plants have evolved two different strategies for Fe acquisition, the acidification-reduction strategy (strategy I) and the chelation strategy (strategy II) [2,7]. The latter is used by grasses. It is based on the solubilization of ferric precipitates through the secretion of strong Fe(III)-chelating molecules. These phytosiderophores of the mugineic acid family are released into the rhizosphere by efflux transporters such as TOM1 [8]. Uptake of Fe(III)-phytosiderophore complexes into the symplast is mediated by YS1/YSL-transporters [9]. Non-graminaceous plants acquire Fe by a combination of rhizosphere acidification, the extracellular reduction of ferric to ferrous iron at the root surface, and subsequent uptake of ferrous iron into epidermal cells. The proteins mainly responsible for these processes in *A. thaliana* are AHA2, FRO2 and IRT1, respectively [10–12].

A major gap in our understanding of strategy I has been the potential role of phenolic compounds secreted by the roots [6]. The release of small molecules into the rhizosphere is an important component of a plant's response to fluctuations in the abiotic and biotic environment [13]. Root exudates can, for instance, function as allelochemicals or alter the surrounding substrate. It is well documented that phenolic compounds including flavonoids comprise a large fraction of the root exudates of strategy I plants under Fe deficiency [14]. They have been hypothesized to mobilize apoplastically bound Fe(III) for uptake into the symplast. Studies on red clover showed that removal of secreted phenols from the roots led to Fe deficiency of the shoot even though acidification and ferric reductase activity were enhanced. These observations suggested a crucial role for secreted phenols in Fe acquisition independent of established strategy I processes [15]. In rice, which is exceptional as it employs both strategy I and strategy II [2], the efflux transporter PEZ1 was recently described as an integral component of strategy I [16]. It mediates the secretion of compounds such as caffeic acid and is essential for the solubilization of apoplastic Fe oxides.

The exact mechanisms underlying the mobilization of Fe(III) are unknown. Phenolic compounds including flavonoids have been discussed both as chelators of Fe(III) and as reductants [14,17,18]. Until recently, neither specific information on the activity of particular compounds nor direct genetic evidence for the importance of phenol secretion in Fe acquisition by non-graminaceous plants was available. Rodriguez-Celma et al. then showed that secretion of phenolics is critical for *A. thaliana* Fe acquisition from low bioavailability sources [19]. Later it was demonstrated through the analysis of mutants defective in the ABC transporter ABCG37 [20] and in coumarin biosynthesis [21], respectively, that the active compounds are coumarins.

Our objective was to identify molecules involved in the acquisition of Fe by strategy I plants through a metabolomics approach. We subjected roots of *A. thaliana* plants grown under Fe-replete and two different Fe-deplete conditions to comprehensive metabolome analysis by gas chromatography-mass spectrometry (GC-MS) as well as ultra-pressure liquid chromatography electrospray ionization quadrupole time-of-flight mass spectrometry (UPLC-ESI-QTOF-MS) and searched for compounds increasing in abundance under Fe deficiency. Several hundred features (*m/z* – retention time pairs) showing significant differences were detected. Among the most prominent changes various coumarins could be identified. A respective biosynthetic mutant was unable to grow on alkaline soil unless treated with extra Fe. Co-cultivation with wild type plants partially rescued the mutant phenotype. Taken together, our data clearly confirm the secretion of coumarins as an essential component of *A. thaliana* Fe acquisition and provide more extensive information on metabolome changes elicited by Fe deficiency. The latter can guide future studies aiming at a systems level understanding of plant responses to Fe-deplete conditions.

Materials and Methods

Plant material

Arabidopsis thaliana accession Columbia (Col-0) was used as wild type background (wt). T-DNA insertion lines *f6'h1-1* and *f6'h1-5* (SALK_132418c and SALK_050137) were obtained from the Nottingham Arabidopsis Stock Centre (University of Nottingham, UK) [22]. The *f6'h1-1* mutant carries a T-DNA insertion in exon 1 of At3g13610 and was described before as coumarin-deficient [23]. The *f6'h1-5* line carries a T-DNA insertion in exon 2. This was confirmed by genotyping (File S1). Plants were cultivated in a growth cabinet (Percival Scientific) at a temperature cycle of 23°C (day)/18°C (night) and a photoperiod of 8 h light (110 µE $m^{-2}s^{-1}$) and 16 h dark. Plants were grown on normal soil or on soil that was alkalinized by addition of CaO resulting in a pH of 7.7. Fe fertilization of alkaline soil was performed by watering with 0.5% Fetrilon, which contains Fe-EDTA (BASF, Germany). For hydroponic culture, 1/10 Hoagland Solution 2 (0.28 mM $Ca(NO_3)_2$, 0.6 mM KNO_3, 0.1 mM $NH_4H_2PO_4$, 0.2 mM $MgSO_4$, 4.63 µM H_3BO_3, 32 nM $CuSO_4$, 915 nM $MnCl_2$, 77 nM $ZnSO_4$, 11 nM MoO_3) with or without Fe-HBED (5 µM) as Fe source at pH 5.7 was used [24,25]. Seeds were germinated on solid medium-filled PCR tubes. Ten days after germination, plants were transferred to cultivation vessels with liquid medium. We either used 50 ml Falcon tubes for cultivation of single plants or 1.6 l pots for cultivation of three plants. Fe limitation was imposed in two different ways. Fe-free medium was prepared by omitting Fe-HBED. For alkaline growth conditions, medium was buffered with 10 mM $NaHCO_3$ and adjusted with KOH to pH 7.7. Medium was changed weekly and pH was checked. The metabolome analysis is based on two sets of three independent experiments (medium +Fe vs. medium –Fe; medium pH 5.7 vs. medium 7.7) performed over a period of approximately fifteen months. Three plants were pooled for one sample. Roots were harvested and blotted dry with paper towels, flash-frozen in liquid nitrogen and stored at −80°C. Prior to metabolite extraction root tissue was ground to a fine powder in liquid nitrogen.

Collection of exudates

Exudates were collected from hydroponically grown plants (50 ml tubes) through transfer into 50 ml distilled water for 24 h. Samples were freeze-dried and the metabolites re-dissolved in 0.5 ml 80% methanol per tube. Pooled exudates from 45 plants were centrifuged and 5 µl were analyzed as described for the root extracts. Three independent experiments were performed and analyzed.

Elemental analysis via inductively coupled plasma-optical emission spectroscopy (ICP-OES)

Root and leaf material was freeze-dried and digested in 4 ml 65% HNO_3 and 2 ml 30% H_2O_2 using a microwave (START 1500, MLS GmbH). Fe concentrations were measured with an iCAP 6500 (Thermo Scientific).

Metabolite profiling by GC-MS

For GC-MS measurements, metabolites were extracted and samples derivatized as described [26]. The GC-MS setup consisted of a Gerstel MPS autosampler, an Agilent 7890A GC system and a 5975C inert MSD (Gerstel GmbH, Mülheim/Ruhr, Germany). Chromatographic separation was performed on a Zebron Guardian ZB-5 (40 m×0.25 mm, 25 µm, 10 m integrated pre-column, Phenomenex Aschaffenburg, Germany). Data were analyzed via AMDIS (Ver. 2.71) and SpectConnect using the default settings of the respective software [27–30]. The resulting SpectConnect matrix was imported into Microsoft Excel. Entries were normalized to the internal standard ribitol and filtered according to their mean fold-change ($<$0.66 or $>$1.5) and P value ($<$0.05) in a Student's t-test. Only entities above a relative abundance of 1% of the ribitol peak were further characterized. A compound was regarded as identified when matched to the in house library (ΔRI$<$10, R-match $>$800).

Metabolite profiling by UPLC-ESI-QTOF-MS

A Waters Aquity UPLC system equipped with a HSS T3 column (1.8 µm, 2.1×100 mm) coupled to a Q-TOF Premier mass spectrometer was used for metabolite profiling (Waters Corporation, Milford, MA). Extraction and analysis of plant metabolites was essentially performed as described [31,32]. A linear gradient at a flow of 0.5 ml·min^{-1} from water (A) to acetonitrile (B), both acidified with 0.1% formic acid, was applied as follows: 0 min 99.5% A, 1 min 99.5% A, 16 min 8.5% A, 19 min 0.5% A, 22 min 0.5% A, 23 min 99.5% A, 24 min 99.5%

A. Raw data were converted to the netCDF format prior to analysis and visualization via XCMS online [33–35]. MS2Ts of pooled root samples were recorded as described [36,37]. The recorded MSMS spectra were compared to the primeE-MS2T database and Massbank [38].

Direct infusion mass spectrometry

To study the interaction of ferrous and ferric iron with coumarins, 10 mM aqueous solutions of $FeCl_3$ and $FeCl_2$ were prepared. Methanolic solutions (10 mM) of the ligands esculetin, fraxetin and scopoletin were added in different stoichiometric ratios to an aqueous solution of the respective iron salt. The final Fe concentration in solution was 1 mM. The mixtures (Fe:ligand ratio varying from 1:1 to 1:3) were injected into the mass spectrometer via a syringe pump. Source settings corresponded to those used for LC-MS analysis and flow rate was adjusted to achieve maximum signal intensities. Collision energy in MS-MS experiments was set to 15 V.

Spectral analysis of Fe-coumarin complexes

We prepared, under exclusion of air and moisture, acetonitrile solutions that contained three equivalents of any one of these ligands, six equivalents of the base triethylamine, and one equivalent of either $FeCl_2$ or $FeCl_3$. After stirring for 30 min the solutions were transferred under argon atmosphere to a UV cuvette and the optical spectra were recorded at wavelengths ranging from 300 to 900 nm.

Overexpression of F6′H1

For the complementation of *f6′h1-5* the *F6′H1* coding sequence (cds) was amplified from root cDNA (F6-H1-cds-fw: 5′-atggctccaacactcttgacaacc-3′; F6-H1-cds-wo-Stop-rev: 5′-gatcttggcgtaatcgacggtt-3′) and cloned into pCR8/GW/TOPO (Invitrogen Life Technologies). Using gateway technology (Invitrogen Life Technologies) the cds was subcloned into pMDC83 which adds a C-terminal GFP-tag [39]. Both cloning steps were performed according to the manufacturer's instructions. The final construct was Agro-transformed into SALK_050137 (*f6′h1–5*) by the floral dip method.

Chemicals

Standards of fraxin and scopolin were obtained from Phytolab GmbH & Co. KG (Vestenbergsgreuth, Germany). Scopoletin was synthesized based on Demyttenaere et al. [40,41]. All other standards were obtained from Sigma-Aldrich (Taufkirchen, Germany).

Results

A. thaliana Col-0 wild type plants were cultivated hydroponically for easy access to root tissue. In order to allow stringent filtering of the highly complex metabolomics data, we imposed Fe deficiency conditions in two different ways in separate sets of three independent experiments each. First, four week old plants were grown for additional two weeks in medium without added Fe-HBED. Second, plants were cultivated for six weeks in medium with the pH adjusted to 7.7 (instead of 5.7). Elemental profiles of roots and shoots were determined by ICP-OES. Both the omission of Fe for two weeks and a medium pH of 7.7 resulted in significant reductions of root and shoot Fe concentrations indicating Fe deficiency (Fig. 1).

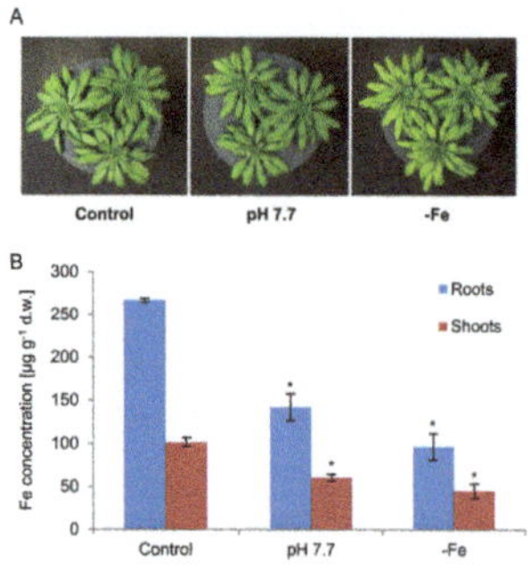

Figure 1. *A. thaliana* Col-0 plants were exposed to two different conditions causing Fe deficiency. (A) Plants were grown hydroponically in 1/10 Hoagland Solution for six weeks. Plants were cultivated either at a pH of 5.7 with Fe-HBED as Fe source (Control), at a pH of 7.7 with Fe-HBED as Fe source (pH 7.7), or the final two weeks at a pH of 5.7 without Fe-HBED (−Fe). (B) Fe concentrations in roots (blue bars) and shoots (red bars) were determined by ICP-OES. The means of three independent biological experiments are displayed. Error bars indicate standard deviation. Significant differences to plants grown under control conditions were determined by Student's t-test, $^{*}P<0.05$.

GC-MS metabolite profiling

GC-MS analysis of root extracts and relative quantification detected in total 12 significant changes (>1.5fold, $P<0.05$) in response to Fe-free conditions and 30 in response to alkaline conditions (Fig. 2A; Tables 1 and 2). The two dominant metabolic changes in plants grown in Fe-free medium relative to plants grown in control medium were increases in the abundance of the organic acids citrate and malate. Quantification based on standard curves showed 5.6-fold and 3.1-fold higher concentrations, respectively (Fig. 3). Similarly, in root metabolite profiles of plants grown in alkaline medium, signals for these two compounds were again the most prominent changes (Table 2). Concentrations were 29.3-fold (citrate) and 4.1-fold (malate) higher than in profiles of plants grown under control conditions (Fig. 3).

The overlap in responses contained three additional metabolites (Fig. 2A). Amino acids asparagine and threonine were found to be up-regulated with a 30-fold higher abundance of asparagine under alkaline conditions representing the most prominent change. Overall, the signal intensities were far less pronounced than those for the organic acids (Tables 1 and 2). A tentatively identified metabolite showing robust differences in abundance was methyl-3-hydroxy-pentandioic acid (more abundant under Fe deficiency).

Importantly, because the up-regulation of citrate and malate synthesis is a well-established root metabolic marker for Fe depletion [42,43], the GC-MS profiling results confirmed the Fe deficiency indicated by the ICP-OES measurements (Fig. 1) and further validated our assay conditions. Growth in Fe-free medium at pH 5.7 as well as growth in hydroponic medium at pH 7.7 imposed Fe deficiency and elicited a respective root response.

UPLC-ESI-QTOF-MS profiling

Most of our analyses focused on LC-MS-based profiling which covers other compound classes than GC-MS and has the potential to provide structural information on unknown compounds [36,44]. Methanolic extracts of roots were analyzed in negative and positive ionization mode. For both sets of three independent experiments hundreds of significant ($P<0.05$) changes associated with Fe deficiency were detected. The total numbers of features with >2-fold changes were 162 and 167 for Fe-free medium in positive and negative mode, respectively, and 678 and 323 for alkaline medium. In order to identify the metabolic changes most

Table 1. Metabolic changes in *A. thaliana* roots upon cultivation in hydroponic medium without added Fe as identified by GC-MS metabolite profiling.

Metabolite	relative abundance −Fe	relative abundance +Fe	fold change	P-value
Citric acid	0.72±0.3	0.13±0.03	5.6	<0.001
Malic acid	0.65±0.36	0.21±0.06	3.1	0.006
Fructose	0.08±0.05	0.2±0.09	0.4	0.005
Alanine	0.05±0.04	0.08±0.03	0.6	0.048
Asparagine	0.05±0.02	0.02±0.01	3.1	0.002
Threonine	0.04±0.01	0.02±0.01	1.7	0
n. i. (Methyl-3-hydroxy-pentandioic acid, R-Match: 930, RI: 1405)	0.02±0.03	<0.01	28.6	0.034
Galactinol	<0.01	0.02±0.01	0.1	<0.001
n. i. (Aspartic acid, R-Match: 861, RI: 1537)	0.01±0	0.02±0.01	0.6	0.037
n. i. (Lysine, R-Match: 831; RI: 1945)	0.01±0.01	<0.01	n. d.	0.002
n. i. (2-Ketoglutaric acid, R-Match: 831, RI: 1579)	0.01±0.01	<0.01	4.3	0.025
n. i. (Phosphoric acid, R-Match: 833, RI: 1813)	0.01±0.01	<0.01	2.4	0.014

Polar metabolites were extracted with methanol, derivatized and subjected to GC-MS analysis. Listed are compounds that showed a significant ($P<0.05$, Student's t-test) difference (>1.5-fold) in three independent biological experiments. Entries are ordered according to their maximum relative abundance under –Fe conditions; n. i.: not unambiguously identified (no comparison with authentic standard), RI: retention index, R-Match: reverse match (only values above 800 are given).

closely associated with Fe deficiency we filtered out all features that showed significant >2-fold changes in signal intensity under both tested conditions. Fifty-three and 36 signals met these criteria in positive and negative mode, respectively (Fig. 2B). The corresponding lists are displayed in Tables S1 and S2 in File S6.

In order to annotate the selected features, MS-MS data were obtained for approximately two thirds of them. Recorded MS-MS-spectra (provided as MS2Tags in a format compatible with Massbank in Files S2 and S3) were compared with Massbank [38] and the Riken MS2T database [36]. We were able to assign several peaks to known MS2Ts. However, in most cases, there was no structural data for the respective compound available yet. Only for a limited number of features, MS2T and Massbank hits led to a reasonable structure prediction. Whenever possible, we then obtained the respective compounds as standards and compared retention times and MS-MS spectra. Following this strategy we were able to identify the main coumarin known in *Arabidopsis thaliana*, scopoletin, and its respective glycoside scopolin as two molecules showing major changes in abundance under Fe-deplete conditions (Fig. 4). The scopoletin standard we had to synthesize. The recrystallized product was checked by ESI-MS. A mass of 193.0522 was found (calculated for C53H76NO7 [M+ H]$^{+}$193.0501). All physical and spectroscopic data of the product were in accordance with the literature [40,41]. Another highly hydroxylated coumarin, fraxetin, and its corresponding glycoside fraxin could be identified as significantly up-regulated too (Fig. 4). The chemical structures of the described coumarins are shown in Fig. 5 (**2**, **3**, **5**, **6**). An unidentifed compound co-eluted with scopolin. The detected marker 225.040 ESI+ at 3.95 min most likely resulted from an in-source fragmentation of the respective hexoside with a molecular weight of 386.088 (experimental) and an elemental composition of C16H18O11. The MSMS could be matched to the MS2T ATH64p07367 and, based on the most probable elemental composition, fraxin substituted with an additional OH-group is a likely candidate. A group of markers at 5.14 min was assigned to a compound with a molecular weight of 522.210. Three MS2Ts could be matched to the compound, and based on the CHNOPS elemental composition we assigned a molecular formula (C26H34O11) to the compound.

A coumarin biosynthetic mutant under Fe-limited alkaline conditions

Biosynthesis of scopoletin has been molecularly elucidated [45] and the enzyme catalyzing a key step, the *ortho*-hydroxylation of cinnamates, is known as F6′H1 [23]. This enabled us to directly test a possible role of coumarins in Fe acquisition. We obtained two mutant alleles of the respective *F6′H1* gene (At3g13610) in Col-0 background, *f6′h1-1* [23] and *f6′h1–5*. For the latter the T-DNA insertion in exon 2 was confirmed (File S1). When grown on normal soil *f6′h1* mutants showed no obvious phenotypes. On alkaline soil, however, a dramatic effect on development was observed (Fig. 6A). While Col-0 plants showed only a slight impairment of growth due to limited Fe availability, *f6′h1* mutant plants were chlorotic and barely grew. Most plants did not survive six weeks of cultivation under these conditions. Expression of *F6′H1* under control of the 35S promoter fully restored wild–type growth in *f6′h1-5* mutants as shown in Fig. 6B for two independent transgenic lines. This established a lack of functional F6′H1 as the cause of the growth defect on alkaline soil. Since the two mutant alleles behaved indistinguishable we performed further experiments with only one of them (*f6′h1–5*).

The alkaline soil phenotype is reminiscent of previously reported ones for mutants with defects in Fe acquisition [46]. Correspondingly, Fe fertilization of alkaline soil, i.e. watering with Fe-EDTA solution (0.5% Fetrilon), attenuated the symptoms of *f6′h1* plants (Fig. 6C). This clearly demonstrated Fe deficiency as the cause of the strong growth inhibition displayed by plants lacking coumarin biosynthesis.

In hydroponic culture at alkaline pH, *f6′h1-5* mutants also showed impaired growth relative to wild-type plants and displayed severe chlorosis, thus again indicating Fe deficiency (Fig. 6D, File S4). No growth phenotype was apparent when Col-0 and *f6′h1-5* were grown hydroponically in Fe-free medium at pH 5.7 (File S4), indicating that coumarin biosynthesis is required for Fe acquisition predominantly under Fe-limited conditions. When grown under the same conditions as Col-0 plants for the metabolome analysis, *f6′h1-5* plants showed shoot and root Fe concentrations that were slightly higher than those measured for wild-type plants. Specifically under conditions of limited Fe availability due to alkaline

Table 2. Metabolic changes in *A. thaliana* roots upon cultivation in hydroponic medium with alkaline pH as identified by GC-MS metabolite profiling.

Metabolite	relative abundance pH7.7	relative abundance pH 5.7	fold change	P-value
Citric acid	2.22±0.26	0.08±0.06	31.8	<0.001
Malic acid	1.2±0.14	0.3±0.34	4.4	<0.001
Threonine	0.36±0.24	0.07±0.05	5.4	0.006
n. i. (RI: 1103)	0.17±0.04	0.05±0.06	3.3	<0.001
Glutamic acid	0.16±0.03	0.09±0.05	2	<0.001
Asparagine	0.15±0.1	0.01±0.01	30.2	0.003
n. i. (3-Methyl-3-Hydroxy -Pentandioic acid R-Match: 930, RI: 1624)	0.12±0.08	0.01±0.02	9.6	0.005
n. i. (Aspartic acid, R-Match: 859, RI: 1536)	0.1±0.05	0.03±0.03	3.9	0.002
n. i. (3-Cyanoalanine, R-Match: 879, RI: 1348)	0.08±0.05	0±0.01	22.9	0.001
n. i. (Asparagine [−H2O] (2TMS), R-Match: 879, RI: 1507)	0.06±0.05	0.01±0.01	7.9	0.007
n. i. (Galactonic acid, R-Match: 901, RI: 2042)	0.06±0.01	0.01±0.01	5.8	<0.001
Valine	0.05±0.03	0.01±0.01	4.3	0.001
n. i. (Urea, R-Match: 904, RI: 1243)	0.05±0.03	<0.01	700	0.001
n. i. (Methylenbutanedioic acid, R-Match: 943, RI: 1353)	0.05±0.01	0.01±0.01	10.3	<0.001
n. i. (Arabinofuranose, R-Match 834, RI 1799)	0.05±0.02	0.01±0.01	3.8	0.001
n. i. (RI: 1552)	0.04±0.02	0.01±0	7.2	0.001
n. i. (RI: 1354)	0.04±0.02	0.01±0.01	4.4	0.007
n. i. (Glyceric acid, R-Match: 840, RI: 1347)	0.03±0.02	0.01±0.01	2.4	0.016
n. i. (RI: 1086)	0.03±0.02	<0.01	392.9	0.001
Leucine	0.02±0.01	<0.01	5.6	0.001
n. i. (RI: 1693)	0.02±0.01	<0.01	45.3	0.001
n. i. (RI: 1791)	0.02±0.01	<0.01	4.5	<0.001
n. i. (2-Butenedioic acid, R-Match: 854, RI:1313)	0.02±0	0.01±0.01	2.1	0.007
n. i. (RI:1345)	0.01±0	<0.01	4.1	0.001
n. i. (Aconitic acid, R-Match: 903, RI: 1770)	0.01±0.01	<0.01	136.3	0.001
n. i. (RI: 1787)	0.01±0	<0.01	10000	<0.001
n. i. (2-Piperidinecarboxylic acid, R-Match: 974, RI: 1348)	0.01±0.01	<0.01	3	0.014
n. i. (RI: 1131)	0.01±0.01	<0.01	17.5	0.005
Phenylalanine	<0.01	<0.01	4.5	0.001
Cysteine	<0.01	<0.01	10.4	<0.001

Polar metabolites were extracted with methanol, derivatized and subjected to GC-MS analysis. Listed are compounds that showed a significant ($P<0.05$, Student's t-test) difference (>1.5-fold) in three independent biological experiments. Entries are ordered according to their maximum relative abundance under alkaline conditions; n. i.: not unambiguously identified (no comparison with authentic standard), RI: retention index, R-Match: reverse match (only values above 800 are given).

pH, however, reductions in shoot Fe concentrations were even stronger than in Col-0 (File S4, compare to Fig. 1B). Root Fe concentrations of *f6'h1-5* plants grown under these conditions were higher than those of Col-0 plants, possibly indicating larger apoplastic Fe pools.

Together these observations strongly suggested an important role of coumarin biosynthesis for Fe acquisition under alkaline conditions. In order to test whether coumarins exert their effects extracellularly or intracellularly we performed hydroponic co-cultivation experiments. One *f6'h1-5* mutant plant was grown together with either two other mutant plants or with two Col-0 plants in 1.6 l containers with alkaline medium. The pH was monitored throughout and did not change over the course of the experiment. Interestingly, *f6'h1-5* plants co-cultivated with Col-0 plants grew much bigger and were less chlorotic when compared to mutant plants grown without Col plants (Fig. 7). This clearly indicated at least a partial contribution of secreted coumarins to Fe acquisition and prompted us to analyze root exudation.

Metabolite profiling of root exudates

Exudates of wild type and *f6'h1-5* mutant plants grown hydroponically under control conditions (pH 5.7) – in order to achieve equal growth rates of the two genotypes - were collected, concentrated and analyzed by UPLC-ESI-QTOF-MS. The resulting metabolite profiles were compared and significant differences determined to identify compounds that are secreted by Col-0 and not by plants with a defect in coumarin biosynthesis. Results are listed in Tables S3 and S4 in File S7. Scopoletin was identified as one of the most intense signals in the exudates of wild-type plants even under control conditions. Only traces were detectable in the exudates of the mutant, confirming the lack of synthesis in *f6'h1-5* mutant plants [23]. As an additional metabolite downstream of F6'H1 we detected esculetin (Fig. 5,

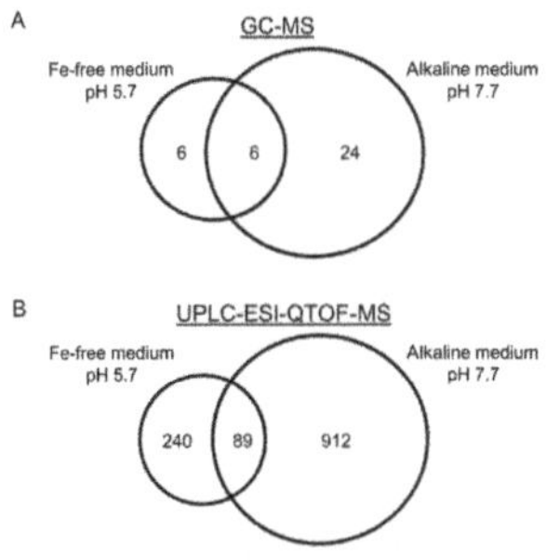

Figure 2. The root metabolome changes triggered by two different conditions of Fe deficiency partially overlap. Venn diagrams display the total number of significant metabolic changes detected by GC-MS (A) and UPLC-ESI-QTOF-MS (B) when comparing growth in the presence of Fe with growth in Fe-free medium for two weeks, or growth at pH 5.7 with growth at pH 7.7. Detailed analysis focused on the metabolites and features (*m/z* – retention time pairs) that were shared by the two conditions of Fe deficiency (see Tables 1 and 2, Tables S1 and S2 in File S6).

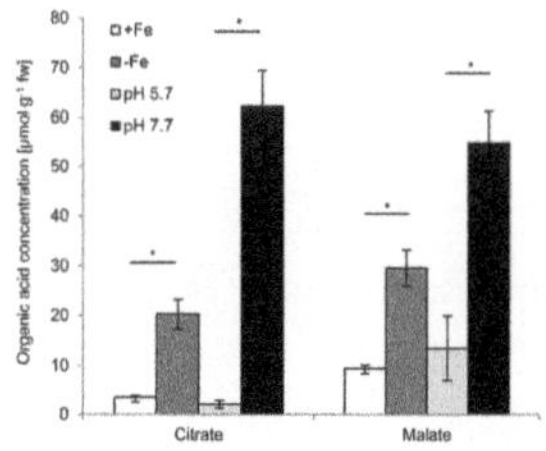

Figure 3. Citrate and malate showed strong increases of root concentrations in response to Fe deficiency. *A. thaliana* Col-0 plants were cultivated hydroponically and in separate sets of experiments exposed to two different conditions of Fe deficiency. First, root metabolomes of plants cultivated in control conditions (+Fe, white bars) were compared to those grown in Fe-free medium for two weeks (−Fe, dark grey bars). Second, plants were cultivated at pH 5.7 (light grey bars) and at pH 7.7 (black bars). Shown is the quantification of citrate and malate, the most prominent changes detected by GC-MS (see Tables 1 and 2). The means of three independent biological experiments are displayed. Error bars indicate standard deviation. Significant differences between respective control and Fe deficiency conditions were determined by Student's t-test, *P<0.05.

1) in the exudates. Thus, coumarins appear to be secreted by *A. thaliana* roots and could indeed be involved in the mobilization of extracellular insoluble Fe(III).

Fe(II)/Fe(III) complexing and Fe(III) reducing capacity of candidate coumarins

Fe reducing as well as Fe chelating activities have been ascribed to phenolic compounds [14,17]. In order to further investigate the mechanism underlying the Fe solubilizing effect of scopoletin and possibly other secreted coumarins we attempted to identify the Fe complexes that most likely form under basic conditions and in the presence of the ligands esculetin (**1**), fraxetin (**2**), and scopoletin (**3**) on the basis of their optical spectra. Fig. 8A depicts these spectra as well as control spectra of solutions of the ligands, of the ligands plus NEt_3, and of the Fe salts. In line with the literature [47] the absorption maxima of the free ligands (ca. 370 nm) were red-shifted by ca. 50–80 nm upon addition of the base and formation of the catecholate dianions of esculetin and fraxetin, or of the phenolate monoanion in the case of scopoletin. The maxima in both the neutral ligands and the catecholate/phenolate anions originate from ligand $\pi \rightarrow \pi^*$ transitions.

Solutions of mixtures of the ligands esculetin (**1**), fraxetin (**2**) and scopoletin (**3**), base NEt_3 and $FeCl_2$ gave rise to UV/vis curves with long, almost horizontal plateaus with maxima around 630–670 nm and tailing off until ca. 800 nm, originating from ligand-to-metal charge-transfer bands [47,48] which are typical of Fe-triscatecholate complexes.

Interestingly, the optical spectra of solutions containing the ligands **1–3**, base NEt_3 and $FeCl_3$ were of similar shape, yet with maxima and tails distinctly shifted to greater wavelengths when compared with the Fe(II) systems, e.g. shifted by ca. 120 nm in the case of esculetin, by ca. 60 nm for fraxetin, and by ca. 30 nm in the case of scopoletin (Fig. 8A). Fig. 8B depicts the interpretation of the spectra shown in Fig. 8A.

To independently assess interaction of the coumarins with Fe and to determine more accurately the stoichiometry, the ligands dissolved in methanol were added to aqueous solutions of ferric or ferrous iron. These mixtures were analyzed by ESI-QTOF-MS in positive and negative ionization mode via direct infusion. The free ligand was visible in all spectra recorded. Astonishingly, only in the combination of Fe(II) and scopoletin the formation of new spectral peaks could be observed independent of the stoichiometric ratio and the methanol concentration (Fig. 8C). For the main peak at *m/z* 316.02 a scopoletin: Fe ratio of 3:1 was calculated. The isotopic pattern of Fe matched well with the respective computed model (File S5). MS-MS experiments confirmed the presence of the respective ligands and Fe in this adduct (Fig. 8D).

Discussion

Our metabolome analysis aimed at elucidating the substantial changes in various metabolic pathways that occur upon Fe deficiency [49–51]. For instance, root secretion of phenols has long been hypothesized to be a biochemical part of the Fe acquisition strategy in higher plants other than grasses [52]. Phenols belong to the main constituents of root exudates and numerous studies have documented an increase in their synthesis under conditions of limited Fe availability (reviewed in [14]). This response has been implicated in the mobilization of Fe bound in the apoplast. However, the mechanisms underlying the re-utilization of Fe are unknown [53], and direct evidence for the biological importance of this process was scarce until recent work demonstrated a role of

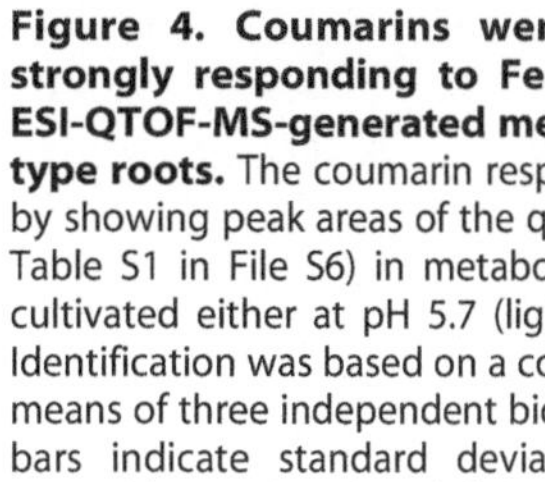

Figure 4. Coumarins were among the compounds most strongly responding to Fe deficiency as identified in UPLC-ESI-QTOF-MS-generated metabolite profiles of *A. thaliana* wild-type roots. The coumarin response to Fe deficiency is illustrated here by showing peak areas of the quantifier ions (ESI+ ionization mode, see Table S1 in File S6) in metabolite profiles of *A. thaliana* Col-0 plants cultivated either at pH 5.7 (light grey bars) or at pH 7.7 (black bars). Identification was based on a comparison with authentic standards. The means of three independent biological experiments are displayed. Error bars indicate standard deviation. Significant differences between control (pH 5.7) and Fe deficiency (pH 7.7) conditions were determined by Student's t-test, *P<0.05.

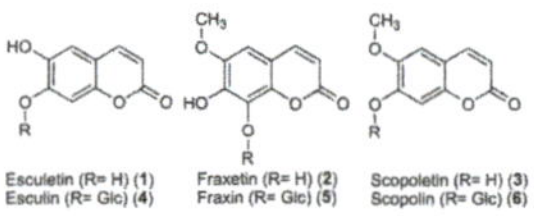

Figure 5. Structures of coumarins and their respective glycosides investigated in this study.

coumarin biosynthesis and secretion for Fe acquisition in *A. thaliana* [19–21].

We combined GC-MS- and UPLC-ESI-QTOF-MS-based metabolite profiling to cover molecules of different polarity. Our analyses detected a large number of metabolic alterations triggered by Fe depletion in *A. thaliana* roots. This is in agreement with the pronounced complexity of physiological plant adaptations to low Fe availability [50]. Monitoring responses using two different conditions helped tremendously in ascertaining the molecules that showed the most robust changes in association with Fe deficiency.

Among sugars, amino acids and organic acids, the compound classes usually covered when analyzing methanolic extracts by GC-MS, strong increases in citrate and malate signals were by far the dominant responses. This confirmed a large body of work on various strategy I plants [42] and at the same time provided strong evidence that our experimental conditions indeed triggered an Fe deficiency response. Citrate is one of the main Fe chelators in plants. It forms complexes with Fe(III) in the xylem. Therefore, sufficient loading of citrate into the xylem is essential for Fe translocation [54–56]. Increases observed in the abundance of a few amino acids on the other hand are in contrast to published reports that found rather a decrease in the abundance of the majority of detected amino acids in *Cucumis sativus* roots exposed to Fe deficiency [57]. On the other hand, Fe deficiency appears to activate N cycling and protein catabolism in *Medicago truncatula* roots [58]. In the absence of comparative kinetic analyses of metabolome changes under Fe deficiency in different plant species we cannot explain these differences. Other changes identified by our GC-MS analyses lack obvious connections to Fe homeostasis but can become informative in future studies.

Metabolome analysis via UPLC coupled to ESI-QTOF-MS has great potential to unravel the dynamics of plant secondary metabolism because wide coverage of relevant compound classes as well as high resolution can be achieved [59]. Among a large number of significant changes in the metabolome of plants exposed to Fe-deplete conditions, the increase in coumarin levels was particularly striking. Peaks representing scopolin and fraxin as well as their respective agylcones scopoletin and fraxetin were among those showing the highest fold changes detected (Fig. 4; Tables S1 and S2 in File S6). This is in agreement with the previously reported analysis of UV-fluorescent metabolites accumulating in *A. thaliana* roots under Fe-deplete conditions [20].

These coumarins could be unequivocally identified owing to the availability of reference spectra and authentic standards. It remains a challenge, however, to annotate peaks detected in LC-MS-derived metabolite profiles [38]. Thus, most of the detected features remain unidentified. Still, with the help of rapidly growing databases the results listed in Tables S1 and S2 in File S6 are expected to represent a valuable resource for future system level analyses of root metabolome dynamics under Fe deficiency conditions, especially in combination with MS-MS data provided in Files S2 and S3.

Strong up-regulation of coumarin biosynthesis as indicated by our data is consistent with several studies that analyzed global responses at the transcriptome, proteome and metabolome level.

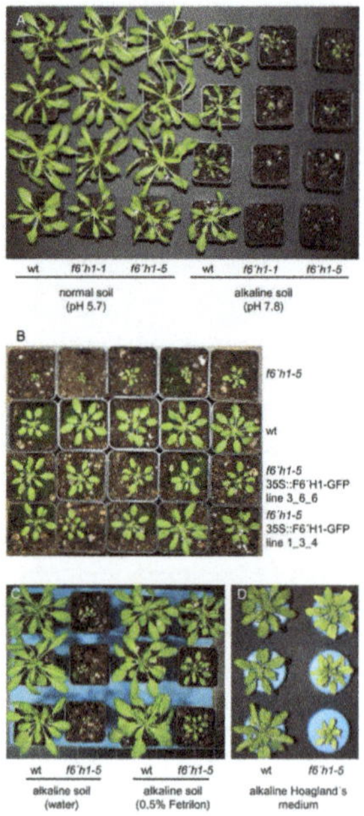

Figure 6. Growth of coumarin-deficient *f6'h1* T-DNA insertion mutants is strongly impaired under Fe-limited alkaline conditions. (A) *A. thaliana* wild type plants (wt) and *f6'h1* T-DNA insertion mutants *f6'h1-1* and *f6'h1-5* were grown on normal soil (left) and on soil alkalinized through the addition of CaO (right). (B) Overexpression of *F6'H1* under control of the 35S promoter in *f6'h1-5* fully rescues the mutant phenotype on alkaline soil. Shown are two independent transgenic lines grown alongside the wild type and the *f6'h1-5* mutant on alkaline soil. (C) The mutant phenotype on alkaline soil can be partially rescued by Fe fertilization through watering with 0.5% Fetrilon (Fe-EDTA solution). (D) Col-0 wild type plants (wt, left) and *f6'h1-5* mutant plants (right) were cultivated for six weeks in hydroponic medium with a pH of 7.7 instead of 5.7. All experiments were repeated three times independently with nearly identical outcome. The individual plants shown represent the range of phenotypes observed.

Microarray experiments showed transcriptional up-regulation of the phenylpropanoid pathway [50]. Following a proteomics approach Lan et al. reported higher levels of enzymes in this pathway under Fe deficiency. The list of identified proteins included F6'H1 [60]. Furthermore, our observations are similar to recently reported findings. Fourcray et al. identified several coumarins including scopoletin and fraxetin as being secreted in a ABCG37-dependent fashion by *A. thaliana* roots [20]. Schmid et al. showed accumulation of scopolin and scopoletin in root extracts of Fe-deficient roots [21]. Unlike the results reported here

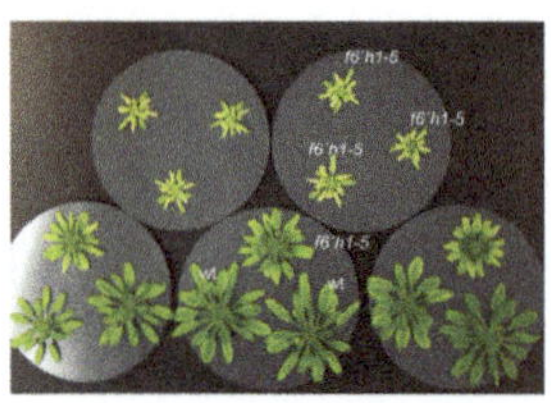

Figure 7. Partial rescue of the *f6'h1-5* growth defect in alkaline medium by co-cultivation with wild-type plants. *F6'H1* knock-out plants (*f6'h1–5*) were co-cultivated for four weeks in alkaline Hoagland's solution (pH 7.7) either with plants of the same mutant genotype (top row) or with *A. thaliana* Col-0 plants (wt) (bottom row). Experiments were repeated three times independently with nearly identical outcome.

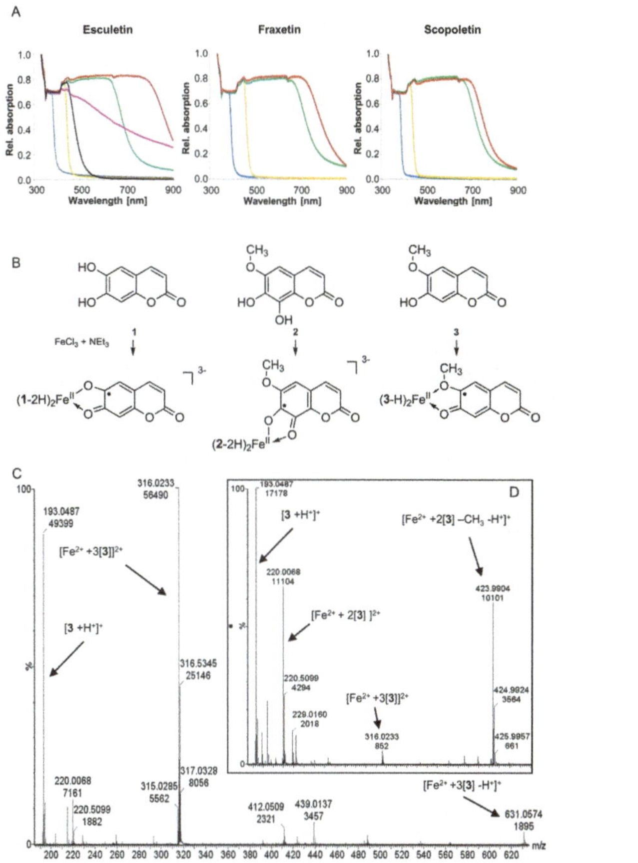

Figure 8. UV/vis spectroscopy and direct-infusion ESI-QTOF-MS demonstrate reduction of Fe(III) by coumarins and the formation of Fe(II)-coumarin complexes *in vitro*. (A) Optical spectra of solutions (CH_3CN) of ligands esculetin (**1**), fraxetin (**2**) and scopoletin (**3**), of iron salts, of mixtures of ligands and 2 equiv of NEt_3, and of mixtures containing 3 equiv of ligand, 6 equiv of NEt_3, and 1 equiv of $FeCl_2$ or $FeCl_3$. Left: **1** (blue); **1**+ NEt_3 (orange); **1**+ NEt_3+ $FeCl_2$ (green); **1**+ NEt_3+ $FeCl_3$ (red); $FeCl_3$ (black); $FeCl_2$ (magenta). Center: **2** (blue); **2**+ NEt_3 (orange); **2**+ NEt_3+ $FeCl_2$ (green); **2**+ NEt_3+ $FeCl_3$ (red). Right: **3** (blue); **3**+ NEt_3 (orange); **3**+ NEt_3+ $FeCl_2$ (green); **3**+ NEt_3+ $FeCl_3$ (red). (B) Interpretation of the UV/vis spectra depicted in (A). (C) Results of direct-infusion ESI-QTOF-MS of a mixture of Fe(II) with synthesized and purified scopoletin. (D) MS-MS spectrum of the main signal at *m/z* 316.02.

and by Fourcray et al., however, Schmid et al. also detected esculin and esculetin in root extracts.

Growth experiments with Col-0 wild type, *f6′h1* mutants and complemented lines clearly demonstrated an essential role of molecules downstream of the *ortho*-hydroxylation of cinnamates catalyzed by F6′H1 [23] for Fe acquisition both when cultivated on soil and in hydroponics (Figs. 6 and 7). Under alkaline conditions lack of this enzyme resulted in severe Fe deficiency as indicated by pronounced leaf chlorosis and strongly reduced shoot Fe levels (File S4). This again is in agreement with recently published observations for *f6′h1* mutant plants exposed to Fe deficiency at the seedling stage *in vitro* [19] or on soil [21] as well as mutant seedlings defective in the presumed coumarin export system ABCG37 [20]. Thus, we further support the conclusion that coumarin biosynthesis represents an integral part of strategy I. It is crucial under alkaline conditions, which represent a major limiting factor for agricultural productivity worldwide. Furthermore, it is interesting to note that the specific adaptations of calcicole plants to calcareous substrates have been hypothesized to be at least in part dependent on a pronounced shift from classic strategy I responses towards phenolics secretion specifically under alkaline conditions [61]. This was observed for *Parietaria diffusa*, an Fe-efficient plant that can be found on walls and similar substrates in the Mediterranean, when effects elicited by Fe-free medium were compared to those of an alkaline carbonate medium.

The partial rescue we observed upon co-cultivation with wild-type plants was reported in a study published while this manuscript was in preparation [19], albeit in a different experimental setup, i.e. with younger plants. Co-cultivation effects suggested that a lack of secreted coumarins accounts for the *f6′h1* phenotype (Fig. 7). Comparative analysis of root exudates derived from Col-0 and *f6′h1* plants showed indeed unequivocally and in agreement with Schmid et al. [21] that the aglycones scopoletin and esculetin are released by *A. thaliana* wild type roots, but not by *f6′h1* roots. The identification of esculetin was surprising as neither esculetin nor its hexoside esculin could be found in root extracts. Possibly, scopoletin can be extracellulary demethylated to esculetin. Alternatively, our analysis and the one performed by Fourcray et al. [20] may have missed the comparatively small signals (relative to scopoletin) for esculetin and esculin reported by Schmid et al. [21]. A large number of other F6′H1 dioxygenase-dependent features were detected in Col-0 root exudates. Their identities could not be determined. However, the data set reported here (Tables S3 and S4 in File S7) can be helpful in further dissecting the coumarin pathway in a fashion similar to, for instance, the elucidation of reactions upstream and downstream of chalcone synthase [31]. This will aid in meeting the challenge of identifying other coumarins potentially involved in Fe acquisition [21].

Given the essential role of secreted scopoletin one has to postulate the existence of efflux transporters similar to rice PEZ1 [2,16]. The ABC transporter ABCG37 has been proposed as a candidate because of its strong expression in Fe-deficient roots [50,51] and lack of functional ABCG37 indeed compromises growth of *A. thaliana* under alkaline conditions [19]. Indeed, the recently reported growth impairment of *pdr9–2* seedlings in the presence of pH conditions limiting Fe availability associated with a lack of coumarin secretion strongly supports this hypothesis [20]. Phenols of the catechol type exudated into the rhizosphere are considered to mobilize ferric iron by complexation and/or reduction. Indeed, Fe chelating activity of coumarins at neutral pH was already demonstrated [62]. We attempted to further characterize the mechanism underlying the demonstrated beneficial effect of coumarins through *in vitro* studies. For that we used a non-aqueous system to avoid the formation of oxo-, hydroxyl- and aquo-Fe complexes. While the conditions applied were with the necessary use of organic solvents non-physiological, they still led us to tentatively propose that scopoletin, esculetin and fraxetin can solubilize apoplastic Fe(III) because they can act both as reductants of Fe(III) and as ligands for Fe(II) under basic conditions.

There was little difference between the UV/vis spectra of mixtures of base NEt_3 and $FeCl_2$ containing the catechols esculetin and fraxetin, and those containing the *o*-hydroxyanisole scopoletin (Fig. 8A). Careful studies with heteroleptic Fe complexes bearing monodentate phenolate or *o*-chlorophenolate ligands versus optionally bisdentate *o*-hydroxyanisole ligands showed that Fe complexes with monodentate phenolate ligands have UV maxima at distinctly shorter wavelengths around 430–450 nm [63]. Hence, we conclude that scopoletin in $[(\text{scopoletin-H})_n\text{Fe(II)}]^{m-}$ complexes also acts as a bisdentate ligand with the methoxy oxygen providing a dative bond to Fe.

A conceivable explanation for the UV/vis curves of our Fe(III)–ligand systems in acetonitrile could lie in the oxidation of the catecholates of ligands esculetin and fraxetin by Fe(III) to give the respective *o*-semiquinonates that coordinate to the concomitantly formed Fe(II). Jones et al. [47] recorded UV/vis spectra of water-free solutions (Me_2SO or MeCN) containing Fe(II) or Fe(III) plus electrochemically generated 3,5-di-tert-butylchatecholate dianions, or *o*-semiquinonate anions in various stoichiometric ratios. They found that solutions containing Fe(III) and catecholate dianions in a 1:3 ratio yield the complex species $[Fe^{III}(\text{catecholate})_3]^{3-}$ showing a band with a sharp maximum at ca. 490 nm and steeply tailing off. Curves with very long plateaus reaching to wavelengths of ca. 800–900 nm and so greater than those of the Fe(II)-catecholate complexes were observed by them for complexes with *o*-semiquinonate anions. The mixed complexes of type $[Fe^{II}(o\text{-semiquinonate})(\text{catecholate})_{1-2}]^{1- \text{ or } 3-}$ should be stable and show UV/vis bands as observed (Fig. 8A). It is plausible that scopoletin gives rise to a similar complex (Fig. 8B). The relatively small red-shift of only 30 nm when compared with the $[(\text{scopoletin-H})_3Fe(II)]^-$ analog can be rationalized by a less extensive change of the ligand than in the case of esculetin and fraxetin.

While it is difficult to study complexes of Fe with phenols under alkaline conditions by ESI-MS [64], we did observe that scopoletin in contrast to esculetin readily forms stable adducts with Fe(II) ions. Such interactions might prevent Fe from re-oxidation and keep it available for uptake into the symplast under physiological conditions. However, we cannot at this stage explain the failure to detect adducts with esculetin and fraxetin.

The Fe(III) mobilizing activity found by Schmid et al. [21] for esculetin but not scopoletin suggests a chelating activity of this catechol-type molecule with neighbouring hydroxyl groups as being responsible for the beneficial effect of coumarin secretion under alkaline conditions. On the other hand, scopoletin and esculin were as efficacious as esculetin in rescuing the growth defect of *f6′h1* mutant seedlings [21]. Thus, more detailed studies and a comprehensive picture of root exudation upon Fe deficiency as well as possible conversions of secreted coumarins will be needed to unravel the exact mechanism.

In conclusion, we lend further support to the recently established crucial role of coumarin secretion for Fe acquisition by the strategy I plant *A. thaliana* under alkaline conditions. We show that coumarin biosynthesis in roots is enhanced under conditions of Fe deficiency. Coumarins are found in root exudates and appear to contribute to Fe acquisition extracellulary. Our *in vitro* evidence suggests a Fe(III) reducing and Fe(II) complexing activity of coumarins as the underlying mechanism. The metabolome data represent a potentially valuable resource for future system level analyses of Fe deficiency responses.

Supporting Information

File S1 Genotyping of T-DNA insertion line SALK_050137 (=*f6′h1-5*).

File S2 MS2Tags_positive mode_Massbank.

File S3 MS2Tags_negative mode_Massbank.

File S4 *A. thaliana f6′h1-5* plants were exposed to two different conditions causing Fe deficiency and used for the metabolite profiling experiments with Col-0 plants. (A) Plants were grown hydroponically in 1/10 Hoagland Solution for six weeks. Plants were cultivated either at a pH of 5.7 with Fe-HBED as Fe source (Control), at a pH of 7.7 with Fe-HBED as Fe source (pH 7.7), or the final two weeks at a pH of 5.7 without Fe-HBED (−Fe). (B) Fe concentrations in roots (blue bars) and shoots (red bars) were determined by ICP-OES. The means of three independent biological experiments are displayed. Error bars indicate standard deviation. Significant differences to plants grown under control conditions were determined by Student's t-test, $^*P<0.05$.

File S5 Isotopic pattern of iron for the main peak at *m/z* 316.02 shown in Figure 8C. A scopoletin: Fe ratio of 3:1 was calculated.

File S6 Tables S1 and S2 listing markers consistently up-regulated upon hydroponic cultivation in Fe-free and alkaline medium condition in *A. thaliana* as detected by UPLC-ESI-QTOF-MS in either positive ionization mode (Table S1) or negative ionization mode (Table S2). Markers from three biological replicates were chosen when they met the following criteria in both sets of three biologically independent experiments each: Fold-change >2 and P<0.05 (Student's t-test). Annotation level (Ann. Level): 1. compound identified using a synthesized standard; 2. compound putatively annotated by interpretation of mass spectrometry data; 3. compound class putatively annotated; 4. unknown compounds. *m/z*: Mass to charge ratio. Annotation: MS2T identifiers, elemental composition of the uncharged compound, adducts or the identified compounds are given. Molecular Mass: Molecular mass of the respective compound (i.e. precursor or M) is given.

File S7 Tables S3 and S4 listing markers identified in a comparison of root exudates harvested from *A. thaliana* wild type and *f6′h1-5* mutant plants as detected by UPLC-ESI-QTOF-MS in either positive ionization mode (Table S3) or negative ionization mode (Table S4). Markers accumulating in the wild-type exudates were chosen when they met the following criteria: Fold-change >2 and P<0.05 (Student's t-test; 3 independent biological experiments). Annotation level (Ann. Level): 1. compound identified using a synthesized standard; 2. compound putatively annotated by interpretation of mass spectrometry data; 3. compound class putatively annotated; 4. unknown compounds. *m/z*: Mass to charge ratio. Annotation: adducts or the identified compounds are given. Molecular Mass: Molecular mass of the respective compound (i.e. precursor or M) is given. Entries are ordered according to their fold-change.

Acknowledgments

We thank Blen Beyene for valuable discussions, Silke Matros for excellent technical assistance and Manuel Braun and Willi Riber for contributions to implementing the GC-MS data analysis workflow.

Author Contributions

Conceived and designed the experiments: RS SC. Performed the experiments: HS CG MW CS SL CB. Analyzed the data: HS MW CS SL RS SC. Wrote the paper: SC.

References

1. Thomine S, Vert G (2013) Iron transport in plants: better be safe than sorry. Curr Opin Plant Biol 16: 322–327.
2. Kobayashi T, Nishizawa NK (2012) Iron uptake, translocation, and regulation in higher plants. Annu Rev Plant Biol 63: 131–152.
3. WHO (2002) World Health Report 2002. Available: http://www.who.int/whr/2002/en/whr02_en.pdf.
4. White PJ, Broadley MR (2009) Biofortification of crops with seven mineral elements often lacking in human diets - iron, zinc, copper, calcium, magnesium, selenium and iodine. New Phytol 182: 49–84.
5. Schroeder JI, Delhaize E, Frommer WB, Guerinot ML, Harrison MJ, et al. (2013) Using membrane transporters to improve crops for sustainable food production. Nature 497: 60–66.
6. Morrissey J, Guerinot ML (2009) Iron uptake and transport in plants: the good, the bad, and the Ionome. Chem Rev 109: 4553–4567.
7. Römheld V, Marschner H (1986) Evidence for a specific uptake system for iron phytosiderophores in roots of grasses. Plant Physiol 80: 175–180.
8. Nozoye T, Nagasaka S, Kobayashi T, Takahashi M, Sato Y, et al. (2011) Phytosiderophore efflux transporters are crucial for iron acquisition in graminaceous plants. J Biol Chem 286: 5446–5454.
9. Curie C, Panaviene Z, Loulergue C, Dellaporta S, Briat J, et al. (2001) Maize yellow stripe1 encodes a membrane protein directly involved in Fe(III) uptake. Nature 409: 346–349.
10. Santi S, Schmidt W (2009) Dissecting iron deficiency-induced proton extrusion in Arabidopsis roots. New Phytol 183: 1072–1084.
11. Robinson NJ, Procter CM, Connolly EL, Guerinot ML (1999) A ferric-chelate reductase for iron uptake from soils. Nature 397: 694–697.
12. Vert G, Grotz N, Dedaldechamp F, Gaymard F, Guerinot M, et al. (2002) IRT1, an Arabidopsis transporter essential for iron uptake from the soil and for plant growth. Plant Cell 14: 1233–1243.
13. Badri DV, Vivanco JM (2009) Regulation and function of root exudates. Plant Cell Environ 32: 666–681.
14. Cesco S, Neumann G, Tomasi N, Pinton R, Weisskopf L (2010) Release of plant-borne flavonoids into the rhizosphere and their role in plant nutrition. Plant Soil 329: 1–25.
15. Jin CW, You GY, He YF, Tang C, Wu P, et al. (2007) Iron deficiency-induced secretion of phenolics facilitates the reutilization of root apoplastic iron in red clover. Plant Physiol 144: 278–285.
16. Ishimaru Y, Kakei Y, Shimo H, Bashir K, Sato Y, et al. (2011) A rice phenolic efflux transporter is essential for solubilizing precipitated apoplasmic iron in the plant stele. J Biol Chem 286: 24649–24655.
17. Römheld V, Marschner H (1986) Mobilization of iron in the rhizosphere of different plant species. Adv Plant Nutr 2: 155–204.
18. Tomasi N, Weisskopf L, Renella G, Landi L, Pinton R, et al. (2008) Flavonoids of white lupin roots participate in phosphorus mobilization from soil. Soil Biol Biochem 40: 1971–1974.
19. Rodríguez-Celma J, Lin W-D, Fu G-M, Abadia J, López-Míllán A-F, et al. (2013) Mutually exclusive alterations in secondary metabolism are critical for the uptake of insoluble iron compounds by Arabidopsis and Medicago truncatula. Plant Physiol. 162: 1473–1485.
20. Fourcroy P, Sisó-Terraza P, Sudre D, Savirón M, Reyt G, et al. (2014) Involvement of the ABCG37 transporter in secretion of scopoletin and derivatives by Arabidopsis roots in response to iron deficiency. New Phytol 201: 155–167.
21. Schmid NB, Giehl RFH, Doll S, Mock H-P, Strehmel N, et al. (2014) Feruloyl-CoA 6′-hydroxylase1-dependent coumarins mediate iron acquisition from alkaline substrates in Arabidopsis. Plant Physiol 164: 160–172.
22. Alonso JM, Stepanova AN, Leisse TJ, Kim CJ, Chen H, et al. (2003) Genome-wide insertional mutagenesis of Arabidopsis thaliana. Science 301: 653–657.
23. Kai K, Mizutani M, Kawamura N, Yamamoto R, Tamai M, et al. (2008) Scopoletin is biosynthesized via ortho-hydroxylation of feruloyl CoA by a 2-oxoglutarate-dependent dioxygenase in Arabidopsis thaliana. Plant J 55: 989–999.
24. Hoagland DR, Arnon DI (1950) The water-culture method for growing plants without soil. Circular. California Agricultural Experiment Station 347, 1–32.
25. Chaney R (1988) Plants can utilize iron from Fe-N,n'-Di-(2-Hydroxybenzoyl)-Ethylenediamine-N,n'-Diacetic Acid, a ferric chelate with 106 greater formation constant than Fe-EDDHA. J Plant Nutr 11: 1033–1050.
26. Erban A, Schauer N, Fernie AR, Kopka J (2007) Nonsupervised construction and application of mass spectral and retention time index libraries from time-of-flight gas chromatography–mass spectrometry metabolite profiles. Metabolomics - Methods and Protocols. Methods in Molecular Biology. Humana Press Inc. 19–38.
27. Stein SE (1999) An integrated method for spectrum extraction and compound identification from gas chromatography/mass spectrometry data. J Am Soc Mass Spectrom 10: 770–781.
28. Barupal DK, Kind T, Kothari SL, Lee DY, Fiehn O (2010) Hydrocarbon phenotyping of algal species using pyrolysis-gas chromatography mass spectrometry. BMC Biotechnol 10: 40.
29. Styczynski MP, Moxley JF, Tong LV, Walther JL, Jensen KL, et al. (2007) Systematic identification of conserved metabolites in GC/MS data for metabolomics and biomarker discovery. Anal Chem 79: 966–973.
30. SpectConnect (n.d.). Available: http://spectconnect.mit.edu/.
31. Böttcher C, von Roepenack-Lahaye E, Schmidt J, Schmotz C, Neumann S, et al. (2008) Metabolome analysis of biosynthetic mutants reveals a diversity of metabolic changes and allows identification of a large number of new compounds in arabidopsis. Plant Physiol 147: 2107–2120.
32. Khandal D, Samol I, Buhr F, Pollmann S, Schmidt H, et al. (2009) Singlet oxygen-dependent translational control in the tigrina-d.12 mutant of barley. Proc Natl Acad Sci U S A 106: 13112–13117.
33. Tautenhahn R, Patti GJ, Rinehart D, Siuzdak G (2012) XCMS Online: A web-based platform to process untargeted metabolomic data. Anal Chem 84: 5035–5039.
34. Tautenhahn R, Cho K, Uritboonthai W, Zhu Z, Patti GJ, et al. (2012) An accelerated workflow for untargeted metabolomics using the METLIN database. Nat Biotechnol 30: 826–828.
35. Patti GJ, Tautenhahn R, Rinehart D, Cho K, Shriver LP, et al. (2013) A view from above: cloud plots to visualize global metabolomic data. Anal Chem 85: 798–804.
36. Matsuda F, Yonekura-Sakakibara K, Niida R, Kuromori T, Shinozaki K, et al. (2009) MS/MS spectral tag-based annotation of non-targeted profile of plant secondary metabolites. Plant J 57: 555–577.
37. Sakurai T, Yamada Y, Sawada Y, Matsuda F, Akiyama K, et al. (2013) PRIMe update: Innovative content for plant metabolomics and integration of gene expression and metabolite accumulation. Plant Cell Physiol 54: e5.
38. Horai H, Arita M, Kanaya S, Nihei Y, Ikeda T, et al. (2010) MassBank: a public repository for sharing mass spectral data for life sciences. J Mass Spectrom 45: 703–714.
39. Curtis MD, Grossniklaus U (2003) A gateway cloning vector set for high-throughput functional analysis of genes in planta. Plant Physiol 133: 462–469.
40. Demyttenaere J, Van Syngel K, Markusse AP, Vervisch S, Debenedetti S, et al. (2002) Synthesis of 6-methoxy-4H-1-benzopyran-7-ol, a character donating component of the fragrance of Wisteria sinensis. Tetrahedron 58: 2163–2166.
41. Demyttenaere J, Vervisch S, Debenedetti S, Coussio J, Maes D, et al. (2004) Synthesis of virgatol and virgatenol, two naturally occurring coumarins from Pterocaulon virgatum (L.) DC, and 7-(2,3-epoxy-3-methylbutoxy)-6-methoxy-coumarin, isolated from Conyza obscura DC. Synth-Stuttg: 1844–1848.
42. Abadia J, Lopez-Millan AF, Rombola A, Abadia A (2002) Organic acids and Fe deficiency: a review. Plant Soil 241: 75–86.
43. Schuler M, Rellán-Álvarez R, Fink-Straube C, Abadía J, Bauer P (2012) Nicotianamine functions in the phloem-based transport of iron to sink organs, in pollen development and pollen tube growth in Arabidopsis. Plant Cell 24: 2380–2400.
44. Saito K, Matsuda F (2010) Metabolomics for functional genomics, systems biology, and biotechnology. Annu Rev Plant Biol 61: 463–489.
45. Kai K, Shimizu B, Mizutani M, Watanabe K, Sakata K (2006) Accumulation of coumarins in Arabidopsis thaliana. Phytochemistry 67: 379–386.
46. Jeong J, Cohu C, Kerkeb L, Pilon M, Connolly EL, et al. (2008) Chloroplast Fe(III) chelate reductase activity is essential for seedling viability under iron limiting conditions. Proc Natl Acad Sci 105: 10619–10624.
47. Jones S, Leon L, Sawyer D (1982) Redox chemistry of metal-catechol complexes in aprotic media.3. 3,5-di-tert-butylcatecholato and ortho-semiquinonato complexes of iron(III). Inorg Chem 21: 3692–3698.
48. Palaniandavar M, Viswanathan R (1996) Iron(III) complexes of phenolate ligands as models for catechol dioxygenases. Proc Indian Acad Sci-Chem Sci 108: 235–249.
49. Buckhout TJ, Thimm O (2003) Insights into metabolism obtained from microarray analysis. Curr Opin Plant Biol 6: 288–296.
50. Yang TJ, Lin W-D, Schmidt W (2010) Transcriptional profiling of the Arabidopsis iron deficiency response reveals conserved transition metal homeostasis networks. Plant Physiol 152: 2130–2141.
51. Abadia J, Vazquez S, Rellan-Alvarez R, El-Jendoubi H, Abadia A, et al. (2011) Towards a knowledge-based correction of iron chlorosis. Plant Physiol Biochem 49: 471–482.
52. Römheld V, Marschner H (1983) Mechanism of iron uptake by peanut plants.1. FeIII reduction, chelate splitting, and release of phenolics. Plant Physiol 71: 949–954.
53. Pavlovic J, Samardzic J, Maksimovic V, Timotijevic G, Stevic N, et al. (2013) Silicon alleviates iron deficiency in cucumber by promoting mobilization of iron in the root apoplast. New Phytol 198: 1096–1107.
54. Rellán-Álvarez R, Giner-Martínez-Sierra J, Orduna J, Orera I, Rodríguez-Castrillón JÁ, et al. (2010) Identification of a tri-iron(III), tri-citrate complex in the xylem sap of iron-deficient tomato resupplied with iron: New insights into plant iron long-distance transport. Plant Cell Physiol 51: 91–102.
55. Durrett TP, Gassmann W, Rogers EE (2007) The FRD3-mediated efflux of citrate into the root vasculature is necessary for efficient iron translocation. Plant Physiol 144: 197–205.
56. Roschzttardtz H, Séguéla-Arnaud M, Briat J-F, Vert G, Curie C (2011) The FRD3 citrate effluxer promotes iron nutrition between symplastically disconnected tissues throughout Arabidopsis development. Plant Cell 23: 2725–2737.
57. Borlotti A, Vigani G, Zocchi G (2012) Iron deficiency affects nitrogen metabolism in cucumber (*Cucumis sativus* L.) plants. BMC Plant Biol 12: 189.

58. Rodriguez-Celma J, Lattanzio G, Grusak MA, Abadia A, Abadia J, et al. (2011) Root Responses of *Medicago truncatula* plants grown in two different iron deficiency conditions: Changes in root protein profile and riboflavin biosynthesis. J Proteome Res 10: 2590–2601.
59. Matsuda F, Hirai MY, Sasaki E, Akiyama K, Yonekura-Sakakibara K, et al. (2010) AtMetExpress development: A phytochemical atlas of Arabidopsis development. Plant Physiol 152: 566–578.
60. Lan P, Li W, Wen T, Shiau J, Wu Y, et al. (2011) iTRAQ protein profile analysis of Arabidopsis roots reveals new aspects critical for iron homeostasis. Plant Physiol 155: 821–834.
61. Donnini S, De Nisi P, Gabotti D, Tato L, Zocchi G (2012) Adaptive strategies of Parietaria diffusa (M. & K.) to calcareous habitat with limited iron availability. Plant Cell Environ 35: 1171–1184.
62. Mladenka P, Macakova K, Zatloukalova L, Rehakova Z, Singh BK, et al. (2010) In vitro interactions of coumarins with iron. Biochimie 92: 1108–1114.
63. Heistand R, Lauffer R, Fikrig E, Que L (1982) Catecholate and phenolate iron complexes as models for the dioxygenases. J Am Chem Soc 104: 2789–2796.
64. Guo M, Perez C, Wei Y, Rapoza E, Su G, et al. (2007) Iron-binding properties of plant phenolics and cranberry's bio-effects. Dalton Trans Camb Engl 2003: 4951–4961.

15

Vitamin D Deficiency Aggravates Nephrotoxicity, Hypertension and Dyslipidemia Caused by Tenofovir: Role of Oxidative Stress and Renin-Angiotensin System

Daniele Canale, Ana Carolina de Bragança, Janaína Garcia Gonçalves, Maria Heloisa Massola Shimizu, Talita Rojas Sanches, Lúcia Andrade, Rildo Aparecido Volpini, Antonio Carlos Seguro*

Nephrology Department, University of São Paulo School of Medicine, São Paulo, Brazil

Abstract

Vitamin D deficiency (VDD) is prevalent among HIV-infected individuals. Vitamin D has been associated with renal and cardiovascular diseases because of its effects on oxidative stress, lipid metabolism and renin-angiotensin-aldosterone system (RAAS). Tenofovir disoproxil fumarate (TDF), a widely used component of antiretroviral regimens for HIV treatment, can induce renal injury. The aim of this study was to investigate the effects of VDD on TDF-induced nephrotoxicity. Wistar rats were divided into four groups: control, receiving a standard diet for 60 days; VDD, receiving a vitamin D-free diet for 60 days; TDF, receiving a standard diet for 60 days with the addition of TDF (50 mg/kg food) for the last 30 days; and VDD+TDF receiving a vitamin D-free diet for 60 days with the addition of TDF for the last 30 days. TDF led to impaired renal function, hyperphosphaturia, hypophosphatemia, hypertension and increased renal vascular resistance due to downregulation of the sodium-phosphorus cotransporter and upregulation of angiotensin II and AT1 receptor. TDF also increased oxidative stress, as evidenced by higher TBARS and lower GSH levels, and induced dyslipidemia. Association of TDF and VDD aggravated renovascular effects and TDF-induced nephrotoxicity due to changes in the redox state and involvement of RAAS.

Editor: Dulce Elena Casarini, Federal University of São Paulo (UNIFESP), Escola Paulista de Medicina, Brazil

Funding: This study was supported by grants from Conselho Nacional de Desenvolvimento Científico e Tecnológico (CNPq, 309947/2009-0) and Fundação de Amparo à Pesquisa do Estado de São Paulo (FAPESP, 2012/50227-9; 2011/50409-7; 2010/52294-0). The funders had no role in the study design, data collection and analysis, decision to publish, or preparation of the manuscript.

Competing Interests: The authors confirm that co-author Antonio Carlos Seguro is a PLOS ONE Editorial Board Member and this does not alter their adherence to PLOS ONE Editorial policies and criteria.

* Email: trulu@usp.br

Introduction

Tenofovir disoproxil fumarate (TDF) is a nucleotide reverse transcriptase inhibitor commonly used for treatment of HIV infection and hepatitis B on the basis of its effectiveness in clinical trials [1–4]. However, the long-term use of TDF has been associated with hypophosphatemia due to proximal renal tubular dysfunction, renal failure [5] and enhancement of oxidative stress by disruption of mitochondrial DNA in proximal tubule cells [6]. In addition to the renal impairment caused by TDF-induced nephrotoxicity it has been recently shown that low vitamin D levels are associated with the progression of HIV-related diseases in patients receiving antiretroviral therapy [7,8].

Vitamin D is an indispensable nutrient for mineral homeostasis [9] and is also responsible for kidney protection and the regulation of several renal physiological activities [10]. Thus, vitamin D deficiency (VDD) (<10 ng/mL) or insufficiency (10–30 ng/mL) can accelerate the progression of kidney disease [10–13].

Vitamin D has been associated with renal and cardiovascular diseases because of its effects on oxidative stress, lipid metabolism and renin-angiotensin-aldosterone system (RAAS). *Tarcin et al* demonstrated that vitamin D deficient individuals presented higher plasma levels of Thiobarbituric Acid Reactive Substances (TBARS) [14]. Besides the effects of VDD on oxidative stress, studies have demonstrated that HIV-infected individuals exhibit a deficiency of total glutathione (GSH) [15] aggravating the redox state. Furthermore, several studies have shown that vitamin D is a negative endocrine regulator of RAAS [16] and its concentration has been inversely associated with the prevalence of metabolic syndrome [17].

Given that VDD is highly prevalent among HIV-infected individuals, the aim of this study was to investigate the effects of VDD on TDF-induced nephrotoxicity, mainly focused on the role of oxidative stress and RAAS.

Materials and Methods

All experimental procedures were approved by the local Research Ethics Committee (CEP-FMUSP – Comitê de Ética em Pesquisa da Faculdade de Medicina da Universidade de São Paulo), protocol number 086/11). All experiments were developed in strict conformity with local institutional guidelines and with well-established international standards for manipulation and care of laboratory animals.

Animals and experimental protocol

Male Wistar rats, weighing 200–250 g, were obtained from the animal facilities of the University of São Paulo School of Medicine, housed in standard cages, and given *ad libitum* access to water and

Table 1. Body weight, renal function and hemodynamic measurements in normal (control) rats, in rats maintained 60 days on vitamin D free diet (VDD), in rats on normal diet treated for additional 30 days with tenofovir (TDF) and in rats on vitamin D free diet for 60 days, to which tenofovir was added on day 30 and continued throughout (VDD+TDF).

	C	VDD	TDF	VDD+TDF
BW	498±12	476±7	461±6	463±14
GFR	0.88±0.04	0.61±0.06^{b}	0.63±0.04^{c}	0.45±0.04^{c,d}
MAP	117±3	127±4	134±2^{b}	148±5^{c,e}
RBF	5.58±0.03	5.82±0.04	5.59±0.05	5.72±0.08
RVR	19.8±0.4	21.1±0.8	24.1±0.5^{c}	26.9±1.0^{c,e}

BW, body weight (g); GFR, inulin clearance (mL/min/100 g); MAP, mean arterial pressure (mmHg); RBF, renal blood flow (mL/min); RVR, renal vascular resistance (mmHg/mL/min). Values are means ± SEM. $^{a}p<0.05$, $^{b}p<0.01$, $^{c}p<0.001$ vs. C; $^{d}p<0.05$; $^{e}p<0.01$ vs. TDF.

commercial rodent chow, standard (Cat.# 960397) or vitamin D-free (Cat.# 960074), both obtained from *MP Biomedicals* (MP Biomedicals, Irvine, CA, USA). Rats were randomly allocated to the following groups: control (C, n = 10), receiving a standard diet for 60 days; VDD (n = 7), receiving a vitamin D-free diet for 60 days; TDF (n = 10), receiving a standard diet for 60 days with the addition of TDF (50 mg/kg food) for the last 30 days; and VDD+TDF (n = 8) receiving a vitamin D-free diet for 60 days with the addition of TDF (50 mg/kg food) for the last 30 days. The dose of TDF was based on a previous study from our laboratory [5] and is compatible with the dosage administered to humans.

Metabolic cage studies and analysis of urine samples

At the end of the protocol, rats were moved to metabolic cages (one rat per cage), maintained on a 12-h light/dark cycle and given free access to drinking water. The rats were acclimated to the housing conditions for 1 day before the experimental procedures, which began with the collection of 24-h urine samples. The volume of each 24-h urine sample was measured gravimetrically. Urine samples were centrifuged in aliquots to remove suspended material, and the supernatants were analyzed. Urine concentrations of sodium and potassium were determined with specific electrodes (ABL800Flex - Radiometer, Brønshøj, Denmark). Urinary potassium/sodium ratio was calculated (U_K/U_{Na}). Urine concentrations of phosphorus, calcium and protein were measured by a colorimetric system using a commercial kit (Labtest Diagnóstica – Minas Gerais, Brazil). Urinary excretions of phosphorus (U_PV), calcium ($U_{Ca}V$) and protein ($U_{Prot}V$) were determined.

Hemodynamic studies

To determine glomerular filtration rate (GFR), inulin clearance studies were conducted at the end of the protocol. On the day of the experiment, the animals were anesthetized intraperitoneally with sodium pentobarbital (50 mg/kg BW). The trachea was cannulated with a PE-240 catheter, and spontaneous breathing was maintained. To control mean arterial pressure (MAP) and allow blood sampling, a PE-60 catheter was inserted into the right

Table 2. Biochemical parameters measurements in normal (control) rats, in rats maintained 60 days on vitamin D free diet (VDD), in rats on normal diet treated for additional 30 days with tenofovir (TDF) and in rats on vitamin D free diet for 60 days, to which tenofovir was added on day 30 and continued throughout (VDD+TDF).

	C	VDD	TDF	VDD+TDF
25(OH)D	15.4±1.0	<1.5 (undetectable)^{c}	14.8±1.3	<1.5 (undetectable)^{c,e}
PTH	120±11	1261±33^{c}	83±15	516±151^{b,e}
Aldosterone	116±15	243±46	316±57^{a}	479±83^{c,d}
P_P	9.38±0.40	5.03±0.11^{c}	6.47±0.34^{c}	6.29±0.39^{c}
P_{Ca}	1.13±0.01	0.94±0.05^{c}	1.14±0.02	0.94±0.03^{c,f}
P_{Na}	136±1	139±3	136±1	138±1
P_K	3.9±0.3	4.3±0.2	3.7±0.2	4.1±0.2
Cholesterol	39±1	53±4^{a}	54±3^{a}	80±7^{c,f}
Triglycerides	17±4	34±5	59±9^{b}	74±13^{c}
U_PV	14.9±1.1	17.0±0.9	18.7±0.8^{a}	21.5±0.7^{c,d}
$U_{Ca}V$	0.08±0.01	0.13±0.01	0.11±0.02	0.13±0.01
U_K/U_{Na}	3.27±0.17	3.39±0.16	3.07±0.18	4.46±0.49^{a,e}
$U_{Prot}V$	5.3±0.3	11.3±0.8^{c}	10.8±0.3^{c}	11.8±0.5^{c}

25(OH)D, 25 hydroxyvitamin D (ng/mL); PTH, parathormone (pg/mL); Aldosterone (pg/mL); P_P, plasma phosphate concentration (mg/dL); P_{Ca}, plasma calcium concentration (mmol/L); P_{Na}, plasma sodium concentration (mEq/L); P_K, plasma potassium concentration (mEq/L); Cholesterol, total cholesterol (mg/dL); Triglycerides (mg/dL); U_PV, urinary phosphorus excretion (mg/day); $U_{Ca}V$, urinary calcium excretion (mg/day); U_K/U_{Na}, urinary concentration of potassium and sodium ratio; $U_{Prot}V$, urinary protein excretion (mg/day). Values are means ± SEM. $^{a}p<0.05$, $^{b}p<0.01$, $^{c}p<0.001$ vs. C; $^{d}p<0.05$; $^{e}p<0.01$, $^{f}p<0.001$ vs. TDF.

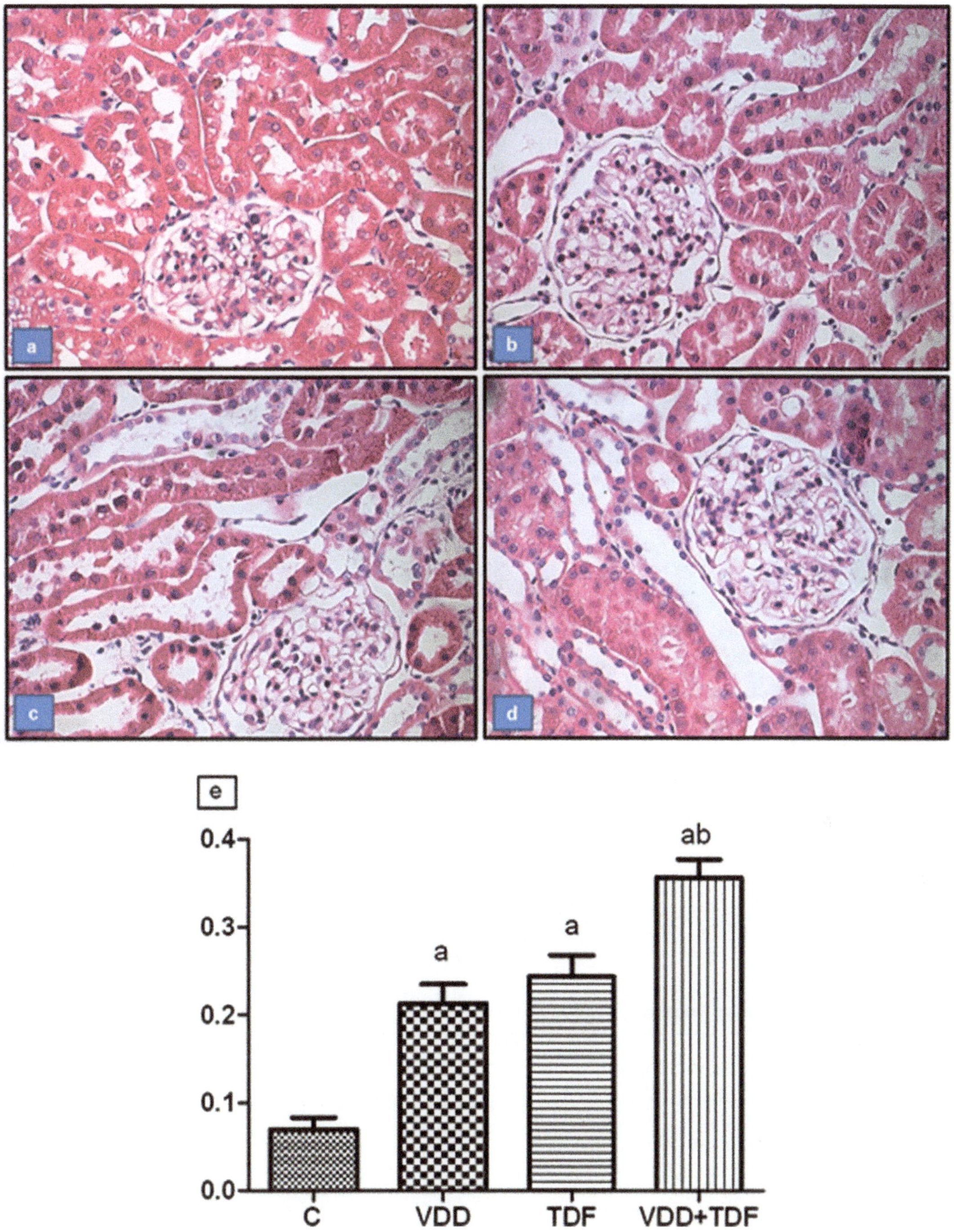

Figure 1. Representative photomicrographs of the tubular injury. (a) control, (b) VDD, (c) TDF and (d) VDD+TDF. Magnification, 400x. (e) Score of tubular injury of C, VDD, TDF and VDD+TDF. Values are means ± SEM. $^{a}p<0.001$ vs. C; $^{b}p<0.001$ vs. TDF.

carotid artery. MAP was assessed using Biopac Systems Inc MP100 (Santa Barbara, CA, USA). For the infusion of inulin and fluids, another PE-60 catheter was inserted into the left jugular vein. In order to collect urine samples, a suprapubic incision was made, and the urinary bladder was cannulated with a PE-240 catheter. After the surgical procedure has been completed, a loading dose of inulin (100 mg/kg BW diluted in 0.9% saline) was administered through the jugular vein. Subsequently, a constant infusion of inulin (10 mg/kg BW in 0.9% saline) was started and kept at 0.04 ml/min throughout the experiment. Three urine samples were collected at 30-min intervals. Blood samples were obtained at the beginning and at the end of the experiment. Blood and urine inulin were determined using the anthrone method. GFR data are expressed as ml/min/100 g.

To measure renal blood flow (RBF), a midline incision was made. Then, we carefully dissected the left renal pedicle and isolated the renal artery, taking precautions to avoid disturbing the renal nerves. An ultrasonic flow probe was placed around the exposed renal artery. RBF was measured using an ultrasonic flowmeter (T402; Transonic Systems, Bethesda, MD, USA) and is

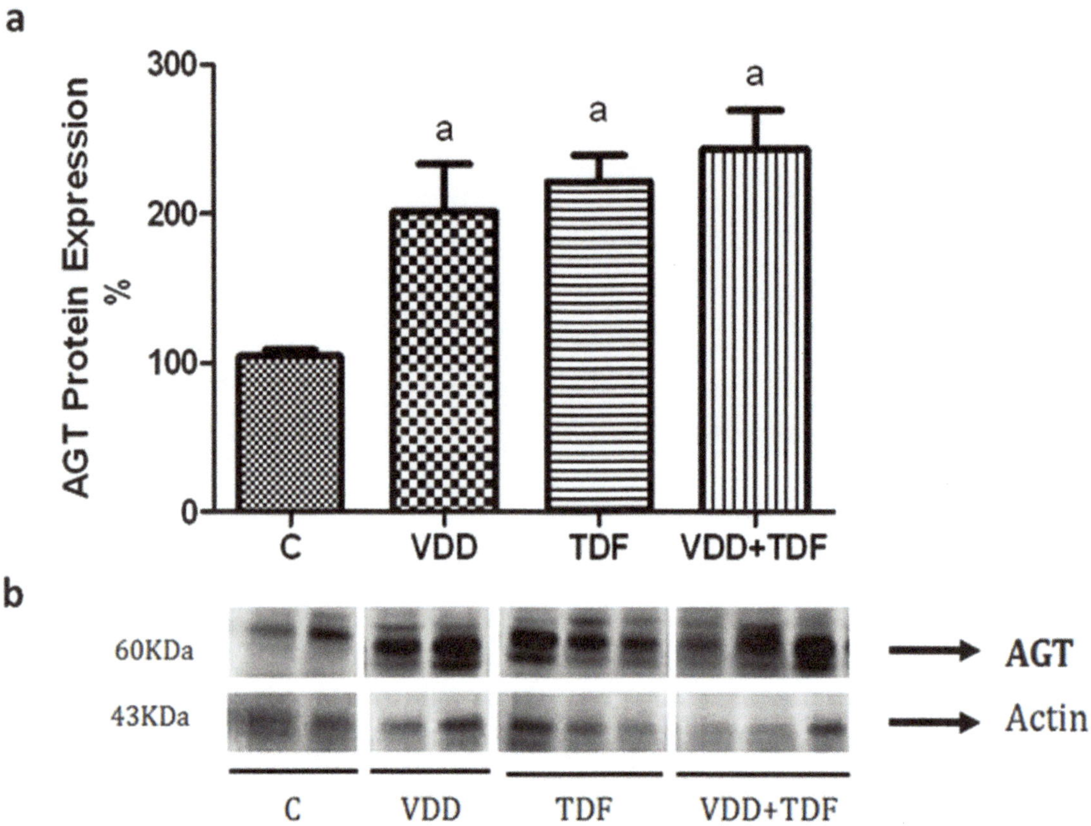

Figure 2. Semiquantitative immunoblotting of kidney fractions. (a) A densitometric analysis of samples from control (n = 4), VDD (n = 6), TDF (n = 6) and VDD+TDF (n = 6) rats is shown. (b) Immunoblots reacted with anti-angiotensinogen revealing a 60-kDa band. Values are means ± SEM. [a]p<0.05 vs. C.

expressed as ml/min. Renal vascular resistance (RVR) was calculated by dividing the blood pressure by RBF and is expressed as mmHg/ml/min.

Evaluation of 25-hydroxyvitamin D [25(OH)D]

For assessment of plasma levels of circulating vitamin D [25(OH)D], we used a radioimmunoassay (RIA) commercial kit from DiaSorin (DiaSorin, MN, USA). Briefly, this method consists of two-step procedure: (1) a rapid extraction of 25(OH)D from plasma with acetonitrile; (2) following extraction, the treated sample is then assayed using an equilibrium RIA procedure, based on an antibody with specificity to 25(OH)D.

Assessment of plasma biochemical parameters

For evaluation of PTH, aldosterona, sodium (P_{Na}), potassium (P_K), phosphate (P_P), calcium (P_{Ca}), cholesterol and triglycerides blood samples were collected. PTH was assessed by Enzyme-Linked Immunosorbent Assay (ELISA) using a commercial kit (Rat Bioactive Intact PTH (Immutopics - California, USA), aldosterone was determined by radioimmunoassay (RIA) using a commercial kit (Immunotech, Marseille, FR), P_P was evaluated by a colorimetric system using a commercial kit (Labtest Diagnóstica – Minas Gerais, Brazil) and P_{Na}, P_K and P_{Ca} were determined with specific electrodes (ABL800Flex – Radiometer, Brønshøj, Denmark). Cholesterol and triglycerides were evaluated by a colorimetric system using a commercial kit (Cobas C111 - Roche, São Paulo, Brazil).

Tissue sample collection/preparation

At the end of the experiments, the organs were perfused with PBS solution (0.15 M NaCl and 0.01 M sodium phosphate buffer, pH 7.4). The left kidney were removed and weighed. For histological/immunohistochemical examination, a fragment of the right kidney was fixed in 10% neutral-buffered formalin solution. The kidney block was dehydrated in graded alcohol, embedded in paraffin and cut at 4-µm sections. Another fragment of the right kidney was frozen in liquid nitrogen and stored at −80°C for assessment of endothelial nitric oxide syntase (eNOS), sodium-phosphate cotransporter subtype IIa (NaPi-IIa), AT1 receptor (AT1r) and angiotensinogen/angiotensin I and II (Ang) protein expression.

Light microscopy studies

Four-µm histological sections of renal tissue were stained with hematoxylin-eosin and examined under light microscope. For the evaluation of renal damage, 40–60 grid fields (×400 magnification) measuring 0.245 mm^2 were evaluated by graded scores according to the following criteria: (0), less than 5% of the field showing tubular epithelial swelling, vacuolar degeneration, necrosis, and desquamation; (I), 5–25% of the field presenting renal lesions; (II), involvement of 25–50% with renal damage; (III), 50–75% of damaged area; and (IV), more that 75% of the grid field presenting renal lesions. The morphometric examination was blinded to minimize observer bias, i.e. the observer was unaware of the treatment group from which the tissue originated. The mean score for each rat and the mean score for each group were calculated.

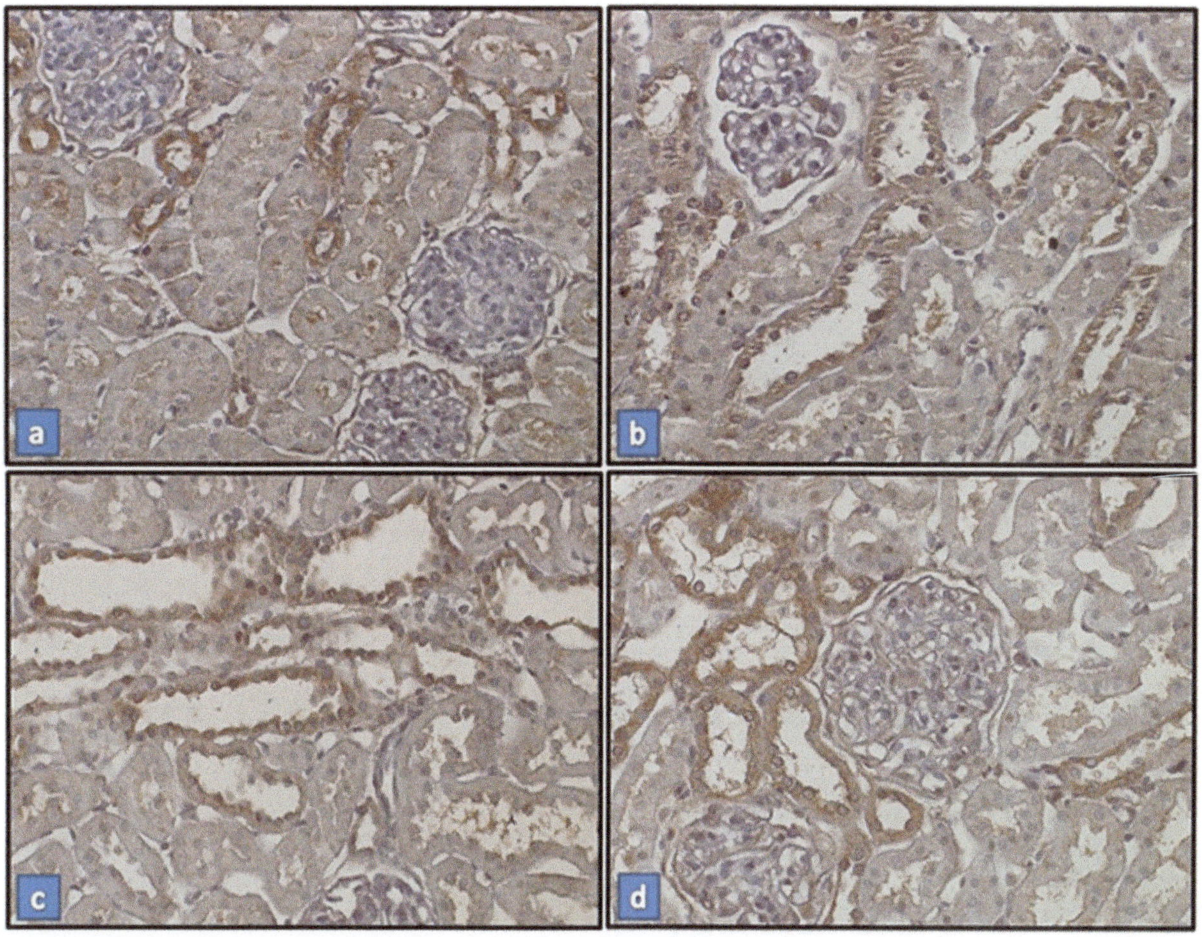

Figure 3. Expression of Angiotensin II in renal tissue. Immunostaining for angiotensin II (brown) in kidney cortex samples from C (a), VDD (b), TDF (c) and VDD+TDF (d). Magnification, ×400. Note that the staining is more extensive and intense in the sample from the VDD, TDF and VDD+TDF.

Immunohistochemistry studies

Four-µm sections of kidney were incubated 60 min at room temperature (1/1,000) with a polyclonal primary antibody anti-angiotensin II (Santa Cruz Biotechnology). The reaction product was detected with an avidin-biotin-peroxidase complex (Vector Laboratories, Burlingame, CA). The color reaction was developed with 3,3-diaminobenzidine (Sigma), and the material was counterstained with Harris hematoxilin, dehydrated, and mounted.

Preparation of samples for the determination of eNOS, NaPi-IIa, AT1r and Angiotensinogen (AGT) protein expression

In order to quantify eNOS, NaPi-IIa, AT1r and AGT protein expression, kidney sections were prepared. The sections were homogenized using a Teflon pestle glass homogenizer (Schmidt and Co.) in an ice-cold isolation solution of 200 mM mannitol, 80 mM HEPES and 41 mM KOH, pH 7.5, also containing a protease inhibitor cocktail (Sigma). The homogenates were centrifuged at a low speed (3000×g) for 15 min at 4°C to remove nuclei and cell debris. The pellets were suspended in an isolation solution with protease inhibitors. Protein quantities were determined using the Bradford assay method (Bio-Rad Protein Assay kit, Bio-Rad Laboratories, Hercules, CA, USA).

Electrophoresis and immunoblotting

Kidney samples were run on 8% polyacrylamide minigels (for eNOS) or 10% polyacrylamide minigels (for NaPi-IIa, AT1r and Ang). After transfer by electroelution to nitrocellulose membranes (PolyScreen, PVDF Transfer, Life Science Products, Boston, MA, USA), blots were blocked with 5% skin milk and 0.1% Tween 20 in TBS for 1 hour. Blots were then incubated overnight with an anti-eNOS antibody (1:2,000), anti-NaPi-IIa antibody (0.54 µg/mL), anti-AT1r antibody (1:500) and anti-AGT antibody (1:1,000). The labeling was visualized with a horseradish peroxidase-conjugated secondary antibody (anti-mouse IgG diluted 1:2,000, anti-rabbit IgG, diluted 1:2,000 or anti-goat IgG diluted 1:10,000) using the enhanced chemiluminescence detection system ECL Western blotting detection reagents (GE Healthcare, Buckinghamshire, UK). The specific polyclonal antibody to NaPi-IIa was kindly supplied by Dr Mark Knepper (NHLBI/NIH, Bethesda, MD, USA). The specific polyclonal antibody to eNOS was obtained from BD Transduction Laboratories (CA, USA) and specific polyclonal antibody to AT1 and angiotensin II were obtained from Santa Cruz Biotechnology (CA, USA). As a loading control, blots were incubated with an actin antibody (Santa Cruz, CA, USA; 1:2,000 with anti-goat 1:10,000).

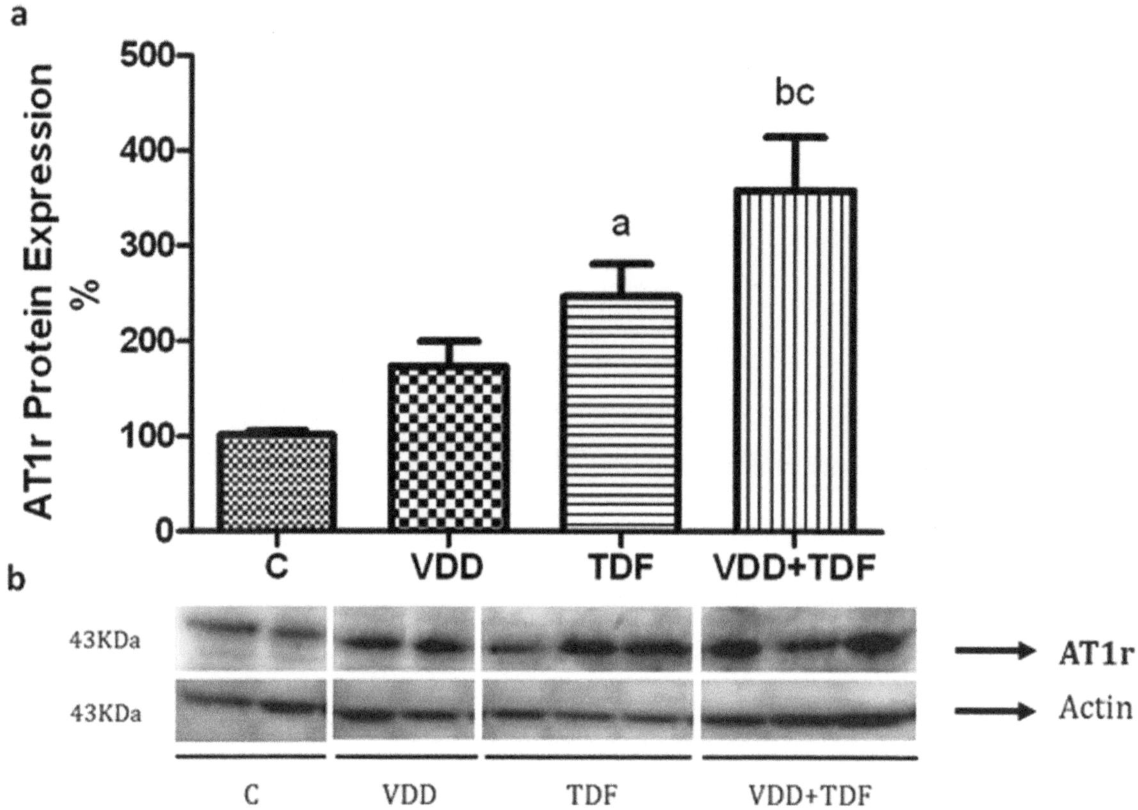

Figure 4. Semiquantitative immunoblotting of kidney fractions. (a) A densitometric analysis of samples from control (n = 4), VDD (n = 6), TDF (n = 6) and VDD+TDF (n = 6) rats is shown. (b) Immunoblots reacted with anti-AT1 revealing a 43-kDa band. Values are means ± SEM. ^{a}p<0.05 vs. C; ^{b}p<0.01 vs. C and ^{c}p<0.05 vs. TDF.

Quantification of renal levels of eNOS, NaPi-IIa, AT1r and AGT

The images were obtained using chemiluminescence imaging system Alliance 4.2 (Uvitec, Cambridge, UK) and performed quantitative analysis of antibodies using densitometry, normalizing the bands to actin expression.

Gene expression of renin-angiotensin components

Quantitative real-time PCR (qPCR) was performed in frozen renal tissue to analyze the expression of genes deemed likely to be related to the development of hypertension in rats. The following genes were assessed: renin (Rn00561847_m1), angiotensinogen (AGT – Rn00593114_m1), angiotensin converting enzyme (ACE – Rn00561094_m1) and angiotensin II receptor type a (AT1a – Rn02758772_s1). The extraction and preparation of total RNA were performed. For cDNA synthesis, total RNA and a Superscript VILO MasterMix (Invitrogen Technologies, CA, USA) were employed. Real-time PCR was performed using TaqMan (Applied Biosystem, CA, USA) on Step One Plus (Applied Biosystem, CA, USA). All primers were purchased from Invitrogen Technologies. Relative gene expression values were evaluated with the $2^{-\Delta\Delta Ct}$ method [18] using GAPDH as housekeeping gene.

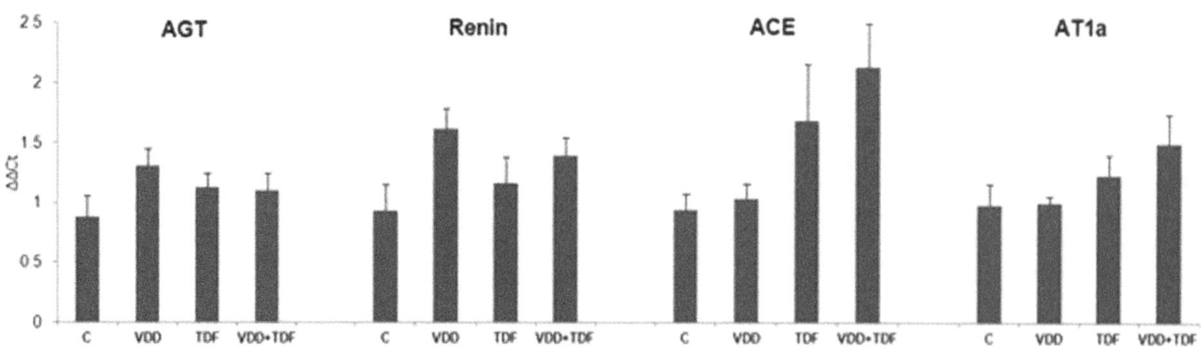

Figure 5. Bar graph representation of the renal mRNA expression of components of renin-angiotensin system in C (n = 5), VDD (n = 6), TDF (n = 5) and VDD+TDF (n = 6).

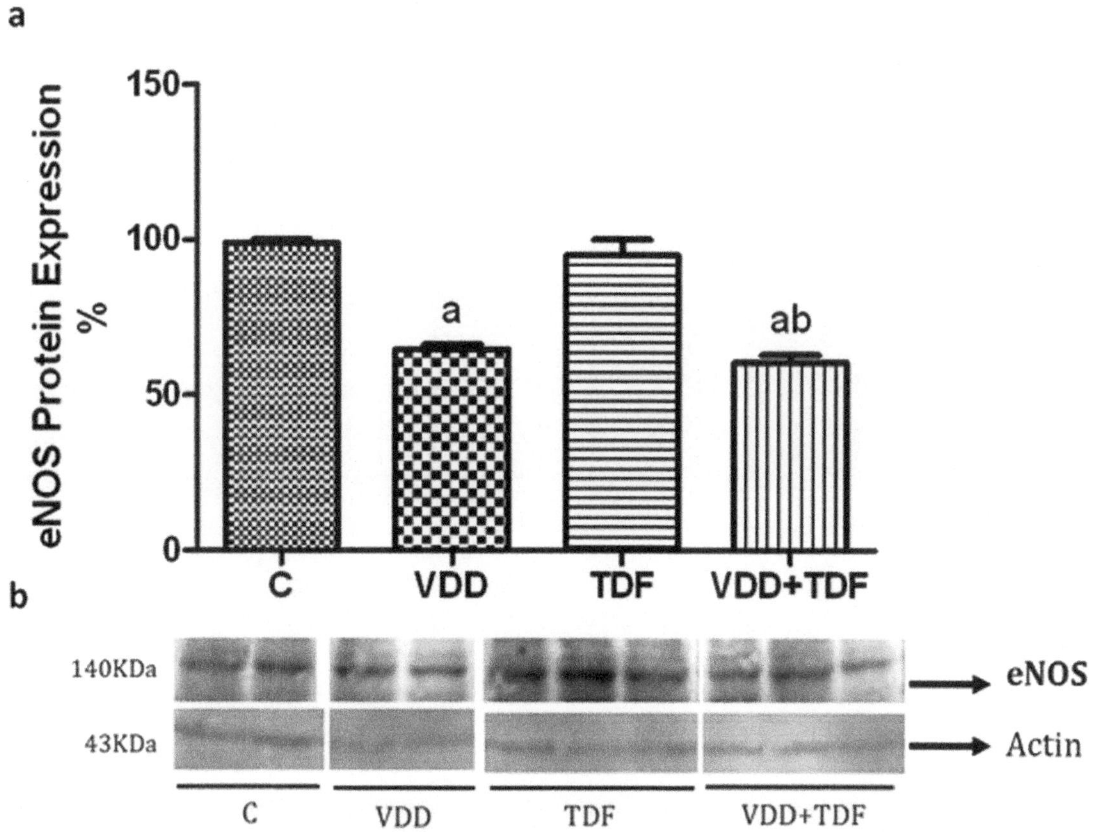

Figure 6. Semiquantitative immunoblotting of kidney fractions. (a) A densitometric analysis of samples from control (n = 4), VDD (n = 6), TDF (n = 6) and VDD+TDF (n = 6) rats is shown. (b) Immunoblots reacted with anti-eNOS revealing a 140-kDa band. Values are means ± SEM. $^{a}p<0.001$ vs. C; $^{b}p<0.001$ vs. TDF.

Reactive oxygen metabolites

Urinary and plasma levels of thiobarbituric acid reactive substances (TBARS), which are markers of lipid peroxidation, were determined using the thiobarbituric acid assay. In brief, a 0.2-ml sample was diluted in 0.8 ml of distilled water. Immediately thereafter, 1 ml of 17.5% trichloroacetic acid was added. Following the addition of 1 ml of 0.6% thiobarbituric acid, pH 2, the sample was placed in a boiling water bath for 15 min, after which it was allowed to cool. Subsequently, 1 ml of 70% trichloroacetic acid was added, and the mixture was incubated for 20 min. The sample was then centrifuged for 15 min at 2000 rpm. The optical density of the supernatant was read at 534 nm against a blank reagent using a spectrophotometer. The concentration of lipid peroxidation products was calculated as malondialdeide (MDA) equivalent using a molar extinction coefficient for the MDA-thiobarbituric acid complex of $1.56\times105\ mol^{-1}/cm^{-1}$. Urinary and plasma levels of TBARS were expressed as nM/24 hours and nM/mL, respectively [19].

Renal reduced glutathione (GSH) was determined in total blood by the method of Sedlak and Lindsay [20]. Whole blood was processed by addition of four volumes of ice-cold 5% (W/V) metaphosphoric acid (MPA) (Sigma) and centrifuged at 14,000×g for 3 min. This assay consists of reacting the supernatants of the total blood with Ellman's reagent to produce a yellow pigment measured spectrophotometrically at 412 nm. The GSH was quantified by mean of standard curve and reported as µmol of GSH/mL [21].

Statistical analysis

All quantitative data are expressed as mean ± SEM. Differences among the means of multiple parameters were analyzed by one-way analysis of variance followed by the Student–Newman–Keuls test. Values of $P<0.05$ were considered statistically significant.

Results

The animals were maintained on a standard or a free-vitamin D diet for 30 days. After this time, VDD animals had low levels of 25(OH)D (4.10±0.8 ng/mL) compared to respective control animals (14.79±0.9 ng/mL), demonstrating that these animals were already deficient before treatment with TDF.

As described in Table 1, there were no significant changes in body weight among groups since all animals showed similar food ingestion during 60 days (approximately 25 g/day). Rats treated with TDF presented a higher blood pressure and significantly impaired renal function, evidenced by lower inulin clearance compared to control group. These alterations were accompanied by a renal vasoconstriction. VDD animals showed a decreased inulin clearance compared to control rats, without alterations in blood pressure and renal vascular resistance. Treatment of VDD with TDF resulted in an even greater elevation of blood pressure than in the TDF-group associated with a greater decrease in inulin clearance and an intense vasoconstriction, indicating that vitamin D deficiency is an aggravating factor in the progression of TDF-induced renal injury.

Another marker of renal impairment is proteinuria. As shown in Table 2, rats that received TDF, deficient or not in vitamin D,

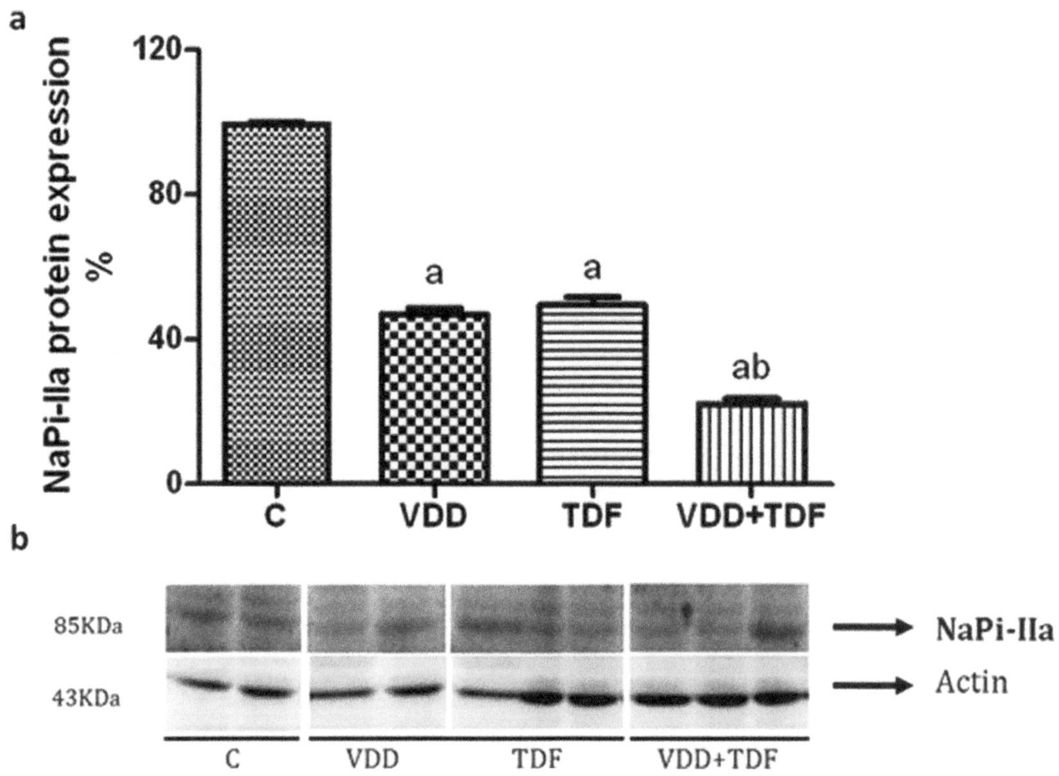

Figure 7. Semiquantitative immunoblotting of kidney fractions. (a) A densitometric analysis of samples from control (n = 4), VDD (n = 6), TDF (n = 6) and VDD+TDF (n = 6) rats is shown. (b) Immunoblots reacted with anti-NaPi-IIa revealing a 85 kDa band. Values are means ± SEM. $^{a}p<0.001$ vs. C; $^{b}p<0.001$ vs. TDF.

showed a greater loss of urinary protein compared to the control group. Urinary protein excretion was also increased in the VDD group. It is worth considering that if we had evaluated urinary fraction excretion of proteins of VDD+TDF group, it would be higher due to decreased glomerular filtration rate with subsequent lower protein filtered load.

The histological study showed alterations characteristic of mild acute tubular necrosis in the renal cortex from the VDD (0.21±0.02) and TDF (0.24±0.02) groups compared to control (0.07±0.01). Tubular cell necrosis, focal areas of denuded basement membrane, flattening of proximal tubular cells with brush border loss and tubular atrophy or dilatation were observed. Vitamin D deficient animals treated with TDF (0.36±0.02) exhibited a higher tubular injury score compared to groups VDD and TDF (Figure 1).

Renal protein expression of angiotensinogen (Figure 2) was up-regulated in groups VDD (201±32%), TDF (222±18%) and VDD+TDF (244±26%) compared to control (104±45%). The immunohistochemical study showed an increased intensity of the immunoreaction of angiotensin II in the renal cortex of VDD, TDF and VDD+TDF (Figure 3). To support data previously shown, renal protein expression of AT1 receptor (Figure 4) was also up-regulated in TDF rats (247±33%) compared to control and VDD (101±5% and 173±27%). Treatment of VDD with TDF resulted in a more intense up-regulation of AT1 protein expression (359±56%).

The renal expression of renin-angiotensin system components assessed by qPCR are given in Figure 5. AGT, renin, ACE and AT1a exhibited a tendency for upregulation in all experimental groups compared to control. As can be seen in Table 2, plasma aldosterone increased significantly and progressively in VDD, TDF and VDD+TDF groups compared to control animals. In addition, the U_K/U_{Na} ratio was significantly higher in VDD+TDF in agreement with the more elevated aldosterona level in this group (Table 2). Altogether, this data confirms a possible involvement of the RAAS in the increase of MAP in vitamin D deficient rats treated with TDF.

The e-NOS expression (Figure 6) was downregulated in VDD groups (VDD = 65±2%; VDD+TDF = 60±2%) compared with control (99±1%) and TDF rats (95±5%). These findings may explain the more elevated blood pressure, the intense renal vasoconstriction, and the decrease in glomerular filtration rate in VDD+TDF, and it may be an additional mechanism responsible for the increased TDF toxicity induced by vitamin D deficiency.

Serum calcium and phosphate concentrations were lower in groups that were fed a vitamin D-free diet. Decreased serum calcium and phosphate levels were also expected since the diet composition has lower calcium and phosphorus concentration (0.4% Ca and 0.4% P) compared to the standard diet. However, group TDF showed diminished serum phosphate concentration, indicating that treatment with TDF alone leads to hypophosphatemia. Association of treatment with TDF and vitamin D deficiency did not aggravate serum phosphate concentration (Table 2).

Proximal tubule function was impaired in TDF rats, as was evidenced by increased urinary excretion of phosphorus (Table 2). Association of vitamin D deficiency and treatment with TDF showed a greater impairment of proximal tubule function. To support this data, renal protein expression of NaPi-IIa was decreased by approximately 50% in VDD and TDF rats and 78% in VDD+TDF animals. Renal protein expression of NaPi-IIa is shown in Figure 7.

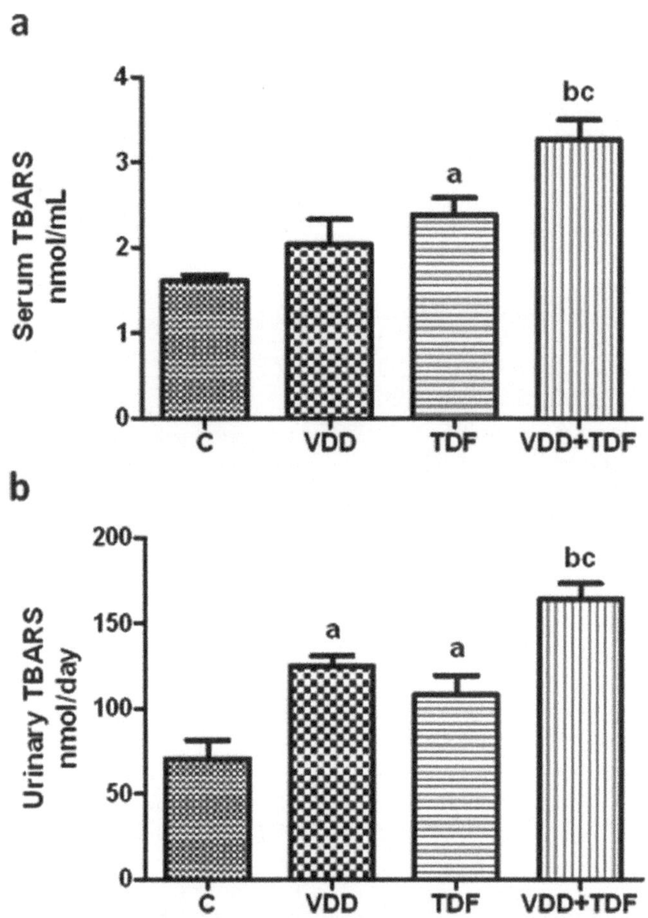

Figure 8. Serum and urinary TBARS. (a) Serum TBARS concentration of C, VDD, TDF and VDD+TDF groups and (b) urinary TBARS excretion of C, VDD, TDF and VDD+TDF groups. Values are means ± SEM. $^{a}p<0.05$, $^{b}p<0.001$ vs. C; $^{c}p<0.01$ vs. TDF.

VDD rats showed an increased plasma PTH concentration compared to control. TDF group did not exhibit alteration in PTH level. Combination of vitamin D deficiency and TDF increased PTH compared to groups C and TDF, but this elevation was moderate compared to VDD (Table 2).

As illustrated in Table 2, TDF animals showed higher levels of total cholesterol and triglycerides compared to control group.

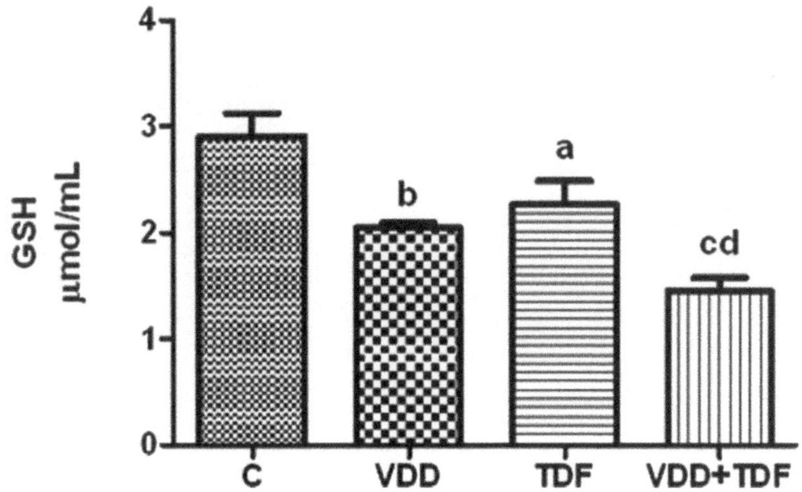

Figure 9. Whole blood glutathione concentration of C, VDD, TDF and VDD+TDF groups. Values are means ± SEM. $^{a}p<0.05$, $^{b}p<0.01$, $^{c}p<0.001$ vs. C; $^{d}p<0.01$ vs. TDF.

When compared with control group, VDD animals showed higher levels of total cholesterol and triglycerides, although the latter parameter was not statistically significant. Association of vitamin D deficiency to treatment with TDF aggravated levels of both total cholesterol and triglycerides compared to groups C, VDD and TDF.

The oxidative stress was initially evaluated by TBARS plasma concentration and urinary excretion measurements. The results are presented in Figures 8a and b. Plasma TBARS concentration (2.38±0.20 nmol/mL) and urinary TBARS excretion (107±11 nmol/24 h) was higher in group TDF when compared with control rats (serum TBARS = 1.61±0.07; urinary TBARS excretion = 70±11 nmol/24 h, $p<0.05$). VDD rats also exhibited a slight but not statistically significant increase in serum TBARS concentration (2.04±0.29 nmol/mL) and a higher urinary TBARS excretion (125±6 nmol/24 h, $p<0.05$) compared to control group probably due to the effects of vitamin D in the modulation of the oxidative stress mechanism. VDD+TDF rats showed an even more pronounced increase of serum TBARS concentration (3.26±0.23 nmol/mL) and urinary TBARS excretion (164±9 nmol/24 h).

Glutathione is a major intracellular antioxidant agent. As shown in Figure 9, the total gluthatione concentration in control rats was 2.90±0.22 µml/mL, a value statistically higher than VDD group (2.05±0.04 µml/mL, $p<0.01$) and TDF (2.27±0.22 µmol/mL, $p<0.05$). VDD+TDF presented markedly lower glutathione concentration compared to groups C, VDD and TDF (1.46±0.12 µml/mL).

Discussion

Vitamin D deficiency or insufficiency has been increasing in recent years reaching 73% of total HIV-infected patients and has been associated with HIV disease progression and its related complications [7,8,22]. Treatment with TDF led to renal failure, proximal tubule injury, hypertension, abnormal lipid metabolism and oxidative stress. Our data demonstrated that vitamin D deficiency aggravates TDF-induced nephrotoxicity.

Our data showed that circulating vitamin D levels were undetectable in VDD and VDD+TDF groups (<1.5 ng/mL), while C and TDF groups presented 15.4±1.0 and 14.8±1.3 ng/mL respectively. Thus, our vitamin D deficiency model was successfully developed. Previous studies demonstrated that basal levels of vitamin D in rats range from 12 to 20 ng/mL [23,24]. Moreover, Ismail et al [25] using a 6-week-vitamin D deficiency model in Wistar rats showed that the levels of 25(OH)D were approximately 1.0 ng/mL in vitamin D-deficient animals while control group presented around 20.0 ng/mL.

Scherzer et al [26] showed that TDF use was associated with proteinuria and chronic kidney disease. Furthermore, vitamin D deficiency itself has been associated with increased prevalence of proteinuria in adults. Vitamin D is a known negative endocrine regulator of the RAAS, which plays a key role in the development of kidney disease. *Li et al* [27] demonstrated that VDR-null mice presented higher renin and angiotensin II levels leading to hypertension. Moreover, low levels of vitamin D also induce podocyte loss and the development of glomerulosclerosis through direct cellular effects, compromising the integrity of the glomerular filtration membrane [10,28].

Hypertension, renin-angiotensin-aldosterone system and nitric oxide in TDF-induced nephrotoxicity associated with vitamin D deficiency

In this study, vitamin D deficient rats receiving TDF showed higher blood pressure. This alteration was accompanied by a marked increase in protein expression of angiotensinogen and AT1 receptor. In addition, gene expression of some RAS compounds such as renin, AGT, ACE and AT1a were also augmented. Furthermore, we demonstrated a progressive elevation in plasma aldosterone in VDD, TDF and VDD+TDF groups. Previous studies have shown strong evidences that vitamin D deficiency led to an upregulation of the renin-angiotensin system [29,30]. Studies conducted in humans and animals reported that gene expression and plasma renin activity are increased in vitamin D-deficient patients [31] and vitamin D receptor knockout mice [32]. Since our findings also revealed increased activation of RAAS, it is possible to speculate that the more severe hypertension observed in VDD+TDF could be explained by the increased mRNA expression of renin, AGT, ACE, and AT1a associated with augmented levels of aldosterone. In addition, our data showed higher expression of angiotensin II and its receptor in the kidney of VDD+TDF animals, reinforcing the role of vitamin D on blood pressure control. Moreover, it is important to point out that vitamin D deficient rats treated with TDF exhibited a higher urinary concentration of potassium and sodium ratio suggesting an increased potassium secretion in the distal tubule due to more elevated levels of aldosterone [33].

It is well known that oxidative stress is also implicated in the development of hypertension. Angiotensin II activates NADPH oxidase leading to the generation of superoxides [34,35]. Our data demonstrated that vitamin D deficient rats treated with TDF showed hypertension accompanied by elevated RVR and decreased renal eNOS expression, suggesting the possibility of the involvement of nitric oxide (NO) cascade. Within the kidney, e-NOS is the main NOS isoform responsible for NO production in both renal epithelial and endothelial cells. Nitric oxide regulates blood pressure by its effects on vascular tone, renal haemodynamics, sodium balance and extracellular fluid volume. Kopkan el al [36] reported that mice lacking the gene for eNOS developed salt-sensitive hypertension due to oxidative imbalance to keep the optimal production of NO. The decrease in eNOS expression in vitamin D deficient rats treated with TDF may explain the more severe hypertension observed in this group.

The role of PTH and vitamin D deficiency in calcium and phosphorus metabolism associated with TDF

Our study showed that vitamin D deficient rats presented hypophosphatemia, hypocalcemia and higher levels of PTH. These alterations were expected since the lack of vitamin D reduces calcium intestinal absorption leading to a lower level of calcium and higher production of PTH by the parathyroid gland. PTH, in turn, acts on bone tissue in order to attenuate the decrease in serum calcium and the increase in phosphorus excretion.

Treatment with TDF led to proximal tubule injury, evidenced by higher excretion of phosphorus and decreased renal expression of the NaPi-IIa cotransporter leading to hyperphosphaturia and hypophosphatemia. Combination of vitamin D deficiency and treatment with TDF aggravated these tubular alterations. Kurnik *et al* reported that treatment with $1,25(OH)_2D_3$ decreased urinary phosphate excretion in partially vitamin D depleted rats, indicating a physiological stimulatory role of $1,25(OH)_2D_3$ in renal phosphate transport [37].

Vitamin D deficient rats presented high levels of plasma PTH supporting previous studies that reported a relationship between the highest PTH levels and the lowest vitamin D concentrations [38]. It is well known that vitamin D and calcium are potent regulators of PTH, suggesting that hypocalcemia and hypovitaminosis D combined with a slight decrease in renal function, as observed in VDD animals, may be responsible for the increase in PTH. This may occur in order to restore these parameters in CKD. The hyperphosphaturic effect of TDF may explain the lower levels of PTH in VDD+TDF when compared with VDD group.

TDF and vitamin D deficiency lead to metabolic syndrome

TDF rats showed higher levels of triglycerides and total cholesterol. These parameters were aggravated when TDF was administered in association with vitamin D deficiency. *Gagnon et al* [17] demonstrated that vitamin D levels were associated inversely with the risk of developing metabolic syndrome. To support data previously shown, another study reported that mice with type 1 and 2 *diabetes mellitus* treated with doxercalciferol showed a higher renal VDR renal expression and the activation of this receptor led to a reduction in the accumulation of triglycerides and cholesterol. Moreover, dyslipidaemia is a frequent complication among HIV-infected patients on antiretroviral therapy [39,40].

Oxidative stress is associated with renal injury and renovascular alterations

The association of vitamin D deficiency and treatment with TDF led to the increase of lipid peroxidation and the decrease in the major intracellular antioxidant agent, observed by higher TBARS and lower GSH levels respectively, showing the influence of oxidative stress in the development of renal injury and the onset of hypertension. *Borges-Santos et al* [15] reported that HIV-infected individuals presented an antioxidant deficit, evidenced by higher levels of oxidized glutathione (GSSG), contributing to disease progression. Furthermore, there are several studies regarding the indirect effects of vitamin D on the protection against oxidative stress. *Tarcin et al* [14] showed a negative correlation between 25(OH)D_3 levels and TBARS in vitamin D deficient patients and the protective effect of vitamin D on endothelial function. Experimental studies reported that treatment with calcitriol led to an increase of VDR expression and decrease in malondialdehyde levels, supporting the role of vitamin D in protecting DNA against oxidative damage [41].

Final considerations

In summary, our data confirms that vitamin D deficiency aggravates TDF nephrotoxicity at least in part by the increase of oxidative stress and the involvement of renin-angiotensin system and nitric oxide cascade, demonstrating that vitamin D has an essential role in the development and progression of kidney and cardiovascular diseases in HIV-infected subjects. Hence, it is important to monitor vitamin D levels in HIV-infected patients treated with TDF. Further studies are required for the clarification of specific mechanisms involved in the progression of HIV-related diseases in vitamin D deficient individuals.

Acknowledgments

Portions of this paper were presented in abstract form at the (1) 49th ERA-EDTA Congress, Paris, France, May 24–27, 2012. Tenofovir-induced nephrotoxicity in vitamin D-deficient rats: the role of oxidative stress. Nephrology Dialysis Transplantation 27, 337–337; (2) 50th ERA-EDTA Congress, Istanbul, Turkey, May 18–21, 2013. Vitamin D deficiency aggravates tenofovir induced metabolic syndrome and renal failure. Nephrology Dialysis Transplantation 28, 115–116.

Author Contributions

Conceived and designed the experiments: DC ACS. Performed the experiments: DC ACB JGG MHMS TRS LA RAV. Analyzed the data: DC RAV LA ACS. Contributed reagents/materials/analysis tools: LA RAV ACS. Wrote the paper: DC RAV ACS.

References

1. Boyd SD (2011) Management of HIV infection in treatment-naive patients: a review of the most current recommendations. Am J Health Syst Pharm 68: 991–1001.
2. Deeks ED, Perry CM (2010) Efavirenz/emtricitabine/tenofovir disoproxil fumarate single-tablet regimen (Atripla(R)): a review of its use in the management of HIV infection. Drugs 70: 2315–2338.
3. Gish R, Jia JD, Locarnini S, Zoulim F (2012) Selection of chronic hepatitis B therapy with high barrier to resistance. Lancet Infect Dis 12: 341–353.
4. Zhao SS, Tang LH, Dai XH, Wang W, Zhou RR, et al. (2011) Comparison of the efficacy of tenofovir and adefovir in the treatment of chronic hepatitis B: a systematic review. Virol J 8: 111.
5. Liborio AB, Andrade L, Pereira LV, Sanches TR, Shimizu MH, et al. (2008) Rosiglitazone reverses tenofovir-induced nephrotoxicity. Kidney Int 74: 910–918.
6. Izzedine H, Launay-Vacher V, Deray G (2005) Antiviral drug-induced nephrotoxicity. Am J Kidney Dis 45: 804–817.
7. Mehta S, Giovannucci E, Mugusi FM, Spiegelman D, Aboud S, et al. (2010) Vitamin D status of HIV-infected women and its association with HIV disease progression, anemia, and mortality. PLoS One 5: e8770.
8. Sudfeld CR, Wang M, Aboud S, Giovannucci EL, Mugusi FM, et al. (2012) Vitamin D and HIV progression among Tanzanian adults initiating antiretroviral therapy. PLoS One 7: e40036.
9. Baeke F, Gysemans C, Korf H, Mathieu C (2010) Vitamin D insufficiency: implications for the immune system. Pediatr Nephrol 25: 1597–1606.
10. Li YC (2011) Podocytes as target of vitamin D. Curr Diabetes Rev 7: 35–40.
11. Cuppari L, Garcia Lopes MG, Kamimura MA (2011) Vitamin D biology: from the discovery to its significance in chronic kidney disease. J Ren Nutr 21: 113–116.
12. Gonzalez EA, Sachdeva A, Oliver DA, Martin KJ (2004) Vitamin D insufficiency and deficiency in chronic kidney disease. A single center observational study. Am J Nephrol 24: 503–510.
13. Ulerich L (2010) Vitamin D in chronic kidney disease–new insights. Nephrol Nurs J 37: 429–431.
14. Tarcin O, Yavuz DG, Ozben B, Telli A, Ogunc AV, et al. (2009) Effect of vitamin D deficiency and replacement on endothelial function in asymptomatic subjects. J Clin Endocrinol Metab 94: 4023–4030.
15. Borges-Santos MD, Moreto F, Pereira PC, Ming-Yu Y, Burini RC (2012) Plasma glutathione of HIV(+) patients responded positively and differently to dietary supplementation with cysteine or glutamine. Nutrition 28: 753–756.
16. Petchey WG, Johnson DW, Isbel NM (2011) Shining D′ light on chronic kidney disease: mechanisms that may underpin the cardiovascular benefit of vitamin D. Nephrology (Carlton) 16: 351–367.
17. Gagnon C, Lu ZX, Magliano DJ, Dunstan DW, Shaw JE, et al. (2012) Low serum 25-hydroxyvitamin D is associated with increased risk of the development of the metabolic syndrome at five years: results from a national, population-based prospective study (The Australian Diabetes, Obesity and Lifestyle Study: AusDiab). J Clin Endocrinol Metab 97: 1953–1961.
18. Livak KJ, Schmittgen TD (2001) Analysis of relative gene expression data using real-time quantitative PCR and the 2(-Delta Delta C(T)) Method. Methods 25: 402–408.
19. Nath KA, Salahudeen AK (1990) Induction of renal growth and injury in the intact rat kidney by dietary deficiency of antioxidants. J Clin Invest 86: 1179–1192.
20. Sedlak J, Lindsay RH (1968) Estimation of total, protein-bound, and nonprotein sulfhydryl groups in tissue with Ellman's reagent. Anal Biochem 25: 192–205.
21. Vogt BL, Richie JP, Jr. (2007) Glutathione depletion and recovery after acute ethanol administration in the aging mouse. Biochem Pharmacol 73: 1613–1621.
22. Childs K, Welz T, Samarawickrama A, Post FA (2012) Effects of vitamin D deficiency and combination antiretroviral therapy on bone in HIV-positive patients. AIDS 26: 253–262.

23. Kelly J, Lin A, Wang CJ, Park S, Nishimura I (2009) Vitamin D and bone physiology: demonstration of vitamin D deficiency in an implant osseointegration rat model. J Prosthodont 18: 473–478.
24. Salum E, Kals J, Kampus P, Salum T, Zilmer K, et al. (2013) Vitamin D reduces deposition of advanced glycation end-products in the aortic wall and systemic oxidative stress in diabetic rats. Diabetes Res Clin Pract 100: 243–249.
25. Ismail A, Namala R (2000) Impaired glucose tolerance in vitamin D deficiency can be corrected by calcium. J Nutr Biochem 11: 170–175.
26. Scherzer R, Estrella M, Li Y, Deeks SG, Grunfeld C, et al. (2012) Association of tenofovir exposure with kidney disease risk in HIV infection. AIDS 26: 867–875.
27. Li YC, Kong J, Wei M, Chen ZF, Liu SQ, et al. (2002) 1,25-Dihydroxyvitamin D(3) is a negative endocrine regulator of the renin-angiotensin system. J Clin Invest 110: 229–238.
28. Kuhlmann A, Haas CS, Gross ML, Reulbach U, Holzinger M, et al. (2004) 1,25-Dihydroxyvitamin D3 decreases podocyte loss and podocyte hypertrophy in the subtotally nephrectomized rat. Am J Physiol Renal Physiol 286: F526–533.
29. Li YC (2003) Vitamin D regulation of the renin-angiotensin system. J Cell Biochem 88: 327–331.
30. Tamez H, Kalim S, Thadhani RI (2013) Does vitamin D modulate blood pressure? Curr Opin Nephrol Hypertens 22: 204–209.
31. Schroten NF, Ruifrok WP, Kleijn L, Dokter MM, Sillje HH, et al. (2013) Short-term vitamin D3 supplementation lowers plasma renin activity in patients with stable chronic heart failure: an open-label, blinded end point, randomized prospective trial (VitD-CHF trial). Am Heart J 166: 357–364 e352.
32. Kong J, Qiao G, Zhang Z, Liu SQ, Li YC (2008) Targeted vitamin D receptor expression in juxtaglomerular cells suppresses renin expression independent of parathyroid hormone and calcium. Kidney Int 74: 1577–1581.
33. Hene RJ, Koomans HA, Boer P, Roos JC, Dorhout Mees EJ (1984) Relation between plasma aldosterone concentration and renal handling of sodium and potassium, in particular in patients with chronic renal failure. Nephron 37: 94–99.
34. Finch JL, Suarez EB, Husain K, Ferder L, Cardema MC, et al. (2012) Effect of combining an ACE inhibitor and a VDR activator on glomerulosclerosis, proteinuria, and renal oxidative stress in uremic rats. Am J Physiol Renal Physiol 302: F141–149.
35. Patzak A, Persson AE (2007) Angiotensin II-nitric oxide interaction in the kidney. Curr Opin Nephrol Hypertens 16: 46–51.
36. Kopkan L, Hess A, Huskova Z, Cervenka L, Navar LG, et al. (2010) High-salt intake enhances superoxide activity in eNOS knockout mice leading to the development of salt sensitivity. Am J Physiol Renal Physiol 299: F656–663.
37. Kurnik BR, Hruska KA (1984) Effects of 1,25-dihydroxycholecalciferol on phosphate transport in vitamin D-deprived rats. Am J Physiol 247: F177–184.
38. Masia M, Padilla S, Robledano C, Lopez N, Ramos JM, et al. (2012) Early changes in parathyroid hormone concentrations in HIV-infected patients initiating antiretroviral therapy with tenofovir. AIDS Res Hum Retroviruses 28: 242–246.
39. Kanjanavanit S, Puthanakit T, Vibol U, Kosalaraksa P, Hansudewechakul R, et al. (2011) High prevalence of lipid abnormalities among antiretroviral-naive HIV-infected Asian children with mild-to-moderate immunosuppression. Antivir Ther 16: 1351–1355.
40. McGee KC, Shahmanesh M, Boothby M, Nightingale P, Gathercole LL, et al. (2012) Evidence for a shift to anaerobic metabolism in adipose tissue in efavirenz-containing regimens for HIV with different nucleoside backbones. Antivir Ther 17: 495–507.
41. Banakar MC, Paramasivan SK, Chattopadhyay MB, Datta S, Chakraborty P, et al. (2004) 1alpha, 25-dihydroxyvitamin D3 prevents DNA damage and restores antioxidant enzymes in rat hepatocarcinogenesis induced by diethylnitrosamine and promoted by phenobarbital. World J Gastroenterol 10: 1268–1275.

16

Abnormal Brain Iron Metabolism in *Irp2* Deficient Mice Is Associated with Mild Neurological and Behavioral Impairments

Kimberly B. Zumbrennen-Bullough[1], Lore Becker[2,3], Lillian Garrett[2,4], Sabine M. Hölter[2,4], Julia Calzada-Wack[2,5], Ilona Mossbrugger[2,5], Leticia Quintanilla-Fend[2,5], Ildiko Racz[2,6], Birgit Rathkolb[2,7], Thomas Klopstock[8,13,14], Wolfgang Wurst[4,11,12,13,14], Andreas Zimmer[6], Eckhard Wolf[7], Helmut Fuchs[2,3], Valerie Gailus-Durner[2,3], Martin Hrabě de Angelis[2,3,9,10], Steven J. Romney[15], Elizabeth A. Leibold[15]*

1 Program in Anemia Signaling Research, Division of Nephrology, Program in Membrane Biology, Center for Systems Biology, Massachusetts General Hospital, Harvard Medical School, Boston, Massachusetts, United States of America, **2** German Mouse Clinic, Helmholtz-Zentrum München, German Research Center for Environmental Health, Neuherberg, Germany, **3** Institute of Experimental Genetics, Helmholtz-Zentrum München, German Research Center for Environmental Health, Neuherberg, Germany, **4** Institute of Development Genetics, Helmholtz-Zentrum München, German Research Center for Environmental Health, Neuherberg, Germany, **5** Institute of Pathology, Helmholtz-Zentrum München, German Research Center for Environmental Health, Neuherberg, Germany, **6** Institute of Molecular Psychiatry, Life & Brain Center, University of Bonn, Bonn, Germany, **7** Institute of Molecular Animal Breeding and Biotechnology, Gene Center, Ludwig-Maximilians-Universitat, Munich, Germany, **8** Department of Neurology, Friedrich-Baur-Institute, Klinikum der Ludwig-Maximilians-Universitat, Munich, Germany, **9** Chair of Experimental Genetics, Center of Life and Food Sciences Weihenstephan, Technische Universitat München, Freising, Germany, **10** German Center for Diabetes Research, Neuherberg, Germany, **11** Chair of Developmental Genetics, Technische Universitat München, Freising-Weihenstephan, Germany, **12** Max Planck Institute of Psychiatry, Munich, Germany, **13** Deutsches Zentrum für Neurodegenerative Erkrankungen, Munich, Germany, **14** Munich Cluster for Systems Neurology, Munich, Germany, **15** University of Utah, Department of Medicine, Division of Hematology and Hematological Malignancies, Salt Lake City, Utah, United States of America

Abstract

Iron Regulatory Protein 2 (Irp2, Ireb2) is a central regulator of cellular iron homeostasis in vertebrates. Two global knockout mouse models have been generated to explore the role of Irp2 in regulating iron metabolism. While both mouse models show that loss of Irp2 results in microcytic anemia and altered body iron distribution, discrepant results have drawn into question the role of Irp2 in regulating brain iron metabolism. One model shows that aged Irp2 deficient mice develop adult-onset progressive neurodegeneration that is associated with axonal degeneration and loss of Purkinje cells in the central nervous system. These mice show iron deposition in white matter tracts and oligodendrocyte soma throughout the brain. A contrasting model of global Irp2 deficiency shows no overt or pathological signs of neurodegeneration or brain iron accumulation, and display only mild motor coordination and balance deficits when challenged by specific tests. Explanations for conflicting findings in the severity of the clinical phenotype, brain iron accumulation and neuronal degeneration remain unclear. Here, we describe an additional mouse model of global Irp2 deficiency. Our aged $Irp2^{-/-}$ mice show marked iron deposition in white matter and in oligodendrocytes while iron content is significantly reduced in neurons. Ferritin and transferrin receptor 1 (TfR1, Tfrc), expression are increased and decreased, respectively, in the brain from $Irp2^{-/-}$ mice. These mice show impairments in locomotion, exploration, motor coordination/balance and nociception when assessed by neurological and behavioral tests, but lack overt signs of neurodegenerative disease. Ultrastructural studies of specific brain regions show no evidence of neurodegeneration. Our data suggest that Irp2 deficiency dysregulates brain iron metabolism causing cellular dysfunction that ultimately leads to mild neurological, behavioral and nociceptive impairments.

Editor: Kostas Pantopoulos, Lady Davis Institute for Medical Research/McGill University, Canada

Funding: This work was supported by the NIH grant R01GM45201 to EAL and the NIH Hematology training grant T32DK007115 to KZB. German Mouse Clinic researchers (SMH, WW, BR, EW, LG, LB, IM, JCW, LQF, IR and AZ) were supported by the German Federal Ministry of Education and Research (Infrafrontier grant 01KX1012); the German Center for Vertigo and Balance Disorders (grant 01EO 0901); by the Helmholtz Alliance HelMA-Helmholtz Alliance for Mental Health in an Ageing Society, through the Initiative and Network Fund of the Helmholtz Association; by the Helmholtz Portfolio Theme 'Metabolic Dysfunction and disease', by the DFG grant 'DJ-1 Linked Neurodegeneration Pathways in New Mouse Models of Parkinson's Disease'(WU 164/5-1). TK was supported by the Seventh Framework Programme of the European Commission (FP7/2007-2013, HEALTH-F2-2011), grant agreement no. 277984 to TIRCON (Treat Iron-Related Childhood-Onset Neurodegeneration). The funders had no role in study design, data collection and analysis, decision to publish, or preparation of the manuscript.

Competing Interests: The authors have declared that no competing interests exist.

* E-mail: betty.leibold@genetics.utah.edu

Introduction

Iron is essential for growth and proliferation of mammalian cells due to its role as a protein cofactor for hemoglobin synthesis, DNA synthesis and mitochondrial respiration. Regulation of cellular iron content is crucial since excess cellular iron catalyzes the generation of reactive oxygen species that damage DNA and proteins, while cellular iron deficiency causes cell cycle arrest and cell death. Dysregulation of iron homeostasis caused by iron excess or iron deficiency leads to hematological, metabolic and neurodegenerative diseases [1–3].

The central nervous system is particularly vulnerable to altered iron metabolism. Iron deficiency perinatally or postnatally can cause permanent neurocognitive and motor impairments in humans [4–6] and in rodent models [7]. Abnormally high brain iron is associated with common neurodegenerative disorders, including Parkinson's and Alzheimer's diseases, as well as rare inherited diseases known as Neurodegeneration with Brain Iron Accumulation (NBIA) [3,8], which manifest as movement disorders. Whether brain iron accumulation is the primary pathologic event causing neurodegeneration or whether iron accumulation is a secondary event caused by neuronal death is unclear. However, two NBIA diseases, hereditary ferritinopathy and aceruloplasminemia, caused by mutations in the ferritin-L subunit gene (*FTL*) [9] and in the ceruloplasmin (*CP*) gene [10], respectively, suggest that abnormal iron metabolism is the pathologic event leading to neurodegeneration in these disorders. These studies highlight the importance of maintaining brain iron within a physiological range to avoid the adverse consequences of iron depletion or excess.

Vertebrate cellular iron metabolism is regulated post-transcriptionally by iron regulatory protein 1 (Irp1, also known as Aco1) and Irp2 [11,12]. Irps are cytosolic RNA-binding proteins that bind to iron-responsive elements (IREs) located in the 5′ or 3′ untranslated regions of mRNAs encoding proteins involved in iron sequestration (ferritin) and iron uptake (TfR1), respectively. When cells are iron-deficient, Irps bind IREs with high affinity inhibiting ferritin translation while stabilizing TfR1 mRNA. When cells are iron-sufficient, Irp1 is converted to an [4Fe-4S]-containing aconitase and Irp2 is degraded by iron-mediated proteasomal degradation [13–15], increasing ferritin translation and promoting TfR1 mRNA degradation. Irps thus regulate the amount of iron sequestered by ferritin and acquired by TfR1 ensuring that cells acquire adequate iron for their needs without it reaching toxic levels. Ferritin and TfR1 are the primary Irp-regulated target mRNAs; however, Irps regulate other IRE-containing mRNAs that encode proteins involved in the tricarboxylic acid cycle, heme biosynthesis, iron export, hypoxia and the cell cycle [12,16].

Mouse models of Irp1 and Irp2 deficiency have been generated [17–19]. *Irp1*$^{-/-}$ mice display polycythemia due to derepression of the Irp1-specific target mRNA hypoxia-inducible factor 2α (Hif-2α; also known as Epas1) [20–22]. Two mouse models of global Irp2 deficiency display dysregulation of ferritin and TfR1and abnormal iron content in several tissues, and develop microcytic anemia and erythropoietic protoporphyria [17,19,23,24]. *Irp2*$^{-/-}$ mice generated by LaVaute et al. [17] developed a progressive late-onset neurodegenerative disorder (>6 months old) characterized by tremors, abnormal gait, subtle kyphosis and hind-limb weakness. Neurological tests showed impaired neuromuscular performance and grooming activity in these mice and histochemical studies showed evidence of axonpathy in white matter that is associated with increased ferric iron and ferritin expression [17]. The severity of neurodegeneration and microcytic anemia is worse in *Irp2*$^{-/-}$ mice lacking one copy of Irp1 (*Irp2*$^{-/-}$;*Irp1*$^{+/-}$), indicating a dosage effect [25]. In contrast, fourteen month old *Irp2* $^{-/-}$ mice generated by Galy et al. [26] showed no overt signs of neurodegeneration, abnormal brain iron accumulation or evidence of neuronal degeneration, and displayed only mild motor coordination/balance impairments and reduced grooming activity when assessed by neurological and behavioral tests [26]. The cause of the differences in the severity of clinical phenotypes and neuropathology in these two *Irp2*$^{-/-}$ mouse models remains unclear.

Here, we describe neurological, behavioral and brain iron phenotypes in an additional global Irp2 deficient mouse model. We find that our *Irp2* $^{-/-}$ mice recapitulate the salient features of other *Irp2*$^{-/-}$ models, including microcytic anemia, erythropoietic protoporphyria, altered body iron distribution and dysregulation of ferritin and TfR1 in several tissues. Our aged *Irp2*$^{-/-}$ mice do not display overt signs of neurodegeneration, but show mild impairments in motor coordination/balance, locomotion and nociception. *Irp2*$^{-/-}$ mice have marked iron deposition in white matter and in oligodendrocytes, and iron deficiency in neurons without pathological evidence of neurodegeneration. We conclude that alterations in brain iron caused by Irp2 deficiency likely disrupts cellular function, and causes neurological, behavioral and nociception impairments.

Materials and Methods

Mice

The generation of *Irp2*$^{-/-}$ mice is described in Figure S1. *Irp2*$^{-/-}$ mice were generated on a C57BL/6J and 129/Sv background and backcrossed with C57BL/6J for five generations. *Irp2*$^{-/-}$ and WT littermates were obtained from intercrosses from *Irp2*$^{+/-}$ parents. Only male mice were used for this study. Mice used for neurological and behavioral experiments were 57–63 weeks (WT) and 38–45 weeks (*Irp2*$^{-/-}$) and mice used for hematological/clinical analysis were 64–75 weeks (WT) and 49–71 weeks (*Irp2*$^{-/-}$). Mice were kept in accordance with the recommendations in the Guide for the Care and Use of Laboratory Animals of the National Institutes of Health. The protocol was approved by the Institutional Animal Care and Use Committee (IACUC) of the University of Utah (Protocol Number: 13-02012). All mice were housed in a pathogen free environment with water and fed mouse breeder diet containing 270 mg Fe/kg (Teklad 8626) provided ad libitum. Mice were euthanized according to AVMA Guidelines for the Euthanasia of Animals. At the German Mouse Clinic, mice were maintained in IVC cages with free access to water and standard mouse chow containing 183 mg Fe/kg (Altromin no.1324) according to the GMC housing conditions and German laws. All tests performed at the GMC were approved by the responsible authority of the Regierung von Oberbayern.

Immunoblot analysis and RNA electrophoretic mobility shift assay (RNA-EMSA)

Tissues were homogenized in lysis buffer (150 mM NaCl, 10 mM EDTA, 10 mM Tris-HCl pH 7.4, 1% Triton X-100, 1 mM DTT and Cocktail Protease Inhibitor (Roche)) and whole-cell lysates were prepared. Protein concentration was determined using Coomassie Plus Protein Assay Reagent (Thermo Scientific). Lysates were analyzed by NuPAGE 4–12% Bis-Tris Gel with MES SDS-running buffer (Invitrogen). Proteins were transferred to a Hybond-ECL nitrocellulose membrane (Amersham) and probed with the following antibodies: chicken anti-Irp1 polyclonal antibody [27]; rabbit anti-Irp2 antibody [28]; rabbit anti-ferritin-L (Ftl1) antibody (Santa Cruz); TfR1 monoclonal antibody (Zymed); β-actin monoclonal antibody (Calbiochem). Horseradish peroxidase-conjugated secondary antibodies were bound and proteins were visualized using Western Lighting Chemiluminescence Reagent Plus (PerkinElmer Life Sciences). RNA-EMSA was performed by incubating tissue lysate (12 ug) isolated from *Irp2*$^{-/-}$ and WT mice with a ^{32}P-labeled ferritin-L IRE probe (pGL-66 linearized with *Sma*I) followed by analysis of the RNA-protein complexes on nondenaturing 5% polyacrylamide gels according to Leibold and Munro [29]. The gels were dried and exposed to a PhosphorImager screen for analysis.

Tissue iron content

Tissue iron content was determined by digesting tissue (20–30 mg) in 40% metal-free nitric acid at 95°C. Samples were diluted in water and analyzed by PerkinElmer Optima 3100XL ICP-OES Spectrometer.

Immunohistochemistry

Male WT mice at 68–78 weeks old (n = 8) and *Irp2*$^{-/-}$ mice at 52–73 weeks old (n = 10) were perfused with Wash Buffer (0.8% NaCl, 0.4% dextrose, 0.8% sucrose, 0.023% $CaCl_2$, and 0.034% sodium cacodylate) until liver was cleared, and then fixed with Fix Buffer (4% paraformaldehyde, 4% sucrose, and 1.4% sodium cacodylate, pH 7.4) by cardiac perfusion. Heads were amputated and stored overnight in Fix buffer. Brains were removed and stored in Cacodylate buffer (14.3% sodium cacodylate, pH 7.4) before all 18 brains were embedded together in a solid block matrix using Multi-Brain Technology (NeuroScience Associates (NSA), Knoxville, TN). Cryostat sections (35 um) were stained with 3,3′-diaminobenzidine (DAB)-enhanced Perls' iron stain to detect ferric iron. Whole brain images were viewed with a Zeiss Stemi SV6 microscope and captured with a MTI 3CCD camera. Perls' stained brain sections were imaged with the EVOS-FL imaging system (Life Technologies). Quantification of Perls' stain in CA1 pyramidal cells and Purkinje cells was carried out by measuring staining intensity in a defined subsection of brain sections from *Irp2*$^{-/-}$ (n = 10) and WT (n = 8) mice using Image J software.

Immunofluorescence

For immunofluorescence, cryostat sections were mounted on slides and incubated in a boiled citrate-based antigen retrieval solution (10 mM citrate pH 6.0, 0.05% Tween-20) until cooled (20 min). Sections were blocked using 5% goat serum in Tris-buffered saline plus 0.3% Triton X-100 for 1 h. Double immunofluorescence staining was performed by costaining sections with rabbit anti-rat ferritin antibody (UT106, generated in our laboratory against rat-H- and -L liver ferritin) overnight at 4°C and the following antibodies: mouse anti-NeuN for neuronal nuclei (1:500, MAB377, Millipore) and mouse calbindin for Purkinje cells (1:1000, Sigma). Sections were incubated with secondary antibodies Alexa Fluor 488 goat anti-rabbit IgG and Alexa Fluor 594 goat anti-mouse for 1 h at room temperature. Images were viewed with an Olympus IX81 microscope and captured with a DP71 camera.

Quantitative RT-PCR (qRT-PCR)

Total RNA was extracted from 9.5–10.5 day embryos using TRIzol reagent (Invitrogen). cDNA synthesis was performed with total RNA (200 ng) using Super SuperScript III First -Strand synthesis SuperMix for qRT-PCR (Invitrogen). qRT-PCR was performed using TaqMan assay probes (Table S6) on an Applied Biosystems 7900HT Sequence Detection System. All experiments were performed using 8–10 mice/genotype with each sample assayed in triplicate. The fold change for each gene was calculated using the ΔΔCt method normalized to Actin with data represented as average ± SEM. Statistical significance was determined using a Student's *t*-test.

Hematology and clinical chemistry

Blood samples were collected under isoflurane anesthesia by retrobulbar puncture. Blood samples were divided in two portions collected Li-heparin-coated sample tubes (Kabe, Nümbrecht-Elsenroth, Germany) for clinical chemistry of plasma samples and EDTA-coated sample tubes (Kabe, Nümbrecht-Elsenroth, Germany) for hematological analyses, respectively.

EDTA-blood samples were analyzed for the complete blood count using an abc-animal blood counter (Scil animals care company, Viernheim, Germany) using predefined settings for C57BL/6 mice. Number and size of red blood cells, white blood cells, and platelets were measured by electrical impedance and hemoglobin by spectrophotometry. Mean corpuscular volume (MCV), mean platelet volume (MPV) and red blood cell distribution width (RDW) were calculated directly from the cell volume measurements. The hematocrit (HCT) was assessed by multiplying the MCV with the red blood cell count. Mean corpuscular hemoglobin (MCH) and mean corpuscular hemoglobin concentrations (MCHC) were calculated from hemoglobin/red blood cell count (MCH) and hemoglobin/hematocrit (MCHC), respectively. Li-Heparin plasma was separated from cells by centrifugation within two hours after collection. Samples were diluted 1:2 with deionized water and analyzed for 24 clinical-chemical parameters using an AU400 autoanalyzer (Olympus Germany, Hamburg, Germany) and reagents for human samples provided Olympus Germany (Hamburg, Germany) or Wako Chemicals GmbH (Neuss, Germany) in case of non-esterified fatty acid concentrations (NEFA). Parameters measured included plasma iron concentration, ferritin levels, transferrin concentration and unsaturated iron binding capacity (UIBC). Transferrin saturation was calculated from iron and UIBC values as percentage of iron level on total iron binding capacity (TIBC = iron+UIBC). Data were statistically analyzed with the level of significance set at $p<0.05$ by pair-wise comparisons of the means by Welsh-Student's *t*-test.

Protoporphyrin IX (PPIX) analysis

Tissue samples were collected in 150 µL water, sonicated, and then an equal volume of 3 M HCl was added for a final concentration of 1.5 M HCl. Acidified samples were then incubated for 1 h at 37°C, spun at 13,000 RPM for 10 min, and the supernatant quantified by HPLC using the method for regular porphyrins [30].

Modified Hole Board (mHB)

The mHB experiments were carried out as previously described [31,32]. In brief, for each trial an unfamiliar (a blue plastic tube lid, diameter 2 cm, height 1 cm) and a copy of a familiar object (metal cube, diameter 2 cm, height 1.5 cm; remaining for 48 h in the home cage, removed 24 h before testing) were placed into the same corner of the arena at a distance of 2 cm. Each mouse was placed at the start position in the same corner diametrical to the corner where the two objects were placed, facing the board diagonally and was tested for 5 min in moderate light conditions (150 lux in the corners to

200 lux in the middle of the test arena). After each trial, the arena was cleaned and disinfected. All trials were videotaped and tracked by Ethovision 2.3 (Noldus, Wageningen, NL) for calculation of horizontal locomotor activity parameters. The movement detection threshold was set at a shift of the center of gravity of the animal for at least 1 cm in a horizontal direction. A hand-held computer was used by a trained observer to assess line crossings, board entries, rearings on board, rearings in the box, hole exploration, familiar and unfamiliar object exploration, immobility, stretched attends (i.e. risk assessment behaviour), defecation and grooming. Data were analysed by use of the Observer software 4.1 (Noldus, Wageningen, NL) with respect to frequency, latency of first occurrence and duration in % of total observation time. Any behaviour that did not occur within the 5 min observation time was given the maximal latency of 300 s. The object index was calculated as total investigation time (s) at the unfamiliar object divided by the sum of the total investigation time (s) at both objects.

Neurological testing

Neurological analysis was performed as previously described [33]. Grip strength was measured by measuring maximal force the mice applied to grid attached a force-meter (Bioseb, France) in three consecutive trials. Fore paws and combined fore and hind paw measurements were performed by allowing the mice to grasp the grid before being slowly pulled away. Motor coordination was evaluated by the latencies the animals stayed on a rotating rod, acceleration from 4 to 40 rpm in five minutes. Mice were tested four times with 15 minutes in between. For statistical analysis linear models were used also considering body mass variations.

Nociception methods

In nociception, 18 *Irp2*$^{-/-}$ mice (9 males, 9 females) and 20 WT animals (10 males and 10 females) were screened using a hot-plate assay. A mouse was placed on a 28 cm diameter metal surface maintained at 52+0.2°C surrounded by a 20 cm high Plexiglass wall (TSE, Bad Homburg, Germany). Mice remained for 30 seconds on the plate or until they performed one of three behaviors regarded as indicative of nociception: hind paw licking, hind paw shake/flutter or jumping [34]. The latency of the first sign of pain was compared for sex and genotype using a factorial ANOVA.

Transmission electron microscopy

Animals (a subset of 5 *Irp2KO* and 4 WT mice) were transcardially perfused with 50 ml ice cold PBS, prior to perfusion with 70 ml of fixing solution (2.5% PFA, 2.5% glutaraldehyde in PBS). Different brain regions were removed and cut into 1 mm^3 cubes, which were postfixed in 2.5% glutaraldehyde containing 0.1 M sodium cacodylate buffer (pH 7.4) at 4°C overnight. Tissues were fixed in 2.5% electron microscopy grade glutaraldehyde in 0.1 M sodium cacodylate buffer pH 7.4 (Science Services, Munich, Germany), postfixed in 2% aqueous osmium tetraoxide, dehydrated in gradual ethanol (30–100%) and propylene oxide, embedded in Epon (Merck, Darmstadt, Germany) and baked for 24 hours at 60°C. Semi thin sections were cut and stained with toluidine blue. Ultrathin sections of 50 nm were collected onto 200 mesh copper grids, contrasted with uranyl acetate and lead citrate before examination by transmission electron microscopy (Zeiss EM 10 CR electron microscope, Carl Zeiss NTS GmbH, Oberkochen, Germany).

Results and Discussion

Phenotypic characterization of *Irp2*$^{-/-}$ mice

Irp2$^{-/-}$ mice were generated by inserting a self-excision cassette containing neomycin (*Neo*^{r}) linked to Cre-recombinase (*Cre*) into exon 3 of the mouse *Irp2* gene (Figure S1). *Irp2*$^{-/-}$ mice were fertile and indistinguishable from wildtype (WT) littermates in weight or appearance (data not shown). *Irp2*$^{-/-}$ mice showed mild microcytic anemia characterized by reduced hemoglobin, hematocrit and mean corpuscular volume (Table S1). Transferrin saturation, serum iron levels and total iron binding capacity were unchanged in *Irp2*$^{-/-}$ and WT mice while serum ferritin levels were markedly increased in *Irp2*$^{-/-}$ mice (WT, 58.1±12.5 ng/ml (n = 9); *Irp2*$^{-/-}$, 218.6±7.3 ng/mL (n = 10), $p<0.001$) (Table S2). *Irp2*$^{-/-}$ mice also showed elevated levels of serum and liver protoporphyrin IX (PPIX) and PPIX-containing aggregates in the cystic, hepatic, and common bile ducts (Table S3 and Figure S2). *Irp2*$^{-/-}$ mice displayed altered body iron distribution with total iron content increased in duodenum, kidney and liver and decreased in heart while total brain iron content is unchanged (Table 1).

Ferritin and TfR1 have been shown to be dysregulated in liver, duodenum and brain in two other distinct *Irp2*$^{-/-}$ mouse strains [17,23,24]. Similarly, we find increased ferritin-L chain (Ftl1) levels in brain (forebrain and cerebellum), liver, kidney and duodenum and decreased TfR1 levels in brain, heart, liver and kidney in *Irp2*$^{-/-}$ mice compared to WT mice (Figure 1A). Ferritin-L and TfR1 levels are similar in *Irp2*$^{-/-}$ and WT spleen. Irp2 RNA-binding activity and protein are not detected in *Irp2*$^{-/-}$ tissue lysates (Figure 1 A and B). A non-specific band is seen by Western blot analysis that migrates close to Irp2 in some tissue lysates (Figure 1A). Taken together, these phenotypes are in agreement with those described for other *Irp2*$^{-/-}$ mouse strains in which Irp2 deficiency causes microcytic anemia, erythropoietic protoporphyria, and altered body iron distribution and expression of ferritin and TfR1 [18,19,23].

Motor coordination/balance, locomotion and nociception are impaired in *Irp2*$^{-/-}$ mice

The *Irp2*$^{-/-}$ strain generated by LaVaute et al. [17,35] developed an adult-onset neurodegenerative movement disorder at >6 months of age characterized by tremors, hind-limb weakness, subtle kyphosis and abnormal gait. These mice displayed poor self-grooming activity, and impaired muscular strength and motor coordination when assayed by the hang test and rotarod [17,35]. In contrast, *Irp2*$^{-/-}$ mice generated by Galy et al. [19] showed no overt signs of neurodegeneration or impaired muscle strength at 13–14 months of age. These mice displayed reduced self-grooming activity consistent with a tendency toward reduced rearings (vertical locomotor activity) and impaired motor coordination/balance when challenged by the modified-Hole Board and rotarod tests, respectively [26].

As our *Irp2*$^{-/-}$ mice at 45–63 weeks old did not display tremors, kyphosis, or abnormal gait, we performed a battery of tests to assess behavioral and neurological function. We used the modified-Hole Board test to assay locomotor and exploratory activities, arousal, memory and social affinity, the modified SHIRPA test to assess neurological function, the grip strength test to quantify muscular strength and the accelerating rotarod to measure motor coordination and balance (Tables S4–S5). *Irp2*$^{-/-}$ mice displayed an overall reduction in forward locomotion, speed of movement and reduced vertical exploratory activities (rearing frequency and latency) (Figure 2A and B). Rotarod performance was slighty impaired in aged *Irp2*$^{-/-}$

Table 1. Tissue iron content of aged male *Irp2*$^{-/-}$ and WT mice.

Tissue	*WT* (n = 8)	*Irp2*$^{-/-}$ (n = 10)
Brain	1.98±0.08	1.84±0.07
Duodenum	6.01±1.68	15.41±1.76*
Liver	2.77±0.21	5.81±0.39***
Spleen	15.39±2.44	12.54±1.09
Heart	5.49±0.05	4.92 ±0.13*
Kidney	2.25±0.10	3.37±0.15***
Lung	3.01±0.40	2.80±0.35

Total iron content was determined by inductively-coupled plasma optical emission spectroscopy (ICP-OES). Statistical analysis performed by Student's paired t-test (*$p<0.05$; ***$p<0.001$, mean (μg Fe/mg wet tissue weight) ×100± SEM). Ages of mice: WT, 64–75 weeks; *Irp2*$^{-/-}$, 49–71 weeks.

mice compared to WT mice, which was not observed in 20-week old *Irp2*$^{-/-}$ mice, suggesting a progressive phenotype (Figure 2C and data not shown). The grip strength test (2-paws and 4-paws) revealed that muscular strength was not impaired in *Irp2*$^{-/-}$ mice (Figure 2D).

Nociception was also assessed in *Irp2*$^{-/-}$ and WT mice. *Irp2*$^{-/-}$ mice showed no significant difference in the first pain reaction (hind paw shaking) since they present with the same reaction latency to heat stimuli as WT mice (Figure 2E). However, *Irp2*$^{-/-}$ mice displayed a significantly longer reaction latency in the second pain reaction (hind paw licking) (Figure 2E). This finding indicated that *Irp2*$^{-/-}$ mice tolerated heat better than WT mice when it was used as noxious stimulus. Increased hind paw licking was also observed in 20-week old *Irp2*$^{-/-}$ mice, indicating that this reaction was independent of age (data not shown). Retarded reaction to thermal stimuli on the hotplate could be a secondary effect of reduced motor abilities. If impaired motor abilities influenced the pain reaction, however, the same effect in both reactions, or at least in the first reaction and not in the second reaction, would be observed. Altered nociception heat tolerance was not reported for other *Irp2*$^{-/-}$ mice.

Impaired motor coordination and balance are consistent with the *Irp2*$^{-/-}$ neurological phenotypes reported by Galy et al. [26] and LaVaute et al. [17], although *Irp2*$^{-/-}$ mice generated by Galy et al. [26] did not display horizontal locomotor impairments that we observed in our *Irp2*$^{-/-}$ mice. Taken together, our data show that Irp2 deficiency is associated with mildly impaired horizontal locomotion, exploration, motor coordination/balance and nociceptive heat tolerance.

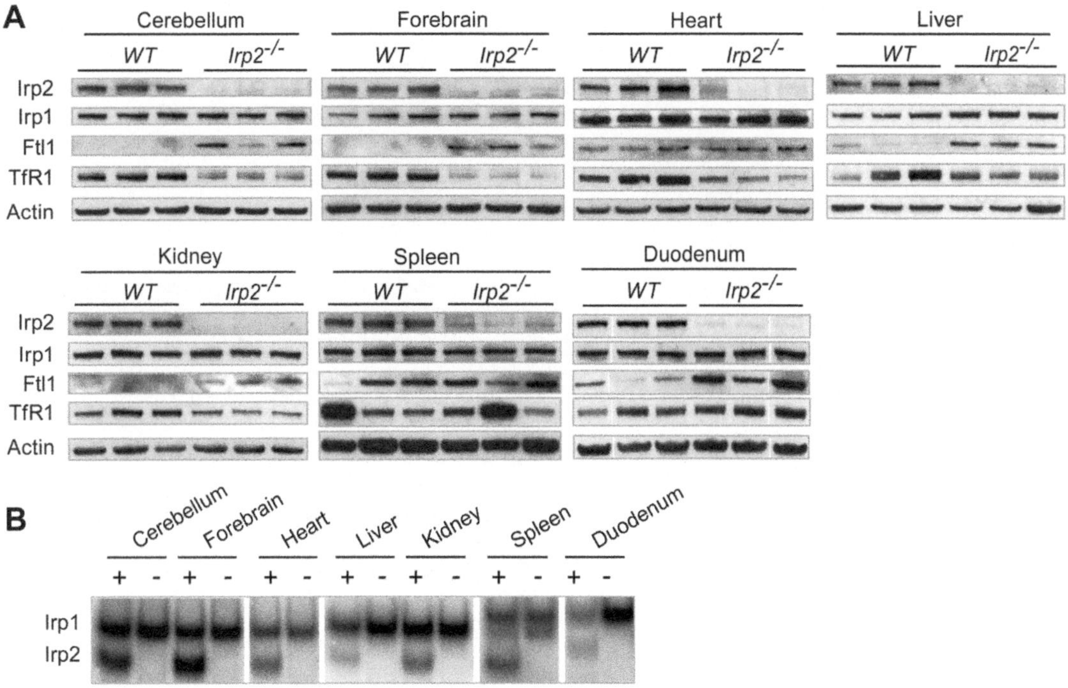

Figure 1. Expression of iron homeostasis proteins in *Irp2*$^{-/-}$ and WT mice. *A)* Western blot analysis of tissue extracts from male *Irp2*$^{-/-}$ and WT mice (n = 3 mice/genotype) using antibodies to detect Irp2, Irp1, ferritin (Ftl1), TfR1 and β-actin (loading control). A non-specific band migrating near Irp2 is observed in some *Irp2*$^{-/-}$ lysates. *B)* Irp1 and *Irp2* RNA-binding activity in lysates was assayed by RNA electrophoretic mobility shift assay using a ^{32}P-labeled ferritin IRE as a probe. 0.5% β-mercaptoethanol was added to samples to assay total RNA-binding activity.

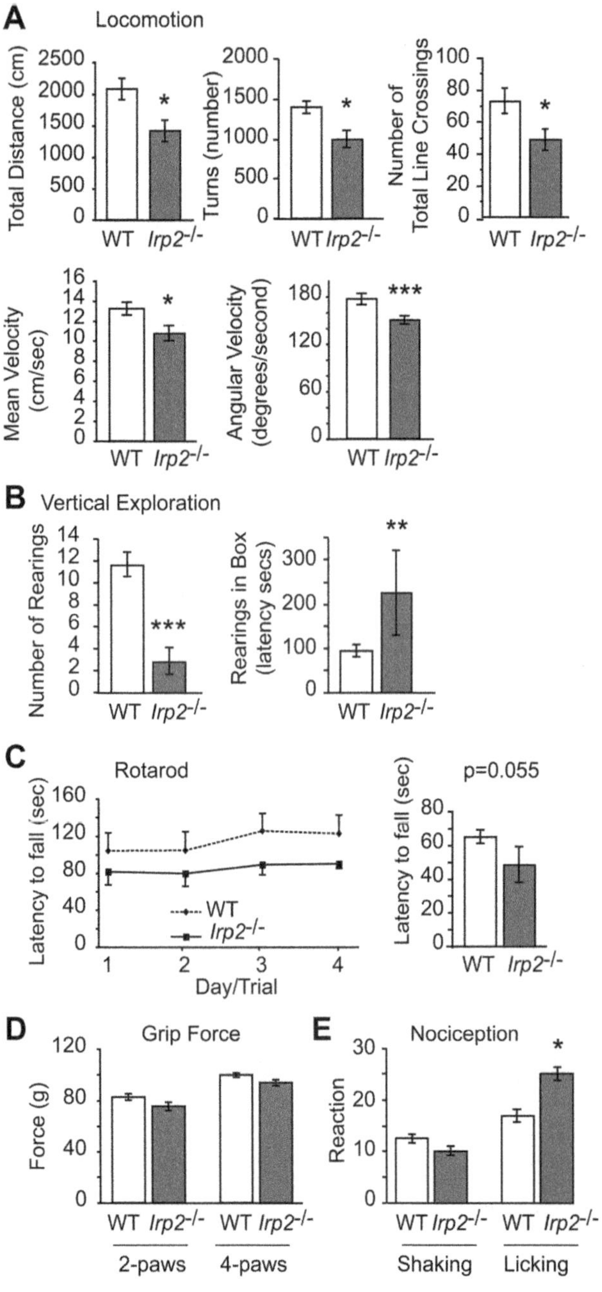

Figure 2. Locomotion, motor coordination and nociception are impaired in *Irp2*$^{-/-}$ mice. *Irp2*$^{-/-}$ mice display reduced horizontal locomotor activity (total distance traveled, number of turns, number of total line crossings, mean velocity and angular velocity), and *B*) reduced vertical exploratory activity (number of rearing and rearing latency) assessed by the modified-Hole Board test [31]. *C) Left panel,* performance of *Irp2*$^{-/-}$ and WT mice on the accelerating rotarod in four trials on four consecutive trials with 15 min inter-trial-interval; *right panel,* decreased mean latency of *Irp2*$^{-/-}$ mice to fall off the rotarod (n = 4 trial; $p = 0.055$). *D)* 4-paw grip force test shows no difference in muscular strength between *Irp2*$^{-/-}$ and WT mice. *E)* Hot plate test shows increased hind paw licking in *Irp2*$^{-/-}$ mice. Data are given as the mean ± SEM; **p*<0.05; ***p*<0.01, ****p*<0.001, relative to WT; WT (n = 9) and *Irp2*$^{-/-}$ (n = 10).

Iron accumulation in oligodendrocytes and axons in the brain of *Irp2*$^{-/-}$ mice

Marked ferric iron accumulation was observed in oligodendrocyte soma and white matter axons in aged *Irp2*$^{-/-}$ mice generated by LaVaute et al. [17,25]. Iron accumulated in the cerebellum, caudate putamen, thalamus, substantia nigra and colliculi, while the frontal cortex, globus pallidus and corpus callosum were not affected [17,25,36]. Iron accumulation in axons in cerebellar white matter was associated with axonopathy. Iron was also detected in neuronal cell bodies in gray matter, including the thalamus, colliculi and deep cerebellar neurons, and in Purkinje axons. In contrast, Galy et al. [26] did not detect abnormal brain iron accumulation in their aged *Irp2*$^{-/-}$ mice. Both groups analyzed aged mice (12–14 months old) and used DAB-enhanced Perls' iron staining method to detect ferric iron. Both groups also reported no significant differences in total brain iron [23] or total non-heme iron [26] between *Irp2*$^{-/-}$ and WT mice.

Similar to previously reported global *Irp2*$^{-/-}$ mice, we found no significant differences in total brain iron content between *Irp2*$^{-/-}$ and WT mice using inductively-coupled optical emission spectroscopy (Table 1). We next assessed ferric iron histochemically in serial brain sections prepared from *Irp2*$^{-/-}$ (n = 10) and WT (n = 8) mice using DAB-enhanced Perls' stain (Files S1 and S2). Marked iron deposition was observed in cortex, caudate putamen, thalamus, superior colliculus and cerebellum as well as in other brain regions in *Irp2*$^{-/-}$ mice (Figure 3 and Files S1 and S2). In cortex, iron accumulated in small cells that have an eccentric nucleus characteristic of oligodendrocyte morphology [37] and in axons (Figure 4A). Iron accumulation was also observed in axon tracts and in oligodendrocyte soma associated with striosomes, as well as in oligodendrocytes scattered throughout the caudate putamen (Figure 4B). Significant iron deposition was observed in the superior colliculus (Figure 4C) and in the cerebellar white matter and oligodendrocytes associated with white matter in *Irp2*$^{-/-}$ mice (Figure 4E). Iron deposition in caudate putamen, cerebellar white matter and colliculus, as well as other regions (Files S1 and S2), is in agreement with *Irp2*$^{-/-}$ mice generated by LaVaute et al. [17,25]. Unlike *Irp2*$^{-/-}$ mice generated by LaVaute et al. [17,25], we did not detect increased iron deposition in the substantia nigra of our *Irp2*$^{-/-}$ mice (Figure 4D). WT and *Irp2*$^{-/-}$ mice used in our study were older than mice used by Smith et al. [25] (<12 months old), and it is possible that the high iron content in the substantia nigra of our WT mice made it difficult to discern iron differences between WT and *Irp2*$^{-/-}$ mice. We also found significant iron deposition in the cerebral cortex and corpus collosum of *Irp2*$^{-/-}$ mice, which was not observed by LaVaute et al. [17] (Figures 3C and 4A).

Iron content is reduced in CA1 pyramidal neurons and in Purkinje neurons of *Irp2*$^{-/-}$ mice

We next assessed Perls' iron staining in hippocampal CA1 pyramidal neurons and in cerebellar Purkinje neurons in *Irp2*$^{-/-}$ and WT mice. Perls' staining was significantly reduced in CA1 pyramidal neuronal soma and in their apical dendrites (Figure 5 and Figure S3). Purkinje neuronal soma in *Irp2*$^{-/-}$ mice showed a slight, but significant reduction in iron content compared to WT mice (Figure 5 and Figure S3).

A reported phenotype of *Irp2*$^{-/-}$ mice generated by LaVaute et al. [17] is the degeneration and partial loss of Purkinje neurons although this was not found in *Irp2*$^{-/-}$ mice generated by Galy

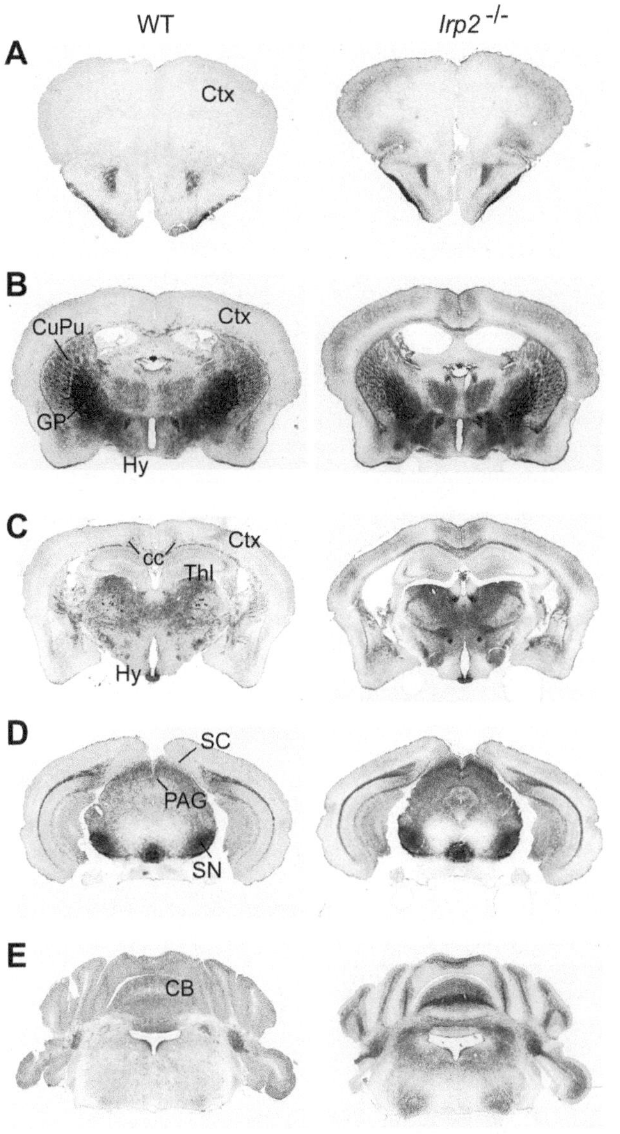

Figure 3. Iron accumulates in specific brain regions of *Irp2*$^{-/-}$ mice. Coronal sections from male *Irp2*$^{-/-}$ and WT brains from rostral (*top*) to caudal (*bottom*) were selected to show iron accumulation in specific regions of brain. Ferric iron was detected using DAB-enhanced Perls' stain. *Ctx* cortex, *CB* cerebellum, *CPu* caudate putamen, *cc* corpus collosum, *Gp* globus pallidus, *Hy* hypothalamus, *PAG*, periaqueductal gray; *SC* superior colliculus, *SN* substantia nigra and *Thl* thalamus.

et al. [26]. We stained *Irp2*$^{-/-}$ and WT cerebellar sections with calbindin antibody (Purkinje cell specific) and found no abnormalities in Purkinje cell morphology or cell number in *Irp2*$^{-/-}$ mice (WT, 3.16 cells/inch ±0.267; *Irp2*$^{-/-}$, 3.57 cells/inch ±0.232; $p = 0.264$) (Figure 6A). Ultrastructural analysis of substantia nigra, caudate putamen, cerebellum, cortex, hippocampus and hypothalamus did not reveal pathological alterations in these regions except for the presence of age-related lipofuscin deposits in neurons that are detected in aged WT and *Irp2*$^{-/-}$ mice (Figure S4 and data not shown). Myelinization also appeared normal in *Irp2*$^{-/-}$ mice evaluated by Luxol Fast Blue staining (Figure S5).

The reduction in Perls' staining in *Irp2*$^{-/-}$ CA1 pyramidal and Purkinje neurons suggests that these neurons may be iron deficient. Because neurons acquire iron primarily by TfR1 [38,39], the reduction in TfR1 abundance in *Irp2*$^{-/-}$ cerebellar and forebrain lysates compared to WT is consistent with reduced transferrin-dependent iron uptake (Figure 1A). In contrast to TfR1, ferritin expression is increased in *Irp2*$^{-/-}$ cerebellar and forebrain lysates (Figure 1A). We next assessed ferritin expression in neurons in *Irp2*$^{-/-}$ and WT sections from cerebellum, caudate putamen and hippocampus by double immunofluorescence using a ferritin antibody in combination with antibodies specific to neurons (NeuN) and to Purkinje neurons (calbindin). Ferritin immunoreactivity was similar in *Irp2*$^{-/-}$ and WT Purkinje neurons (Figure 6B), but was increased in *Irp2*$^{-/-}$ CA1 pyramidal neurons and in neurons in the caudate putamen (Figure 6C and D). We were not able to assess TfR1 immunostaining in these sections due to technical difficulties. Taken together, these data suggest that the reduction in TfR1 expression and increased ferritin expression in *Irp2*$^{-/-}$ mice could lead to reduced iron uptake and increased iron storage, thus causing cellular iron deficiency. While notable neuronal pathology was not observed in *Irp2*$^{-/-}$ brain, we suggest that neuronal iron deficiency may cause cellular dysfunction that contributes to the neurological and behavioral deficits in *Irp2*$^{-/-}$ mice.

Conclusions

In conclusion, our data show that mice with a global *Irp2* deficiency recapitulate the main features of other Irp2 deficient mouse models such as microcytic anemia, erythropoietic protoporphyria, altered body iron distribution and altered expression of ferritin and TfR1 in tissues. Our aged *Irp2*$^{-/-}$ mice did not exhibit, tremor, ataxia, bradykinesia and postural abnormalities as described by LaVaute et al. [17], but did display mild impairments in horizontal locomotion, rearing activity, balance/motor coordination and nociceptive heat tolerance when assayed by specific tests. Our data are consistent with impaired motor and balance coordination reported for the other two strains of *Irp2*$^{-/-}$ mice and with reduced rearing activity reported for *Irp2*$^{-/-}$ mice generated by Galy et al. [26]. The reduced rearing activity in our *Irp2*$^{-/-}$ mice is consistent with a slight reduction in self-grooming (which could imply a reduction in vertical locomotion), although this did not reach statistical significance, and is similar to other *Irp2*$^{-/-}$ mice that exhibited a significant reduction in self-grooming activity [17,26].

Our *Irp2*$^{-/-}$ mice showed distinctive features not reported for other *Irp2*$^{-/-}$ mice. The modified hole board test revealed that *Irp2*$^{-/-}$ mice displayed an overall reduction in locomotor activity characterized by decreased total distance moved, line crossings, turning frequency and movement velocity. This combination of mild hypoactivity and reduced rearing in our *Irp2*$^{-/-}$ mice suggests reduced exploratory motivation. Galy et al. [26] also used the modified hole board test, but did not observe impaired horizontal locomotion in their 13–14 month old *Irp2*$^{-/-}$ mice. We also found that *Irp2*$^{-/-}$ mice showed a hypoalgesic phenotype as assessed by the hot plate test that was independent of age. Our *Irp2*$^{-/-}$ mice develop diabetes (EAL, SN, CPA and KBZ, unpublished observation), and it is possible that hypoalgesia is a consequence of impaired glucose tolerance. Another novel phenotype in our *Irp2*$^{-/-}$ mice is the presence of PPIX containing aggregates in the cystic, hepatic, and common bile ducts. Cooperman et al. [23] showed increased synthesis of the heme biosynthetic enzyme erythroid aminolevulinate synthase 2 (Alas2), which contains an IRE in the 5′ untranslated region, and reduced expression of TfR1 in *Irp2*$^{-/-}$ erythroid

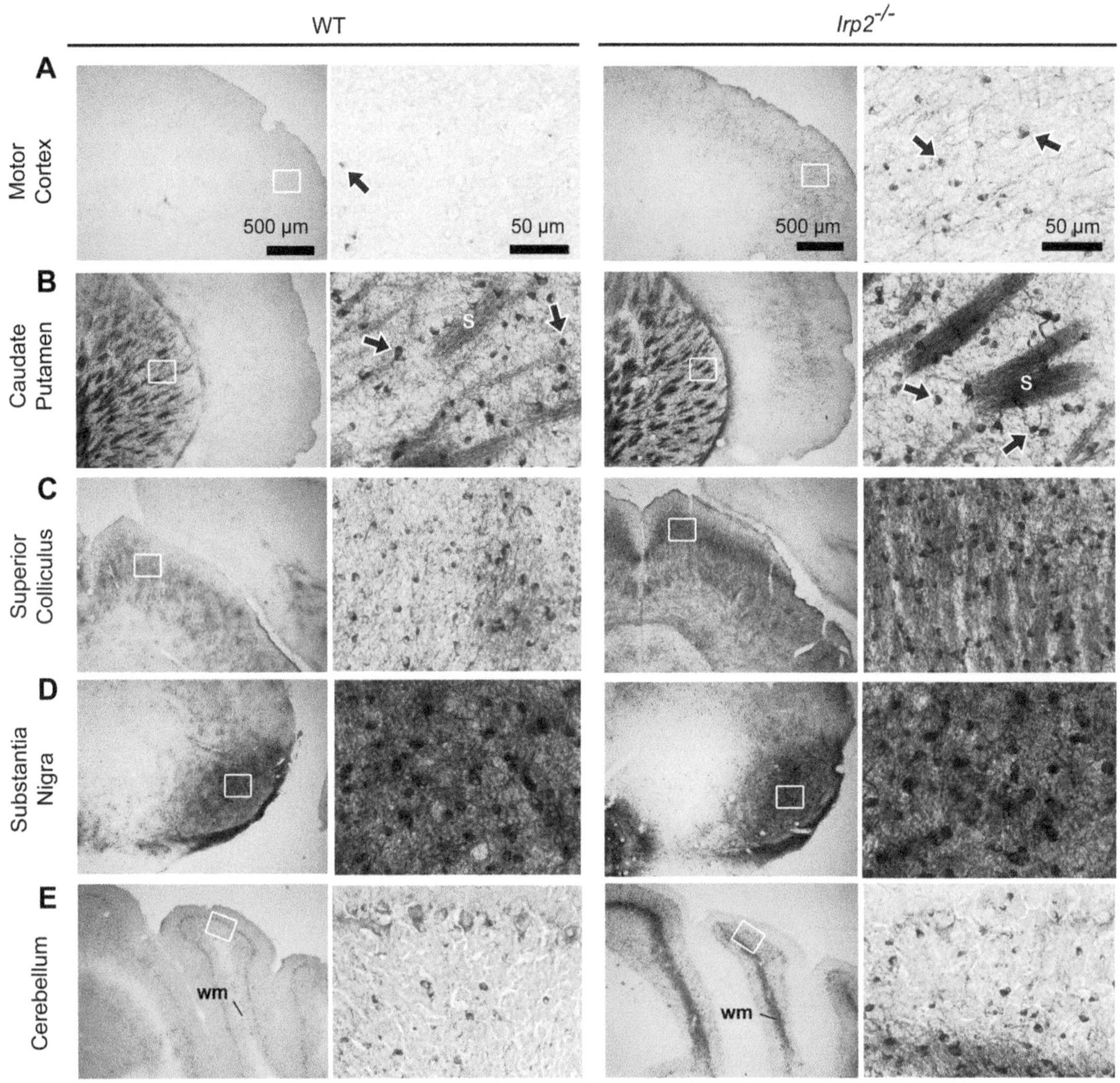

Figure 4. Iron accumulates in axons and oliogodendrocyte cell bodies of *Irp2*$^{-/-}$ mice. Increased DAB-enhanced Perls' iron stain is observed in small cells that have an eccentric nucleus characteristic of oliogodendrocyte morphology [37] and in axons in *A)* cerebral cortex, *B)* caudate putamen, *C)* superior colliculus, *D)* substantia nigra, and *E)* cerebellum. *Arrows*, oligodendrocytes; *S*, striosomes; *wm*, white matter; *gl*, granule layer. Scale bars: 50 µm and 500 µm.

precursor cells. Loss of translational repression of Alas2 by Irp2 deficiency and reduced Tf-dependent iron uptake likely results in elevated PPIX levels we observed in the serum, liver and bile ducts. Whether other *Irp2*$^{-/-}$ mice show PPIX aggregates in the bile ducts remains to be determined.

An explanation for the varied neurodegenerative phenotypes in the different *Irp2*$^{-/-}$ models is not clear, but it is known that neurological and behavioral phenotypes can be sensitive to genetic background differences and gene targeting strategies [40–42]. Our mice were generated using 129/Sv-CP ES cell line and were backcrossed to C57BL/6J mice for five generations, and those of Galy et al. [19,26] were generated using the 129P2/OlaHsd ES cell line and backcrossed to C57BL/6J mice for three generations. *Irp2*$^{-/-}$ mice generated by LaVaute et al. [17] are mixed genetic background consisting of C57BL/6 and B129S4/SVJ. In addition, different targeting approaches were used to generate *Irp2*$^{-/-}$ mice. LaVaute et al. [17] generated a global model of Irp2 deficiency by insertion of a PGK-neomycin gene into exon 3/4 of *Irp2* gene. Galy et al. [19] generated conditional alleles of *Irp2* by insertion of a β-Geo cassette flanked by Frt sites into intron 2 of the *Irp2* gene and was co-inserted with LoxP sites flanking exon 3. Cre-mediated excision of exon 3 generated a null allele. Our *Irp2*$^{-/-}$ mice were generated by the insertion of a self-excision cassette containing neomycin linked to Cre-recombinase into exon 3 of the mouse *Irp2* gene. Targeting strategies can lead to different phenotypes due to silencing or activation of flanking genes caused by the retention of selection cassettes, generation of truncated gene products with biological activity or inactivation of non-coding RNAs with the targeted locus [43,44]. The expression of neighboring genes close to the *Irp2* locus was not altered in *Irp2*$^{-/-}$ mice [19] and we did not identify annotated non-coding RNAs located within the *Irp2* locus. The differences in neurological and behavioral phenotypes in *Irp2*$^{-/-}$ mice could also be affected by environmental conditions (food, altitude or environmental stimulation) [44] and natural variation

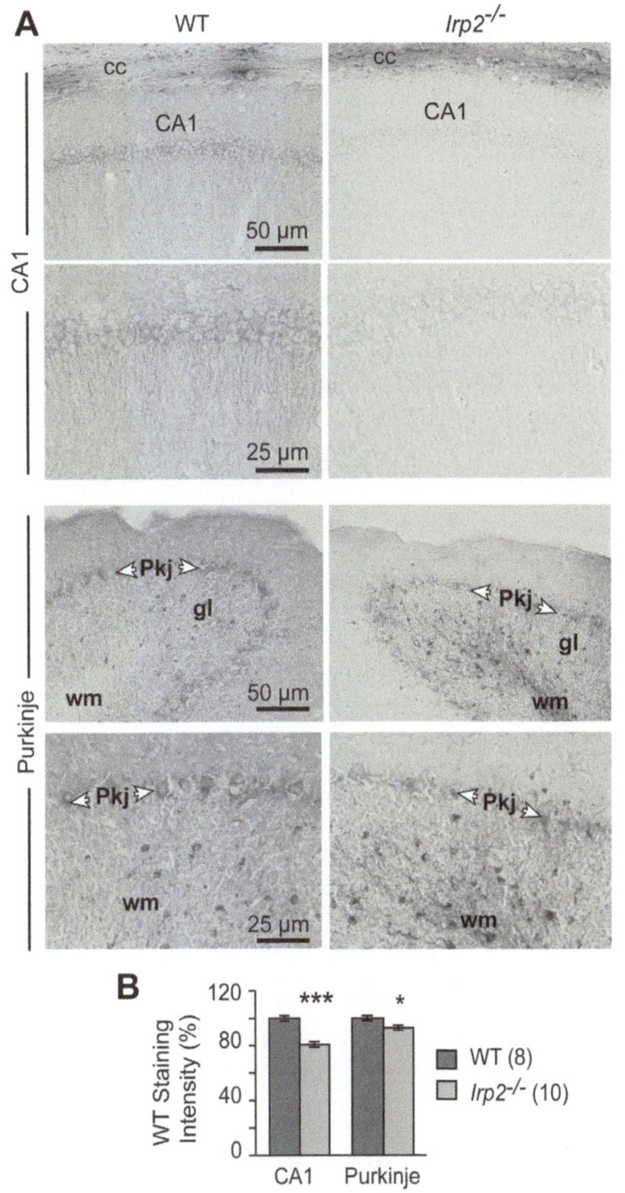

Figure 5. Iron is reduced in Purkinje neurons and in CA1 pyramidal neurons of *Irp2*$^{-/-}$ mice. *A)* Perls' DAB-enhanced iron staining in CA1 pyramidal neurons and Purkinje neurons in *Irp2*$^{-/-}$ and WT mice (*Pkj*, Purkinje; *gl*, granular layer; *wm*, white matter). *B)* Quantification of Perls' staining of images in *(A)* was carried out by measuring staining intensity in a defined subsection of brains from *Irp2*$^{-/-}$ (n = 10) and WT (n = 8) (Figure S3). Data are given as the mean ± SEM; **p*<0.05; ****p*<0.001 relative to WT. Scale bars: 25 μm and 50 μm.

in iron metabolism in different strains of inbred mice [45]. The reasons for the different neurological and behavioral phenotypes observed in *Irp2*$^{-/-}$ mice are not completely understood, but it is likely that the genetic background and the targeting strategies used to generate *Irp2*$^{-/-}$ are important components.

Ultrastructural analyses of several regions of brain from *Irp2*$^{-/-}$ mice reveal normal neuronal morphology and calbindin staining of cerebellar sections show no loss of Purkinje cells. However, marked iron accumulation is observed in white matter and in oligodendrocytes associated with white matter throughout the

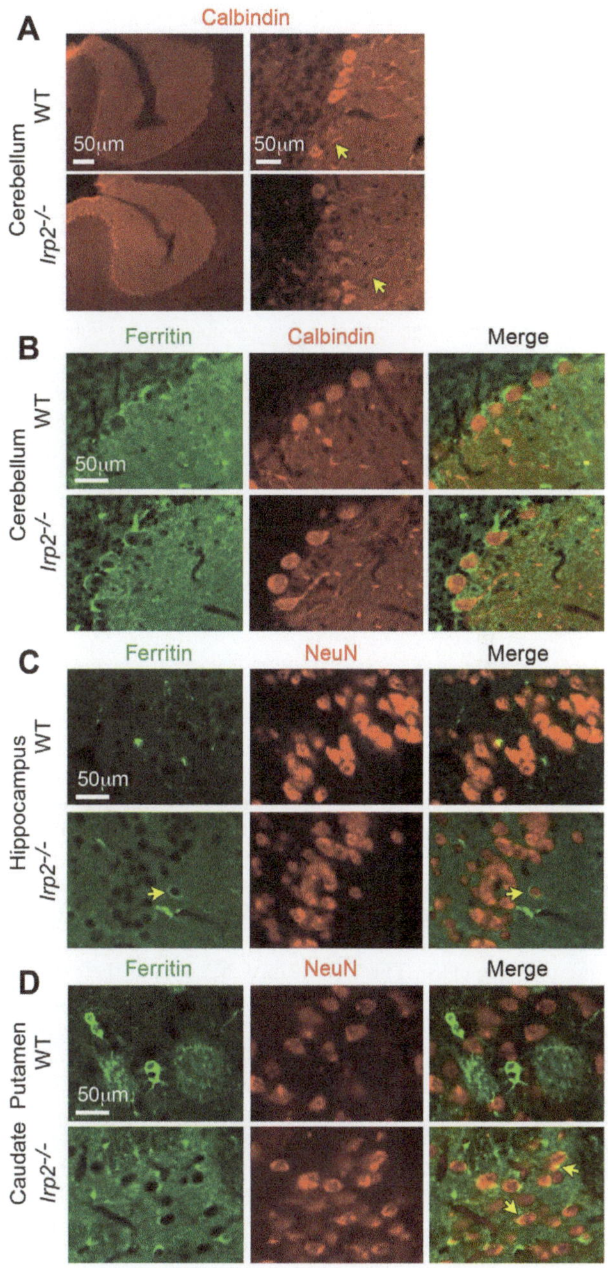

Figure 6. Ferritin expression is increased in *Irp2*$^{-/-}$ neurons. Double immunofluorescence labeling of brain sections from male *Irp2*$^{-/-}$ and WT mice using ferritin antibody with either calbindin (Purkinje specific) or NeuN (neuronal nuclei) antibodies. *A)* Calbindin immunofluorescence shows that Purkinje cell number and morphology (*yellow arrows*, processes), are normal in *Irp2*$^{-/-}$ cerebellum. *B)* Ferritin and calbindin double immunofluorescence of cerebellum shows similar ferritin expression in *Irp2*$^{-/-}$ and WT Purkinje neurons. *C)* Ferritin and NeuN double immunofluorescence of hippocampal CA1 pyramidal cell layer, and *D)* caudate putamen shows increased ferritin expression in neuronal cell bodies (*yellow arrows*) of *Irp2*$^{-/-}$ mice compared to WT mice. Increased ferritin staining is observed in the neuropil in the hippocampus and caudate putamen of *Irp2*$^{-/-}$ mice. Scale bars: 50 μm.

brain consistent with studies from LaVaute et al. [17]. Oligodendrocytes normally contain high levels of iron and express high levels of ferritin. The high iron content of oligodendrocytes is thought to be required for myelin production [46]. Myelinization is not affected in *Irp2*$^{-/-}$ brain, suggesting that high iron content is not detrimental to oligodendrocyte function.

A notable difference between our *Irp2*$^{-/-}$ mice and those of LaVaute et al. [17] is the significant iron accumulation in oligodendroycytes in the cortex of *Irp2*$^{-/-}$ mice. We also found that CA1 pyramidal neurons and Purkinje neurons are iron deprived. Since neurons primarily acquire iron by TfR1, reduced TfR1 and increased ferritin expression in *Irp2*$^{-/-}$ brain would reduce transferrin-dependent iron uptake in parallel with an increase ferritin iron sequestration, eventually leading to cellular iron deficiency. Although we did not find pathological evidence of neurodegeneration, it is possible that cellular iron deficiency in neurons causes cellular dysfunction that leads to mild deficits in locomotion, motor coordination and nociception. This idea is consistent with a recent study showing that *Irp2*$^{-/-}$ mice develop motor neuron disease characterized by increased ferritin and decreased TfR1 expression in motor neurons, reduced spinal cord iron and impaired mitochondrial function [47]. Taken together, these studies suggest that abnormal brain iron metabolism due to Irp2 deficiency disrupts cellular function and leads to mild neurological, behavioral and nociception impairments.

Supporting Information

Figure S1 Generation of *Irp2*$^{-/-}$ mice. (A1) Schematic representation of exons I-VII of the murine *Irp2* (*Ireb2*) gene. Exons (black boxes) and introns (black lines). (A2) Schematic diagram of the targeting vector. A genomic clone (p11.1) containing exons III-VII encoding amino acids 37–233 in Irp2 was isolated from a mouse 129 genomic library. A *ScaI-PstI* fragment from p11.1 (dotted lines) was subcloned into Bluescript SK to generate the targeting vector. A self-excision cassette containing neomycin (*Neo*^{r}) linked to Cre-recombinase (*Cre*) was inserted into exon III of the mouse *Irp2* gene [48]. This cassette (pACN) contains the *Cre* gene (driven by the testes-specific angiotensin-converting enzyme (tACE promoter) linked to the *Neo*^{r} gene (driven by the polymerase II promoter), and is flanked by loxP sites allowing for excision of *Neo*^{r} as it passes through the male germ line. This cassette also contains human *hIrp1-Flag* sequence fused in-frame to exon III of *Irp2* for experiments related to functional replacement of Irp2 with Irp1. For reasons discussed below, Irp1-Flag was not detected in any tissues examined. Thymidine kinase (*Tk1* and *Tk2*) genes were inserted at the 5′ and 3′ ends of the targeting vector to select against random insertion. (A3) Predicted structure of the *Irp2* replacement allele after homologous recombination and germ-line induced self-excision. The targeting vector was electroporated into R1 ES cell line (129/Sv-CP) and heterozygous cells in which a homologous recombination event occurred were identified by PCR and Southern blot analysis of *ScaI*-digested DNA probed with 3′ EXT and Neo probes (Figure S1B, left panels). A targeted ES cell clone (F4) was microinjected into C57BL/6J blastocysts to generate chimeric animals. A chimera was bred to C57BL/6J mice and resulting chimeric progeny was identified by coat color and for the presence of the *Irp2*$^{+/-}$ allele by PCR and Southern blotting. Heterozygous offspring were backcrossed five times to the C57BL/6J background and intercrossed to generate homozygous *Irp2*$^{-/-}$ mice. (B) Germline transmission of the *Neo*-deleted allele was confirmed by Southern blot analysis of *Sca*1-digested genomic DNA from *Irp2*$^{+/+}$, *Irp2*$^{+/-}$ and *Irp2*$^{-/-}$ mice probed with the 3′ EXT probe and shows a WT band (10 kb) in *Irp2*$^{+/+}$, a WT and a mutant band (7 kb) in *Irp2*$^{+/-}$ and a mutant band in *Irp2*$^{-/-}$ (7 kb). The absence of the *Neo*^{r}/*Cre* cassette was confirmed by probing the blot with a Neo probe (not shown). PCR genotyping was performed using tail DNA biopsies (Table S9). (C) Quantitative RT-PCR showed *Irp2* mRNA was not detected in *Irp2*$^{-/-}$ E9.5-E10.5 lysates and reduced 2-fold in *Irp2*$^{+/-}$ lysates compared to WT lysates (TaqMan assay: *Irp2* exons 3–4). *hIrp1-Flag* mRNA was not expressed in *Irp2*$^{+/+}$ lysates, but is expressed in *Irp2*$^{+/-}$ and *Irp2*$^{-/-}$ lysates (TaqMan assay: *hIrp1*). A TaqMan assay corresponding to exons 1–2 (common to both *Irp2* and *hIrp1-Flag*) showed that *hIrp1-Flag* mRNA expression is ~ 80% of endogenous *Irp2* mRNA. (D) Although *hIrp1-Flag* mRNA was detected in *Irp2*$^{-/-}$ lysates, no hIrp1-Flag protein or RNA-binding activity was detected by Western blot analysis or by RNA-EMSA, respectively, in E9.5-E10.5 lysates or any tissue examined (data not shown). The lack of hIrp1-Flag expression is likely due to faulty translation and/or increased turnover of the hIrp1-Flag protein. If hIrp1-Flag is expressed at low levels, the RNA-binding activity of this recombinant protein is not sufficient to compensate for loss of Irp2 protein since *Irp2*$^{-/-}$ mice display altered body iron distribution (Table 1), microcytic anemia (Table S1), and inappropriate regulation of Irp2 targets ferritin and TfR1 (Figure 1) in agreement with published phenotypes of *Irp2*$^{-/-}$ mice [17,23,24]. TaqMan assays used in these experiments can be found in Table S6.

Figure S2 Presence of PPIX-containing granules in the common bile duct of *Irp2*$^{-/-}$ mice. Black arrows indicate PPIX-containing granules in *Irp2*$^{-/-}$ (C) mice. B and D are magnified images of A and C. PPIX-containing granules are found in all male and female *Irp2*$^{-/-}$ mice examined at 2.5- to 18-months of age.

Figure S3 DAB-enhanced Perls' iron staining of hippocampus and cerebellum of aged *Irp2*$^{-/-}$ and WT mice. Coronal sections of hippocampus (A) (slide 41) and cerebellum (B) (slide 58) used for quantification of iron in CA1 pyramidal neurons and in Purkinje neurons in Figure 5. Dotted boxes indicate the WT (6B-4) and the *Irp2*$^{-/-}$ (6A-3) mice used for DAB-enhanced Perls' staining in File S1 and File S2. Ages of male mice: WT, 65–71 weeks; *Irp2*$^{-/-}$, 46–53 weeks.

Figure S4 Ultrastructural analysis of brain regions of aged *Irp2*$^{-/-}$ and WT mice shows no evidence of neurodegeneration. Electron micrographs of the caudate putamen, substantia nigra and cerebellum of *Irp2*$^{-/-}$ and WT mice. Myelinized (white arrows) and non-myelinized (black arrow) axons are shown. No pathological alterations were evident in these brain regions. Similar amounts of lipofuscin deposits (L) were detected in both *Irp2*$^{-/-}$ and WT mice. This can be accounted as a normal finding since lipofuscin accumulates with age in many organs including brain. Representative images are shown from WT (n = 4) and *Irp2*$^{-/-}$ (n = 5) mice. Ages of male mice: WT, 65–71 weeks; *Irp2*$^{-/-}$ 46–53 weeks. Scale bars are indicated.

Figure S5 Luxol Fast Blue staining of brains of aged *Irp2*$^{-/-}$ and WT mice shows no difference in myelinization. Representative images are shown from WT (n = 4) and *Irp2*$^{-/-}$ (n = 5) mice. Ages of male mice: WT, 65–71 weeks; *Irp2*$^{-/-}$, 46–53 weeks.
(TIF)

Table S1 Hematological parameters of aged male WT and *Irp2*$^{-/-}$ mice.

Table S2 Serum iron parameters of aged male WT and *Irp2*$^{-/-}$ mice.

Table S3 Protoporphyrin IX (PPIX) levels of 12-month old male WT and *Irp2*$^{-/-}$ mice.

Table S4 Results of behavioral observation in the modified-Hole Board test.

Table S5 Video-tracking results regarding locomotor behavior.

Table S6 List of primers and TaqMan assays used for genotyping and qRT-PCR.

File S1 DAB-enhanced Perls' iron staining of coronal sections of WT (6B-4) brains. Images (10–66) are from rostral to caudal. High resolution files are available from the corresponding author.

File S2 DAB-enhanced Perls' iron staining of coronal sections of *Irp2*$^{-/-}$ (6A-3) brains. Images (10–66) are from rostral to caudal. High resolution files are available from the corresponding author.

Acknowledgments

We thank Dr. Scott Rogers and Dr. Lorise Gahring for assistance with mouse perfusions and brain imaging, and neuroanatomy and Dr. John Phillip for assistance with PPIX assays. We also thank Ms. Diana Lim for assistance with manuscript and image preparation.

Author Contributions

Conceived and designed the experiments: EAL KZB MHA VGD HF SMH WW. Performed the experiments: KZB SJR BR LB. Analyzed the data: EAL KZB SJR BR EW LG SMH LB IM JCW LQF IR TK. Wrote the paper: EAL KZB. Reviewed the manuscript: TK EW AZ.

References

1. Ganz T, Nemeth E (2012) Hepcidin and iron homeostasis. Biochim Biophys Acta 1823: 1434–1443.
2. Simcox JA, McClain DA (2013) Iron and diabetes risk. Cell Metab 17: 329–341.
3. Rouault TA (2013) Iron metabolism in the CNS: implications for neurodegenerative diseases. Nat Rev Neurosci.
4. Rao R, Georgieff MK (2007) Iron in fetal and neonatal nutrition. Semin Fetal Neonatal Med 12: 54–63.
5. Lozoff B, Georgieff MK (2006) Iron deficiency and brain development. Semin Pediatr Neurol 13: 158–165.
6. Youdim MB (2008) Brain iron deficiency and excess; cognitive impairment and neurodegeneration with involvement of striatum and hippocampus. Neurotox Res 14: 45–56.
7. Fretham SJ, Carlson ES, Wobken J, Tran PV, Petryk A, et al. (2012) Temporal manipulation of transferrin-receptor-1-dependent iron uptake identifies a sensitive period in mouse hippocampal neurodevelopment. Hippocampus 22: 1691–1702.
8. Dusek P, Jankovic J, Le W (2012) Iron dysregulation in movement disorders. Neurobiol Dis 46: 1–18.
9. Burn J, Chinnery PF (2006) Neuroferritinopathy. Semin Pediatr Neurol 13: 176–181.
10. Kono S, Miyajima H (2006) Molecular and pathological basis of aceruloplasminemia. Biol Res 39: 15–23.
11. Hentze MW, Muckenthaler MU, Galy B, Camaschella C (2010) Two to tango: regulation of Mammalian iron metabolism. Cell 142: 24–38.
12. Anderson CP, Shen M, Eisenstein RS, Leibold EA (2012) Mammalian iron metabolism and its control by iron regulatory proteins. Biochim Biophys Acta 1823: 1468–1483.
13. Vashisht AA, Zumbrennen KB, Huang X, Powers DN, Durazo A, et al. (2009) Control of iron homeostasis by an iron-regulated ubiquitin ligase. Science 326: 718–721.
14. Salahudeen AA, Thompson JW, Ruiz JC, Ma HW, Kinch LN, et al. (2009) An E3 ligase possessing an iron-responsive hemerythrin domain is a regulator of iron homeostasis. Science 326: 722–726.
15. Moroishi T, Nishiyama M, Takeda Y, Iwai K, Nakayama KI (2011) The FBXL5-IRP2 axis is integral to control of iron metabolism in vivo. Cell Metab 14: 339–351.
16. Sanchez M, Galy B, Schwanhaeusser B, Blake J, Bahr-Ivacevic T, et al. (2011) Iron regulatory protein-1 and -2: transcriptome-wide definition of binding mRNAs and shaping of the cellular proteome by iron regulatory proteins. Blood 118: e168–179.
17. LaVaute T, Smith S, Cooperman S, Iwai K, Land W, et al. (2001) Targeted deletion of the gene encoding iron regulatory protein-2 causes misregulation of iron metabolism and neurodegenerative disease in mice. Nat Genet 27: 209–214.
18. Meyron-Holtz EG, Ghosh MC, Iwai K, LaVaute T, Brazzolotto X, et al. (2004) Genetic ablations of iron regulatory proteins 1 and 2 reveal why iron regulatory protein 2 dominates iron homeostasis. EMBO J 23: 386–395.
19. Galy B, Ferring D, Hentze MW (2005) Generation of conditional alleles of the murine iron regulatory protein (Irp)-1 and -2 genes. Genesis 43: 181–188.
20. Anderson SA, Nizzi CP, Chang YI, Deck KM, Schmidt PJ, et al. (2013) The IRP1-HIF-2alpha axis coordinates iron and oxygen sensing with erythropoiesis and iron absorption. Cell Metab 17: 282–290.
21. Ghosh MC, Zhang DL, Jeong SY, Kovtunovych G, Ollivierre-Wilson H, et al. (2013) Deletion of iron regulatory protein 1 causes polycythemia and pulmonary hypertension in mice through translational derepression of HIF2alpha. Cell Metab 17: 271–281.
22. Wilkinson N, Pantopoulos K (2013) IRP1 regulates erythropoiesis and systemic iron homeostasis by controlling HIF2alpha mRNA translation. Blood 122: 1658–1668.
23. Cooperman SS, Meyron-Holtz EG, Olivierre-Wilson H, Ghosh MC, McConnell JP, et al. (2005) Microcytic anemia, erythropoietic protoporphyria, and neurodegeneration in mice with targeted deletion of iron-regulatory protein 2. Blood 106: 1084–1091.
24. Galy B, Ferring D, Minana B, Bell O, Janser HG, et al. (2005) Altered body iron distribution and microcytosis in mice deficient in iron regulatory protein 2 (IRP2). Blood 106: 2580–2589.
25. Smith SR, Cooperman S, Lavaute T, Tresser N, Ghosh M, et al. (2004) Severity of neurodegeneration correlates with compromise of iron metabolism in mice with iron regulatory protein deficiencies. Ann N Y Acad Sci 1012: 65–83.
26. Galy B, Holter SM, Klopstock T, Ferring D, Becker L, et al. (2006) Iron homeostasis in the brain: complete iron regulatory protein 2 deficiency without symptomatic neurodegeneration in the mouse. Nat Genet 38: 967–969; discussion 969–970.
27. Guo B, Yu Y, Leibold EA (1994) Iron regulates cytoplasmic levels of a novel iron-responsive element-binding protein without aconitase activity. J Biol Chem 269: 24252–24260.
28. Yu Y, Radisky E, Leibold EA (1992) The iron-responsive element binding protein. Purification, cloning, and regulation in rat liver. J Biol Chem 267: 19005–19010.
29. Leibold EA, Munro HN (1988) Cytoplasmic protein binds in vitro to a highly conserved sequence in the 5′ untranslated region of ferritin heavy- and light-subunit mRNAs. Proc Natl Acad Sci U S A 85: 2171–2175.
30. Phillips JD, Bergonia HA, Reilly CA, Franklin MR, Kushner JP (2007) A porphomethene inhibitor of uroporphyrinogen decarboxylase causes porphyria cutanea tarda. Proc Natl Acad Sci U S A 104: 5079–5084.
31. Ohl F, Holsboer F, Landgraf R (2001) The modified hole board as a differential screen for behavior in rodents. Behav Res Methods Instrum Comput 33: 392–397.
32. Kallnik M, Elvert R, Ehrhardt N, Kissling D, Mahabir E, et al. (2007) Impact of IVC housing on emotionality and fear learning in male C3HeB/FeJ and C57BL/6J mice. Mamm Genome 18: 173–186.
33. Neff F, Flores-Dominguez D, Ryan DP, Horsch M, Schroder S, et al. (2013) Rapamycin extends murine lifespan but has limited effects on aging. J Clin Invest 123: 3272–3291.
34. Mogil JS (1999) The genetic mediation of individual differences in sensitivity to pain and its inhibition. Proc Natl Acad Sci U S A 96: 7744–7751.
35. Ghosh MC, Tong WH, Zhang D, Ollivierre-Wilson H, Singh A, et al. (2008) Tempol-mediated activation of latent iron regulatory protein activity prevents symptoms of neurodegenerative disease in IRP2 knockout mice. Proc Natl Acad Sci U S A 105: 12028–12033.
36. Grabill C, Silva AC, Smith SS, Koretsky AP, Rouault TA (2003) MRI detection of ferritin iron overload and associated neuronal pathology in iron regulatory protein-2 knockout mice. Brain Res 971: 95–106.
37. Todorich B, Pasquini JM, Garcia CI, Paez PM, Connor JR (2009) Oligodendrocytes and myelination: the role of iron. Glia 57: 467–478.

38. Dickinson TK, Connor JR (1998) Immunohistochemical analysis of the transferrin receptor: regional and cellular distribution in the hypotransferrinemic (hpx) mouse brain. Brain Research 801: 171–181.
39. Leitner DF, Connor JR (2012) Functional roles of transferrin in the brain. Biochim Biophys Acta 1820: 393–402.
40. Gerlai R (1996) Gene-targeting studies of mammalian behavior: is it the mutation or the background genotype? Trends Neurosci 19: 177–181.
41. Watase K, Zoghbi HY (2003) Modelling brain diseases in mice: the challenges of design and analysis. Nat Rev Genet 4: 296–307.
42. Yoshiki A, Moriwaki K (2006) Mouse phenome research: implications of genetic background. Ilar J 47: 94–102.
43. Pham CT, MacIvor DM, Hug BA, Heusel JW, Ley TJ (1996) Long-range disruption of gene expression by a selectable marker cassette. Proc Natl Acad Sci U S A 93: 13090–13095.
44. Crusio WE (2004) Flanking gene and genetic background problems in genetically manipulated mice. Biol Psychiatry 56: 381–385.
45. Leboeuf RC, Tolson D, Heinecke JW (1995) Dissociation between tissue iron concentrations and transferrin saturation among inbred mouse strains. J Lab Clin Med 126: 128–136.
46. Connor JR, Menzies SL (1996) Relationship of iron to oligodendrocytes and myelination. Glia 17: 83–93.
47. Jeong SY, Crooks DR, Wilson-Ollivierre H, Ghosh MC, Sougrat R, et al. (2011) Iron insufficiency compromises motor neurons and their mitochondrial function in Irp2-null mice. PLoS One 6: e25404.
48. Bunting M, Bernstein KE, Greer JM, Capecchi MR, Thomas KR (1999) Targeting genes for self-excision in the germ line. Genes Dev 13: 1524–1528.

17

Genome-Wide Association Studies Identifies Seven Major Regions Responsible for Iron Deficiency Chlorosis in Soybean (*Glycine max*)

Sujan Mamidi[1,2], Rian K. Lee[1,2], Jay R. Goos[3], Phillip E. McClean[1,2]*

1 Genomics and Bioinformatics Program, North Dakota State University, Fargo, North Dakota, United States of America, **2** Department of Plant Sciences, North Dakota State University, Fargo, North Dakota, United States of America, **3** Department of Soil Science, North Dakota State University, Fargo, North Dakota, United States of America

Abstract

Iron deficiency chlorosis (IDC) is a yield limiting problem in soybean (*Glycine max* (L.) Merr) production regions with calcareous soils. Genome-wide association study (GWAS) was performed using a high density SNP map to discover significant markers, QTL and candidate genes associated with IDC trait variation. A stepwise regression model included eight markers after considering LD between markers, and identified seven major effect QTL on seven chromosomes. Twelve candidate genes known to be associated with iron metabolism mapped near these QTL supporting the polygenic nature of IDC. A non-synonymous substitution with the highest significance in a major QTL region suggests soybean orthologs of *FRE1* on Gm03 is a major gene responsible for trait variation. NAS3, a gene that encodes the enzyme nicotianamine synthase which synthesizes the iron chelator nicotianamine also maps to the same QTL region. Disease resistant genes also map to the major QTL, supporting the hypothesis that pathogens compete with the plant for Fe and increase iron deficiency. The markers and the allelic combinations identified here can be further used for marker assisted selection.

Editor: Swarup Kumar Parida, National Institute of Plant Genome Research (NIPGR), India

Funding: This work is supported by North Central Soybean Research Program. The funders had no role in study design, data collection and analysis, decision to publish, or preparation of the manuscript.

Competing Interests: The authors have declared that no competing interests exist.

* Email: Phillip.Mcclean@ndsu.edu

Introduction

Iron (Fe) is an essential element for multiple plant functions including photosynthesis, respiration, chlorophyll biosynthesis, and redox reactions in plants, and is a structural component in heme, the Fe-sulfur cluster, and Fe-binding sites. To avoid toxicity, plants control the uptake, utilization, and storage in response to Fe availability [1]. Despite its abundance in the soil, Fe is only slightly soluble under aerobic conditions, especially in high-pH and calcareous soils [2]. Under these conditions, iron deficiency leads to developmental defects, including chlorosis, growth retardation, and reduced crop productivity [3]. Iron deficiency chlorosis (IDC) is an important yield-limiting factor for soybeans (*G. max*) grown on calcareous soils that have a high percentage of calcium carbonate and soluble salts. This soil type is common in the north-central regions of the United States [4] where soybean is widely grown. In these soils, interactions of high pH, carbonate and high field moisture content at planting leads to early IDC symptoms that effect yield. It is estimated that the current revenue losses due to IDC in soybean are $260 million [5].

IDC results from the inability of susceptible genotypes to efficiently mobilize iron into the plant when it is growing in high pH calcareous soils. In these soils, ferrous iron is not readily released from soil particles, and subsequently iron availability is limited. Based on its response to Fe availability, soybean is considered a Strategy I plant [6] that reduces ferric chelates at the root surface and absorbs ferrous ions across the plasma membrane of the root [2]. Other processes involved in Strategy I include excretion of proton and phenolic compounds from the roots to the rhizosphere, which increases the solubility of ferric ions and support the reducing capacity of ferric Fe on the root surface [2]. Strategy I plants also increase root hair formation, thereby increasing the surface area available for iron uptake [7]. Once iron enters the root, membrane transporters move Fe into the xylem where it chelates with citrate. The chelated form of iron then moves through the xylem stream to growing leaves. Iron is then remobilized from the leaves, forms a complex with nicotianamine, and is transported via the phloem to younger leaves and seeds. Excess water leads to an elevated concentration of bicarbonates in the root apoplast that impedes the Fe^{3+}– chelate reductase activity necessary for the conversion of Fe^{3+} to Fe^{2+}. Bicarbonates also immobilize the movement of iron to young leaves once it is absorbed at the root level [8].

Given the many physiological mechanisms associated with iron metabolism, it is not surprising that IDC is a complex quantitative trait with multiple genetic factors [9]. In addition to the genes involved in Fe acquisition, translocation and compartmentalization within the organelles, there are other genes involved in Fe transcriptional and post transcriptional changes that are expressed/repressed under deficient and excess conditions or affect iron homeostasis pathways [10–17].

Genetic experiments using bi-parental mapping populations have identified multiple quantitative trait loci (QTL) associated with IDC in soybean [11–12]. O'Rourke et al. [13] identified several genes induced under iron-limiting conditions using a microarray study. Severin et al. [14] discovered multiple introgressed genomic regions responsible for IDC in near isogenic lines, and Stec et al. [15] further refined these introgression regions. Recently, Peiffer et al. [5] evaluated candidate genes on Gm03.

A genome-wide association study (GWAS) is an excellent approach to discover genetic factors in a population because of the high number of recombinant events the population represents. GWAS uses the linkage disequilibrium (LD) pattern in a large population of unrelated individuals [16] to map significant effect loci. Since IDC is a complex trait, utilizing GWAS can identify major factors controlling the IDC response in soybean. Previously, Wang et al. [17] used GWAS to identify simple sequence repeat (SSR) markers associated with IDC in two independent populations. Later, nine shared SNP were discovered and confirmed by Mamidi et al. [9] in two separate populations. The objective of this study was to identify QTL and genes involved in IDC of soybean using a GWAS population and a new high density SNP map obtained through genotype-by-sequencing (GBS). Those results were then translated into SNP markers that can be used for marker assisted selection (MAS).

Materials and Methods

Phenotype and genotyping

Two plant populations consisting of unique set of advanced soybean breeding lines developed for the north-central region of the US were grown in years 2005 (n = 132) and 2006 (n = 138). IDC screening protocols and DNA isolation procedures were described previously [9]. The trait was rated on a scale of 1 to 5, where 1 indicates no chlorosis and a normal green plant, 2 indicates slight yellowing of upper leaves and the leaf veins, 3 indicates interveinal chlorosis in the upper leaves with no stunning of growth or death of tissue (necrosis), 4 indicates interveinal chlorosis of the upper leaves along with some apparent stunning of growth or necrosis of tissue, and 5 indicates severe chlorosis plus stunned growth and necrosis in the youngest leaves and growing points [9]. Phenotypic data was adjusted based on least squares means for each population independently.

GBS libraries were prepared and analyzed at the Institute for Genomic Diversity (IGD), Cornell University, according to Elshire et al. [18], using the enzyme *Ape*KI. The GBS analysis pipeline [3.0.128], an extension of the Java program TASSEL [19], was used to call SNPs from the sequenced GBS library. Reads were aligned to the soybean reference genome v1.1 [20] using BWA 0.6.1 [21]. VCFtools (v0.1.8) [22] was used to summarize the SNP data.

The data was analyzed by combining the two populations (which are of similar size) to account for unique alleles that are at a low frequency in one or both populations. These low frequency alleles can have a significant phenotypic effect in a small set of genotypes, but that effect cannot be detected in a normal statistical framework [16].

Genome-wide association study

Imputation. fastPHASE 1.3 [23], a likelihood-based imputation software, was used with default settings to impute missing data for the combined population. Imputation analysis was performed to increase the power of the study and fine map the causal variant [24]. A minor allele frequency (MAF) of 0.05 was used as cutoff, since variants at low frequency have little power to detect association with the phenotype [16].

Linkage disequilibrium (LD). The LD between markers was estimated as the partial squared allele frequency correlation (r^2) using CORR procedure in SAS 9.3. Three principal components (PC) that explain about 25% of cumulative variation were used as cofactors. We used a partial correlation because unlinked loci can be in LD simply because of population structure [25–26]. The decay of r^2 with physical and/or genetic distance between loci is often used to determine the density of markers to use in whole genome association scans [27] whereas local LD on chromosomes is used to account for genes/QTL associated with trait variation. Overestimation of LD can lead to misinterpretations either on the extent of LD decay or on the size of the QTL [26]. LD decay graphs were plotted with physical distance (Mbp) vs. r^2 for all intra-chromosomal comparisons using nonlinear regression as described by Remington et al. [28]. The expected decay of LD was estimated as described by Pyhajarvi et al. [29]. We fit this equation into a nonlinear regression model using NLIN procedure in SAS 9.3.

Population structure, kinship, and model testing. A principal component analysis was utilized to control for population structure [30]. PCs were estimated using the PRINCOMP procedure in SAS 9.3. The PCs that explained 25% (PC_{25}) and 50% (PC_{50}) cumulative variation were selected for the analysis. In addition an identity-by-state matrix [31] was used to control for relatedness estimated as a centered relatedness matrix in Gemma 0.92 [32]. Gower's similarity coefficient was calculated using the DISTANCE procedure in SAS 9.3 to measure the relatedness by state of the individuals.

To test for marker-trait associations, the MIXED procedure in SAS for the three linear models that do not have kinship (Naïve, PC_{25} and PC_{50}) was used. Since approximate tests compromise the analysis of complex genetic architectures when one genetic factor masks another [33], we used the exact test implemented in Gemma 0.92 to estimate marker significance [32] for the other three models with kinship (Kinship, PC_{25}+kinship, PC_{50}+kinship). As the standard errors follow a uniform distribution [34], we used a rank based mean squared difference (MSD) for model selection as described in Mamidi et al [9].

Marker-trait associations. Markers are defined as significant at two levels, within 0.01 percentile, and 0.1 percentile tails of the empirical p-value distribution of 10,000 bootstraps. This method of using an empirical distribution of data as a replacement for a population with an unknown distribution has the advantage of simplicity and provides an efficient and precise estimation [35–36]. This approach is similar to choosing an arbitrary value but instead it is based on choosing a predefined percentile tail from an empirical distribution. Here, the confidence intervals for an empirical distribution were obtained from 10,000 bootstraps over ~35,000 markers distributed throughout the genome. We chose this approach over a cutoff because p-value is dependent on the distribution of phenotype, the variation explained by the marker, structure and relatedness of the population, and heritability of the trait.

The means for the alleles were calculated using MEANS procedure in SAS. The percent of variation explained by the marker is calculated using a simple regression (GLM procedure) in SAS. The additive effect of the variant allele is calculated as half the difference between IDC mean of the variant allele and IDC mean of the reference allele.

To determine the minimal number of SNPs independently associated with IDC, stepwise regression analysis was applied to all significant markers from a single-SNP analysis at a significance level of 0.1 percentile [37]. In addition, a multiple R^2 value for all these loci was also estimated [9]. A significant p-value of 0.05 was necessary for both marker and model for stepwise inclusion of the marker in REG procedure in SAS 9.3.

Annotation of SNP. To characterize SNPs as intergenic, UTR, intron, or coding site, snpEFF 3.3 [38] was used. Coding sites were further differentiated into synonymous or non-synonymous substitutions based on amino acid changes. Coding regions were also differentiated into transitions and transversions based on changes between or among purines and pyrimidines.

Significant QTL and genes. A QTL region is defined as the region around significant stepwise markers that has a partial LD (r^2) >0.6 with the adjacent marker (corresponds to partial correlation of 0.77). Adjacent blocks were combined if the distance is less than 10 kb and includes up to four markers that are not in LD with either of the block. Candidate genes for iron homeostasis were identified from the research literature, and gene symbols are used from the annotation file available at phytozome (http://www.phytozome.net/soybean.php). A candidate iron gene is considered to be significant in our population if the gene is within the QTL region.

Epistatic interactions. To detect epistatic interactions between significant markers, we used a general linear model with both significant markers and their interaction term in the model. We used PC_{25} as covariates in the regression model and an interaction term was considered significant at a p-value of≤1E-03. Genes that are in LD with these significant markers are used to identify the gene-by-gene interactions.

Significant allelic combinations. We compared the allelic combinations of the significant markers (0.1 percentile) that were included in stepwise regression. Allelic combinations with a mean IDC<2.5 were termed tolerant, and those with a mean IDC>3.5 were considered susceptible. We chose these values based on standard genotypes grown in the field instead of a statistical approach of mean differentiation, because not all allelic combinations are present in the population. With this approach, the phenotypic distribution does not need to be continuous, where statistically two allelic combinations can be considered significantly different in the absence of intermediate phenotypes.

Results

Phenotype and genotyping

For the combined population, the range of IDC is 1.46 to 3.84 with an average of 2.76. IDC scores were normally distributed with a p-value of 0.15 for Kolmogorov–Smirnov test (Figure 1). An average of 1,645,563 reads was obtained for each genotype, and ~92% of reads mapped to the reference genome. A total of 79,000 putative SNPs that are bi-allelic were identified in the population using the TASSEL-GBS analysis pipeline after removing SNPs that have greater than 50% missing data. The mean coverage depth for each identified SNP was 6.85±2.72.

Association Mapping

Imputation. Missing data (37.5%) was estimated using imputation. Of the 79,000 SNPs, 34,428 had a MAF>0.05 (Table S1). Based on the genome size of *Glycine max*, a polymorphic marker was located, on average, every 31 kbp. In addition, the maximum distance between two adjacent markers did not exceed 500 Kbp providing a good coverage of the SNPs. Of these polymorphic SNPs, 6,520 mapped to a coding region, 6,898 are located in the non-coding region of a gene model and 21,010 are in an intergenic region. The transition to transversions ratio was 1.67.

Linkage Disequilibrium Decay. A nonlinear regression model that fits the partial r^2 of pairwise intra-chromosomal comparisons to physical distance was developed. The average decay of LD (r^2) in terms of physical distance declined to $r^2 = 0.7$ at ~500 kb (Figure S1). The physical distance at which $r^2 = 0.2$ is 3.2 Mbp and at $r^2 = 0.1$ was 8.0 Mbp.

Population structure, Kinship and model selection. For the population, three and 13 PC explained 26.8% and 50.5% of the cumulative genotypic variation. Based on the first two PCs, two distinct clusters of populations were observed which indicated the presence of a subpopulation structure (Figure 2). In the population, 80% of the Gowers similarity coefficients are within the range of 0.6 to 0.7 (Figure 3) indicating the presence of relatedness among individuals. This is expected given the narrow genetic base of the breeding population. For the six models tested, the best linear model for the population included 13 PCs (PC_{50}) and kinship matrix (MSD = 6.06E-06; Figure 4).

Marker Trait associations. Five markers were significant at the 0.01 percentile level (p≤4.0E-05). One located on Gm03 at 45.03 Mbp, one on Gm05 at 8.82 Mbp and three on Gm11 at 0.53 Mbp (Table 1, Fig. 5). The variation explained by these markers ranged from 5% to 16%, and the mean allelic difference is between 0.31 and 0.38. Stepwise regression included three markers (one from each of the chromosome). Together these three markers explained 23.2% of phenotypic variation.

At a significance level of 0.1 percentile (p≤2.12E-04), 33 significant markers were distributed on 10 of the 20 chromosomes (Table 1, Figure 5). Eight of these markers included in stepwise regression are on Gm03 (45.03 Mbp), Gm05 (8.87 Mbp), Gm07 (6.39 Mbp), Gm11 (0.53 Mbp), Gm16 (27.30 Mbp), Gm17 (25.85 Mbp), Gm18 (28.14 Mbp), and Gm19 (40.19 Mbp). These markers together explained 46.3% variation.

Annotation of SNP. Of the significant markers at 0.1 percentile, five SNP are present in a coding region (three are transitions and two are transversions), 11 in introns, two in 3′UTR regions, and 15 in intergenic regions. Of the five SNPs from a coding region, two are non-synonymous substitutions. For FRE1 (Glyma03G38620), one of these amino acid changes is associated with both a polarity and a charge change of the protein. This SNP at position 44,927,455 bp of Gm03 changes an asparagine to aspartic acid. The R-square explained by this marker alone is 15.2% for the population. The variant allele ‘A’ is more tolerant than reference allele. The other non-synonymous substitution is located in the gene model (Glyma03g39151) close to the above non-synonymous substitution at 45,343,612 bp. This SNP explains about 18.85% of the phenotypic variation in the population and has a partial r^2 of 0.80 with the above marker. These two markers together explain 19.0% of phenotypic variation.

Significant QTL and genes. At the significance level of 0.01 percentile, three markers were included in the stepwise regression. One of these marker is in LD (r^2≥0.6) with the adjacent markers, and the QTL is located on Gm03 between 44.798 Mbp and 47.140 Mbp (Table 2; Figure 5; Figure 6). The two major candidate genes in this QTL are phytochrome A (FRE1; Glyma03g38620) and nicotianamine synthase 3 (NAS3; Glyma03g39050). In addition to these genes, nitrate transporter 1:2 (NRT1:2; Glyma03g38640) and ammonium transporter 2 (AMT2; Glyma03g40700), each with a role in iron homeostasis, are also located within the QTL region. The QTL around the significant marker on Gm05 is between 7.837 and 10.627 Mbp (Table 2; Figure 5; Figure 6). The candidate genes in this QTL

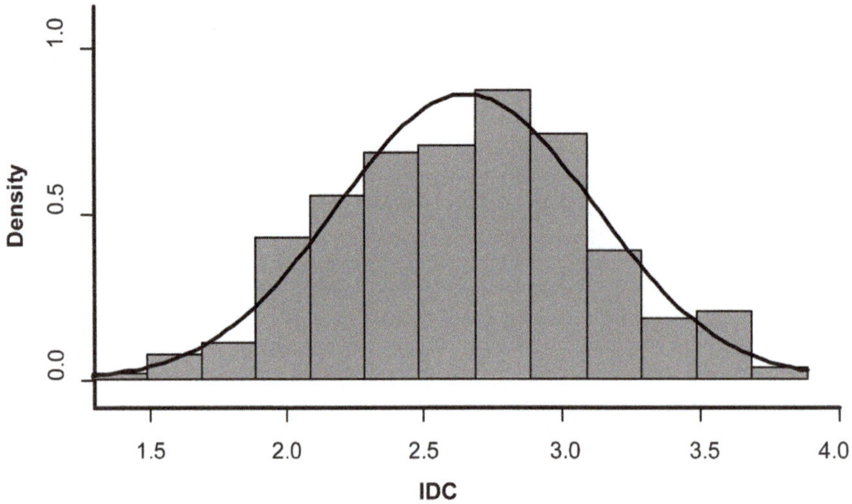

Figure 1. Phenotypic distribution of iron deficiency chlorosis (IDC). The rating of IDC (1–5) is on x-axis and the number of genotypes having the IDC score (represented as density) are presented as y-axis. The curve over the histogram represents the normal distribution of the IDC scores in the population.

include stabilizer of iron transporter (AGO10, PNH, ZLL; Glyma05g08170), RAS-related nuclear protein-1 (RAN1; Glyma05g08260) and H (+)-ATPase 11 (AHA11; Glyma05g01460). The third significant marker on Gm11 is located in the 5′ UTR region of the CVP2 like 1 gene (CVL1; Glyma11g00990). The marker is not in LD with any of the adjacent markers.

At a significance level of 0.1 percentile, eight markers are included in the stepwise regression model. These eight markers are located in eight QTL regions. The QTL on Gm03, Gm05 and Gm11 are the same as the ones identified at the 0.01 percentile level. The other QTL at this significance level include Gm07 (6.074 Mbp–7.101 Mbp), Gm16 (26.914–27.597 Mbp), Gm17 (25.629–27.007 Mbp), Gm18 (27.547–29.978 Mbp), and Gm19 (39.831–41.320 Mbp) (Table 2; Figure 5; Figure 6). On Gm07, the significant candidate genes include ferric reduction oxidase 2 (FRO2; Glyma07g07380), and signal recognition particle receptor

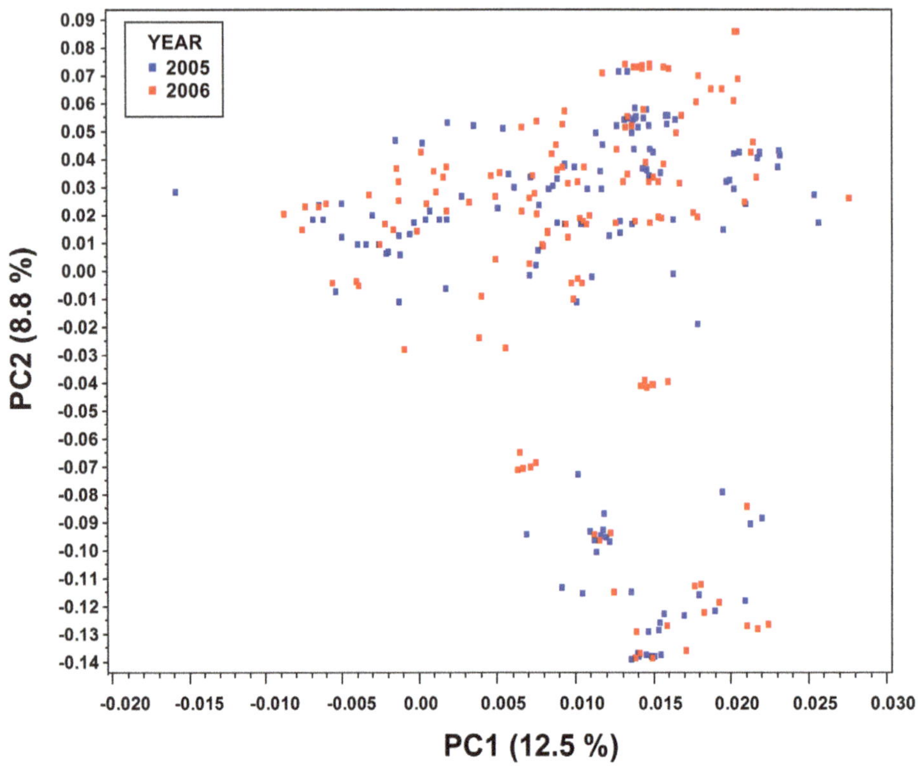

Figure 2. A graph of the first two principal components obtained from all the 34,428 polymorphic SNPs. This graph explains the similarities between the two independent populations and the overall population structure.

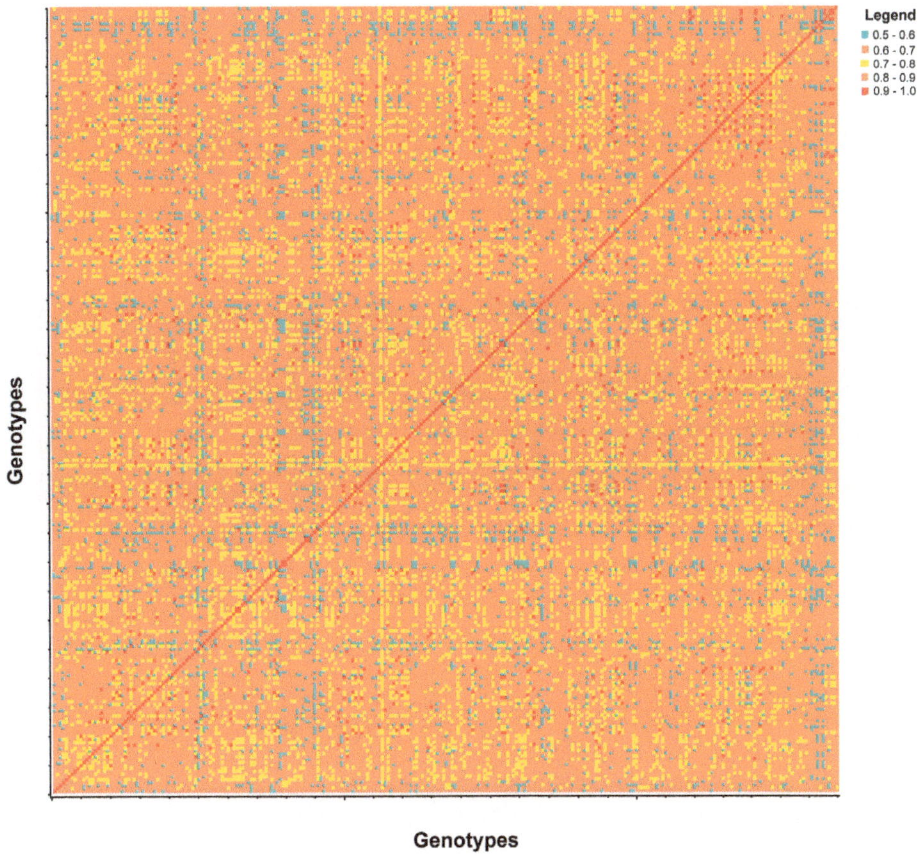

Figure 3. Heatmap of Gower's similarity distance among the individuals of the population. Based on the colors distribution, it is evident that relatedness can have a major effect on identifying associations to IDC in the population.

protein on chloroplast (FRD4; Glyma07g08240). On Gm16, the significant candidate gene ferrodoxin NADP (+) oxidoreductase 1 (FNR1, Glyma16g23710) is within the QTL region. On Gm19, heavy metal atpase-5 (HMA5; Glyma19g32190), and oligopeptide transporter-5 (OPT5; Glyma19g32401) are significant.

Other than the genes involved in iron metabolism, several genes involved in disease resistance are also identified in the QTL regions. For example, QTL on Gm03 has two RING/U-box superfamily proteins that have a role in plant defense. Similarly on Gm05, two CC-NBS-LRR, one NBS and one LRR genes are present. On Gm07 within the QTL region, three NBS genes are present. On Gm16, seven LRR proteins, and on Gm19, six NBS proteins, two LRR and one RING/U-box superfamily proteins are present.

Epistatic interactions. With 33 significant markers at 0.1 percentile, 528 two way interactions were tested with a population structure component, and five interactions were significant at p-value<0.001. Three of these interactions are between Gm07 (around 6.4 Mbp) and Gm18 (59.28 Mbp). The other significant interactions are between Gm16 (27.30 Mbp) and Gm18 (59.28 Mbp), Gm02 (46.939) and Gm15 (21.42 Mbp). The genes within LD regions include cytochrome P450 like protein (Glyma18g50051) on Gm18 with FRO2 (Glyma07g07380) on Gm07 and FNR1 (Glyma16g23710) on Gm16. The genes on Gm02 include AUX1 (Glyma02g42290) and FER4 (Glyma02g43040) which interact with CCC1 (Glyma15g22520) on Gm15.

Significant Marker Allelic combinations. Allelic combinations of SNPs can be used to infer the tolerant/susceptible phenotype of a genotype. For the significant markers (0.1 percentile) that were included in stepwise regression in the population, 14 allelic combinations are predicted as tolerant (IDC mean≤2.5) and 6 allelic combinations indicate susceptibility (IDC mean≥3.5) (Table 3).

Discussion

A higher marker density facilitates identification of high resolution QTL and gene discovery [39,40]. One method of generating a high frequency of SNPs is next generation sequencing [41,42]. Using GBS, we identified ~35,000 polymorphic markers with a minor allele frequency>0.05. This provided good coverage, one marker at every 31 kb. This density is useful for characterizing most genetic factors responsible for soybean IDC given that LD decayed here to $r^2 = 0.7$ at 500 kbp.

LD decay assesses the depth of markers required for GWAS. Partial LD was calculated using population structure as a cofactor, and as expected we observed a variation in LD decay when including this as a cofactor. For example, LD decay for the population is at 10 Mbp at $r^2 = 0.1$ whereas adjustments for confounding effect of population structure reduced LD decay to 7 Mbp. The use of partial LD (r^2) helps overcome the bias between adjacent markers and leads to smaller QTL regions.

The population consisted of breeding lines developed by public and private programs targeting the north central states of the US. The germplasm is expected to be narrow given the limited range of maturity group (0–1), the short history of soybean breeding in USA, and the limited number of traits selected in the breeding

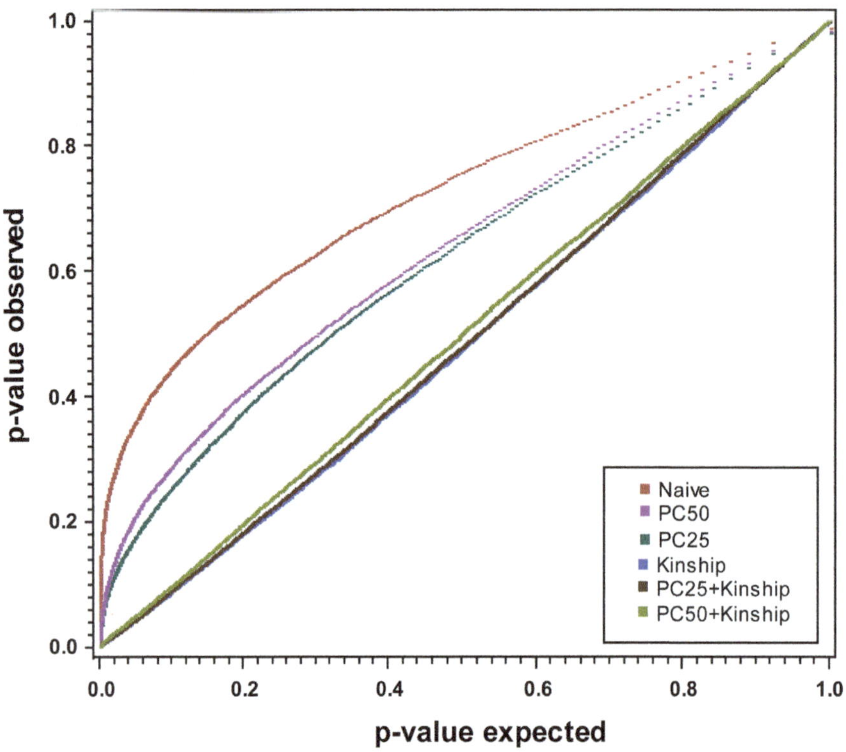

Figure 4. QQ plot for the six models tested. P-value observed is plotted on the y-axis and P-expected is plotted on the x-axis. Each color represents a model of regression used. The best model is the one that is close to the diagonal line.

programs. Here we used multiple mixed models [31,34,43–45] that control for confounding effect of population structure and population relatedness [16,46].

The percentile p-value cutoffs derived from empirical distribution were all within the p = 0.001 error level, and the significant markers were distributed on eleven of the twenty chromosomes. This is expected given the complex nature of iron homeostasis in plants. At a significance level of one percentile ($p \leq 2.12E-04$), many more markers were significant (345 markers) and explained the majority of the phenotypic variation in the population ($R^2 = 85\%$). However, owing to the complexity of the trait, we limited the interpretations to the 0.1 percentile to find the major QTL effects.

To determine if any significant SNP is a potential causal variant, we searched for non-synonymous substitutions. One was discovered in Far red elongated 1 (FRE1) which encodes a protein that increase reductase activity and provides a higher level of tolerance in high pH calcareous soils [47–49]. The other non-synonymous substitution was discovered in a gene with no known function related to iron homeostasis. This can be expected because the functions of many genes are still unknown [50–52].

Stepwise regression facilitates the selection of markers that have a major effect in a QTL region and simultaneously masks the effects of other minor QTL. As an example, the QTL regions on Gm02 and Gm15 that have a significant interaction were not included in the stepwise regression given these QTL have a minor effect. Additionally, the partial LD between the 33 significant markers is 0.09 (±0.247). But for the eight markers included in stepwise regression, partial LD (r^2) is 0.008 (±0.021). This subset of markers included in stepwise regression explains 23.2% and 46.3% of the 0.01 and 0.1 percentile, respectively. This is similar to the variation explained by all significant markers (23.2% and 48.6% at the 0.01 and 0.1 percentile, respectively).

Comparing with independent populations, the combined population analysis was able to identify markers from eight addition QTL regions that are not discovered in independent populations at significance level of 0.1 percentile. Only six QTL regions are common with either one of the population. Further using a stepwise regression to identify major effect QTL, the combined analysis was able to identify three unique QTL regions (On Gm05, Gm17, and Gm18) that were not identified in the independent populations. Of the other five QTL regions, two are common with 2005 population (on Gm03, Gm11) and three are common with 2006 population (Gm07, Gm16, Gm19).

For the population, we identified seven QTL on seven chromosomes. Given the complex quantitative nature of iron metabolism, multiple QTL distributed throughout the genome are expected. The region on Gm03 is in the same region identified earlier by Severin et al. [14] and Stec et al. [15] using an introgression analysis and is a significant QTL in many biparental studies [53–55]. In addition to this major QTL, other QTL regions were also identified earlier. For example, QTL region on Gm05 were identified earlier by Severin et al. [14]. The QTL on Gm16 is close to an introgression region identified earlier [14,15]. Similarly Lin et al. [53] identified QTL on Gm18 and Gm19 and Lin et al.[56] identified QTL on Gm18. Most of these regions were also identified earlier using the same population with about 1000 polymorphic markers [9]. The major difference of this study from the previous one is the ability to narrow the QTL region and the ability to study the entire genome given a polymorphic marker every 31 kb. In addition we were able to identify significant SNP markers within the candidate genes.

Table 1. Significant markers associated with IDC in the population of soybean.

Chromosome	Position	–log10 (p-value)	Reference Allele	Variant Allele	$R^{2§}$	MAF[§§]	Mean Difference	Additive Effect (Variant allele)	Included in stepwise regression[§§§]
Gm02	46,939,135	3.784**	A	T	5.20	21.48	0.26	−0.13	
Gm03	44,927,455	4.165**	A	G	15.20	38.89	0.37	−0.19	
Gm03	44,930,187	4.165**	A	T	15.20	38.89	0.37	−0.19	
Gm03	44,970,860	4.275**	A	G	14.42	39.26	0.36	−0.18	
Gm03	44,985,022	4.165**	G	A	15.20	38.89	0.37	−0.19	
Gm03	45,031,929	5.127***	T	C	15.77	38.89	0.38	−0.19	x
Gm03	45,038,912	3.684**	C	T	14.71	39.26	0.36	−0.18	
Gm03	45,107,141	3.905**	C	A	13.87	45.56	0.35	−0.17	
Gm03	45,343,317	3.689**	G	T	17.28	42.59	0.39	−0.19	
Gm03	45,343,612	4.231**	A	T	18.85	41.48	0.41	−0.20	
Gm05	8,817,714	3.912**	G	A	10.81	49.26	0.30	0.15	
Gm05	8,823,135	4.617***	G	A	11.43	49.63	0.31	0.16	
Gm05	8,877,264	3.855**	G	T	8.30	45.93	0.27	0.13	x
Gm05	17,397,118	3.704**	G	A	0.08	39.63	0.03	0.01	
Gm05	17,397,130	3.704**	T	C	0.08	39.63	0.03	0.01	
Gm05	17,397,135	3.704**	C	T	0.08	39.63	0.03	0.01	
Gm07	6,397,319	3.961**	C	T	8.80	25.56	0.32	−0.16	x
Gm07	6,405,421	3.961**	T	C	8.80	25.56	0.32	−0.16	
Gm07	6,540,541	4.128**	G	A	8.10	26.30	0.30	−0.15	
Gm07	6,575,306	3.961**	A	G	8.80	25.56	0.32	−0.16	
Gm11	530,116	4.401***	A	G	4.73	8.89	0.35	0.18	x
Gm11	530,117	4.401***	A	C	4.73	8.89	0.35	0.18	
Gm11	530,118	4.401***	G	T	4.73	8.89	0.35	0.18	
Gm12	20,406,669	3.697**	T	C	0.02	20.74	0.01	0.01	
Gm15	21,422,057	4.152**	A	G	2.10	20.37	0.17	0.08	
Gm16	27,300,116	3.779**	T	G	4.80	8.52	0.36	0.18	x
Gm17	25,859,992	4.322**	T	C	0.66	6.67	0.15	0.08	x

Table 1. Cont.

Chromosome	Position	-log10 (p-value)	Reference Allele	Variant Allele	R^2§	MAF§§	Mean Difference	Additive Effect (Variant allele)	Included in stepwise regression§§§
Gm17	25,859,995	4.322**	T	C	0.66	6.67	0.15	0.08	
Gm18	15,905,372	3.781**	T	C	3.25	28.52	0.18	0.09	
Gm18	28,141,888	3.786**	G	A	3.78	22.59	0.22	0.11	x
Gm18	59,284,729	4.006**	C	T	0.70	45.93	0.08	0.04	
Gm19	34,914,546	3.769**	A	G	0.81	5.19	0.19	0.09	
Gm19	40,193,564	3.955**	C	A	15.62	44.07	0.37	−0.18	x

***Significant at 0.01 percentile (4.0E-05).
**Significant at 0.1 percentile (2.1E-04).
§R^2– Calculated using a simple linear regression and is represented as percentage.
§§MAF = Minor Allele Frequency.
§§§The markers that have an 'X' are included in stepwise regression. All other significant markers are in LD with one of these eight markers. This is the subset of markers around which QTLs were identified, and allelic combinations that have applications for MAS are characterized.

Iron is a structural component of many important processes in plants, and multiple physiological steps are used by strategy-I plants, such as soybean, to manage plant growth and development in iron-deficient conditions [56]. Protons release results in the acidification of the rhizosphere which increases the solubility of iron. Ferric iron is reduced at the root surface, and ferrous iron uptake increases [57–59]. Here we discovered multiple genes located in major QTL associated with these major activities.

AHA11 (Gm05) is an abundant protein found in the seedlings and leaves [60] and limits the transport of iron to leaves resulting in chlorotic plants. Ferric-chelate reductase oxidase (FRO2; Gm07) is expressed in the epidermal cells of Fe-deficient roots and is one of the main Fe (III) chelate reductase proteins. It reduces iron at the cell surface before transport into roots [61]. FRO2 also interacts with IRT1 under Fe sufficiency conditions to increase iron uptake [62,63]. FRE1 (Gm03) increases reductase activity and tolerance to high pH in calcareous soils [47,48]. Based on transgenic lines in *Oryza*, Ishimaru et al. [47,48] suggested that this gene is regulated by the IRT1 since transgenic lines have a higher level of Fe uptake and enhanced tolerance to low Fe availability in both hydroponic culture and calcareous soils.

Ferric chelate reductase defective (FRD4; Gm07) is a gene that acts post-translationally and reduces Fe (III) chelate reductase activity in response to iron deficiency [56]. In addition, *frd4* mutants are chlorotic, grow more slowly, have smaller chloroplasts, and possess fewer thylakoid membranes and grana stacks. Map-based cloning revealed that this gene encodes a component that is responsible for the insertion of proteins into the thylakoid membranes of the chloroplast [56]. Ferredoxin NADP reductase 1 (FNR1; Gm16) is an enzyme that catalyzes reversible electron transfer in photosynthetic electron transport. In iron stress conditions, its activity is decreased resulting in reduced chlorophyll biosynthesis [64].

Nicotianamine (NA) is an iron chelator involved in iron (Fe) acquisition, transport, and homeostasis [65,66], and NA is synthesized by nicotianamine synthase that is encoded by *NAS3* (Gm03) gene. Overexpression of NAS genes in rice increased Fe and Zn uptake by at least twofold [67,68]. Nicotianamine synthase genes are induced by nitrate levels [69,70]. Ammonium and nitrate transporters (Gm03) increase the uptake of nitrate from rhizosphere and increase the concentration of nitrate in plants and lead to increased growth and extension of roots [71,72]. In addition, nitrates enhance H+ extrusion and acidify the rhizosphere leading to increased bioavailability of Fe [71–75].

Several transporters such as RAN1 (Gm05), OPT5 (Gm19), and HMA (Gm19) are in the significant QTL regions. RAN1 is involved in copper trafficking and iron transport [76]. OPT5, an oligopeptide transporter is highly expressed in multiple organs of adult plants [77], and HMA sequesters Cd, Zn, and Ni in vacuoles under Fe deficiency to maintain metal balance and to detoxify heavy metals [78–80].

Argonaute (AGO) like proteins are down-regulated under conditions of low Fe and phosphorus [81]. Vaucheret [82] suggested that these genes have functions in both development and stress response by regulating gene expression at various levels and has additional functions including chromatin remodeling, DNA methylation, translational repression, and RNA cleavage. One such *AGO* gene, *AGO10* (Gm05) is in a major QTL.

Disease resistant genes (R genes) are distributed throughout the *G.max* genome and are a key component of gene interactions between plants and pathogens [83]. We identified multiple R genes in IDC QTL regions. Iron is an important element for all living organisms and pathogens and hosts actively compete for available metals. Plants need metals for defensive generation of

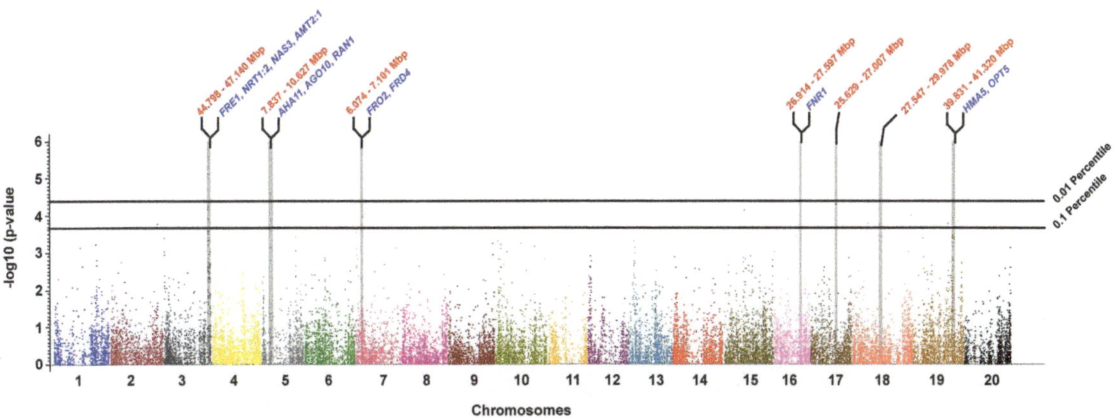

Figure 5. Manhattan plots with significant QTL that are associated with IDC. Chromosomes (1–20) ordered on x-axis and each chromosome is represented by a different color. The $-\log_{10}$(p-value) is presented on the y-axis. The cutoff horizontal lines indicate 0.01 and 0.1 percentile tails of the empirical distribution obtained using 10,000 bootstraps. Vertical grey blocks indicate QTL regions that have major effect on IDC trait identified by stepwise regression. The boundaries of the QTL region (based on the position of markers) and significant candidate genes are represented on the top of QTL.

reactive oxygen species (ROS) and other plant defenses that limit pathogen growth whereas pathogens use low-metal conditions as a signal to recognize and respond to the host environment [84]. Pathogens have developed sophisticated strategies to acquire metal during plant growth that include production of multiple siderophores. Chen et al. [85] studied the interaction IDC and soybean cyst nematode (SCN) resistance and discovered SCN susceptible varieties had higher IDC rating. Since there exists a significant interaction between diseases and IDC, selecting for disease resistance may improve IDC tolerance.

For many traits, estimating epistatic interactions in plants [86,87] has been restricted to bi-parental populations [50,88–90]. For the population, FRO2, a proton with reductase activity interacts with Cytochrome P450 like proteins. Cytochrome P450

Table 2. Significant QTL regions associated with IDC that have Candidate iron genes.

Gene Model*	Chrom	Start	End	Gene symbol*	Annotation*	Function
Gm03: 44.798–47.140						
Glyma03g38620	Gm03	44,925,730	44,930,360	FRE1	Phytochrome A	Increased reductase activity and better tolerance in high pH soils [47–48].
Glyma03g38640	Gm03	44,943,759	44,948,193	NRT1:2	Nitrate Transporter 1:2	Increase concentration of nitrate in plants and lead to increased growth and root extension [71–72].
Glyma03g39050	Gm03	45,279,743	45,281,178	NAS3	Nicotianamine Synthase 3	Synthesis of iron chelator, nicotiamine [67–68].
Glyma03g40700	Gm03	46,372,699	46,374,428	AMT2;1	Ammonium Transporter 2	Increase concentration of nitrate in plants and lead to increased growth and root extension [71–72].
Gm05: 7.837–10.627						
Glyma05g01460	Gm05	960,779	967,307	AHA11	H(+)-ATPase 11	Limits transport of iron in plants [60].
Glyma05g08170	Gm05	8,130,422	8,137,850	AGO10	Stabilizer of iron transporter SufD/Polynucleotidyl transferase	Stress response [82].
Glyma05g08260	Gm05	8,219,986	8,222,377	RAN1	RAS-related nuclear protein-1	Involved in iron transport [76].
Gm07: 6.074–7.101						
Glyma07g07380	Gm07	6,059,979	6,064,461	FRO2	Ferric reduction oxidase 2	Reduce iron at cell surface before transport [61]
Glyma07g08240	Gm07	6,837,072	6,844,618	FRD4	Signal recognition particle receptor protein, chloroplast (FTSY)	Reduces iron in response to iron deficiency [56].
Gm16: 26.914–27.597						
Glyma16g23710	Gm16	27,560,086	27,563,676	FNR1	Ferrodoxin NADP (+) oxidoreductase 1	Decreased chlorophyll biosynthesis [64].
Gm19: 39.831–41.320						
Glyma19g32190	Gm19	39,950,268	39,955,547	HMA5	Heavy Metal Atpase 5	Maintain metal balance under Fe deficiency [78–80].
Glyma19g32401	Gm19	40,141,923	40,144,157	OPT5	Oligopeptide transporter 5	Oligopeptide transporter [77].

*Gene Model, gene symbol and annotation obtained from phytozome (www.phytozome.net/soybean, V8.0).

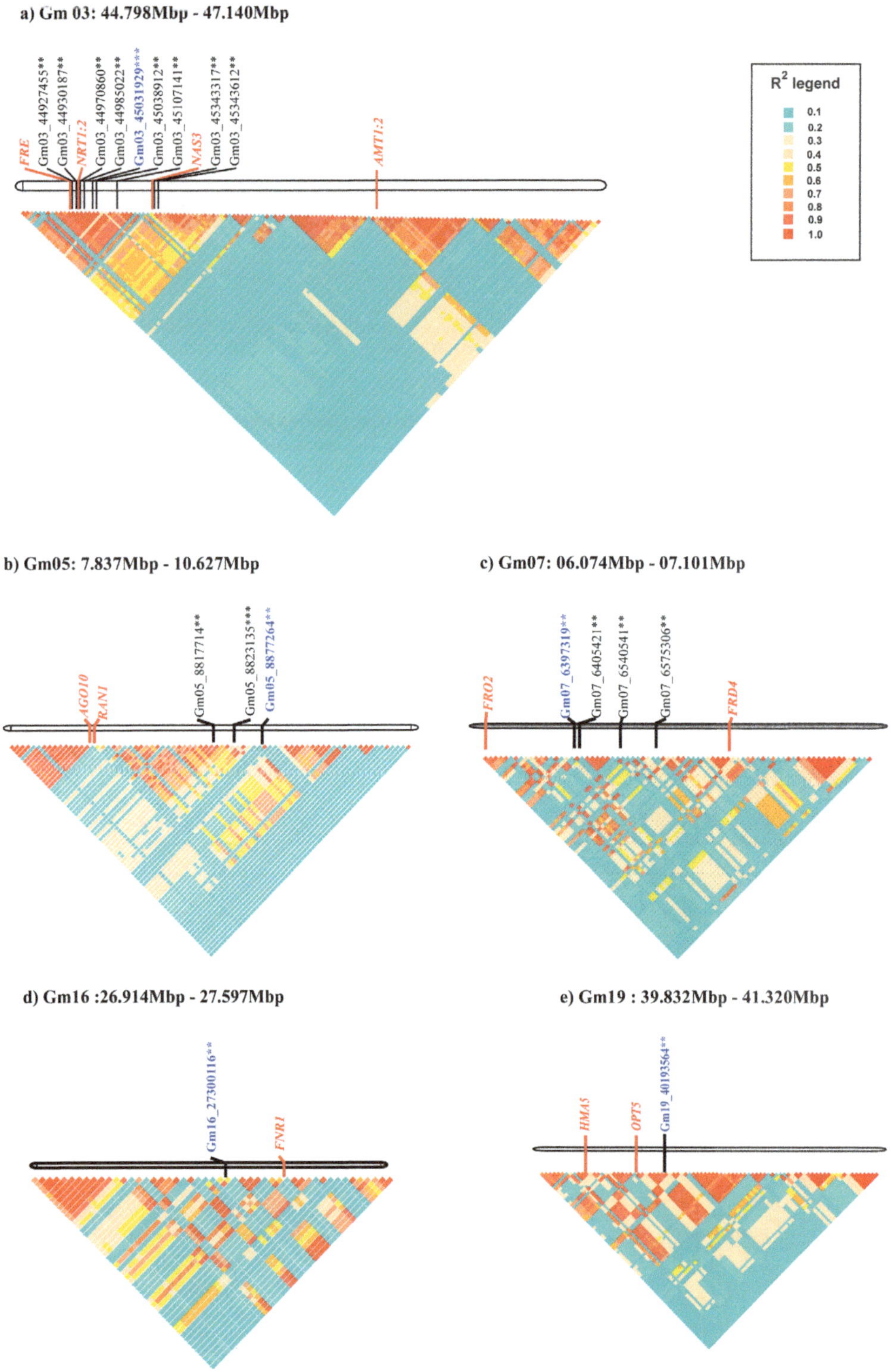

Figure 6. Heatmap of major QTL regions. QTL that has known candidate gene are only represented. Only significant markers at the 0.1 percentile bootstrapped empirical distribution were included in the figure. Significance of the markers is indicated as *** if fall in the 0.01 percentile tail and ** if fall in the 0.1 percentile tail of the bootstrapped empirical distribution. The stepwise included markers are marked in blue. r^2 values are represented in different colors. Marker pairs with r^2 values>0.6 are considered to be in linkage disequilibrium. a) is the QTL on Gm03 (44.798 Mbp–47.140 Mbp), b) is the QTL on Gm05 (7.837 Mbp–10.627 Mbp), c) is the QTL on Gm07 (6.074 Mbp–7.101 Mbp), d) is the QTL on Gm16 (26.914 Mbp–27.597 Mbp) and e) is QTL region on Gm19 (39.832 Mbp–41.320 Mbp).

proteins accumulate in response to iron deficiency [91]. If iron uptake is limited by the function of FRO2, it would lead to iron deficiency and limit AUX1 and initiate cytochrome P450 activities. Similar to Cytochrome P450 proteins, activity of FNR is reduced under iron deficient conditions [64]. AUX1 is a gene that is involved in auxin transport, a plant hormone that

Table 3. Allelic combinations and IDC means for the allele combinations that have a mean<2.5 (Tolerant) and>3.5 (Susceptible).

Allelic combination[§]	# of genotypes	IDC			
		Minimum	Maximum	Mean	Standard Deviation
CTTATTGA	3	1.63	2.23	1.88	0.31
TGTATTGA	7	1.46	2.58	2.17	0.37
CGTAGTGA	2	2.18	2.34	2.26	0.11
CTTATTGC	6	1.96	2.86	2.29	0.33
TTTATTGA	11	1.95	3.25	2.32	0.40
CGCATTGA	9	2.08	2.83	2.38	0.26
CTCGTTAA	1	2.4	2.4	2.40	
CTTATTAA	2	2.16	2.66	2.41	0.35
CTCATTGA	26	1.8	3.01	2.41	0.33
CTTGTTGC	2	2.16	2.69	2.43	0.37
CTCATTGC	9	2.11	3.03	2.44	0.33
CGTATTGA	5	2.31	2.57	2.47	0.13
CTTATCGC	2	2.42	2.52	2.47	0.07
CGTATTGC	1	2.5	2.5	2.50	
TTCGTTAC	1	3.56	3.56	3.56	
TTCAGTAC	1	3.58	3.58	3.58	
TGCAGCGC	1	3.68	3.68	3.68	
TGCGTTGC	1	3.7	3.7	3.70	
TGCGTTAA	1	3.72	3.72	3.72	
TGCGTTAC	1	3.79	3.79	3.79	

[§]The order of the markers for the allelic combination are Gm03_45031929, Gm05_8877264, Gm07_6397319, Gm11_530116, Gm16_27300116, Gm17_25859992, Gm18_28141888, and Gm19_40193564.

accumulates in Fe-deficient Arabidopsis roots and acts upstream of nitric oxide [92]. FER4 is a gene responsible for cellular iron homeostasis and subcellular iron trafficking [93]. CCC is a transporter molecule that transports iron [94]. If the activity of the transporter is reduced, auxin accumulates more and the activity of FER4 is reduced.

Evaluating allelic combinations of markers can define appropriate groups of markers for MAS. It is well understood, that there is no single universal marker that is significant in all populations. This is because of the altered effect of the genes and the QTL. It is the combination of these markers that have a significant difference on the phenotype. Of the many allelic combinations possible for multiple SNP (2^n, where n is the number of biallelic markers), only a few of them represent the extremes of phenotype. We provide allelic combination details for the extreme phenotypes for the significant markers that are included in the stepwise regression.

Conclusion

We used a high density GBS data set with a large plant GWAS population to map genes/QTL involved in IDC of soybean. Stepwise regression was used to select a subset of markers that have a major effect on IDC. We identified several significant QTL and candidate iron genes confirming the polygenic nature of the trait. Among these, a non-synonymous substitution identifies FRE1 as a candidate gene. Stepwise regression was effective for selecting the subset of markers that have major effect. This subset of markers can further be used for validation and testing in other populations. A high throughput study on expression differences of genes and the variants responsible for these differences would further help breeders identify varieties tolerant to IDC.

Supporting Information

Figure S1 Genome-wide linkage disequilibrium (LD) decay plot for the population. Linkage disequilibrium, measured as partial R^2, between pairs of polymorphic marker loci (intra-chromosomal comparisons) is plotted against the physical distance (Mbp).

Table S1 Detailed information of SNPs used in the study. SNP postions, alleles based on soybean reference genome V1.1 (phytozome.org) and minor allele frequency for this population (in %).

Author Contributions

Conceived and designed the experiments: PEM. Performed the experiments: SM RKL JRG. Analyzed the data: SM. Contributed reagents/materials/analysis tools: SM RKL JRG. Contributed to the writing of the manuscript: SM PEM.

References

1. Pil JS, Jungmin P, Mi-Jeong P, Youn-Sung K, Sang-Gyu K, et al. (2012) A Golgi-localized MATE transporter mediates iron homoeostasis under osmotic stress in Arabidopsis. Biochemical Journal 442: 551–561.
2. Kobayashi T, Nishizawa NK (2012) Iron uptake, translocation, and regulation in higher plants. Annual Review of Plant Biology 63: 131–152.
3. Briat J-F, Curie C, Gaymard F (2007) Iron utilization and metabolism in plants. Current Opinion in Plant Biology 10: 276–282.
4. Franzen DW, Richardson JL (2000) Soil factors affecting iron chlorosis of soybean in the Red River Valley of North Dakota and Minnesota. Journal of Plant Nutrition 23: 67–78.
5. Peiffer GA, King KE, Severin AJ, May GD, Cianzio SR, et al. (2012) Identification of candidate genes underlying an iron efficiency quantitative trait locus in soybean. Plant Physiology 158: 1745–1754.
6. Marschner H, Romheld V, Kissel M (1986) Different strategies in higher plants in mobilization and uptake of iron. Journal of Plant Nutrition 9: 695–713.
7. Schmidt W (1999) Mechanisms and regulation of reduction-based iron uptake in plants. New Phytologist 141: 1–26.
8. Barker AV, Pilbeam DJ (2010) Handbook of plant nutrition. CRC press.
9. Mamidi S, Chikara S, Goos RJ, Hyten DL, Annam D, et al. (2011) Genome-wide association analysis identifies candidate genes associated with iron deficiency chlorosis in soybean. The Plant Genome 4: 154–164.
10. Curie C, Briat J-F (2003) Iron transport and signaling in plants. Annual Review of Plant Biology 54: 183–206.
11. Diers BW, Cianzio SR, Shoemaker RC (1992) Possible identification of quantitative trait loci affecting iron efficiency in soybean. Journal of Plant Nutrition 15: 2127–2136.
12. King KE, Peiffer GA, Reddy M, Lauter N, Lin SF, et al. (2013) Mapping of Iron and Zinc Quantitative Trait Loci in Soybean for Association to Iron Deficiency Chlorosis Resistance. Journal of Plant Nutrition 36: 2132–2153.
13. O'Rourke J, Charlson D, Gonzalez D, Vodkin L, Graham M, et al. (2007) Microarray analysis of iron deficiency chlorosis in near-isogenic soybean lines. BMC Genomics 8: 476.
14. Severin AJ, Peiffer GA, Xu WW, Hyten DL, Bucciarelli B, et al. (2010) An integrative approach to genomic introgression mapping. Plant Physiology 154: 3–12.
15. Stec AO, Bhaskar PB, Bolon Y-T, Nolan R, Shoemaker RC, et al. (2013) Genomic heterogeneity and structural variation in soybean near isogenic lines. Frontiers in Plant Science 4: 104.
16. Myles S, Peiffer J, Brown PJ, Ersoz ES, Zhang Z, et al. (2009) Association mapping: critical considerations shift from genotyping to experimental design. The Plant Cell Online 21: 2194–2202.
17. Wang J, McClean PE, Lee R, Goos RJ, Helms T (2008) Association mapping of iron deficiency chlorosis loci in soybean (*Glycine max* L. Merr.) advanced breeding lines. Theoretical and Applied Genetics 116: 777–787.
18. Elshire RJ, Glaubitz JC, Sun Q, Poland JA, Kawamoto K, et al. (2011) A robust, simple genotyping-by-sequencing (GBS) approach for high diversity species. PloS One 6: e19379.
19. Bradbury PJ, Zhang Z, Kroon DE, Casstevens TM, Ramdoss Y, et al. (2007) TASSEL: software for association mapping of complex traits in diverse samples. Bioinformatics 23: 2633–2635.
20. Schmutz J, Cannon SB, Schlueter J, Ma J, Mitros T, et al. (2010) Genome sequence of the palaeopolyploid soybean. Nature 463: 178–183.
21. Li H, Durbin R (2009) Fast and accurate short read alignment with Burrows Wheeler transform. Bioinformatics 25: 1754–1760.
22. Danecek P, Auton A, Abecasis G, Albers CA, Banks E, et al. (2011) The variant call format and VCFtools. Bioinformatics 27: 2156–2158.
23. Scheet P, Stephens M (2006) A fast and flexible statistical model for large-scale population genotype data: applications to inferring missing genotypes and haplotypic phase. The American Journal of Human Genetics 78: 629–644.
24. Marchini J, Howie B (2010) Genotype imputation for genome-wide association studies. Nature Reviews Genetics 11: 499–511.
25. Mangin B, Siberchicot A, Nicolas S, Doligez A, This P, et al. (2011) Novel measures of linkage disequilibrium that correct the bias due to population structure and relatedness. Heredity 108: 285–291.
26. Long Q, Rabanal FA, Meng D, Huber CD, Farlow A, et al. (2013) Massive genomic variation and strong selection in *Arabidopsis thaliana* lines from Sweden. Nature genetics 45: 884–890.
27. Stram DO (2004) Tag SNP selection for association studies. Genetic Epidemiology 27: 365–374.
28. Remington DL, Thornsberry JM, Matsuoka Y, Wilson LM, Whitt SR, et al. (2001) Structure of linkage disequilibrium and phenotypic associations in the maize genome. Proceedings of the National Academy of Sciences 98: 11479–11484.
29. Pyhäjärvi T, García-Gil MR, Knürr T, Mikkonen M, Wachowiak W, et al. (2007) Demographic history has influenced nucleotide diversity in European *Pinus sylvestris* populations. Genetics 177: 1713–1724.
30. Price AL, Patterson NJ, Plenge RM, Weinblatt ME, Shadick NA, et al. (2006) Principal components analysis corrects for stratification in genome-wide association studies. Nature Genetics 38: 904–909.
31. Zhao K, Aranzana MJ, Kim S, Lister C, Shindo C, et al. (2007) An Arabidopsis example of association mapping in structured samples. PLoS Genetics 3: e4.
32. Zhou X, Stephens M (2012) Genome-wide efficient mixed-model analysis for association studies. Nature Genetics 44: 821–824.
33. Rakitsch B, Lippert C, Stegle O, Borgwardt K (2013) A Lasso multi-marker mixed model for association mapping with population structure correction. Bioinformatics 29: 206–214.
34. Yu J, Pressoir G, Briggs WH, Bi IV, Yamasaki M, et al. (2005) A unified mixed-model method for association mapping that accounts for multiple levels of relatedness. Nature Genetics 38: 203–208.
35. Hall P, Miller H (2010) Bootstrap confidence intervals and hypothesis tests for extrema of parameters. Biometrika 97: 881–892.
36. Li J, Tai BC, Nott DJ (2009) Confidence interval for the bootstrap P-value and sample size calculation of the bootstrap test. Journal of Nonparametric Statistics 21: 649–661.
37. Meyer KB, O'Reilly M, Michailidou K, Carlebur S, Edwards SL, et al. (2013) Fine-scale mapping of the FGFR2 breast cancer risk locus: putative functional variants differentially bind FOXA1 and E2F1. The American Journal of Human Genetics 93: 1046–1060.
38. Cingolani P, Platts A, Coon M, Nguyen T, Wang L, et al. (2012) A program for annotating and predicting the effects of single nucleotide polymorphisms, SnpEff: SNPs in the genome of *Drosophila melanogaster* strain w1118; iso-2; iso-3. Fly 6: 80–92.
39. Davey JW, Hohenlohe PA, Etter PD, Boone JQ, Catchen JM, et al. (2011) Genome-wide genetic marker discovery and genotyping using next-generation sequencing. Nature Reviews Genetics 12: 499–510.
40. Deschamps S, Campbell MA (2010) Utilization of next-generation sequencing platforms in plant genomics and genetic variant discovery. Molecular Breeding 25: 553–570.
41. Ganal MW, Durstewitz G, Polley A, Berard A, Buckler ES, et al. (2011) A large maize (*Zea mays* L.) SNP genotyping array: development and germplasm genotyping, and genetic mapping to compare with the B73 reference genome. PloS One 6: e28334.
42. Mandel JR, Nambeesan S, Bowers JE, Marek LF, Ebert D, et al. (2013) Association Mapping and the Genomic Consequences of Selection in Sunflower. PLoS Genetics 9: e1003378.
43. Gurung S, Mamidi S, Bonman JM, Jackson EW, Del Rio LE, et al. (2011) Identification of novel genomic regions associated with resistance to *Pyrenophora tritici-repentis* races 1 and 5 in spring wheat landraces using association analysis. Theoretical and Applied Genetics 123: 1029–1041.
44. Iqbal MJ, Mamidi S, Ahsan R, Kianian SF, Coyne CJ, et al. (2012) Population structure and linkage disequilibrium in *Lupinus albus* L. germplasm and its implication for association mapping. Theoretical and Applied Genetics 125: 517–530.
45. Patel JS, Mamidi S, Bonman JM, Adhikari TB (2013) Genome-wide Association Analysis in Spring Wheat Accessions Identifies QTL Associated with Resistance to a 2 Novel Isolate of *Pyrenophora tritici-repentis* 3. Crop Science 53: 842–852.
46. Astle W, Balding DJ (2009) Population structure and cryptic relatedness in genetic association studies. Statistical Science 24: 451–471.
47. Ishimaru Y, Kim S, Tsukamoto T, Oki H, Kobayashi T, et al. (2007) Mutational reconstructed ferric chelate reductase confers enhanced tolerance in rice to iron deficiency in calcareous soil. Proceedings of the National Academy of Sciences 104: 7373–7378.
48. Oki H, Kim S, Nakanishi H, Takahashi M, Yamaguchi H, et al. (2004) Directed evolution of yeast ferric reductase to produce plants with tolerance to iron deficiency in alkaline soils. Soil Science and Plant Nutrition 50: 1159–1165.
49. Samuelsen AI, Martin RC, Mok DWS, Mok MC (1998) Expression of the yeast FRE genes in transgenic tobacco. Plant Physiology 118: 51–58.
50. Grillo MA, Li C, Hammond M, Wang L, Schemske DW (2013) Genetic architecture of flowering time differentiation between locally adapted populations of *Arabidopsis thaliana*. New Phytologist 197: 1321–1331.
51. Pineau C, Loubet S, Lefoulon C, Chalies C, Fizames C, et al. (2012) Natural Variation at the FRD3 MATE Transporter Locus Reveals Cross-Talk between Fe Homeostasis and Zn Tolerance in *Arabidopsis thaliana*. PLoS Genetics 8: e1003120.
52. Zhang N, Gur A, Gibon Y, Sulpice R, Flint-Garcia S, et al. (2010) Genetic analysis of central carbon metabolism unveils an amino acid substitution that alters maize NAD-dependent isocitrate dehydrogenase activity. PloS One 5: e9991.
53. Lin S, Cianzio S, Shoemaker R (1997) Mapping genetic loci for iron deficiency chlorosis in soybean. Molecular Breeding 3: 219–229.
54. Lin SF, Grant D, Cianzio S, Shoemaker R (2000) Molecular characterization of iron deficiency chlorosis in soybean. Journal of Plant Nutrition 23: 1929–1939.
55. Lin S-F, Baumer JS, Ivers D, de Cianzo SR, Shoemaker RC (1998) Field and nutrient solution tests measure similar mechanisms controlling iron deficiency chlorosis in soybean. Crop Science 38: 254–259.
56. Durrett TP, Connolly EL, Rogers EE (2006) Arabidopsis cpFtsY mutants exhibit pleiotropic defects including an inability to increase iron deficiencyinducible root Fe (III) chelate reductase activity. The Plant Journal 47: 467–479.
57. Eide D, Broderius M, Fett J, Guerinot ML (1996) A novel iron-regulated metal transporter from plants identified by functional expression in yeast. Proceedings of the National Academy of Sciences 93: 5624–5628.

58. Robinson NJ, Procter CM, Connolly EL, Guerinot ML (1999) A ferric-chelate reductase for iron uptake from soils. Nature 397: 694–697.
59. Vert G, Grotz N, Dédaldéchamp F, Gaymard F, Guerinot ML, et al. (2002) IRT1, an Arabidopsis transporter essential for iron uptake from the soil and for plant growth. The Plant Cell Online 14: 1223–1233.
60. Alsterfjord M, Sehnke PC, Arkell A, Larsson H, Svennelid F, et al. (2004) Plasma membrane H+-ATPase and 14-3-3 isoforms of Arabidopsis leaves: evidence for isoform specificity in the 14-3-3/H+-ATPase interaction. Plant and cell physiology 45: 1202–1210.
61. Kim SA, Guerinot ML (2007) Mining iron: iron uptake and transport in plants. FEBS letters 581: 2273–2280.
62. Connolly EL, Campbell NH, Grotz N, Prichard CL, Guerinot ML (2003) Overexpression of the FRO2 ferric chelate reductase confers tolerance to growth on low iron and uncovers posttranscriptional control. Plant Physiology 133: 1102–1110.
63. Connolly EL, Fett JP, Guerinot ML (2002) Expression of the IRT1 metal transporter is controlled by metals at the levels of transcript and protein accumulation. The Plant Cell Online 14: 1347–1357.
64. Miller GW, Pushnik JC, Welkie GW (1984) Iron chlorosis, a world wide problem, the relation of chlorophyll biosynthesis to iron. Journal of Plant Nutrition 7: 1–22.
65. Pich A, Manteuffel R, Hillmer S, Scholz G, Schmidt W (2001) Fe homeostasis in plant cells: does nicotianamine play multiple roles in the regulation of cytoplasmic Fe concentration? Planta 213: 967–976.
66. von Wiren N, Klair S, Bansal S, Briat J-F, Khodr H, et al. (1999) Nicotianamine chelates both FeIII and FeII. Implications for metal transport in plants. Plant Physiology 119: 1107–1114.
67. Lee S, Jeon US, Lee SJ, Kim Y-K, Persson DP, et al. (2009) Iron fortification of rice seeds through activation of the nicotianamine synthase gene. Proceedings of the National Academy of Sciences 106: 22014–22019.
68. Masuda H, Usuda K, Kobayashi T, Ishimaru Y, Kakei Y, et al. (2009) Overexpression of the barley nicotianamine synthase gene HvNAS1 increases iron and zinc concentrations in rice grains. Rice 2: 155–166.
69. Wang R, Okamoto M, Xing X, Crawford NM (2003) Microarray analysis of the nitrate response in Arabidopsis roots and shoots reveals over 1,000 rapidly responding genes and new linkages to glucose, trehalose-6-phosphate, iron, and sulfate metabolism. Plant Physiology 132: 556–567.
70. Wang Y-H, Garvin DF, Kochian LV (2001) Nitrate-induced genes in tomato roots. Array analysis reveals novel genes that may play a role in nitrogen nutrition. Plant Physiology 127: 345–359.
71. Bai H, Euring D, Volmer K, Janz D, Polle A (2013) The Nitrate Transporter (NRT) Gene Family in Poplar. PloS One 8: e72126.
72. Gu R, Duan F, An X, Zhang F, von Wiren N, et al. (2013) Characterization of AMT-Mediated High-Affinity Ammonium Uptake in Roots of Maize (*Zea mays* L.). Plant and Cell Physiology 54: 1515–1524.
73. Bloom AJ, Meyerhoff PA, Taylor AR, Rost TL (2002) Root development and absorption of ammonium and nitrate from the rhizosphere. Journal of Plant Growth Regulation 21: 416–431.
74. Taylor AR, Bloom AJ (1998) Ammonium, nitrate, and proton fluxes along the maize root. Plant, Cell & Environment 21: 1255–1263.
75. Zou C, Shen J, Zhang F, Guo S, Rengel Z, et al. (2001) Impact of nitrogen form on iron uptake and distribution in maize seedlings in solution culture. Plant and Soil 235: 143–149.
76. Woeste KE, Kieber JJ (2000) A strong loss-of-function mutation in RAN1 results in constitutive activation of the ethylene response pathway as well as a rosette-lethal phenotype. The Plant Cell Online 12: 443–455.
77. Stacey MG, Osawa H, Patel A, Gassmann W, Stacey G (2006) Expression analyses of Arabidopsis oligopeptide transporters during seed germination, vegetative growth and reproduction. Planta 223: 291–305.
78. Arrivault S, Senger T, Kramer U (2006) The Arabidopsis metal tolerance protein AtMTP3 maintains metal homeostasis by mediating Zn exclusion from the shoot under Fe deficiency and Zn oversupply. The Plant Journal 46: 861–879.
79. Morel M, Crouzet J, Gravot A, Auroy P, Leonhardt N, et al. (2009) AtHMA3, a P1B-ATPase allowing Cd/Zn/Co/Pb vacuolar storage in Arabidopsis. Plant Physiology 149: 894–904.
80. Schaaf G, Honsbein A, Meda AR, Kirchner S, Wipf D, et al. (2006) AtIREG2 encodes a tonoplast transport protein involved in iron-dependent nickel detoxification in *Arabidopsis thaliana* roots. Journal of Biological Chemistry 281: 25532–25540.
81. Zheng L, Huang F, Narsai R, Wu J, Giraud E, et al. (2009) Physiological and transcriptome analysis of iron and phosphorus interaction in rice seedlings. Plant Physiology 151: 262–274.
82. Vaucheret H (2008) Plant argonautes. Trends in Plant Science 13: 350–358.
83. Kang Y, Kim K, Shim S, Yoon M, Sun S, et al. (2012) Genome-wide mapping of NBS-LRR genes and their association with disease resistance in soybean. BMC Plant Biology 12: 139.
84. Fones H, Preston GM (2012) Reactive oxygen and oxidative stress tolerance in plant pathogenic Pseudomonas. FEMS microbiology letters 327: 1–8.
85. Chen S, Kurle JE, Stetina SR, Miller DR, Klossner LD, et al. (2007) Interactions between iron-deficiency chlorosis and soybean cyst nematode in Minnesota soybean fields. Plant and Soil 299: 131–139.
86. Mackay TFC (2014) Epistasis and quantitative traits: using model organisms to study gene-gene interactions. Nature Reviews Genetics 15: 22–33.
87. Shang J, Zhang J, Sun Y, Liu D, Ye D, et al. (2011) Performance analysis of novel methods for detecting epistasis. BMC Bioinformatics 12: 475.
88. Caicedo AL, Stinchcombe JR, Olsen KM, Schmitt J, Purugganan MD (2004) Epistatic interaction between Arabidopsis FRI and FLC flowering time genes generates a latitudinal cline in a life history trait. Proceedings of the National Academy of Sciences 101: 15670–15675.
89. Jiang Z, Han Y, Teng W, Zhang Z, Sun D, et al. (2010) Identification of QTL underlying the filling rate of protein at different developmental stages of soybean seed. Euphytica 175: 227–236.
90. Lin H, Liang Z-W, Sasaki T, Yano M (2003) Fine mapping and characterization of quantitative trait loci Hd4 and Hd5 controlling heading date in rice. Breeding Science 53: 51–59.
91. Colangelo EP, Guerinot ML (2004) The essential basic helix-loop-helix protein FIT1 is required for the iron deficiency response. The Plant Cell Online 16: 3400–3412.
92. Chen WW, Yang JL, Qin C, Jin CW, Mo JH, et al. (2010) Nitric oxide acts downstream of auxin to trigger root ferric-chelate reductase activity in response to iron deficiency in Arabidopsis. Plant Physiology 154: 810–819.
93. Tarantino D, Santo N, Morandini P, Casagrande F, Braun H-P, et al. (2010) AtFer4 ferritin is a determinant of iron homeostasis in *Arabidopsis thaliana* heterotrophic cells. Journal of Plant Physiology 167: 1598–1605.
94. Conte SS, Walker EL (2011) Transporters contributing to iron trafficking in plants. Molecular Plant 4: 464–476.

Vitamin D Insufficiency in Arabs and South Asians Positively Associates with Polymorphisms in GC and CYP2R1 Genes

Naser Elkum[1,5]*, Fadi Alkayal[2], Fiona Noronha[1], Maisa M. Ali[2], Motasem Melhem[2], Monira Al-Arouj[4], Abdullah Bennakhi[4], Kazem Behbehani[1], Osama Alsmadi[2], Jehad Abubaker[3]

1 Department of Biostatistics & Epidemiology, Dasman Diabetes Institute, Kuwait City, Kuwait, **2** Genetics & Genomics Unit, Dasman Diabetes Institute, Kuwait City, Kuwait, **3** Biochemistry & Molecular Biology Unit, Dasman Diabetes Institute, Kuwait City, Kuwait, **4** Clinical Services, Dasman Diabetes Institute, Kuwait City, Kuwait, **5** Clinical Epidemiology, Sidra Medical and Research Centre, Doha, Qatar

Abstract

Background: A number of genetic studies have reported an association between vitamin D related genes such as group-specific component gene (GC), Cytochrome P450, family 2, subfamily R, polypeptide 1 (CYP2R1) and 7-dehydrocholesterol reductase/nicotinamide-adenine dinucleotide synthetase 1 (DHCR7/NADSYN1) and serum levels of the active form of Vitamin D, 25 (OH) D among African Americans, Caucasians, and Chinese. Little is known about how genetic variations associate with, or contribute to, 25(OH)D levels in Arabs populations.

Methods: Allele frequencies of 18 SNPs derived from CYP2R1, GC, and DHCR7/NADSYN1 genes in 1549 individuals (Arabs, South Asians, and Southeast Asians living in Kuwait) were determined using real time genotyping assays. Serum levels of 25(OH)D were measured using chemiluminescence immunoassay.

Results: GC gene polymorphisms (rs17467825, rs3755967, rs2282679, rs7041 and rs2298850) were found to be associated with 25(OH)D serum levels in Arabs and South Asians. Two of the CYP2R1 SNPs (rs10500804 and rs12794714) and one of GC SNPs (rs1155563) were found to be significantly associated with 25(OH)D serum levels only in people of Arab origin. Across all three ethnicities none of the SNPs of DHCR7/NADSYN1 were associated with serum 25(OH)D levels and none of the 18 SNPs were significantly associated with serum 25(OH)D levels in people from South East Asia.

Conclusion: Our data show for the first time significant association between the GC (rs2282679 and rs7041), CYP2R1 (rs10741657) SNPs and 25(OH)D levels. This supports their roles in vitamin D Insufficiency in Arab and South Asian populations respectively. Interestingly, two of the CYP2R1 SNPs (rs10500804 and rs12794714) and one GC SNP (rs1155563) were found to correlate with vitamin D in Arab population exclusively signifying their importance in this population.

Editor: Masaru Katoh, National Cancer Center, Japan

Funding: This work was funded by Kuwait Foundation for the Advancement of Sciences. The funders had no role in study design, data collection and analysis, decision to publish, or preparation of the manuscript.

Competing Interests: The authors have declared that no competing interests exist.

* Email: nelkum@sidra.org

Introduction

Vitamin D deficiency is a common public health problem worldwide. It is associated with many medical outcomes, including osteoporosis [1], type 1 diabetes [2], cardiovascular diseases [3], asthma [4], and cancer [5]. Vitamin D plays a major role in calcium and phosphate homeostasis, both of which are essential in the mineralization of bone, muscle contraction, nerve conduction, and general cellular function in all cells of the body. Its active form, 1,25-dihydroxyvitamin D [1,25(OH)2D], control the expression of a vitamin D-dependent genes that code for calcium-transporting and bone matrix proteins [6]. The best indicator of vitamin D status is the serum concentration of its main circulating metabolite, 25-hydroxyvitamin D [25(OH)D].

Factors that can potentially affect vitamin D status are dietary intake and exposure to ultraviolet-B (UVB) sunlight. Sunlight exposure catalyzes vitamin D photochemical synthesis from a cholesterol-like precursor in the skin, which is by far the most important source of vitamin D [7,8] and therefore limited exposure to sunlight is thought to be a key factor in vitamin D deficiency [9,10]. In Arabian Gulf countries where there is plentiful sunlight throughout the year, vitamin D could be expected to be adequate. Studies in Saudi Arabia and United

Arab Emirates have nevertheless highlighted a high prevalence of vitamin D deficiency in the local populations [10,11].

A study of a multi-ethnic population in the United Arab Emirates (UAE) [11] found serum 25(OH)D levels to be deficient in the overall population but sufficient among the Europeans contingent living in the same environment. Other studies have also reported wide ethnic differences. One study found a vitamin D insufficiency rate in Moroccans of 91% [12]. In the USA, Arab-American women living in southeast Detroit have been found to have dangerously low vitamin D levels [13]. These finding and others suggest potential genetic influences that predispose people of Arab backgrounds to vitamin D deficiency [14,15].

In this study, we look at which genetic variants underlie 25(OH)D status and how single nucleotide polymorphisms (SNPs) in key genes may be influencing vitamin D status. For example, SNPs in enzymes required for the production or secretion of 25(OH)D and 1,25-dihydroxyvitamin D [1,25(OH)D] could influence serum concentrations and polymorphism (e.g. if it results in more or less efficient enzyme, receptor, or binding protein), could either increase or decrease the concentration of 25(OH)D in sera.

Recent genetic studies have associated vitamin D deficiency with several candidate genes including Cytochrome P450, family 2, R, (CYP2R1), the group-specific component gene (GC) and 7-dehydrocholesterol reductase/NAD synthetase 1 (DHCR7/NADSYN1) [16–19]. These genes are involved in cholesterol synthesis (DHCR7/NADSYN1), hydroxylation (CYP2R1), and vitamin D transport (GC). The association between the polymorphisms of these genes and 25(OH)D has been previously studied in populations of European descent [18,20,21], African Americans [22,23], and Chinese [19,24]. Little is known about these associations in Arab populations. This study set out to (a) measure levels of 25(OH)D in Arabs, South Asians, and Southeast Asians; (b) to estimate the allelic frequencies of 18 SNPs from CYP2R1, GC, and DHCR7/NADSYN1 genes; and to investigate the relationship between these genetic polymorphisms and the level of 25(OH)D in Arab and Asian populations. In this study, we report for the first time the significant association between SNPs from GC (rs2282679 and rs7041), CYP2R1 (rs10741657) genes and 25(OH)D levels which clearly support their roles in vitamin D Insufficiency in Arab and South Asian populations. The lack of association between DHCR7/NADSYN1 SNPs and 25(OH)D levels minimize their role in controlling vitamin D levels in all three ethnic groups. Moreover, the fact that two of the CYP2R1 SNPs (rs10500804 and rs12794714) and one GC SNP (rs1155563) were found to associate with Vitamin D levels exclusively in Arabs signify their role in vitamin D insufficiency within this population.

Materials and Methods

Study population

A cross-sectional population-based survey was conducted with a random representative sample of adults (≥18 years) from multi-ethnic origin across the six governorates (strata) of the State of Kuwait. A full description of the study population, design and data collection of this study have outlined previously [25]. Briefly, a stratified random sampling technique was used for the selection of participants from the computerized register of the Public Authority of Civil Information. This survey was carried out between June 2011 and August 2012. The study conformed to the principles outlined in the Declaration of Helsinki and was approved by the Scientific Advisory Council and Ethical Review Committee at the Dasman Diabetes Institute (DDI) IRB # 1– Biomedical. An informed written consent was obtained from all participants before their enrolment in the study.

Measurement of vitamin D levels

Serum 25(OH)D levels were measured by chemiluminescent competitive immunoassay (CLIA) using a DiaSorin LIAISON analyzer (DiaSorin Inc, MN, USA) and following company instruction. In brief, 25 OH Vitamin D was dissociated from its binding protein and bound to a specific antibody on the solid phase. Then the tracer (vitamin D linked to an isoluminol derivative) was added. Next, the unbound material was removed with a wash cycle. Finally, the starter reagents were added to initiate a flash chemiluminescent reaction. The light signal was measured by a photomultiplier as relative light units (RLU) and was inversely proportional to the concentration of 25(OH)D in the samples. The intra-assay coefficients of variations (CVs) were 5.5% and 4.0% at 10 and 25 ng/mL, respectively. The inter-assay CVs were 8% and 6% at 15 and 40 ng/mL, respectively. Body Mass Index (BMI) was calculated, using the standard BMI formula, as body weight (in kilograms) divided by height (in meters) squared. This study was conducted on adult male and female subjects comprising of Normal (BMI = 20–24.9 kg/m^2), overweight (BMI = 25–29.9 kg/m^2) and obese (BMI≥30 kg/m^2) individuals. Other measurements such age, weight, height, gender and ethnicity were also obtained.

DNA collection, SNP selection, and genotyping

Blood samples were taken from consenting participants in accordance with DDI IRB approved consent form in 4 ml tubes containing EDTA anticoagulant. Gentra Puregene kit (Qiagen, Valencia, CA, USA) was used to extract DNA as per manufacturer's protocols. DNA was quantified, with a requirement that the A260/A280 ratio is in the range of 1.8–2.1, using Epoch Microplate Spectrophotometer. DNA stock aliquots were diluted to a concentration of 50 ng/µl and were frozen until needed for use in PCR assays.

We selected three candidate genes containing 18 SNPs (6 SNPs from each gene) that have been shown in previous GWAS reports [17,18] to have an association with vitamin D level, and are known to have a biological impact in vitamin D metabolism. The genes and SNPs included GC (rs17467825, rs2282679, rs3755967, rs2298850, rs7041, rs1155563), CYP2R1 (rs7116978, rs1993116, rs10500804, 4s12794714, rs10741657, rs206793), and DHCR7/NADSYN1 (rs7944926, rs12785878, rs4944957, rs12800438, rs3794060, and rs3829251).

We employed ready-to-use, manufacturer-validated, pre-designed allele discriminating TaqMan single nucleotide polymorphisms (SNP) assays. PCR amplification reactions were each carried out in clear optical 96-well plates on the Applied Biosystems (ABI) 7500 Real Time PCR system. Each reaction was performed in 20 µl volume, containing 20 ng of DNA template, 1X TaqMan pre-designed SNP assay master mix (Applied Biosystems, Carlsbad, CA, United States), and 1X HOT FIREPol EvaGreen qPCR master mix plus containing ROX reference dye (Solis BioDyne, Tartu, Estonia). Amplification cycling reactions were carried out under the following conditions: an initial incubation step at 95°C for 10 minutes followed by 35 cycles at 95°C for 1 minute, 58°C for 45 seconds, and 72°C for 45 seconds, then a final incubation step at 72°C for 7 minutes. An endpoint "plate read" was then performed using the ABI Sequence Detection System (SDS) Software. The Software detects fluorescence released from the bi-allelic TaqMan probes and plots fluorescence (Rn) signals (FAM & VIC) and generates the genotype calls. In every run, two previously validated DNA controls per genotype were included, in addition to two water (no template) negative controls.

Statistical analysis

We compared the baseline characteristics of the participants using analysis of variance tests (ANOVA) for continuous variables. Categorical variables were analyzed using the chi-square test. Mean serum 25(OH)D values were estimated within each group of homozygous referent (HR), heterozygous (HET), and homozygous variant (HV) genotypes for each SNP. The serum 25(OH)D levels were adjusted by age, gender and BMI using analysis of covariance (ANCOVA) approach. A *P*-value<0.05 was considered to be statistically significant. All analyses were performed using SAS (version 9.2; SAS Institute, Cary, NC). Genotype frequencies were determined according to the Hardy-Weinberg equilibrium (HWE).

Results

Clinical and biochemical characteristics of the participants

The study population (1549 in total) comprised subjects mainly of Arab and Asian background; 907 Arabs, 489 South Asians and 153 Southeast Asians. The descriptive characteristics of all participants are summarized in Table 1. There were substantial ethnic differences in BMI, age, and gender (p<0.0001); Arabs had a significantly higher mean BMI and tended to be older than Asians. Southeast Asians had higher mean levels of 25(OH)D compared to Arabs and South Asians.

Distribution of allele frequencies in different populations

Significant differences were found in the allele frequencies across all three study populations. The distribution of minor alleles frequencies of each SNP in the Arab, South Asia, and Southeast Asia populations are shown in Figure 1. Minor alleles (frequency below 0.20) were less common in the Arab population (5.3%) than in the South Asian (31.6%) and Southeast Asian (26.4%) populations. Hardy-Weinberg equilibrium (HWE) was not met for some SNPs across all three-populations (P<0.05). Three CYP2R1 SNPs in the Arab population and four GC SNPs in the Southeast Asian population had HWE<0.05 (Table 2).

Association between genotypes and 25(OH) D serum concentrations

SNP genotype and mean serum 25(OH)D levels categorized by genotype are presented in Table 3. Only two CYP2R1 SNPs (rs10500804 and rs12794714) in Arab and one SNP (rs10741657) in South Asian populations were positively associated with vitamin D. No association was observed between the CYP2R1 gene and vitamin D in the South East Asian population. As for the GC gene, all the SNPs were significantly associated with serum 25(OH)D levels in the Arab population but not in the South East Asia population. In South Asian group, five SNPs in GC the gene (rs17467825, rs2282679, rs3755967, rs2298850, and rs7041) were significantly associated with vitamin D levels. SNPs in DHCR7/NADSYN1 gene showed no significant association with serum 25(OH)D in any of the three study populations. Table S1 shows unadjusted analysis of the association between genotypes and 25(OH)D serum levels.

Discussion

We conducted this research because different studies have recently shown ethnic differences in the allele frequency of "vitamin D associated SNPs" [22,26,27], but little information is available about the frequency of vitamin D SNPs in Arab and Asian populations. Our data show that the minor allele frequency (MAF<0.20) was higher in Asian populations (South Asians 31.6% and South East Asians 26.3%) compared to Arabs (5.3%); this can be attributed to an ascertainment bias as the SNPs examined were from studies representing European and African ethnicities. In the GC gene, MAFs for South Asians were significantly higher (P<0.05) than Arabs and South East Asians (Figure 1), whereas South East Asians have the lowest frequencies among all the SNPs. The Arab population has shown distinctive significant differences in the allele frequency of the NADSYN1/DHCR7 gene compared to other ethnic groups. Arabs showed the highest MAF among all the SNPs of the NADSYN1/DHCR7

Table 1. Characteristics of participants by ethnicity.

Factors	Ethnicities			*P-value* trend
	Arabs	South-East Asia	South Asia	
	n (%)	n (%)	n (%)	
Age (years)				
20–39	316 (20.3)	90 (5.8)	186 (11.9)	<0.0001
40–60	497 (31.9)	59 (3.8)	276 (17.8)	<0.0001
>60	98 (6.3)	5 (0.32)	28 (1.8)	<0.0001
Gender				
Female	270 (17.4)	104 (6.7)	104 (6.7)	<0.0001
Male	641 (41.2)	50 (3.2)	386 (24.8)	<0.0001
BMI				
Normal (18.5–24.9)	107 (6.9)	62 (3.9)	143 (9.2)	<0.0001
Overweight (25–29.9)	296 (19.0)	65 (4.2)	225 (14.5)	<0.0001
Obese (≥30)	508 (32.7)	27 (1.7)	122 (7.9)	<0.0001
*25 OHD (ng/l)	13.5±0.34	17.8±0.82	13.3±0.46	<0.0001

BMI, body mass index; *Data are presented as mean ± SD.

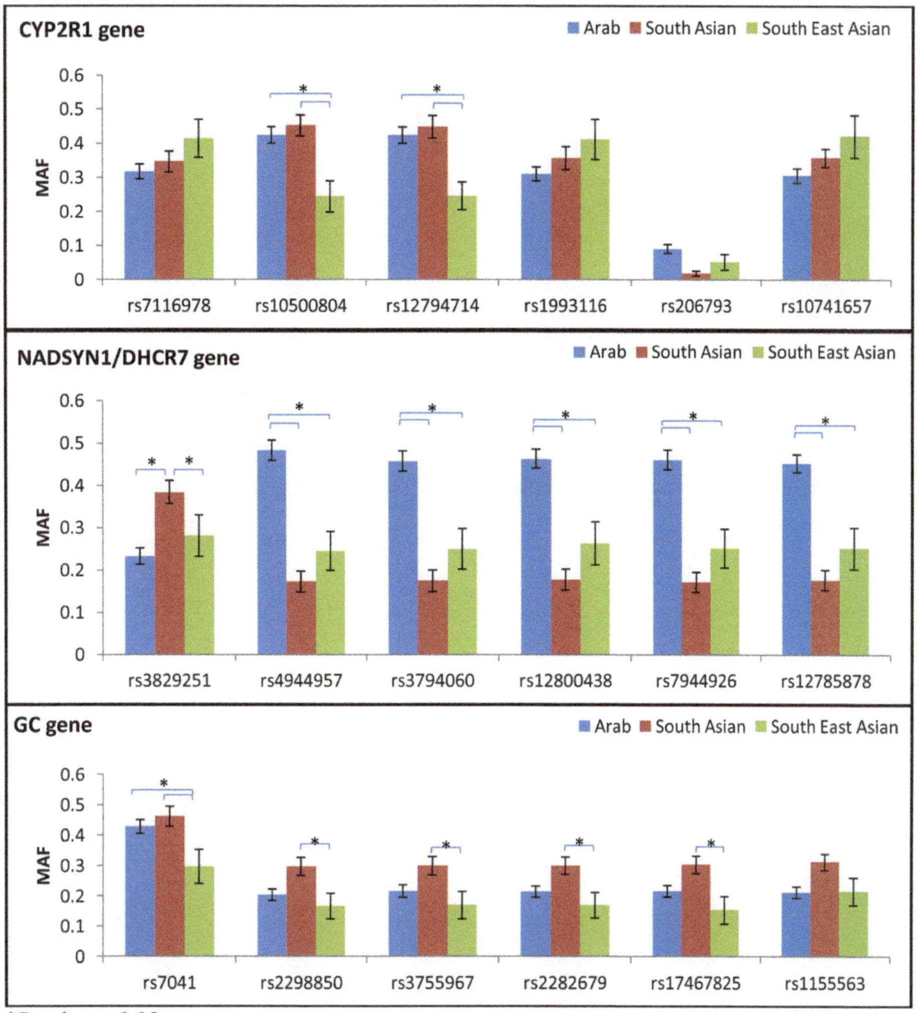

**P-value < 0.05.*

Figure 1. Minor Allele Frequency of SNPs from CYP2R1, DHCR7 & GC genes between Arabs, South Asian and South East Asian ethnicities. The standard deviation was estimated using the.

gene; only the rs3829251 SNP demonstrated higher frequencies in South Asians. Furthermore, analyses showed no significant differences in MAFs between Arab and South Asians populations across the CYP2R1 SNPs (rs206793 was an exception). These differences in allele frequencies are of significant importance in the design of association studies and selecting candidate vitamin D SNPs to investigate.

We were also interested in exploring the relationships between SNPs from the key Vitamin D genes (GC, CYP2R1 and DHCR7/NADSYN1) and 25(OH)D levels. The GC and CYP2R1 genes were found to be significantly associated with 25(OH)D levels. The GC gene encodes the vitamin D binding protein (DBP) that is the key transporter of vitamin D and its metabolites (including 25(OH)D and 1,25(OH)$_2$D) in the circulation [28]. Recent studies have reported an association between SNPs in this gene and 25(OH)D concentrations [22,23,29,30]. Furthermore, other recent studies involving African Americans and Europeans have reported a significant association between SNP rs2282679 of the GC gene and vitamin D insufficiency [17,23]. It is notable that we found a strong association between SNP rs2282679 and 25(OH)D in Arabs and South Asians but not in South East Asians. Similar to the aforementioned studies on different ethnicities [24], rs7041 polymorphism was also associated with 25(OH)D in Arab and South Asian populations, but this was not the case with South East Asians. We also observed that polymorphisms rs17467825, rs3755967, and rs2298850 in the GC gene were associated with serum 25(OH)D levels in Arab and South Asian populations. Interestingly, rs1155563 SNP associated significantly with vitamin D level in Arabs, which suggests a possible involvement in Vitamin D secretion and transportation in this group. A previous study has found that the SNP rs1155563 was associated with vitamin D levels in men of non-Hispanic white background [30]. The significant associations between these GC SNPs and 25(OH)D levels further support the importance of the GC gene in Vitamin D insufficiency.

CYP2R1 is a microsomal vitamin D hydroxylase that hydroxylates vitamin D at the 25-C position for 25(OH)D synthesis (calcidiol) in the liver [31]. Subsequently, calcidiol is converted to calcitriol, the active form of vitamin D3 that binds to the vitamin D receptor (VDR) which arbitrates the majority of vitamin D physiological actions. Previous research has shown the gene CYP2R1 to be associated with several vitamin D related diseases such as type 1 diabetes [21], and in this study we found that rs10741657 SNP, which is a coding SNP that can change the

Table 2. Allele frequencies of 18 Vitamin D associated SNPs by ethnicity.

Gene & SNP	Region	Allele	MAF		Arab n = 907			South Asian n = 489			South East Asian n = 153		
			All[a]	All[b]	MAF	HET	HWE	MAF	HET	HWE	MAF	HET	HWE
CYP2R1													
rs7116978	Ch 11	C/T	0.36	0.33	0.32	0.40	**0.0268**	0.35	0.43	0.2123	0.42	0.44	0.2248
rs10500804	Ch 11	T/G	0.43	0.42	0.42	0.45	**0.0164**	0.45	0.49	0.7610	0.24	0.39	0.6027
rs12794714	Ch 11	G/A	0.43	0.42	0.42	0.45	**0.0169**	0.45	0.48	0.5556	0.25	0.39	0.5849
rs1993116	Ch 11	G/A	0.40	0.33	0.31	0.42	0.6667	0.36	0.44	0.2498	0.41	0.44	0.3073
rs206793	Ch 11	T/C	0.40	0.07	0.09	0.16	0.0710	0.02	0.04	0.6613	0.05	0.10	0.4950
rs10741657	Ch 11	G/A	0.40	0.33	0.31	0.42	0.5537	0.36	0.43	0.1540	0.42	0.44	0.2067
DHCR7/NADSYN1													
rs3829251	Ch 11	G/A	0.24	0.28	0.23	0.36	0.9608	0.38	0.47	0.3126	0.28	0.41	0.9729
rs4944957	Ch 11	A/G	0.23	0.37	0.48	0.49	0.6672	0.17	0.40	0.4225	0.24	0.37	0.9334
rs3794060	Ch 11	C/T	0.23	0.35	0.46	0.49	0.6768	0.18	0.39	0.1186	0.25	0.38	0.8288
rs12800438	Ch 11	G/A	0.23	0.36	0.46	0.49	0.6117	0.18	0.39	0.1430	0.26	0.37	0.5376
rs7944926	Ch 11	A/G	0.23	0.35	0.46	0.49	0.6534	0.17	0.40	0.2068	0.25	0.39	0.7677
rs12785878	Ch 11	G/T	0.23	0.35	0.45	0.49	0.5725	0.18	0.42	0.5105	0.25	0.40	0.4687
GC													
rs7041	Ch 4	**C**/A	0.44	0.47	0.43	0.47	0.1302	0.46	0.47	0.3126	0.30	0.39	0.3394
rs2298850	Ch 4	G/C	0.28	0.23	0.20	0.32	0.6739	0.30	0.40	0.4225	0.17	0.20	**0.0008**
rs3755967	Ch 4	C/T	0.29	0.24	0.22	0.33	0.4866	0.30	0.39	0.1186	0.17	0.21	**0.0014**
rs2282679	Ch 4	T/G	0.29	0.24	0.21	0.33	0.6582	0.30	0.39	0.1430	0.17	0.21	**0.0014**
rs17467825	Ch 4	A/G	0.29	0.24	0.22	0.33	0.6172	0.30	0.40	0.2068	0.15	0.19	**0.0008**
RS1155563	Ch 4	T/C	0.30	0.25	0.21	0.32	0.2397	0.31	0.42	0.5105	0.22	0.31	0.3683

Allele major allele/minor allele; MAF minor allele frequency; HET heterozygosity; HWE *P*-values for Hardy-Weinberg Equilibrium test.
Bold numbers represent significant *P*-values.
[a]Based on GWAS by Wang, et al. 2010;
[b]based on our study.

Table 3. Single nucleotide polymorphisms in GC, CYP2R1, DHCR7/NADSYN1, and their association with serum 25(OH)D among Arabs, South Asian, Southeast Asian participants.

Gene & SNP	Region	HR, HET, HV	Arab n = 907 25(OH)D concentrations				South Asian n = 489 25(OH)D concentrations				South East Asian n = 153 25(OH)D concentrations			
			HR	HET	HV	*P*-values	HR	HET	HV	*P*-values	HR	HET	HV	*P*-values
CYP2R1														
rs7116978	Ch 11	CC, CT, TT	13.5	14.2	14.4	0.5747	13.7	14.4	16.2	0.1068	16.7	18.3	16.1	0.3397
rs1993116	Ch 11	GG, AG, AA	13.3	14.5	14.1	0.2736	13.4	14.6	16.2	0.0555	17.1	17.7	16.8	0.8459
rs10500804	Ch 11	TT, TG, GG	14.4	14.3	12.0	**0.0379**	14.5	14.7	13.3	0.3770	17.8	16.7	16.4	0.6780
rs12794714	Ch 11	GG, AG, AA	14.4	14.3	12.0	**0.0402**	14.5	14.8	13.1	0.2790	17.8	16.7	16.4	0.7009
rs10741657	Ch 11	GG, AG, AA	13.3	14.5	14.1	0.2873	13.4	14.6	16.2	**0.0437**	16.9	17.9	16.7	0.7224
rs206793	Ch 11	TT, CT, CC	13.9	13.7	9.6	0.3804	14.3	13.8	-	0.7915	17.4	16.4	-	0.6456
DHCR7/NADSYN1														
rs7944926	Ch 11	AA, AG, GG	13.2	14.1	14.2	0.5300	13.9	15.5	11.9	0.1096	16.4	18.1	21.9	0.1111
rs12785878	Ch 11	GG, GT, TT	13.2	14.2	14.0	0.5164	14.0	15.4	12.4	0.1660	16.2	18.2	22.2	0.0736
rs4944957	Ch 11	AA, AG, GG	13.0	14.1	14.4	0.3336	14.0	15.5	11.9	0.1234	16.6	17.8	21.9	0.1577
rs12800438	Ch 11	GG, AG, AA	13.3	14.1	14.2	0.6303	14.1	15.2	12.7	0.2761	16.3	18.9	16.0	0.1371
rs3794060	Ch 11	CC, CT, TT	13.3	14.1	14.3	0.5396	14.0	15.5	12.3	0.1364	16.4	18.1	21.9	0.1135
rs3829251	Ch 11	GG, AG, AA	14.4	12.9	14.1	0.1833	13.6	14.9	13.9	0.2599	18.1	16.8	15.0	0.3578
GC														
rs17467825	Ch 4	AA, AG, GG	14.4	13.4	10.3	**0.0165**	15.8	12.9	13.0	**0.0013**	17.7	17.4	12.8	0.2127
rs2282679	Ch 4	TT, GT, GG	14.4	13.3	10.4	**0.0377**	15.8	12.8	13.0	**0.0007**	17.8	17.0	12.8	0.1557
rs3755967	Ch 4	CC, CT, TT	14.4	13.3	10.5	**0.0368**	15.8	12.8	13.0	**0.0007**	17.8	17.0	12.8	0.1557
rs2298850	Ch 4	GG, GC, CC	14.4	13.3	10.3	**0.0374**	15.5	13.2	13.0	**0.0103**	17.9	16.7	13.4	0.2037
rs7041	Ch 4	CC, AC, AA	14.5	14.3	11.7	**0.0110**	15.8	14.4	12.3	**0.0072**	17.3	18.1	16.6	0.5594
rs1155563	Ch 4	TT, TC, CC	14.4	13.3	10.4	**0.0289**	14.8	14.2	12.8	0.3120	18.1	16.2	14.7	0.2541

HR: Homozygous referent, HET: Heterozygous, HV: Homozygous variant. Blue color indicates HV.
P-value for the association between the SNP and 25(OH)D levels from ethnic-stratified ANCOVA models adjusted for sex, age and BMI.

activity of the CYP2R1 enzyme and subsequently cause a relative lack of 25(OH)D, is significantly associate with vitamin D, but only in South Asians [31]. We also found two of the CYP2R1 SNPs (rs10500804 and rs12794714) to associate significantly with Vitamin D level in Arabs signifying their possible roles in vitamin D insufficiency in this population.

Gene DHCR7/NADSYN1 encodes the enzyme 7-dehydrocholesterol (7DHC) reductase, which catalyzes the production of cholesterol from 7 DHC, thereby removing the key substrate necessary for the vitamin D synthesis [18]. Recently, Zhang et al., 2012 have linked some of the DHCR7/NADSYN1 SNPs (rs3829251, rs12785878) to decreased serum 25(OH)D levels in northeastern Han Chinese children [24], while Cooper et al., 2011 has associated rs12785878 T allele carriers with vitamin D deficiency and type 1 diabetes [32]. In contrast, we found that none of the six variant genotypes of DHCR7/NADSYN1 was associated with serum 25(OH)D levels in any of the three population groups that were studied, suggesting minimal involvement of these SNPs or the DHCR7/NADSYN1 gene in mediating vitamin D insufficiency in these populations. However, it is worth noting that in our study the female participant from Arab and South Asian origins were underrepresented which might contribute to the lack of association between DHCR7/NADSYN1 gene and serum 25(OH)D levels. Interestingly, none of the 18 SNPs in this study associated significantly with serum 25(OH)D levels in South East Asians, minimizing the roles of these genes in mediating Vitamin D insufficiency and thus opening the door for the possible involvement of other genes, less common SNPs and/or predisposing factors for Vitamin D insufficiency.

Conclusion

Our study is one of the first to look at genetic determinant of vitamin D levels in Arabs and describes allele frequencies of 18 SNPs localized to three genes related to vitamin D deficiency in Arabs, South Asians and South East Asians. The significant associations between the GC (rs2282679 and rs7041), CYP2R1 (rs10741657) SNPs and 25(OH)D levels clearly support the idea of a role in vitamin D insufficiency in Arab and South Asian populations. The fact that none of the SNPs of the DHCR7/NADSYN1 gene associate with vitamin D levels in the three populations suggests minimized roles in controlling vitamin D release. The finding that GC SNP (rs1155563) and CYP2R1 SNPs (rs10500804 and rs12794714) associated exclusively with vitamin D level in Arabs, suggests the need for further study and possibly sheds light on their mechanism in the context of vitamin D insufficiency. Finally, the lack of association between the selected SNPs and vitamin D levels in South East Asians calls for larger population-based studies that include more genes linked to vitamin D and/or explore the less common SNPs within the existing genes.

Supporting Information

Table S1 Single nucleotide polymorphisms in GC, CYP2R1, DHCR7/NADSYN1, and their association with serum 25(OH)D among Arabs, South Asian, Southeast Asian participants.

Acknowledgments

We would like to thank our study team for their efforts and excellent work. We are grateful to the Clinical Laboratory and the Tissue Bank Core Facility at DDI for their contribution in performing the vitamin D profile analysis and handling samples, respectively. We would also thank Dr William Greer from the Sidra Medical and Research Centre for his proofreading and reviewing of the manuscript. Finally, we are grateful to the senior management, Scientific Advisory Board, and Ethical Review Committee of the Dasman Diabetes Institute for their unwavering support and valuable recommendations.

Author Contributions

Conceived and designed the experiments: NE. Performed the experiments: FA MMA MM OA. Analyzed the data: NE FN. Contributed reagents/materials/analysis tools: KB MA AB. Contributed to the writing of the manuscript: NE JA.

References

1. Simonelli C (2005) The role of vitamin D deficiency in osteoporosis and fractures. Minn Med 88: 34–36.
2. Borkar VV, Devidayal, Verma S, Bhalla AK (2010) Low levels of vitamin D in North Indian children with newly diagnosed type 1 diabetes. Pediatr Diabetes 11: 345–350.
3. Kilkkinen A, Knekt P, Aro A, Rissanen H, Marniemi J, et al. (2009) Vitamin D status and the risk of cardiovascular disease death. Am J Epidemiol 170: 1032–1039.
4. Bosse Y, Lemire M, Poon AH, Daley D, He JQ, et al. (2009) Asthma and genes encoding components of the vitamin D pathway. Respir Res 10: 98.
5. Heist RS, Zhou W, Wang Z, Liu G, Neuberg D, et al. (2008) Circulating 25-hydroxyvitamin D, VDR polymorphisms, and survival in advanced non-small-cell lung cancer. J Clin Oncol 26: 5596–5602.
6. Jones G, Strugnell SA, DeLuca HF (1998) Current understanding of the molecular actions of vitamin D. Physiol Rev 78: 1193–1231.
7. Gannage-Yared MH, Chemali R, Yaacoub N, Halaby G (2000) Hypovitaminosis D in a sunny country: relation to lifestyle and bone markers. J Bone Miner Res 15: 1856–1862.
8. Brustad M, Alsaker E, Engelsen O, Aksnes L, Lund E (2004) Vitamin D status of middle-aged women at 65–71 degrees N in relation to dietary intake and exposure to ultraviolet radiation. Public Health Nutr 7: 327–335.
9. Saliba W, Rennert HS, Kershenbaum A, Rennert G (2012) Serum 25(OH)D concentrations in sunny Israel. Osteoporos Int 23: 687–694.
10. Ardawi MS, Sibiany AM, Bakhsh TM, Qari MH, Maimani AA (2012) High prevalence of vitamin D deficiency among healthy Saudi Arabian men: relationship to bone mineral density, parathyroid hormone, bone turnover markers, and lifestyle factors. Osteoporos Int 23: 675–686.
11. Dawodu A, Absood G, Patel M, Agarwal M, Ezimokhai M, et al. (1998) Biosocial factors affecting vitamin D status of women of childbearing age in the United Arab Emirates. J Biosoc Sci 30: 431–437.
12. Allali F, El Aichaoui S, Khazani H, Benyahia B, Saoud B, et al. (2009) High prevalence of hypovitaminosis D in Morocco: relationship to lifestyle, physical performance, bone markers, and bone mineral density. Semin Arthritis Rheum 38: 444–451.
13. Hobbs RD, Habib Z, Alromaihi D, Idi L, Parikh N, et al. (2009) Severe vitamin D deficiency in Arab-American women living in Dearborn, Michigan. Endocr Pract 15: 35–40.
14. Hunter D, De Lange M, Snieder H, MacGregor AJ, Swaminathan R, et al. (2001) Genetic contribution to bone metabolism, calcium excretion, and vitamin D and parathyroid hormone regulation. J Bone Miner Res 16: 371–378.
15. Shea MK, Benjamin EJ, Dupuis J, Massaro JM, Jacques PF, et al. (2009) Genetic and non-genetic correlates of vitamins K and D. Eur J Clin Nutr 63: 458–464.
16. McGrath JJ, Saha S, Burne TH, Eyles DW (2010) A systematic review of the association between common single nucleotide polymorphisms and 25-hydroxyvitamin D concentrations. J Steroid Biochem Mol Biol 121: 471–477.
17. Ahn J, Yu K, Stolzenberg-Solomon R, Simon KC, McCullough ML, et al. (2010) Genome-wide association study of circulating vitamin D levels. Hum Mol Genet 19: 2739–2745.
18. Wang TJ, Zhang F, Richards JB, Kestenbaum B, van Meurs JB, et al. (2010) Common genetic determinants of vitamin D insufficiency: a genome-wide association study. Lancet 376: 180–188.
19. Zhang Z, He JW, Fu WZ, Zhang CQ, Zhang ZL (2013) An analysis of the association between the vitamin D pathway and serum 25-hydroxyvitamin D levels in a healthy Chinese population. J Bone Miner Res 28: 1784–1792.
20. Kurylowicz A, Ramos-Lopez E, Bednarczuk T, Badenhoop K (2006) Vitamin D-binding protein (DBP) gene polymorphism is associated with Graves' disease and the vitamin D status in a Polish population study. Exp Clin Endocrinol Diabetes 114: 329–335.
21. Ramos-Lopez E, Bruck P, Jansen T, Herwig J, Badenhoop K (2007) CYP2R1 (vitamin D 25-hydroxylase) gene is associated with susceptibility to type 1 diabetes and vitamin D levels in Germans. Diabetes Metab Res Rev 23: 631–636.
22. Engelman CD, Fingerlin TE, Langefeld CD, Hicks PJ, Rich SS, et al. (2008) Genetic and environmental determinants of 25-hydroxyvitamin D and 1,25-

dihydroxyvitamin D levels in Hispanic and African Americans. J Clin Endocrinol Metab 93: 3381–3388.
23. Signorello LB, Shi J, Cai Q, Zheng W, Williams SM, et al. (2011) Common variation in vitamin D pathway genes predicts circulating 25-hydroxyvitamin D Levels among African Americans. PLoS One 6: e28623.
24. Zhang Y, Wang X, Liu Y, Qu H, Qu S, et al. (2012) The GC, CYP2R1 and DHCR7 genes are associated with vitamin D levels in northeastern Han Chinese children. Swiss Med Wkly 142: w13636.
25. Elkum N, Al-Arouj M, Sharifi M, Behbehani K, Bennakhi A (2014) Cardiovascular disease risk factors in the South Asian population living in Kuwait: a cross-sectional study. Diabet Med 31: 531–539.
26. Uitterlinden AG, Fang Y, Van Meurs JB, Pols HA, Van Leeuwen JP (2004) Genetics and biology of vitamin D receptor polymorphisms. Gene 338: 143–156.
27. Larcombe L, Mookherjee N, Slater J, Slivinski C, Singer M, et al. (2012) Vitamin D in a northern Canadian first nation population: dietary intake, serum concentrations and functional gene polymorphisms. PLoS One 7: e49872.
28. Speeckaert M, Huang G, Delanghe JR, Taes YE (2006) Biological and clinical aspects of the vitamin D binding protein (Gc-globulin) and its polymorphism. Clin Chim Acta 372: 33–42.
29. Sinotte M, Diorio C, Berube S, Pollak M, Brisson J (2009) Genetic polymorphisms of the vitamin D binding protein and plasma concentrations of 25-hydroxyvitamin D in premenopausal women. Am J Clin Nutr 89: 634–640.
30. Ahn J, Albanes D, Berndt SI, Peters U, Chatterjee N, et al. (2009) Vitamin D-related genes, serum vitamin D concentrations and prostate cancer risk. Carcinogenesis 30: 769–776.
31. Bu FX, Armas L, Lappe J, Zhou Y, Gao G, et al. (2010) Comprehensive association analysis of nine candidate genes with serum 25-hydroxy vitamin D levels among healthy Caucasian subjects. Hum Genet 128: 549–556.
32. Cooper JD, Smyth DJ, Walker NM, Stevens H, Burren OS, et al. (2011) Inherited variation in vitamin D genes is associated with predisposition to autoimmune disease type 1 diabetes. Diabetes 60: 1624–1631.

19

Protective Vascular and Cardiac Effects of Inducible Nitric Oxide Synthase in Mice with Hyperhomocysteinemia

Sanjana Dayal[1], Ilya O. Blokhin[1,3], Rochelle A. Erger[1,5], Melissa Jensen[1], Erland Arning[6], Jeff W. Stevens[1], Teodoro Bottiglieri[6], Frank M. Faraci[1,2,4], Steven R. Lentz[1]*

1 Department of Internal Medicine, University of Iowa Carver College of Medicine, Iowa City, Iowa, United States of America, **2** Department of Pharmacology, University of Iowa Carver College of Medicine, Iowa City, Iowa, United States of America, **3** Interdisciplinary Graduate Program in Molecular and Cellular Biology, University of Iowa Carver College of Medicine, Iowa City, Iowa, United States of America, **4** Francois M. Abboud Cardiovascular Center, University of Iowa Carver College of Medicine, Iowa City, Iowa, United States of America, **5** Veterans Affairs Medical Center, Iowa City, Iowa, United States of America, **6** Baylor Institute of Metabolic Disease, Dallas, Texas, United States of America

Abstract

Diet-induced hyperhomocysteinemia produces endothelial and cardiac dysfunction and promotes thrombosis through a mechanism proposed to involve oxidative stress. Inducible nitric oxide synthase (iNOS) is upregulated in hyperhomocysteinemia and can generate superoxide. We therefore tested the hypothesis that iNOS mediates the adverse oxidative, vascular, thrombotic, and cardiac effects of hyperhomocysteinemia. Mice deficient in iNOS (*Nos2−/−*) and their wild-type (*Nos2+/+*) littermates were fed a high methionine/low folate (HM/LF) diet to induce mild hyperhomocysteinemia, with a 2-fold increase in plasma total homocysteine ($P<0.001$ vs. control diet). Hyperhomocysteinemic *Nos2+/+* mice exhibited endothelial dysfunction in cerebral arterioles, with impaired dilatation to acetylcholine but not nitroprusside, and enhanced susceptibility to carotid artery thrombosis, with shortened times to occlusion following photochemical injury ($P<0.05$ vs. control diet). *Nos2−/−* mice had decreased rather than increased dilatation responses to acetylcholine ($P<0.05$ vs. *Nos2+/+* mice). *Nos2−/−* mice fed control diet also exhibited shortened times to thrombotic occlusion ($P<0.05$ vs. *Nos2+/+* mice), and iNOS deficiency failed to protect from endothelial dysfunction or accelerated thrombosis in mice with hyperhomocysteinemia. Deficiency of iNOS did not alter myocardial infarct size in mice fed the control diet but significantly increased infarct size and cardiac superoxide production in mice fed the HM/LF diet ($P<0.05$ vs. *Nos2+/+* mice). These findings suggest that endogenous iNOS protects from, rather than exacerbates, endothelial dysfunction, thrombosis, and hyperhomocysteinemia-associated myocardial ischemia-reperfusion injury. In the setting of mild hyperhomocysteinemia, iNOS functions to blunt cardiac oxidative stress rather than functioning as a source of superoxide.

Editor: Partha Mukhopadhyay, National Institutes of Health, United States of America

Funding: This study was supported by research funding from National Institutes of Health grants HL063943 (to SRL) and HL062984 (to SRL and FMF), American Heart Association grants 0860052Z, 13SDG140500021 (to SD) and 14PRE18850045 (to IOB), the Department of Veterans Affairs (BX001399 to FMF), the American Society of Hematology (to SRL), and a grant from the Foundation Leducq (to FMF). The funders had no role in study design, data collection and analysis, decision to publish, or preparation of the manuscript.

Competing Interests: The authors have declared that no competing interests exist.

* Email: steven-lentz@uiowa.edu

Introduction

Hyperhomocysteinemia is an established risk factor for cardiovascular disease and stroke [1,2]. Even relatively mild elevations of plasma total homocysteine (e.g. 10 to 20 μmol/L) are associated with increased cardiovascular risk [1,2]. Several distinct cardiovascular abnormalities, including endothelial and cardiomyocyte dysfunction, and thrombosis, have been demonstrated in animal models of diet-induced hyperhomocysteinemia [3,4]. Hyperhomocysteinemia has been proposed to exert its adverse effects in the vasculature in part by generating vascular oxidative stress that diminishes the bioavailability of endothelial-derived nitric oxide (NO) [3]. NO is normally produced in a highly regulated manner by endothelial NO synthase (eNOS; *Nos3*), which is expressed constitutively in vascular endothelium. An inducible isoform of NOS (iNOS; *Nos2*) is expressed in vascular smooth muscle, endothelium, and myocardium in certain pathological conditions such as atherosclerosis, diabetes, and inflammatory disorders [5–9]. Experimental overexpression of iNOS in isolated murine blood vessels causes endothelial dysfunction [10–12], which may be due to iNOS uncoupling [13,14]. iNOS uncoupling results in the generation of superoxide rather than NO as the predominant reaction product and iNOS-derived superoxide can limit the bioavailability of endothelial NO [15]. Studies in diabetic mice revealed that deficiency of iNOS or reversal of iNOS uncoupling restores endothelium-dependent relaxation [16,17] and tolerance to myocardial ischemia/reperfusion (I/R) injury [18,19]. Collectively, these studies suggest a role for iNOS in the pathophysiology of multiple types of cardiovascular disease.

The potential role of iNOS in the etiology of hyperhomocysteinemia-induced cardiovascular abnormalities has not been directly explored, but several lines of evidence suggest that iNOS expression is upregulated in the setting of elevated homocysteine levels. *In vitro* studies with cultured endothelial and smooth muscle cells treated with homocysteine showed increased expression of iNOS [20,21]. Similarly, upregulation of iNOS has been detected in the coronary and carotid artery, and kidneys of hyperhomocysteinemic rats [22–24]. Additionally, we and others have shown that NOS inhibitors abrogate the increased production of reactive oxygen species (ROS) in carotid and coronary arteries of hyperhomocysteinemic rats or mice [22,25]. These observations suggest that the upregulation and uncoupling of iNOS, with increased production of superoxide, may be a mechanism that contributes to endothelial dysfunction in hyperhomocysteinemia. Consistent with this notion, impaired endothelium-dependent vasomotor responsiveness in the aorta of hyperhomocysteinemic rats could be reversed by tetrahydrobiopterin, an essential cofactor that promotes NOS coupling [26]. It remains unclear, however, whether iNOS directly and mechanistically contributes to the adverse vascular and cardiac effects of hyperhomocysteinemia.

We utilized a genetic approach to examine the mechanistic role of endogenous iNOS in the vascular phenotype of diet-induced hyperhomocysteinemia in mice. Using iNOS-deficient (*Nos2−/−*) mice, we tested the hypothesis that iNOS contributes to endothelial dysfunction, thrombosis, and myocardial ischemia-reperfusion injury in hyperhomocysteinemia. Contrary to our hypothesis, our data suggest that endogenous iNOS protects against, rather than exacerbates, vascular oxidative stress, endothelial dysfunction, and thrombosis. Our findings also indicate that, during hyperhomocysteinemia, endogenous iNOS prevents myocardial injury by blunting cardiac oxidative stress.

Materials and Methods

Mice

This study was carried out in strict accordance with the recommendations in the Guide for the Care and Use of Laboratory Animals of the National Institute of Health. All animal protocols were approved by the University of Iowa Animal Care and Use Committee (approval # 1211243). All surgery was performed under anesthesia (sodium pentobarbital) and all efforts were made to minimize suffering. Male homozygous iNOS deficient (*Nos2−/−*) mice on the C57BL6/J background were obtained from the Jackson Laboratory and were backcrossed to C57BL6/J female mice (Jackson Laboratory) to generate male and female heterozygous iNOS deficient (*Nos2+/−*) breeders. These *Nos2+/−* breeder mice were then intercrossed to generate wild-type (*Nos2+/+*) and *Nos2−/−* littermate mice for study. Genotyping for the wild-type and targeted *Nos2* alleles was performed by polymerase chain reaction (PCR) using the following primer sequences: for the wild-type *Nos2* allele, 5′- TCA ACA TCT CCT GGT GGA AC -3′ and 5′- AGC ACA CAT GCA GAA TGA GTA -3′; for the targeted *Nos2* allele, 5′- AAT ATG CGA AGT GGA CCT CG -3′ and 5′- AGC ACA CAT GCA GAA TGA GTA -3′. Starting from 4 weeks of age, mice were fed either a control diet (LM485, Harlan Teklad) that contains 4.0 g/Kg L-methionine and 6.7 mg/Kg of folic acid, or a high methionine/low folate (HM/LF) diet (TD00205, Harlan Teklad) that contains 8.2 g/Kg L-methionine and 0.2 mg/Kg folic acid [27]. Mice were fed the diets for 5–11 months before study.

Dilator responses in cerebral arterioles

Dilatation of cerebral arterioles was measured as described previously [25]. Briefly, mice were anesthetized with sodium pentobarbital and ventilated mechanically. A cranial window was made over the left parietal cortex, and a segment of a randomly selected pial arteriole (~30 μm in diameter) was studied. The diameter of the cerebral arteriole was measured, using a video microscope coupled to an image-shearing device, under control conditions and during superfusion with acetylcholine (1.0 μmol/L and 10.0 μmol/L), nitroprusside (0.1 μmol/L and 1.0 μmol/L), and papaverine (1.0 μmol/L and 10.0 μmol/L).

Carotid artery thrombosis

Carotid artery thrombosis was induced by photochemical injury as described previously [28]. Mice were anesthetized with sodium pentobarbital (70–90 mg/Kg intraperitoneally) and ventilated mechanically with room air and supplemental oxygen. The right femoral vein was cannulated for the administration of rose bengal. The right common carotid artery was dissected free and carotid artery blood flow was measured with a 0.5 PSB Doppler flow probe (Transonic Systems, Inc) and digital recording system (Gould Ponemah Physiology Platform version 3.33). To induce endothelial injury, the right common carotid artery was transilluminated continuously with a 1.5-mV, 540-nm green laser (Melles Griot) from a distance of 6 cm, and rose bengal (35 mg/

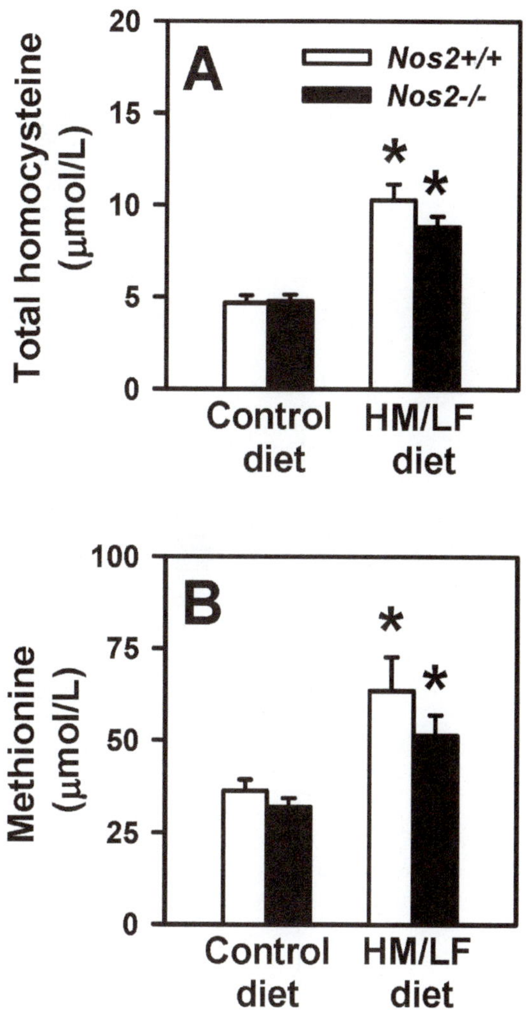

Figure 1. Plasma total homocysteine and methionine levels. Compared with mice fed the control diet, both *Nos2+/+* (open bars) and *Nos2−/−* (filled bars) mice fed the HM/LF diet exhibited elevation in plasma total homocysteine and methionine levels. 15–20 mice were studied in each group. *P<0.01 compared with mice of the same genotype fed the control diet by two-way ANOVA.

Kg) was injected via a femoral vein catheter. Blood flow was monitored continuously for 90 minutes or until stable occlusion occurred, at which time the experiment was terminated. Stable occlusion was defined as the time at which blood flow remained absent for ≥10 minutes.

Myocardial I/R injury

Regional myocardial I/R injury was performed using a procedure modified from Gandhi et al [29]. Male mice were anesthetized with sodium pentobarbital and supplemented every hour (sodium pentobarbital, 20 mg/Kg IP) as needed to maintain adequate depth of anesthesia. Body temperature was monitored with a rectal probe and maintained at 36.5–37.5°C with a heating pad. A tracheotomy was performed and a volume-controlled Harvard respirator (model 681) was used to mechanically ventilate mice with room air (stroke volume 0.24 mL, 105 strokes per minute). A thoracotomy was performed in the fourth intercostal space, and the left coronary artery was ligated 2 mm below the tip of the left atrium using 8.0 Ethicon mounted on a tapered needle. A short (1 mm) section of PE-10 tubing was placed into the ligature to facilitate later reperfusion. Successful occlusion of the left coronary artery was verified by visual inspection (development of paleness of the anterolateral wall of the left ventricle, color change of left coronary artery from bright-red to violet, and regional akinesis). After occlusion for 30 minutes, reperfusion was induced by cutting the ligature on the top of the PE-10 tubing and was visually confirmed by a return of pink-red color of the

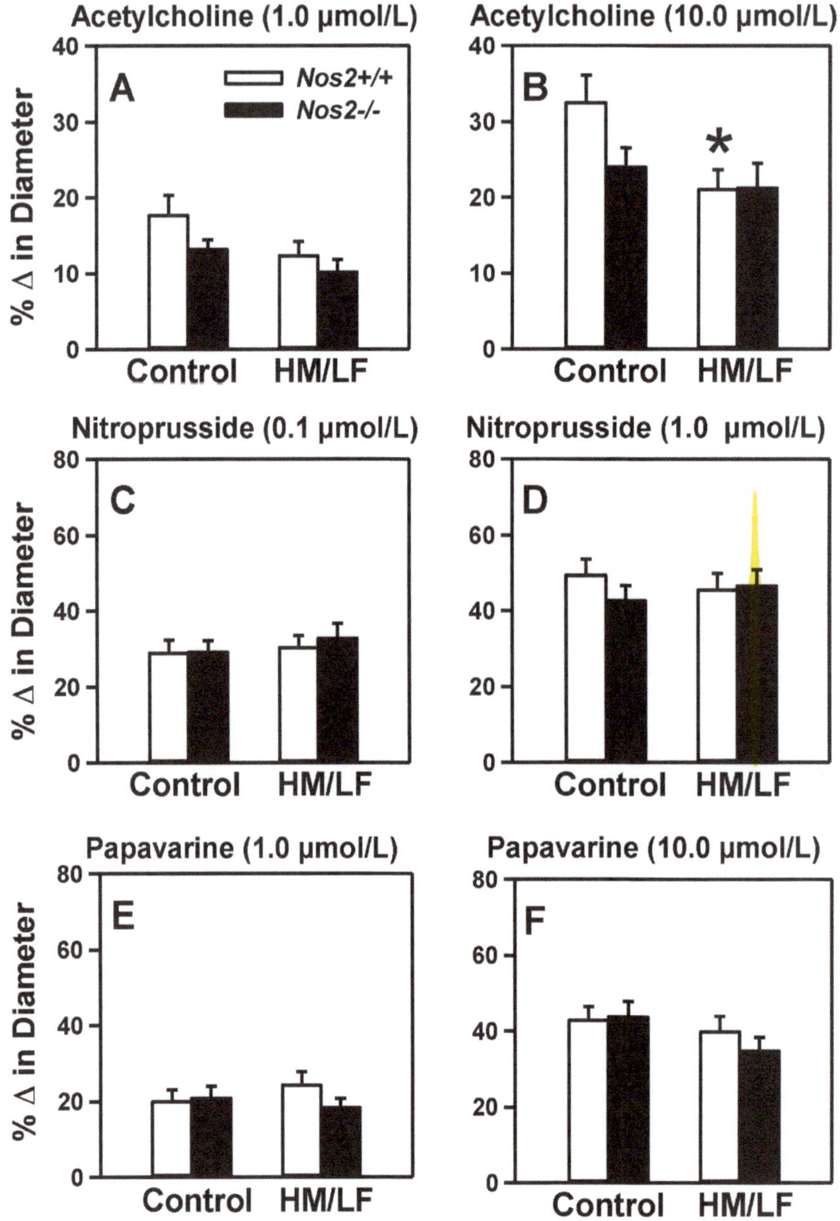

Figure 2. Dilator responses in cerebral arterioles. Dilatation of cerebral arterioles to (A) 1.0 μmol/L acetylcholine, (B) 10.0 μmol/L acetylcholine, (C) 0.1 μmol/L nitroprusside, (D) 1.0 μmol/L nitroprusside, (E) 1.0 μmol/L papaverine and (F) 10.0 μmol/L papaverine were measured in *Nos2+/+* (open bars) or *Nos2−/−* (filed bars) mice. 10–15 mice were studied in each group. *P<0.05 compared with mice of same genotype fed the control diet by two-way ANOVA.

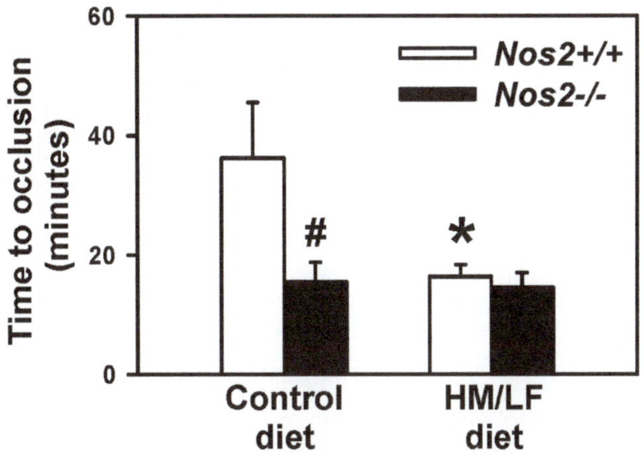

Figure 3. Carotid artery thrombosis. The time to stable occlusion of the carotid artery in *Nos2+/+* (open bars) or *Nos2−/−* (filled bars) mice fed either the control diet or the HM/LF diet was measured following photochemical injury. 6–8 mice were studied in each group. *P<0.05 compared with mice of the same genotype fed the control diet; #P<0.01 compared with *Nos2+/+* mice fed the same diet by two-way ANOVA.

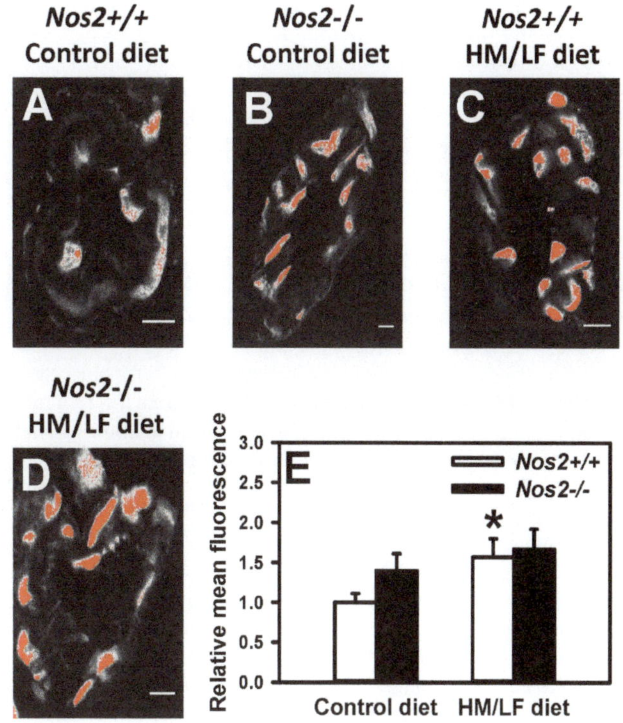

Figure 4. Laser-scanning confocal micrographs of cerebral arterioles stained with DHE. (A) *Nos2+/+* mice fed the control diet. (B) *Nos2−/−* mice fed the control diet. (C) *Nos2+/+* mice fed the HM/LF diet. (D) *Nos2−/−* mice fed the HM/LF diet. (E) Quantification of DHE fluorescence using Image J. Images are representative of 5 separate experiments. Scale bar = 10 μm.

anterolateral wall of the left ventricle and brief period of tachycardia.

After 2 hours of reperfusion, the left coronary artery was re-ligated and 0.5 mL of 3% Evans blue dye (TCI America) was slowly injected into the left ventricle by cardiac puncture to delineate the ischemic area at risk (AR). The heart was then rapidly excised, rinsed in ice-cold saline, and serially sectioned perpendicular to its long axis using an acrylic mouse heart slicer matrix (Zivic Instruments). Heart sections (2 mm) were immediately imaged using a digital camera (Nikon Coolpix 5000) for determination of AR and then incubated with 3.0 mL of 1.5% 2,3,5-triphenyltetrazolium chloride (TTC) (GFS Chemicals) in phosphate buffer (0.1 mol/L NaH_2PO_4/Na_2HPO_4, pH 7.4) for 20 minutes at 37°C to demarcate the viable and nonviable area of necrosis (AN) and imaged. The AR, AN, and total myocardial area (TA) were determined using computer planimetry by a blinded investigator using National Institutes of Health (NIH) Image J (v1.57) software.

Plasma homocysteine and methionine

Blood was collected by cardiac puncture into EDTA (final concentration 5 mmol/L), and plasma was flash frozen. Plasma total homocysteine, defined as the total concentration of homocysteine after quantitative reductive cleavage of all disulfide bonds [30], was measured by high performance liquid chromatography (HPLC) using ammonium 7-fluorobenzo-2-oxa-1,3-diazole-4-sulphonate (SBDF) fluorescence detection [31]. Plasma methionine was measured by HPLC coupled to fluorescence detection after precolumn derivatization using *o*-phthaldialdehyde as described previously [32].

Detection of ROS

The oxidative fluorescent dye dihydroethidium (DHE) (Molecular Probes) was used to detect ROS in sections of cerebral arterioles as described previously [33]. Frozen transverse sections (10 μm) of cerebral arterioles were incubated with 10 μmol/L DHE for 30 minutes at room temperature in a dark chamber. Fluorescence was detected by laser-scanning confocal microscopy. Data were quantified using Image J software and reported as mean fluorescence relative to *Nos2+/+* mice fed the control diet.

Real-time PCR

Levels of mRNA for *Nos2*, neuronal and endothelial nitric oxide synthase (*Nos1* and *Nos3*, respectively), and *18S* were measured by quantitative real-time PCR as described previously [34]. Total RNA was isolated from frozen hearts using Trizol reagent (Invitrogen, Carlsbad, CA) and treated with DNAse I to remove contaminating genomic DNA. RNA (325 ng) was then reverse transcribed using Taqman reverse transcriptase and random hexamer primers. PCR primers and 6-carboxy fluorescein-labeled probes for *18s (Mm03928990_g1)*, *Nos2* (Mm01309892_g1), and *Nos3* (Mm00435204_m1) were purchased from Applied Biosystems. Reverse transcribed cDNA was incubated with TaqMan Universal PCR mix (Applied Biosystems) and PCR primers and probes at 50°C for 2 minutes and then at 95°C for 10 minutes followed by 40 cycles of 95°C for 15 seconds and 60°C for 1 minute using the Applied Biosystems 7700 sequence detection system. For quantitative analysis of mRNA, the comparative threshold cycle ($\Delta\Delta C_T$) method [35] was used, with values normalized to *18S* and expressed relative to levels in *Nos2+/+* mice fed the control diet. Validation experiments were performed to confirm equal amplification efficiency for all primers sets.

Statistical analysis

Two-way analysis of variance (ANOVA) with the Tukey test for multiple comparisons was used to analyze the effects of *Nos2* genotype and diet on endothelial function, occlusion time, ROS levels, infarct size and troponin levels. The data sets for occlusion time and cardiac ROS did not show normal distributions, therefore the analysis was performed on log transformed values. One way ANOVA was used to compare mRNA levels in cardiac tissue. Statistical significance was defined as a P value <0.05. Values are reported as mean±SE.

Results

Deficiency of iNOS does not protect against endothelial dysfunction in hyperhomocysteinemic mice

To investigate the potential contribution of iNOS to endothelial dysfunction during hyperhomocysteinemia, *Nos2−/−* mice deficient in iNOS were placed on a HM/LF diet. Plasma levels of total homocysteine were elevated approximately 2-fold in both *Nos2+/+* and *Nos2−/−* mice fed the HM/LF diet compared with mice fed the control diet (Figure 1, P<0.001). Plasma levels of methionine also were elevated significantly in mice fed the HM/LF diet compared with mice fed the control diet (Figure 1, P<0.05). Deficiency of iNOS had no impact on plasma levels of homocysteine or methionine (P = 0.5).

Hyperhomocysteinemia is a risk factor for small vessel disease in the brain [36]. Thus, we next measured responses of small cerebral arterioles to endothelium-dependent and -independent dilators (Figure 2). Dilator responses to 10.0 µmol/L acetylcholine, an endothelium-dependent dilator, were decreased in *Nos2+/+* mice fed the HM/LF diet compared with *Nos2+/+* mice fed the control diet (P<0.05; Figure 2B). Deficiency of iNOS failed to protect cerebral arterioles from this effect of hyperhomocysteinemia, as demonstrated by the similar dilator responses to acetylcholine in *Nos2+/+* and *Nos2−/−* mice fed the HM/LF diet. These data suggest that iNOS does not play a causative role in the endothelial vasomotor dysfunction associated with hyperhomocysteinemia. In mice without hyperhomocysteinemia, the data suggest a possible protective effect of endogenous *Nos2*, indicated by a strong trend towards decreased dilator responses to acetylcholine in *Nos2−/−* mice compared with *Nos2+/+* mice fed the control diet, (P = 0.053; Figure 2B). The endothelium-independent vasodilators nitroprusside (Figure 2C and 2D) and papaverine (Figure 2E and 2F) also produced dilatation of cerebral arterioles, and the responses were not influenced by either diet or *Nos2* genotype.

Absence of iNOS does not reverse the prothrombotic phenotype produced by HM/LF diet

To further examine the vascular effects of iNOS deficiency in hyperhomocysteinemic mice, experimental thrombosis of the carotid artery was induced by photochemical injury. *Nos2+/+* mice fed the HM/LF diet exhibited a significant shortening in the time to stable occlusion compared with *Nos2+/+* mice fed the control diet (P<0.05, Figure 3). A similar shortening of the time to stable occlusion was observed in *Nos2−/−* mice fed the HM/LF diet, indicating that deficiency of iNOS did not prevent this prothrombotic effect of hyperhomocysteinemia. In mice fed the control diet, the mean time to stable occlusion was significantly shortened in *Nos2−/−* mice compared with *Nos2+/+* mice (P< 0.01), again suggesting a protective effect of endogenous *Nos2*.

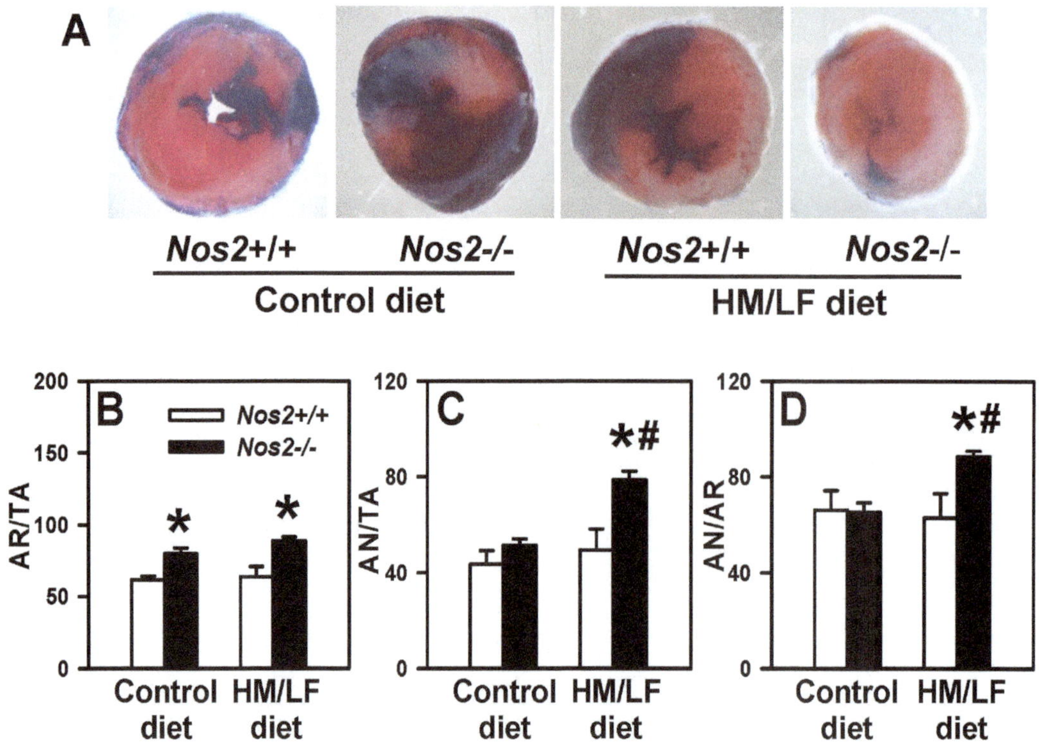

Figure 5. Regional myocardial ischemia-reperfusion injury. The left coronary artery was ligated for 30 minutes and then reperfused for 2 hours. Panel A illustrates representative 2,3,5-triphenyltetrazolium chloride (TTC) stained images for each of the four groups of mice. The percent of (B) area at risk over total area (AR/TA), (C) area of necrosis over total area (AN/TA), and (D) area of necrosis over area at risk (AN/AR) were calculated in *Nos2+/+* (open bars) or *Nos2−/−* mice (filled bars) by staining with Evans blue and TTC. Values are mean ±SE. 8–12 mice were studied in each group. *P<0.01 compared with *Nos2+/+* mice fed the same diet, #P<0.05 compared with mice of the same genotype fed the control diet by two-way ANOVA.

Increased vascular ROS was detected with the HM/LF diet and iNOS deficiency

Previous work has suggested a possible mechanistic role for vascular ROS in both the endothelial vasomotor dysfunction and prothrombotic state of diet-induced hyperhomocysteinemia [3]. Therefore, we utilized laser-scanning confocal microscopy to detect ROS in cerebral arterioles by DHE fluorescence. We found that DHE fluorescence was significantly ($P<0.05$) higher in *Nos2+/+* mice fed the HM/LF diet (Figure 4C) compared with *Nos2+/+* mice fed the control diet (Figure 4A). Deficiency of iNOS tended to increase DHE fluorescence in *Nos2−/−* mice fed the control diet ($P = 0.07$) (Figure 4B) and was increased further in *Nos2−/−* mice fed the HM/LF diet (Figure 4D). The quantitative data are summarized in Figure 4E. These findings suggest that endogenous *Nos2* protects from ROS generation rather than acting as a source of vascular ROS. Our findings also suggest that both iNOS deficiency and hyperhomocysteinemia independently contribute to increased vascular ROS.

Hyperhomocysteinemia exacerbates myocardial I/R injury in iNOS-deficient mice

We next examined the effect of *Nos2* deficiency on regional myocardial I/R injury (Figure 5A). In *Nos2−/−* mice, the ischemic area at risk (AR) following I/R injury was significantly increased compared with *Nos2+/+* littermate mice, regardless of diet ($P<0.01$, Figure 5B). In *Nos2+/+* mice, the HM/LF diet did not alter infarct size, calculated either as area of necrosis per total area (AN/TA) (Figure 5C) or area of necrosis per area at risk (AN/AR) (Figure 5D). In *Nos2−/−* mice, however, the HM/LF diet caused a significant increase in infarct size (Figure 5C and 5D; $P<0.05$ vs. *Nos2+/+* mice fed the HM/LF diet; $P<0.05$ vs. *Nos2−/−* mice fed the control diet). These data suggest that endogenous iNOS protects against reperfusion injury in the setting of hyperhomocysteinemia.

To further explore the relationship between NOS and ROS in the heart, we measured cardiac levels of *Nos1*, *Nos2* and *Nos3* mRNA by quantitative real-time PCR. The data demonstrate a 50% increase in *Nos2* mRNA levels in hearts from *Nos2+/+* mice fed the HM/LF diet compared with the control diet (Figure 6A; $P<0.05$). This finding indicates that hyperhomocysteinemia induces the upregulation of iNOS expression in the heart, as has been previously reported in vascular tissue [22] and kidney [23]. As expected, no *Nos2* mRNA was detected in *Nos2−/−* mice (Figure 6A). There was no significant difference in *Nos3* mRNA expression between *Nos2+/+* mice fed the control diet vs. the HM/LF diet (Figure 6B). We did detect a small but significant increase in *Nos3* mRNA levels in *Nos2−/−* mice fed the HM/LF diet (Figure 6B; $P<0.05$ vs. *Nos2−/−* mice fed the control diet). *Nos1* mRNA was not detected in cardiac tissue from any of the groups of mice (not shown). We next determined whether *Nos2* deficiency during hyperhomocysteinemia alters cardiac ROS production. A significant increase in cardiac ROS was observed in *Nos2−/−* mice fed the HM/LF diet (Figure 6C, $P<0.05$ compared with *Nos2−/−* mice fed the control diet; $P<0.01$ compared with *Nos2+/+* mice fed the HM/LF diet), consistent with the larger infarct size in this group (Figure 5B and 5C). These findings suggest that during hyperhomocysteinemia, endogenous iNOS protects cardiac tissue from oxidative stress and I/R injury.

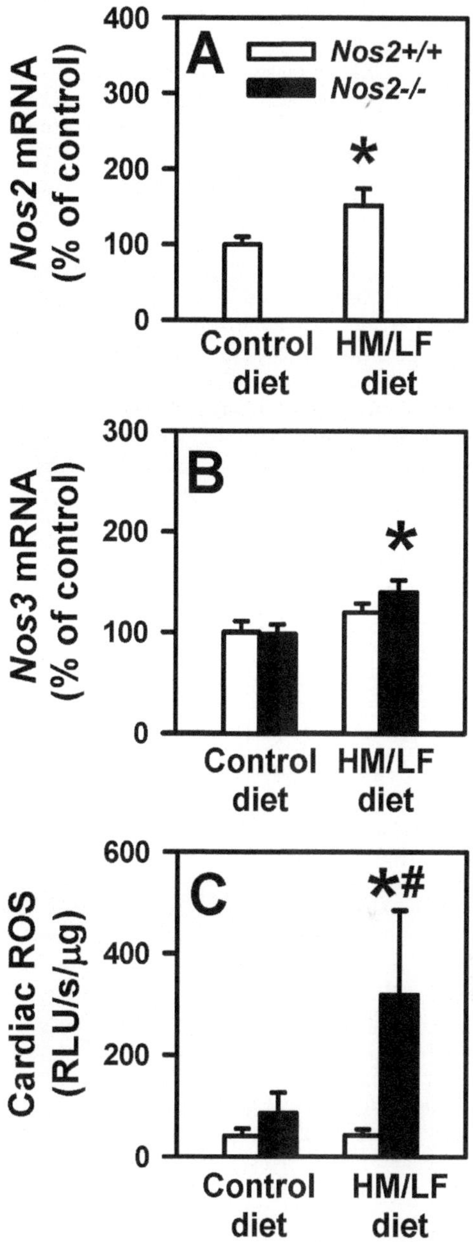

Figure 6. Cardiac levels of *Nos2* and *Nos3* mRNA and ROS. Levels of *Nos2* mRNA (A) and *Nos3* mRNA (B) were measured by real-time PCR in *Nos2+/+* (open bars) or *Nos2−/−* (filled bars) mice. Values were normalized to *18S* mRNA and are expressed as percent of the control values observed in *Nos2+/+* mice fed the control diet. (C) Tiron-quenchable and NADPH-enhanced lucigenin chemiluminescence was measured in cardiac homogenates. Values are mean ±SE. 6–9 mice were studied in each group. *$P<0.05$ compared with mice of the same genotype fed the control diet; #$P<0.05$ compared with *Nos2+/+* mice fed the same diet.

Discussion

In certain pathological conditions such as diabetes and atherosclerosis, iNOS has been proposed to be a mediator of increased oxidative stress and impaired vascular function. In diabetic mice, deficiency of iNOS protects against endothelial dysfunction [16,17] and myocardial I/R injury [18,19]. The absence of iNOS also decreases oxidative stress and protects against atherosclerosis in apolipoprotein E-deficient (ApoE−/−) mice [37]. Because hyperhomocysteinemia causes upregulation of vascular iNOS expression and increases vascular oxidative stress [22,34], we hypothesized that genetic deficiency of iNOS also might protect against hyperhomocysteinemia-induced vascular dysfunction and thrombosis. To address this hypothesis, we examined the mechanistic role of iNOS in endothelial dysfunction, thrombosis and myocardial I/R injury in mice with or without diet-induced hyperhomocysteinemia. The major findings of our study are: 1) the absence of iNOS failed to protect mice against endothelial dysfunction or accelerated thrombosis produced by hyperhomocysteinemia; and 2) deficiency of iNOS exacerbated, rather than protected against myocardial ischemia-reperfusion injury and cardiac oxidative stress in hyperhomocysteinemic mice. These findings demonstrate that, unlike what has been described in models of diabetes or atherosclerosis, iNOS is not a mediator of the adverse vascular and endothelial effects of hyperhomocysteinemia.

Our data also suggest a baseline antithrombotic effect of endogenous iNOS in mice without hyperhomocysteinemia, demonstrated by a marked shortening of the time to thrombotic occlusion of the carotid artery in *Nos2−/−* mice fed the control diet (Figure 3). This observation is consistent with a prior study in which iNOS was found to provide protection against injury-induced thrombosis in female mice [38]. In our study, loss of endogenous iNOS also appeared to decrease dilatation responses to acetylcholine (Figure 2) and increase levels of ROS in cerebral arterioles (Figure 4) in the absence of hyperhomocysteinemia. Interestingly, a previous study found that *Nos2−/−* mice exhibited enhanced oxidative stress after traumatic brain injury [39]. These observations suggest that, rather than contributing to oxidative vascular injury, endogenous iNOS may protect against endothelial dysfunction and thrombosis by suppressing vascular oxidative stress.

Clinical evidence for increased troponin levels after coronary artery bypass in hyperhomocysteinemic patients suggests a relationship between elevated homocysteine and cardiac injury [40]. *Ex vivo* studies in isolated Langendorff-perfused hearts from mice with heterozygous deficiency of cystathionine β-synthase suggested that elevated homocysteine results in impaired relaxation and contractile function and increased apoptosis following I/R injury [4]. Unexpectedly, we did not observe a difference in infarct size in wild-type mice fed control vs. HM/LF diet. Potential reasons for the different findings between the *ex vivo* Langendorff results and our *in vivo* data include the different endpoints for myocardial injury examined, and that the *ex vivo* studies were conducted with a genetic model of hyperhomocysteinemia [4], whereas we used a diet-induced model of hyperhomocysteinemia.

Our findings in the myocardial I/R model are particularly interesting, since prior reports have suggested contrastingly that either deficiency or overexpression of iNOS can protect against I/R injury in mouse models [19,41,42]. We observed that the myocardial area at risk was increased with iNOS deficiency regardless of diet, suggesting that endogenous iNOS may limit the area of myocardial ischemia by promoting vasodilation of collateral blood vessels. We also found that cardiac iNOS mRNA was significantly upregulated by hyperhomocysteinemia in *Nos2+/+* mice (Figure 6A). Our data further suggest that the elevated levels of cardiac iNOS in hyperhomocysteinemic mice are protective against oxidative stress and I/R injury, because *Nos2−/−* mice had increased cardiac ROS production (Figure 6C) and increased infarct size (Figure 5) compared with *Nos2+/+* mice in the setting of hyperhomocysteinemia. This protective effect of iNOS is in accordance with previous studies in which gene transfer of iNOS protected against myocardial injury [42].

Our study has some limitations, including the inherent weaknesses of mouse models of human disease. The mouse model of diet-induced hyperhomocysteinemia, and the experimental models of vascular injury utilized herein may only approximate conditions that occur in human patients. Moreover, it is possible that some or all of the vascular effects observed in this study may be driven by metabolic consequences of the HM/LF diet that are independent of hyperhomocysteinemia. We note that the HM/LF diet produced only modest hyperhomocysteinemia in mice, with levels of plasma tHcy (10.3±0.9 μmol/L) somewhat lower than those seen in human patients with moderate hyperhomocysteinemia (10–20 μmol/L) and vascular diseases [1,2]. It may be interesting in future studies to explore the vascular effects of additional dietary and genetic models of altered homocysteine, methionine and folate metabolism.

In summary, our data suggest a model in which, under normal or minimally pathological conditions (e.g. mild hyperhomocysteinemia, which is common in the general population), iNOS expressed at low levels in vascular cells is primarily protective against vascular oxidative stress and its complications. This vasoprotective effect of iNOS contrasts with its harmful effects in more severe pathological conditions (e.g. diabetes, atherosclerosis, or sepsis), in which upregulation of iNOS can mediate increased oxidative stress and related vascular pathology [16–19,37,43]. Our study design was comprehensive in that we examined the modulating effects of iNOS deficiency in both vascular and cardiac tissues in mice with diet-induced hyperhomocysteinemia. Our findings argue strongly against a role for iNOS as a mediator of the vascular, thrombotic, or cardiac complications of hyperhomocysteinemia in this mouse model.

Acknowledgments

The authors thank Kristina W. Thiel for assistance in manuscript editing.

Author Contributions

Conceived and designed the experiments: SD SRL. Performed the experiments: SD RAE MJ IOB EA JWS. Analyzed the data: SD TB FMF SRL. Contributed to the writing of the manuscript: SD IOB JWS SRL.

References

1. Homocysteine Studies Cillaboration. (2002) Homocysteine and risk of ischemic heart disease and stroke: a meta-analysis. JAMA 288: 2015–2022.
2. Boushey CJ, Beresford SA, Omenn GS, Motulsky AG (1995) A quantitative assessment of plasma homocysteine as a risk factor for vascular disease. Probable benefits of increasing folic acid intakes. JAMA 274: 1049–1057.
3. Dayal S, Lentz SR (2007) Role of redox reactions in the vascular phenotype of hyperhomocysteinemic animals. Antioxid Redox Signal 9: 1899–1909.
4. Wang X, Cui L, Joseph J, Jiang B, Pimental D, et al. (2012) Homocysteine induces cardiomyocyte dysfunction and apoptosis through p38 MAPK-mediated increase in oxidant stress. J Mol Cell Cardiol 52: 753–760.
5. Bardell AL, MacLeod KM (2001) Evidence for inducible nitric-oxide synthase expression and activity in vascular smooth muscle of streptozotocin-diabetic rats. J Pharmacol Exp Ther 296: 252–259.
6. Behr-Roussel D, Rupin A, Simonet S, Bonhomme E, Coumailleau S, et al. (2000) Effect of chronic treatment with the inducible nitric oxide synthase inhibitor N-iminoethyl-L-lysine or with L-arginine on progression of coronary and aortic atherosclerosis in hypercholesterolemic rabbits. Circulation 102: 1033–1038.
7. Detmers PA, Hernandez M, Mudgett J, Hassing H, Burton C, et al. (2000) Deficiency in inducible nitric oxide synthase results in reduced atherosclerosis in apolipoprotein E-deficient mice. J Immunol 165: 3430–3435.
8. Hollenberg SM, Broussard M, Osman J, Parrillo JE (2000) Increased microvascular reactivity and improved mortality in septic mice lacking inducible nitric oxide synthase. Circ Res 86: 774–778.
9. Upmacis RK, Crabtree MJ, Deeb RS, Shen H, Lane PB, et al. (2007) Profound biopterin oxidation and protein tyrosine nitration in tissues of ApoE-null mice on

an atherogenic diet: contribution of inducible nitric oxide synthase. Am J Physiol Heart Circ Physiol 293: H2878–2887.
10. Eguchi D, D'Uscio LV, Wambi C, Weiler D, Kovesdi I, et al. (2002) Inhibitory effect of recombinant iNOS gene expression on vasomotor function of canine basilar artery. Am J Physiol Heart Circ Physiol 283: H2560–2566.
11. Gunnett CA, Lund DD, Chu Y, Brooks RM 2nd, Faraci FM, et al. (2001) NO-dependent vasorelaxation is impaired after gene transfer of inducible NO-synthase. Arterioscler Thromb Vasc Biol 21: 1281–1287.
12. Gunnett CA, Lund DD, Howard MA 3rd, Chu Y, Faraci FM, et al. (2002) Gene transfer of inducible nitric oxide synthase impairs relaxation in human and rabbit cerebral arteries. Stroke 33: 2292–2296.
13. Alderton WK, Cooper CE, Knowles RG (2001) Nitric oxide synthases: structure, function and inhibition. Biochemical Journal 357: 593–615.
14. Shah AM (2000) Inducible nitric oxide synthase and cardiovascular disease. Cardiovascular Research 45: 148–155.
15. Channon KM (2004) Tetrahydrobiopterin: regulator of endothelial nitric oxide synthase in vascular disease. Trends Cardiovasc Med 14: 323–327.
16. Gunnett CA, Heistad DD, Faraci FM (2003) Gene-targeted mice reveal a critical role for inducible nitric oxide synthase in vascular dysfunction during diabetes. Stroke 34: 2970–2974.
17. Kitayama J, Faraci FM, Gunnett CA, Heistad DD (2006) Impairment of dilator responses of cerebral arterioles during diabetes mellitus: role of inducible NO synthase. Stroke 37: 2129–2133.
18. Okazaki T, Otani H, Shimazu T, Yoshioka K, Fujita M, et al. (2011) Reversal of inducible nitric oxide synthase uncoupling unmasks tolerance to ischemia/reperfusion injury in the diabetic rat heart. J Mol Cell Cardiol 50: 534–544.
19. Marfella R, Di Filippo C, Esposito K, Nappo F, Piegari E, et al. (2004) Absence of inducible nitric oxide synthase reduces myocardial damage during ischemia reperfusion in streptozotocin-induced hyperglycemic mice. Diabetes 53: 454–462.
20. Tyagi N, Sedoris KC, Steed M, Ovechkin AV, Moshal KS, et al. (2005) Mechanisms of homocysteine-induced oxidative stress. Am J Physiol Heart Circ Physiol 289: H2649–2656.
21. Welch GN, Upchurch GR Jr, Farivar RS, Pigazzi A, Vu K, et al. (1998) Homocysteine-induced nitric oxide production in vascular smooth-muscle cells by NF-kappa B-dependent transcriptional activation of Nos2. Proc Assoc Am Physicians 110: 22–31.
22. Ungvari Z, Csiszar A, Edwards JG, Kaminski PM, Wolin MS, et al. (2003) Increased superoxide production in coronary arteries in hyperhomocysteinemia: role of tumor necrosis factor-alpha, NAD(P)H oxidase, and inducible nitric oxide synthase. Arterioscler Thromb Vasc Biol 23: 418–424.
23. Zhang F, Siow YL, O K (2004) Hyperhomocysteinemia activates NF-kappaB and inducible nitric oxide synthase in the kidney. Kidney Int 65: 1327–1338.
24. Celotto AC, Fukada SY, Laurindo FR, Haddad R, Eberlin MN, et al. (2010) Chronic hyperhomocysteinemia impairs vascular function in ovariectomized rat carotid arteries. Amino Acids 38: 1515–1522.
25. Dayal S, Arning E, Bottiglieri T, Boger RH, Sigmund CD, et al. (2004) Cerebral vascular dysfunction mediated by superoxide in hyperhomocysteinemic mice. Stroke 35: 1957–1962.
26. Dhillon B, Badiwala MV, Maitland A, Rao V, Li SH, et al. (2003) Tetrahydrobiopterin attenuates homocysteine induced endothelial dysfunction. Mol Cell Biochem 247: 223–227.
27. Devlin AM, Arning E, Bottiglieri T, Faraci FM, Rozen R, et al. (2004) Effect of Mthfr genotype on diet-induced hyperhomocysteinemia and vascular function in mice. Blood 103: 2624–2629.
28. Wilson KM, Lynch CM, Faraci FM, Lentz SR (2003) Effect of mechanical ventilation on carotid artery thrombosis induced by photochemical injury in mice. J Thromb Haemost 1: 2669–2674.
29. Gandhi C, Motto DG, Jensen M, Lentz SR, Chauhan AK (2012) ADAMTS13 deficiency exacerbates VWF-dependent acute myocardial ischemia/reperfusion injury in mice. Blood 120: 5224–5230.
30. Mudd SH, Finkelstein JD, Refsum H, Ueland PM, Malinow MR, et al. (2000) Homocysteine and its disulfide derivatives: a suggested consensus terminology. Arterioscler Thromb Vasc Biol 20: 1704–1706.
31. Ubbink JB, Hayward Vermaak WJ, Bissbort S (1991) Rapid high-performance liquid chromatographic assay for total homocysteine levels in human serum. J Chromatogr 565: 441–446.
32. Bottiglieri T (1987) The effect of storage on rat tissues and human plasma amino acid levels determined by HPLC. Biomed Chromatogr 2: 195–196.
33. Dayal S, Devlin AM, McCaw RB, Liu ML, Arning E, et al. (2005) Cerebral vascular dysfunction in methionine synthase-deficient mice. Circulation 112: 737–744.
34. Dayal S, Wilson KM, Leo L, Arning E, Bottiglieri T, et al. (2006) Enhanced susceptibility to arterial thrombosis in a murine model of hyperhomocysteinemia. Blood 108: 2237–2243.
35. Livak KJ, Schmittgen TD (2001) Analysis of relative gene expression data using real-time quantitative PCR and the 2(-Delta Delta C(T)) Method. Methods 25: 402–408.
36. Hassan A, Hunt BJ, O'Sullivan M, Bell R, D'Souza R, et al. (2004) Homocysteine is a risk factor for cerebral small vessel disease, acting via endothelial dysfunction. Brain 127: 212–219.
37. Kuhlencordt PJ, Chen J, Han F, Astern J, Huang PL (2001) Genetic deficiency of inducible nitric oxide synthase reduces atherosclerosis and lowers plasma lipid peroxides in apolipoprotein E-knockout mice. Circulation 103: 3099–3104.
38. Upmacis RK, Shen H, Benguigui LE, Lamon BD, Deeb RS, et al. (2011) Inducible nitric oxide synthase provides protection against injury-induced thrombosis in female mice. Am J Physiol Heart Circ Physiol 301: H617–624.
39. Bayir H, Kagan VE, Borisenko GG, Tyurina YY, Janesko KL, et al. (2005) Enhanced oxidative stress in iNOS-deficient mice after traumatic brain injury: support for a neuroprotective role of iNOS. J Cereb Blood Flow Metab 25: 673–684.
40. Thiengburanatham S (2009) Hyperhomocysteinemia-induced myocardial injury after coronary artery bypass. Asian Cardiovasc Thorac Ann 17: 483–489.
41. Li Q, Guo Y, Xuan YT, Lowenstein CJ, Stevenson SC, et al. (2003) Gene therapy with inducible nitric oxide synthase protects against myocardial infarction via a cyclooxygenase-2-dependent mechanism. Circ Res 92: 741–748.
42. Li Q, Guo Y, Ou Q, Cui C, Wu WJ, et al. (2009) Gene transfer of inducible nitric oxide synthase affords cardioprotection by upregulating heme oxygenase-1 via a nuclear factor-{kappa}B-dependent pathway. Circulation 120: 1222–1230.
43. Lange M, Nakano Y, Traber DL, Hamahata A, Esechie A, et al. (2010) Role of different nitric oxide synthase isoforms in a murine model of acute lung injury and sepsis. Biochem Biophys Res Commun 399: 286–291.

The Status of Vitamin B12 and Folate among Chinese Women: A Population-Based Cross-Sectional Study in Northwest China

Shaonong Dang, Hong Yan*, Lingxia Zeng, Quanli Wang, Qiang Li, Shengbin Xiao, Xiaojing Fan

Department of Epidemiology and Health Statistics, School of Public Health, Xi'an Jiaotong University Health Science Center, Xi'an, Shaanxi, People's Republic of China

Abstract

Objective: To assess the status of the vitamin B12 and folate of Chinese women living in northwest China.

Methods: A population-based cross-sectional study was conducted in 2008 among Chinese women aged 10–49 years living in Shaanxi province of northwest China. A stratified multistage random sampling method was adopted to obtain a sample of 1170 women. The women were interviewed for collection of their background information and their plasma vitamin B12 and folate were measured with the immunoassay method. The status of both vitamins was evaluated and the prevalence of deficiency was estimated.

Results: The median value of the women was 214.5 pg/mL for vitamin B12 and 4.6 ng/mL for folate. The urban women had a significantly higher vitamin B12 (254.1 vs. 195.9 pg/mL) but lower folate (4.4 vs. 4.7 ng/mL) than rural women. Total prevalence of deficiency was 45.5% (95% CI: 42.6%~48.4%) for vitamin B12 and 14.7% (95% CI: 12.6%~16.8%) for folate. About 36% of women presented vitamin B12 deficiency alone, 5.2% belonged to folate deficiency alone and 9.5% was combined deficiency in both vitamins. More than 25% of the women were in marginal vitamin B12 status (200–299 pg/mL) and 60% in marginal status of folate (3–6 ng/mL). About 75.2% of rural women with folate deficiency were deficient in vitamin B12 and 46% for urban women. Quantile regression model found decreasing coefficient of folate status across 73 different quantiles of vitamin B12, which indicated that the women with folate deficiency had lower vitamin B12 significantly compared with those with no deficiency.

Conclusions: The deficiency of vitamin B12 and folate is still prevalent among the Chinese women in northwest China. Vitamin B12 deficiency could be more serious and the improvement of poor vitamin B12 status should be invoked when practicing the supplementation of folate against the neural tube defects in northwest China.

Editor: Shantanu Sengupta, CSIR-INSTITUTE OF GENOMICS AND INTEGRATIVE BIOLOGY, India

Funding: This work was supported by the National Natural Science Foundation of China (Grant No 81230016, http://www.nsfc.gov.cn), Beijing, China, and the Science and Technology Research and Development Program of Shaanxi Province, China (Grant No. 2006K08-G10(3), http://www.sninfo.gov.cn). The funders had no role in study design, data collection and analysis, decision to publish, or preparation of the manuscript.

Competing Interests: The authors have declared that no competing interests exist.

* Email: yanhonge@mail.xjtu.edu.cn

Introduction

There was a widespread low folate status around China, especially in the region of northern China [1–4]. A previous study showed that the mean plasma folate in the adults of northern China was about 8.4 nmol/L, which was significantly lower than 16.7 nmol/L in southern region controlling for age, gender, season and so on [3]. However, most of studies on folate status focused on specific regions and women of childbearing age so it was difficult to estimate the number of folate deficient people in China. Based on limited data, the prevalence of folate deficiency among Chinese women of childbearing age varied from 1% to 20% [1]. Currently available evidences indicated that folate deficiency was associated with increasing risk of neural tube defects (NTD) [5,6]. Folic acid supplementation during the periconceptional period was regarded as an effective strategy against NTD although the mandatory folic acid fortification to reduce NTD rates was introduced in some countries [5–7]. In China the policy of supplementation of folic acid played an important role in preventing NTD [8]. However, magnitude of reduction in NTD rate much varied with regions of China. In Shaanxi province, a high NTD incidence area of China, NTD rate had been reduced to about 1.3‰ in 2007 but since then the rate persisted [9]. The reason might be complicated. Other micronutrient deficiency such as vitamin B12 could be taken into account in addition to lower compliance of the folate supplementation. Vitamin B12 plays an essential role in folate metabolism and the enzyme methionine synthase catalyzes the vitamin B12-dependent conversion of homocysteine and 5-methyltetrahydrofolate to methionine and tetrahydrofolate [10]. Therefore, vitamin B12 deficiency could impair the folate-mediated one-carbon metabolic pathway to present as folate deficiency or to exacerbate folate deficiency.

There was increasing evidence that poor maternal vitamin B12 status may increase the risk of adverse pregnancy outcomes including NTD [11–14]. A Canadian study found a 3-fold increase in the risk of NTDs in mothers who had vitamin B-12 status in the lower quartile, regardless of folate fortification [13]. It implied that deficiency of vitamin B12 might be an independent factor resulting in NTD. Moreover, folate supplementation could mask vitamin B12 deficiency [10]. Suboptimal vitamin B12 status is common in many parts of the world [11,15]. Scientific evidence on vitamin B12 status of Chinese population was limited. Compared with Chinese adults in southern China, adults from the northern regions presented low vitamin B12 status and prevalence of deficiency was about 21% [16]. Accordingly we measured plasma folate and vitamin B12 status of a representative sample of Chinese women living in Shaanxi province. We tried to profile status of vitamin B12 and folate among Chinese women and investigate the relationship between the two vitamins. These data would be helpful in determination of micronutrient supplementation programs in China.

Methods

Study setting

Shaanxi province is located in northwest China geographically with such three regions as northern, middle and southern Shaanxi. The natural environment, culture and lifestyle vary significantly across the three regions. Northern Shaanxi is in the loess plateau of China with semi-arid temperate climate. Middle Shaanxi is situated in the alluvial plains and north temperate monsoon climate predominates. Southern Shaanxi is located in the south of Qinling Mountain which is the main boundary between the south and north of China. It is humid and sub-tropical typically. The resident population is 37.5 million people in Shaanxi and about 30% of them live in urban areas. Compared with the eastern China, Shaanxi is a developing province in economy and society. In 2012 the provincial GDP amounted to 23.6 billion US dollars, ranking sixteenth in China [17].

Sample and subjects

A population-based cross-sectional study was conducted between August and September, 2008. The subject was the Chinese women aged 10–49 years living in Shaanxi. Women were excluded if they were breastfeeding or had breast-fed within the last 12 months, or had a serious or chronic illness. A stratified multistage random sampling method was adopted to obtain the sample. Women were recruited from the urban and rural areas, respectively. In rural areas, 20 counties were selected randomly from 80 counties of Shaanxi according to population size. For each sampled county, one township was selected randomly and one village selected was randomly from the sampled township. Finally the rural women were selected randomly in sampled village. In urban areas, 10 districts were selected randomly from 24 urban districts. One community was obtained randomly from each sampled district and the urban women were selected in each sampled community. A sample size of 1100 was estimated assuming a prevalence of folate deficiency of 15%, a relative error of 15%, $\alpha = 0.05$, accounting for an expected 20% nonresponse rate. The proportion of urban to rural subjects in the sample was determined as about 30%, which was close to a proportion of urban to rural population in Shaanxi province.

Data collection

The subjects were interviewed face to face by the trained staff with a standard questionnaire to collect the information including social-demographical information of women, household background and the woman's health and reproductive history. Anthropometric data of the women was obtained using standard measuring apparatus. Five milliliters of venous blood was taken by venepuncture on arm into tubes containing EDTA and the plasma was isolated on site. All specimens were transported on dry ice to the laboratory center of college of public health, Xi'an Jiaotong University and kept in the refrigerators with −70°C. Measurement of plasma vitamin B12 and folate were performed with immunoassay method using the kit from MP Biomedicals LLC Ltd within two months after collection of blood specimens. The plasma folate concentration of <3 ng/mL was used to indicate folate deficiency and 3–6 ng/mL for marginal folate status. Vitamin B12 status was defined as deficient based on plasma vitamin B12 concentration of <200 pg/mL and 200–299 pg/mL for marginal vitamin B12 status [18].

Survey quality control

Three field-working teams were established according to geographic distribution of sampled sites. Each team consisted of 4 members who accounted for blood collecting, plasma isolation, subject interview, and anthropometry. Staff from county health bureau or maternal and child health care station coordinated activities of each team in each sampled site. And doctors from village clinics or township hospitals were involved in the field-working. Before the formal survey, a training meeting was launched in Xi'an and all members of the teams were trained. The University Health Science Center made training materials and was in charge of training including discussion and practice. After each interview, investigators checked all information in questionnaire. Key member in the team accounted for checking all questionnaires of each investigating site. If errors happened, repeated interview was carried out. All measuring apparatus were corrected before measurement and standard procedures were followed.

Data analysis

A database was established by duplicate entries using EpiData 3.02 software (The EpiData Association, Odense, Denmark). Prior to data analysis, data cleaning and quality check were performed. Skewed distribution of vitamin B12 and folate was observed, so median and interquartile range was used as descriptive statistics. Differences between groups for the selected variables were determined using x^2 test for categorical variables and Kruskal-Wallis test for continuous variables. Kernel density method was employed to describe the distribution of vitamin B12 and folate. The distribution curves by age were plotted with epanechnikov kernel function and width of 0.5. Quantile regression model was used to investigate the relationship between vitamin B12 and folate controlling for potential affecting factors including age, BMI, education level, geographical region, source of family income and morbidity of cold. The model in this setting would allow the impact of the folate status (deficiency or not) to vary along the whole range of vitamin B12 value. Seventy-three different conditional quantile functions were estimated by the variable of residence (urban vs. rural), starting with the 0.05 quantile and proceeding in 0.0125 increments until the 0.95 quantile (i.e., 0.05, 0.0625, 0.75, 0.875, 0.1 ... 0.95). A Markov chain marginal bootstrap was used to compute 95% confidence intervals (CIs) of coefficient for every quantile estimate. Coefficients with 95% CIs of folate status were plotted across the different quantile of vitamin B12. Negative coefficient at each quantile indicated decreasing amount of vitamin B12 of women with folate deficiency compared with those with normal status. The estimated coefficients for

Table 1. Characteristics of the female participants in the study.

Variables	n	Outcome
Residence (%)		
Rural	794	67.9
Urban	376	32.1
Geography (%)		
North	233	19.9
Central	741	63.3
South	196	16.8
Age group (years) (%)		
10–	276	23.6
15–	280	23.9
20–	117	10.0
30–	267	22.8
40–	230	19.7
BMI by age ($\bar{x}\pm s$)*		
10–	276	18.4±2.75
15–	264	19.8±2.24
20+	614	22.7±3.11
Years of schooling by age ($\bar{x}\pm s$)*		
10–	274	7.44±1.42
15–	261	9.21±1.45
20+	609	9.51±4.16
Source of family income (%)*		
Farm only	285	24.8
Migrant working	270	23.5
Government institutions	139	12.1
State-owned Company	214	18.7
Private company	239	20.8
History of catching a cold within 2 weeks (%)*		
Yes	197	16.8
No	956	81.7
Anemia (%)*		
Yes	317	27.1
No	847	72.4

*Few data were missing.

selected quantile with P-value were reported with the coefficient by a typical regression using ordinary least squares (OLS) to provide a basis for comparison with the quantile regression. A P-value <0.05 was considered statistically significant. All statistical analyses were performed using the STATA statistical software package version 9 (StataCorp, College Station, TX, USA).

Ethics Statement

The study complied with the Declaration of Helsinki and was approved by the Ethical Committee of Science of Medical center, Xi'an Jiaotong University. The written informed consent had been obtained from the study participants, and the mothers of the girls aged less than 18 years provided the written consent on behalf of these girls.

Results

The characteristics of the participants

Totally 1193 women were investigated. Among them 23 women were excluded for incomplete or missing value in the vitamins and 1170 data were used for analysis finally. Demographic characteristics were shown in Table 1. All women were ethnically Han Chinese. Rural participants accounted for 67.9%. Geographically, 63.3% of the participants lived in central Shaanxi. The proportion of participants for each age group was about 20% apart from age group of 20 years. The mean of BMI was 18.4 for the women aged 10–14.99 years, 19.8 for the women aged 15–19.99 years and 22.7 for the women aged over 20 years. The women aged over 20 years had 9.51 years of schooling. Almost one-fourth of participants' family lived on farming and 23.5% on migrant working. In remaining families, working in government institutions or company was main source of income. About health status, 16.8% of the women had caught a cold within 2 weeks before investigating. The prevalence of anemia was about 27.1% (Table 1).

The average status and distribution of vitamin B12 and folate

Table 2 showed that the median value was 214.5 pg/mL for vitamin B12 and 4.6 ng/mL for folate among Chinese women in Shaanxi province. The urban women had a significantly higher vitamin B12 (254.1 vs. 195.9 pg/mL) but lower folate (4.4 vs. 4.7 ng/mL) than rural women. The status of two vitamins varied geographically (P<0.001). The women in south and central Shaanxi presented no difference in vitamin B12, but had higher vitamin B12 level than the women in north Shaanxi. The women living in north and middle Shaanxi had a similar level of folate, which were lower significantly compared with the women in south Shaanxi. Figure 1 indicated that the distribution of folate moved upward with age increase and the women aged over 30 years presented higher folate significantly (P<0.001). However, there might be a complicated relationship between vitamin B12 and age. The women aged over 30 years had significantly lower vitamin B12 (P<0.001). Obviously the adolescent girls had a lower status in both folate and vitamin B12 (P<0.001).

Prevalence of deficiency of vitamin B12 and folate

Figure 2 showed the prevalence of deficiency of two vitamins. Total prevalence of deficiency was 45.5% (95% CI: 42.6%~48.4%) for vitamin B12 and 14.7% (95% CI: 12.6%~16.8%) for folate. About 36% of the women presented vitamin B12 deficiency alone and 5.2% belonged to folate deficiency alone. Prevalence of combined deficiency of both vitamins was about 9.5%. The total prevalence of vitamin B12 deficiency was higher in rural women than urban women (52.0% vs. 31.6%, P = 0.004) but there was no difference in folate deficiency between them (13.7% vs. 16.8%, P = 0.172). Compared with urban women, rural women showed a higher prevalence of vitamin B12 deficiency alone (41.7% vs. 23.9%, P<0.001) but lower prevalence of folate deficiency alone (3.4% vs 9.0%, P = 0.001). There was no difference in prevalence of combined two vitamins deficiency found between rural and urban women (10.3% vs. 7.7%, P = 0.156).

Based on the distribution of vitamin B12 in Table 2, rural women showed significantly lower vitamin B12 than urban women (Table 2, P<0.001). It was not different in distribution of folate between rural and urban women (P = 0.185). The women living in south Shaanxi were in higher status in both vitamins, compared with the women in north and central Shaanxi (P<0.001). It was worth noting that more than 25% of the women were in the

Table 2. The median and distribution of vitamin B12 and folate by the residence, geographical environment and age.

		Vitamin B12 (pg/mL)					Folate (ng/mL)			
		Median (P_{25}, P_{75})	n(%)				Median (P_{25}, P_{75})	n(%)		
	n		<100	100-	200-	300-		<3	3-	6-
All women	1170	214.5	125	407	315	323	4.6	172	694	304
		(148.1,311.4)	(10.7)	(34.8)	(26.9)	(27.6)	(3.5,6.0)	(14.7)	(59.3)	(26.0)
Residence*										
Rural	794	195.9	105	308	208	173	4.7	109	468	217
		(137.4,283.2)	(13.2)	(38.8)	(26.2)	(21.8)	(3.6,6.1)	(13.7)	(58.9)	(27.3)
Urban	376	254.1	20	99	107	150	4.4	63	226	87
		(182.2,359.9)	(5.3)	(26.3)	(28.5)	(39.9)	(3.4,5.9)	(16.8)	(60.1)	(23.1)
Geography†										
North	233	188.7	40	87	64	42	4.5	34	147	52
		(126.5,274.1)	(17.2)	(37.3)	(27.5)	(18.0)	(3.5,5.7)	(14.6)	(63.1)	(22.3)
Central	741	219.6	73	255	190	223	4.4	126	450	165
		(152.2,324.1)	(9.9)	(34.4)	(25.6)	(30.1)	(3.3,5.8)	(17.0)	(60.7)	(22.3)
South	196	226.8	12	65	61	58	5.8	12	97	87
		(164.2,323.0)	(6.1)	(33.2)	(31.1)	(29.6)	(4.2,7.2)	(6.1)	(49.5)	(44.4)
Age group (years)‡										
10-	276	233.7	23	85	84	84	4.4	39	175	62
		(163.3,329.6)	(8.3)	(30.8)	(30.4)	(30.4)	(3.4,5.7)	(14.1)	(63.4)	(22.5)
15-	280	197.7	37	110	59	74	4.0	57	183	40
		(140.9,304.4)	(13.2)	(39.3)	(21.1)	(26.4)	(3.1,5.3)	(20.4)	(65.3)	(14.3)
20-	117	229.8	8	41	33	35	4.3	22	71	24
		(154.4,333.9)	(6.8)	(35.0)	(28.3)	(29.9)	(3.2,5.5)	(18.8)	(60.7)	(20.5)
30-	267	216.8	29	88	83	67	5.0	30	134	103
		(144.3,302.4)	(10.9)	(33.0)	(31.1)	(25.1)	(3.9,6.7)	(11.2)	(50.2)	(38.6)
40-	230	204.9	28	83	56	63	5.1	24	131	75
		(144.2,309.2)	(12.2)	(36.1)	(24.3)	(27.4)	(4.0,6.6)	(10.4)	(57.0)	(32.6)

*Compared with rural women, urban women had higher vitamin B12 ($P<0.001$) and lower folate ($P=0.029$).
†The vitamin B12 in south and central Shaanxi was not different statistically ($P=0.379$) but higher than that of north Shaanxi ($P<0.001$). The folate in north and central Shaanxi was not different statistically ($P=0.576$) but lower than that of south Shaanxi ($P<0.001$).
‡There were significantly lower vitamin B12 and folate among the women aged 15-19.99 years ($P<0.001$).

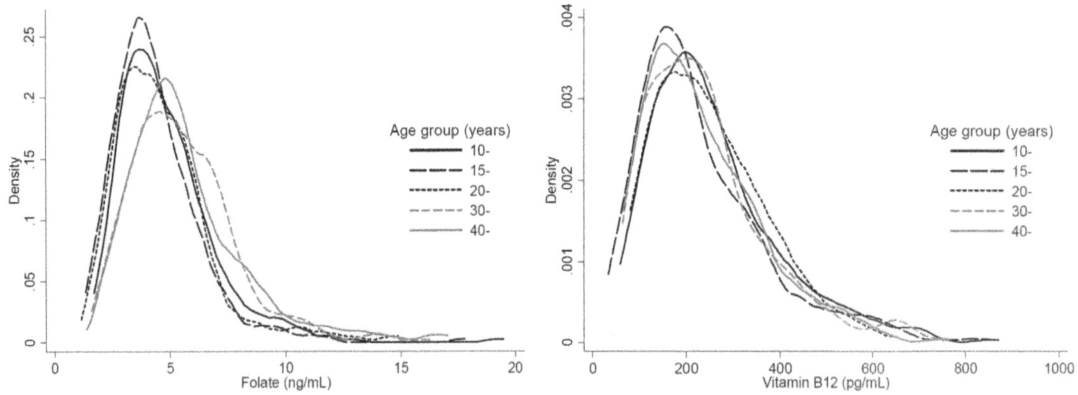

Figure 1. Distribution of vitamin B12 and folate by age among Chinese women in Shaanxi province.

marginal vitamin B12 status and almost 60% of the women in the marginal status of folate.

Relationship between vitamin B12 and folate

Figure 3 showed that the women with folate deficiency might be a high risk of being deficient in vitamin B12. About 75.2% of the rural women with folate deficiency were vitamin B12 deficiency. Among urban women with the folate deficiency, about 46% was deficient in vitamin B12 and 31.7% belonged to the marginal vitamin B12 status. Quantile regression model was used to investigate quantitatively the relationship between vitamin B12 and folate status controlling for the potential affecting factors. Figure 4 indicated the change of coefficient of folate status across 73 different quantiles of vitamin B12. In rural areas, the coefficients were negative and decreased with quantiles and even at higher quantiles the women with folate deficiency had lower vitamin B12 significantly compared with those with no deficiency. In urban areas, the similar trend for the coefficients was observed but at higher quantiles (>85% quantile) there was no significant difference found in vitamin B12 between women with folate deficiency and those without deficiency. Table 3 presented the results for a selected set of quantiles: 0.05, 0.10, 0.25 (lower vitamin B12 level), 0.45, 0.50 (medium vitamin B12 level), 0.75, 0.85, 0.95 (higher vitamin B12 level). Table 3 also showed the multiple linear regression (OLS) estimates at last column. In the rural women with lower vitamin B12 level, vitamin B12 decreased by 15–47 pg/mL in the women with folate deficiency compared with those without deficiency. Even in the rural women with higher vitamin B12 level, the women with folate deficiency had a significant decrease of 88–125 pg/mL in vitamin B12 compared with those without deficiency. The similar situation was found in the urban women but there was no significant difference in vitamin B12 between the women with and without folate deficiency when they were at higher vitamin B 12 level. OLS model estimated that mean difference in vitamin B12 was about 65 pg/mL between the women with and without folate deficiency regardless of urban or rural women.

Discussion

This study was conducted in Shaanxi province of China with a stratified multistage random sampling method based on population distribution, so the sample was a representative of the Shaanxi women and the results from the study also reflected the status of folate and vitamin B12 of Chinese women to some extent. The study outlined the epidemiological features about folate and vitamin B12 among the women in Shaanxi, which implied that the deficiency of folate and vitamin B12 was still prevalent among the Chinese women.

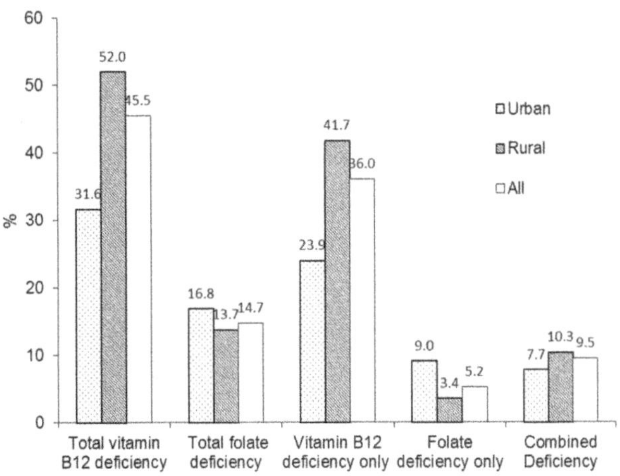

Figure 2. Prevalence of deficiency in vitamin B12 and folate among Chinese women in Shaanxi province.

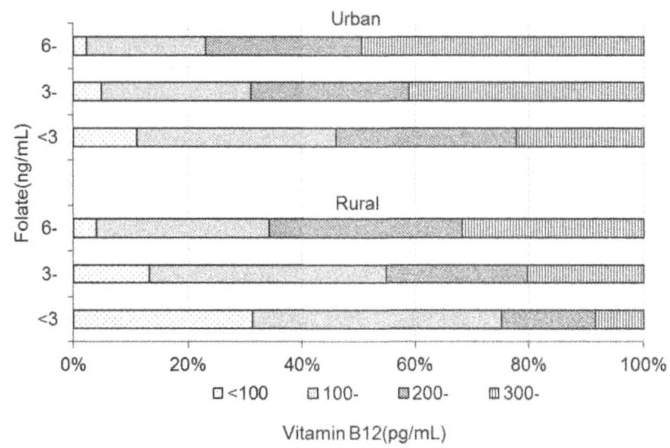

Figure 3. The relationship between the vitamin B12 and folate among Chinese women in Shaanxi province.

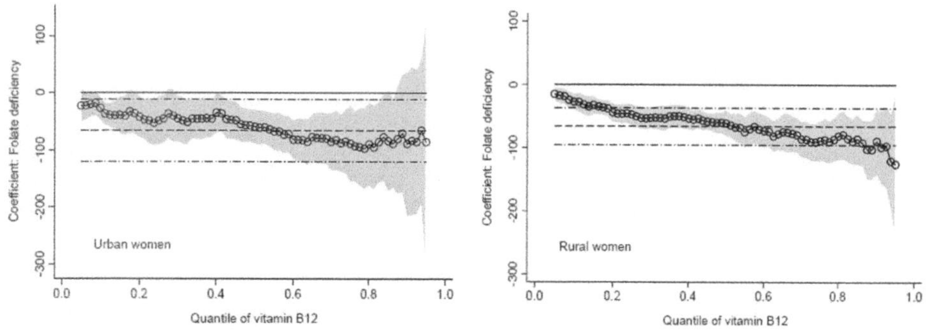

Figure 4. Quantile regression and ordinary least squares (OLS) estimates by residence (urban vs rural): folate deficiency and vitamin B12. Circles represent quantile regression estimates, and the shaded areas around the quantile regression estimates were the 95% confidence intervals. The dashed line was OLS estimate, and the dash-dotted lines showed the OLS 95% confidence interval. Estimates shown here compared folate deficiency with no-deficiency.

Levels of folate and vitamin B12 were low among the women in Shaanxi, and about 14.7% of the women were deficient in folate and 45.5% of the women were deficient in vitamin B12. Significant regional differences were found. Firstly, the urban women had a significantly higher vitamin B12 (254.1 vs. 195.9 pg/mL) but lower folate (4.4 vs. 4.7 ng/mL) than rural women. Such urban-rural difference was also observed among other Chinese woman population [3]. Secondly, geographical difference in folate and vitamin B12 was also obvious, which showed that the women living in southern Shaanxi presented higher folate and vitamin B12 level significantly than those in northern areas. Southern Shaanxi is located in the south of Qinling Mountain which is a boundary between the south and north of China, and the climate and lifestyle in southern Shaanxi is close to typical areas of southern China such as Sichuan [17]. Therefore, this result supported partly the fact of significant difference in the folate and vitamin B12 between the northern and southern China [3]. The geographical difference in folate and vitamin B12 status was consistent with the local lifestyle of Shaanxi and there were the greater availability of fresh vegetables and animal-source foods in the south than the north [17]. Compared with other areas of China, the prevalence of deficiency in folate among Shaanxi women was not very higher, which might be in the middle level. However, notably more than half of women (59.3%) were exposed to lower status of folate (3–6 ng/mL) and the plasma folate in the Shaanxi women was only one third of the American women [19], which suggested that supplementation of folate to the Shaanxi women should be recommended strongly. Around the world, the prevalence of vitamin B12 deficiency varied much from 14.8% to 54.5% [20–23]. Clearly Shaanxi women had a very higher prevalence of deficiency in vitamin B12; especially it was worse in the rural women. Now no national data could be available about vitamin B12 status in China and the magnitude of vitamin B12 deficiency had not been clear. Based on the current local data [4], the prevalence of vitamin B12 deficiency in the Chinese adults was about 4% in the south and 21% in the north. Our study implied that Shaanxi women might be in worse status of vitamin B12.

We also found that the status of folate and vitamin B12 was significantly related to the age. The results showed that the old women had a higher status of folic acid than younger women. The women aged 15–19.99 years had a lowest folate (the median: 4.0 ng/mL) and the women aged 20–29.99 years followed (the median: 4.3 ng/mL). These two groups of women were in child-bearing period when enough folate was required for preparation of pregnancy. So low folate level made them being high risk of NDTs. As for vitamin B12, the age distribution was different. Both younger and older women were in lower status of vitamin B12. Vitamin B12 absorption tended to decrease with age, which might explain some of the difference between age groups [24]. However, we found that younger women, especially adolescent girls, were at the higher risk of being lower status of both folate and vitamin B12. Adolescent girls were in the stage of growth and lower level of vitamins might affect their health adversely. And it suggested that the supplementation of folate and vitamin B12 should focus on the younger female population.

In Shaanxi, only 5.2% of women presented folate deficiency alone but 36% of women were deficient alone in vitamin B12, which suggested that the vitamin B12 deficiency might be predominant and serious, especially in the rural women. Nearly 10% of the women were deficient in both folate and vitamin B12. And among the women with folate deficiency, more than half of the women were deficient in vitamin B12. Further, we investigated quantitative difference in vitamin B12 between the women with and without folate deficiency by using quantile regression model. Compared with the women without folate deficiency, the women with folate deficiency were down 15–125 pg/mL in vitamin B12 level, and averagely about 65 pg/mL. It meant that the women with folate deficiency might be in higher risk of being low vitamin B12. The periconceptional supplementation of folic acid had been practiced in the many countries including China and consequently NTDs were prevented or controlled significantly. Since mid-1990s China has encouraged supplementation of folic acid during the periconceptional period against NTDs and began to provide all women who plan to have a child of free supplements in 2009 [8]. The overall prevalence of NTDs had been decreased from 1.2‰ in 2000 to 0.45‰ in 2011 [25]. But up to now Shaanxi province had still a prevalence of NTDs of 1.3‰ [9] and low vitamin B12 could account for it to some extent. Vitamin B12 played an essential role in folate metabolism and vitamin B12 deficiency could impair the folate-mediated one-carbon metabolic pathway to present as folate deficiency or to exacerbate folate deficiency [10]. The study by Molloy AM et al. found that the mothers of children affected by NTDs had significantly lower B12 status and blood vitamin B12 concentrations of <250 pg/mL during pregnancy was associated with the highest risks [14]. Literatures reported that the hyperhomocysteinemia, which was caused by deficiency in folate and vitamin B12, might be associated with neural tube defects, cardiovascular disease, and mental disorders [6,19,26–29]. A study in China by Ling Hao et al. found that

Table 3. Estimated coefficients from and multiple liner regression quantile regression for selected quantiles: vitamin B12 and folate status by residence.*

Folate deficiency	Quantile 0.05	0.10	0.25	0.45	0.50	0.75	0.85	0.95	OLS
Rural									
Coefficient†	−15.00	−27.19	−47.36	−57.98	−60.69	−88.24	−85.34	−125.08	−65.74
P-value	0.011	<0.001	<0.001	<0.001	<0.001	<0.001	<0.001	0.037	<0.001
Urban									
Coefficient†	−22.40	−26.97	−48.40	−48.17	−58.87	−88.65	−83.95	−85.53	−65.61
P-value	0.136	0.013	0.026	0.006	<0.001	0.01	0.065	0.458	0.018

*Quantile regression model and ordinary least squares (OLS) were used for estimates. In the models the dependent variable was vitamin B12 concentration and folate status (deficiency or not) were regarded as the independent variable controlling for potential affecting factors including age, BMI, education level, geographical region, source of family income and morbidity of cold.
†The coefficient here meant the change of vitamin B12 of women with folate deficiency compared with those with normal status of folate.

vitamin B12 deficiency alone was associated with 4-fold increased risk of being hyperhomocysteinemia and the individuals deficient in both folate and vitamin B-12, had 38-fold higher risk of the hyperhomocysteinemia [16]. Therefore, higher prevalence of vitamin B12 deficiency was associated possibly with NTDs in Shaanxi and further assessment should be required. Moreover, vitamin B12 deficiency often presented as folate deficiency and elevated intakes of folate could interfere with a clinical diagnosis of vitamin B12 deficiency, which implied that folate supplementation could mask vitamin B12 deficiency [10]. This problem also should be paid more attention in the practice of supplementation of folic acid in Shaanxi women.

One of the important causes about lower status of folate and vitamin B12 could be poor dietary pattern [23,30]. Based on our dietary survey among rural women in Shaanxi, the intake of animal protein intake was very low among Shaanxi women [31]. And the intake of fresh vegetables (296.2 g/day) and fruits (25g/day), and animal-source foods (19.4 g/day) was lower significantly than Chinese RNI/AI [32]. Simple diet rich in carbohydrate was a predominant pattern among Shaanxi women [33]. So enriching the dietary pattern and increasing intake of animal foods might be an important way to improve the status of vitamin B12 and folate of Chinese women.

In this study, one limitation had to be addressed. Our survey was about the health status of Shaanxi women and only such blood indicators as folate, vitamin B12 and hemoglobin were measured. Unfortunately, the metabolic markers of folate and vitamin B12, homocysteine (tHcy), methylmalonic acid (MMA) and holotranscobalamin (holoTC), had not been measured. Studies indicated that these markers increased or decreased when the status of plasma folate and vitamin B12 were low [16,34,35]. The elevated tHcy and MMA were found to be related to cognitive decline but high holoTC level was protective against cognitive decline [36,37]. However, tHcy and MMA started to increase at vitamin B12 levels above the typical cut-off value (200 pg/mL), and they increased quickly when vitamin B12 decreased from 400 to 200 pmol/L [38], which suggested that the change of the markers related to the impairment of functioning of the nervous system had already begun before the occurrence of deficiency in vitamin B12 or folate. Therefore, in the view of public health, the detection of such metabolic markers might have an important significance to the control and prevention of neurological disease although more epidemiological evidence still were required [36,39]. Our study found that about 60% of the women were in marginal folate status and 27% in marginal vitamin B12 status and so these women should be paid more attention. Further assessment of the metabolic markers of folate and vitamin B12 could be essential among such female population. Another limitation was that the findings from this study could not be extrapolated to the rest of China, although the sample was representative of Shaanxi province. China is a country that is geographically, climatically and ethnically diverse. Clearly these differences could affect food supply, dietary practices, and consequently folate and vitamin B12 intakes. Geographical difference in folate and vitamin B12 was significant between south and north of China, which might result from different dietary patterns and climate. Moreover, we did not test red blood cell folate in this survey, which could influence accurate estimation of folate level. Nevertheless, our findings provided strong evidence that the deficiency in folate and vitamin B12 was prevalent among Shaanxi women, and especially vitamin B12 deficiency was more serious. Younger women were a high-risk population of being deficient in folate and vitamin B12. We suggested that the control of vitamin B12 deficiency should be considered when practicing the supplementation of folate against NTD in China.

Acknowledgments

We would like to thank all participants of the survey. We are grateful to Health and Family Planning Commission of Shaanxi, and the doctors from the village clinics and community hospitals for their efforts in the coordination of the fieldwork. We are also grateful to all staff for their contribution to data collection.

Author Contributions

Conceived and designed the experiments: HY SD. Performed the experiments: SD LZ QW QL SX. Analyzed the data: SD XF. Wrote the paper: SD HY.

References

1. De Steur H, Gellynck X, Storozhenko S, Liqun G, Lambert W, et al. (2010) Health impact in China of folate-biofortified rice. Nat Biotechnol 28: 554–556.
2. Zhang BY, Zhang T, Lin LM, Wang F, Xin RL, et al. (2008) Correlation between birth defects and dietary nutrition status in a high incidence area of china. Biomed Environ Sci 21(1): 37–44.
3. Hao L, Ma J, Stampfer MJ, Ren A, Tian Y, et al. (2003) Geographical, Seasonal and Gender Differences in Folate Status among Chinese Adults. J Nutr 133: 3630–3635.
4. Hao L, Ma J, Zhu J, Stampfer MJ, Tian Y, et al. (2007) High Prevalence of Hyperhomocysteinemia in Chinese Adults Is Associated with Low Folate, Vitamin B-12, and Vitamin B-6 Status. J Nutr 137: 2407–413 .
5. Wolff T, Witkop CT, Miller T, Syed SB (2009) Folic Acid Supplementation for the Prevention of Neural Tube Defects: An Update of the Evidence for the U.S. Preventive Services Task Force. Ann Intern Med 150(9): 632–639.
6. Berry RJ, Li Z, Erickson JD, Li S, Moore CA, et al. (1999) Prevention of neural-tube defects with folic acid in China. N Engl J Med 341(20): 1485–1490.
7. De Wals P, Tairou F, Van Allen MI, Uh SH, Lowry RB, et al. (2007) Reduction in neural-tube defects after folic acid fortification in Canada. N Engl J Med 357, 135–142.
8. Ministry of Health of China. Management policy on supplementation of folic acid against neural tube defects. Available: http://www.moh.gov.cn/mohbgt/s9510//41532.shtml. Accessed 2013 Aug 25.
9. Li P, Zhou X, Gan L, Yang Y (2012) Analysis of monitoring results for birth defects in Shaanxi province from 2006–2010. Chinese Journal Child Health Care (In Chinese) 20(3): 259–263.
10. Stover PJ (2004) Physiology of Folate and Vitamin B12 in Health and Disease. Nutr Rev 62(6): 3S–12S.
11. Ray JG, Wyatt PR, Thompson MD, Vermeulen MJ, Meier C, et al. (2007) Vitamin B12 and the risk of neural tube defects in a folic-acid-fortified population. Epidemiology 18(3): 362–366.
12. Muthayya S, Kurpad AV, Duggan CP, Bosch RJ, Dwarkanath P, et al. (2006) Low maternal vitamin B12 status is associated with intrauterine growth retardation in urban South Indians. Eur J Clin Nutr 60(6): 791–801.
13. Thompson MD, Cole DE, Ray JG (2009) Vitamin B-12 and neural tube defects: the Canadian experience. Am J Clin Nutr 89(2): 697S–701S.
14. Molloy AM, Kirke PN, Troendle JF, Burke H, Sutton M, et al. (2009) Maternal vitamin B12 status and risk of neural tube defects in a population with high neural tube defect prevalence and no folic acid fortification. Pediatrics 123(3): 917–923.
15. Benson J, Phillips C, Kay M, Webber MT, Ratcliff AJ, et al. (2013) Low vitamin B12 levels among newly-arrived refugees from Bhutan, Iran and Afghanistan: a multicentre Australian study. PLoS One 8(2): e57998.
16. Hao L, Ma J, Zhu J, Stampfer MJ, Tian Y, et al. (2007) High prevalence of hyperhomocysteinemia in Chinese adults is associated with low folate, vitamin B-12, and vitamin B-6 status. J Nutr 137(2): 407–413.
17. Shaanxi Provincial Bureau of Statistics (2012) Statistical yearbook of Shaanxi, 2012. China Statistics Press.
18. Allen LH (2004) Folate and vitamin B12 status in the Americas. Nutr Rev 62: S29–S33.
19. Ganji V, Kafal MR (2006) Trends in serum folate, RBC folate, and circulating total homocysteine concentrations in the United States: analysis of data from National Health and Nutrition Examination Surveys, 1988–1994, 1999–2000, and 2001–2002. J Nutr 136(1): 153–158.
20. McLean E, de Benoist B, Allen LH (2008) Review of the magnitude of folate and vitamin B12 deficiencies worldwide. Food Nutr Bull 29: S38–51.
21. Laillou A, Pham TV, Tran NT, Le HT, Wieringa F, et al. (2012) Micronutrient deficits are still public health issues among women and young children in Vietnam. PLoS One 7: e34906.
22. Seshadri S (2001) Prevalence of micronutrient deficiency particularly of iron, zinc and folic acid in pregnant women in South East Asia. Br J Nutr .85 Suppl 2S87–92
23. WHO (2012) World Health Organization. Nutrition: Micronutrients. Available: http://www.who.int/nutrition/topics/micronutrients/en/.
24. Hughes CF, Ward M, Hoey L, McNulty H (2013) Vitamin B12 and ageing: current issues and interaction with folate. Ann Clin Biochem 50(4): 315–29.
25. Ministry of Health of China (2012) The national report on prevention and treatment of birth defects. Ministry of Health of China, September, 2012. Available: http://www.gov.cn/gzdt/2012-09/12/content_2223371.htm. Accessed 2013 May 5.
26. Schnyder G, Roffi M, Pin R, Flammer Y, Lange H, et al. (2001) Decreased rate of coronary restenosis after lowering of plasma homocysteine levels. N Engl J Med 345: 1593–600.
27. Quadri P, Fragiacomo C, Pezzati R, Zanda E, Forloni G, et al. (2004) Homocysteine, folate and vitamin B-12 in mild cognitive impairment, Alzheimer disease, and vascular dementia. Am J Clin Nutr 80: 114–22.
28. Ellinson M, Thomas J, Patterson A (2004) A critical evaluation of the relationship between serum vitamin B, folate and total homocysteine with cognitive impairment in the elderly. J Hum Nutr Diet 17(4): 371–383.
29. Veena SR, Krishnaveni GV, Srinivasan K, Wills AK, Muthayya S, et al. (2010) Higher maternal plasma folate but not vitamin B-12 concentrations during pregnancy are associated with better cognitive function scores in 9- to 10- year-old children in South India. J Nutr 140(5): 1014–22.
30. Nguyen PH, Nguyen H, Gonzalez-Casanova I, Copeland E, Strizich G, et al. (2014) Micronutrient Intakes among Women of Reproductive Age in Vietnam. PLoS One 9(2): e89504.
31. Liu R, Dang S, Yan H, Wang D, Zhao Y, et al. (2013) Association between dietary proteins intake and risk of hypertension: a cross-sectional study from rural western China. Hypertens Res 36: 972–979.
32. Liu R, Dang S, Yan H, Li Q, Zhao Y, et al. (2012) Dietary patterns and nutrients intakes in rural residents in Hanzhong of Shaanxi Province. Wei Sheng Yan Jiu 41(6): 997–1003.
33. Liu RR, Dang SN, Wang WH, Fan XJ, Yan H, et al. (2013) Study on the diet quality and its relative effect factors among rural residents, using the Chinese Diet Balance Index (CDBI) in Hanzhong, Shaanxi province. Zhonghua Liu Xing Bing Xue Za Zhi 34(3): 225–30.
34. Herrmann W, Obeid R, Schorr H, Geisel J (2005) The usefulness of holotranscobalamin in predicting vitamin B12 status in different clinical settings. Curr Drug Metab 6(1): 47–53.
35. Selhub J, Jacques PF, Dallal G, Choumenkovitch S, Rogers G (2008)The use of blood concentrations of vitamins and their respective functional indicators to define folate and vitamin B12 status. Food Nutr Bull 29: S67–73.
36. Hooshmand B, Solomon A, Kareholt I, Rusanen M, Hänninen T, et al. (2011) Serum homocysteine, holotranscobalamin, folate and cognition in the elderly: a longitudinal study. J Intern Med 271: 204–12.
37. Clarke R, Birks J, Nexo E, Ueland PM, Schneede J, et al. (2007) Low vitamin B-12 status and risk of cognitive decline in older adults. Am J Clin Nutr 86: 1384–91.
38. Vogiatzoglou A, Oulhaj A, Smith AD, Nurk E, Drevon CA, et al. (2009) Determinants of plasma methylmalonic acid in a large population: implications for assessment of vitamin B12 status. Clin Chem 55: 2198–206.
39. Smith AD, Refsum H (2012) Do we need to reconsider the desirable blood level of vitamin B12? J Intern Med 271(2): 179–82.

Vitamin D Deficiency Aggravates Chronic Kidney Disease Progression after Ischemic Acute Kidney Injury

Janaína Garcia Gonçalves, Ana Carolina de Bragança, Daniele Canale, Maria Heloisa Massola Shimizu, Talita Rojas Sanches, Rosa Maria Affonso Moysés, Lúcia Andrade, Antonio Carlos Seguro, Rildo Aparecido Volpini*

Nephrology Department, University of São Paulo School of Medicine, São Paulo, Brazil

Abstract

Background: Despite a significant improvement in the management of chronic kidney disease (CKD), its incidence and prevalence has been increasing over the years. Progressive renal fibrosis is present in CKD and involves the participation of several cytokines, including Transforming growth factor-β1 (TGF-β1). Besides cardiovascular diseases and infections, several studies show that Vitamin D status has been considered as a non-traditional risk factor for the progression of CKD. Given the importance of vitamin D in the maintenance of essential physiological functions, we studied the events involved in the chronic kidney disease progression in rats submitted to ischemia/reperfusion injury under vitamin D deficiency (VDD).

Methods: Rats were randomized into four groups: Control; VDD; ischemia/reperfusion injury (IRI); and VDD+IRI. At the 62 day after sham or IRI surgery, we measured inulin clearance, biochemical variables and hemodynamic parameters. In kidney tissue, we performed immunoblotting to quantify expression of Klotho, TGF-β, and vitamin D receptor (VDR); gene expression to evaluate renin, angiotensinogen, and angiotensin-converting enzyme; and immunohistochemical staining for ED1 (macrophages), type IV collagen, fibronectin, vimentin, and α-smooth mucle actin. Histomorphometric studies were performed to evaluate fractional interstitial area.

Results: IRI animals presented renal hypertrophy, increased levels of mean blood pressure and plasma PTH. Furthermore, expansion of the interstitial area, increased infiltration of ED1 cells, increased expression of collagen IV, fibronectin, vimentin and α-actin, and reduced expression of Klotho protein were observed. VDD deficiency contributed to increased levels of plasma PTH as well as for important chronic tubulointerstitial changes (fibrosis, inflammatory infiltration, tubular dilation and atrophy), increased expression of TGF-β1 and decreased expression of VDR and Klotho protein observed in VDD+IRI animals.

Conclusion: Through inflammatory pathways and involvement of TGF-β1 growth factor, VDD could be considered as an aggravating factor for tubulointerstitial damage and fibrosis progression following acute kidney injury induced by ischemia/reperfusion.

Editor: Makoto Makishima, Nihon University School of Medicine, Japan

Funding: Fundação de Amparo à Pesquisa do Estado de São Paulo - FAPESP (www.fapesp.br) Grant number: 2010/52294-0. The funders had no role in study design, data collection and analysis, decision to publish, or preparation of the manuscript.

Competing Interests: The authors have declared that no competing interests exist.

* Email: rildovolpini@yahoo.com.br

Introduction

In most countries, the incidence and prevalence of chronic kidney disease (CKD) have been increasing over the years mainly due to the aging population and the presence of diabetic nephropathy [1,2]. It is well established that acute kidney injury (AKI) after ischemia/reperfusion injury (IRI) is a major cause of AKI [3]. IRI physiology involves a complex interaction among vascular, tubular and inflammatory factors followed by a repair process that can restore function and epithelial differentiation or result in CKD with progressive development of fibrosis [4,5].

It has been shown that the mortality of patients with CKD is directly related to renal function associated with cardiovascular diseases and infections [6]. However, such traditional risks explain only about half of mortality and various studies are being directed to non-traditional risk factors, such as vitamin D [6].

Vitamin D [25(OH)D] is a circulating hormone in the body indispensable for mineral homeostasis [7] and responsible for kidney protection and regulation of several physiological activities as well [8]. Thus, vitamin D deficiency (VDD) (<10 ng/mL) or insufficiency (10–30 ng/mL) can accelerate the progression of kidney disease [9–11]. The biologically active form of vitamin D is produced in the kidney by mitochondria of the renal proximal convoluted tubules, where 1α-hydroxylase converts 25-hydroxyvitamin D [25(OH)D] to 1,25-dihydroxyvitamin D3 [1,25 $(OH)_2D_3$] or calcitriol [12]. The classical 1,25 $(OH)_2D_3$ pathway requires the nuclear vitamin D receptor (VDR), which is a transcription factor for 1,25 $(OH)_2$ D_3 target genes [4,5,13].

The renal conversion of vitamin D into biologically active form is tightly regulated by several factors, including parathormone (PTH), phosphorus levels and fibroblast growth factor 23 (FGF-23) [12]. FGF-23 is a phosphatonin produced by osteocytes which promotes renal phosphate excretion [8,14–16] and a close relationship between FGF-23 and Klotho is described [17]. The lack of Klotho gene expression (α-klotho) is associated with premature phenotypes related to aging as well as to hyperphosphatemia and low levels of vitamin D [18]. Klotho protein forms binary complexes with fibroblast growth factor receptors (FGFR), increasing Klotho affinity and selectivity for FGF-23 [17], playing an important role in vitamin D synthesis.

Given the importance of vitamin D in essential physiological functions and the respective low levels of this hormone observed in CKD, our aim was to study the vitamin D deficiency in a murine model of CKD progression after AKI induced by ischemia/reperfusion.

Materials and Methods

Experimental Animals and Induction of I/R Injury

The study was approved by the Research Ethics Committee of the University of São Paulo – School of Medicine, protocol numbered 088/12. All procedures were developed in strict accordance with local institutional guidelines and with well-established international standards for the care and use of laboratory animals. All surgery was performed under appropriate anesthesia, and all efforts were made to minimize suffering.

Male Wistar rats (180–200 g) were provided by the University of São Paulo - School of Medicine animal facility. During the 90-day experiment, rats were maintained under standard laboratory conditions, receiving vitamin D-free or standard diets (MP Biomedicals, Irvine, CA, USA) and free access to tap water for 90 days. Rats were divided into four groups: (C) Control (n = 11), received a standard diet for 90 days and submitted to sham surgery; (VDD) Vitamin D Deficiency (n = 8), received a vitamin D-free diet for 90 days and submitted to sham surgery; (IRI) Ischemia/Reperfusion Injury (n = 10), received a standard diet for 90 days and submitted to ischemia/reperfusion injury; and (VDD+IRI) Vitamin D Deficiency plus Ischemia/Reperfusion Injury (n = 9), received a vitamin D-free diet for 90 days and submitted to ischemia/reperfusion injury.

Sham Surgery. On day 28, rats from Control and VDD groups were anesthetized with 2,2,2-Tribromoethanol (250 mg/Kg body weight), and a suprapubic incision was made and then sutured immediately.

Induction of Ischemia/Reperfusion Injury. As described above, on day 28, rats from IRI and VDD+IRI groups were anesthetized, a suprapubic incision was made for induction of ischemic renal injury by clamping both renal arteries for 45 min, followed by reperfusion.

Analysis of Urine Samples

On day 89, all rats were placed in individual metabolic cages, on a 12/12-h light/dark cycle, with free access to drinking water. We collected 24-h urine samples, centrifuged them and analyzed the supernatants. We measured urinary concentrations of sodium and calcium by ion-selective electrodes (ABL800 Flex Analyzer – Radiometer, Brønshøj, Denmark) and urinary phosphorus by automated enzymatic colorimetric assay (COBAS C111 Analyzer – Roche, USA). Urinary protein excretion was measured by a colorimetric system using a commercial kit (Labtest Diagnóstica, Minas Gerais, Brazil).

Inulin Clearance and Hemodynamic Studies

On day 90, the animals were anesthetized with sodium thiopental (50 mg/Kg BW) and placed on a temperature-regulated surgical table. The trachea was cannulated (PE-240 catheter) and spontaneous breathing was maintained. The jugular vein was cannulated (PE-60 catheter) for infusion of inulin and fluids. To monitor mean arterial pressure (MAP) and collect blood samples, the right carotid artery was catheterized with a PE-50 catheter. We assessed MAP with a data acquisition system (MP100; Biopac Systems, Santa Barbara, CA, USA). To collect urine samples, the urinary bladder was cannulated (PE-240 catheter) by suprapubic incision. After completion of the cannulation surgical procedure, a loading dose of inulin (100 mg/Kg body weight diluted in 1 mL of 0.9% saline) was administered through the jugular vein. Subsequently, a constant infusion of inulin (10 mg/kg body weight in 0.9% saline) was started and continued at 0.04 mL/min throughout the whole experiment. Three urine samples were collected at 30-min intervals. Blood samples were obtained at the beginning and at the end of the experiment. Inulin clearance values represent the mean of three periods. Blood and urine inulin were determined by the anthrone method, and the glomerular filtration rate (GFR) data is expressed as ml/min/100 g BW. To measure the renal blood flow (RBF), an ultrasonic flow probe was placed around the exposed renal artery (T402; Transonic Systems, Bethesda, MD, USA) and RBF was expressed as ml/min. To calculate renal vascular resistance (RVR, in mmHg/ml/min), we divided blood pressure by RBF.

Evaluation of Biochemical Parameters

To assess plasma levels of 25-hydroxyvitamin D [25(OH)D], parathormone (PTH), fibroblast growth factor 23 (FGF-23), sodium (P_{Na}), potassium (P_K), phosphate (P_P) and calcium (P_{Ca}), we collected blood samples after the clearance studies. We assessed 25(OH)D by radioimmunoassay (RIA) using a commercial kit (25-Hydroxyvitamin D^{125}, DiaSorin, Vercelli, Italy) and PTH by Enzyme-Linked Immunosorbet Assay (ELISA) using a commercial kit (Rat Bioactive Intact PTH, Immunotopics, CA, USA). FGF-23 levels were assessed by ELISA using a commercial kit (FGF-23 ELISA Kit, Kainos Laboratories, Tokyo, Japan). P_P and P_{Ca} were evaluated by automated enzymatic colorimetric assay (COBAS C111 Analyzer – Roche, USA) while P_{Na} and P_K were measured by ion-selective electrodes (ABL800 Flex Analyzer – Radiometer, Brønshøj, Denmark).

Tissue Sample Collection/Preparation

After blood samples collection, we perfused kidneys with phosphate-buffered solution (PBS, pH 7.4). Right kidneys were frozen in liquid nitrogen and stored at −80°C for Western blotting and real-time quantitative polymerase chain reaction (qPCR). Left kidneys were removed and weighed. Fragments of left kidney were fixed in 10% neutral-buffered formalin or methacarn's solution for 24 hours and in 70% alcohol thereafter. Kidney blocks were embedded in paraffin and cut into 4-µm sections for histological and immunohistochemical examination.

Preparation of Samples for Western Blotting

Kidney samples were homogenized in ice-cold isolation solution (200 mM manitol, 80 mM HEPES and 41 mM KOH, pH 7.5) containing a protease inhibitors cocktail (Sigma Chemical Company, St. Louis, MO, USA) using a homogenizer (Polytron - PT 10–35, Brinkmann Instruments, Westbury, NY, USA). Homogenates were centrifuged at low speed (2000×g) for 15 min at 4°C to remove nuclei and cell debris. Supernatants were isolated, and protein was determined by Bradford assay (BioAgency Laboratórios, São Paulo, Brazil).

Electrophoresis and Immunoblotting

Proteins were separated on SDS-polyacrylamide minigels by electrophoresis [19]. After transfer by electroelution to polyvinylidene difluoride (PVDF) membranes (GE Healthcare Limited, Little Chalfont, UK), blots were blocked for 60 minutes with 5% non-fat dry milk in Tris-buffered saline solution. Blots were then incubated overnight with antibodies against Actin (1:5,000), VDR (1:500), Klotho (1:500) and TGF-beta (1:200) (Santa Cruz Biotechnology, CA, USA). The labeling was visualized with horseradish peroxidase-conjugated secondary antibody (anti-rabbit IgG, diluted 1:2,000, or anti-goat, diluted 1:10,000, Sigma Chemical, St. Louis, MO, USA) and enhanced chemiluminescence (ECL) detection system (GE Healthcare Limited, Little Chalfont, UK).

Kidney protein levels. The images were obtained using an imaging system (Alliance 4.2; Uvitec, Cambridge, UK). We used densitometry to quantitatively analyze the protein levels, normalizing the bands to actin expression.

Gene Expression

We performed real-time qPCR in frozen renal tissue, assessing the following genes: renin (Rn00561847_m1), angiotensinogen (Rn00593114_m1), and angiotensin converting enzyme (Rn00561094_m1), (Applied Biosystems, Foster City, CA, USA). We extracted and prepared total RNA. For cDNA synthesis, we used total RNA and a Superscript VILO MasterMix (Invitrogen Technologies, Carlsbad, CA, USA). We performed real-time PCR using TaqMan on Step One Plus (Applied Biosystems, Foster City, CA, USA). All primers were purchased from Invitrogen. Relative gene expression values were evaluated with the $2^{-\Delta\Delta Ct}$ method [20] using GAPDH (Rn01775763_g1) as housekeeping gene.

Light Microscopy

Four-µm histological sections of kidney tissue were stained with Masson's trichome and examined under light microscope. The fractional interstitial area (FIA) of the renal cortex was determined by morphometry with a light camera connected to an image analyzer (Axiovision, Carl Zeiss, Eching, Germany). We analyzed 30 grid fields (0.087 mm^2 each) per kidney cortex. The interstitial areas were demarcated manually on a video screen, and the proportion of the field they occupied was determined by computerized morphometry [21].The morphometric examination was blinded to minimize observer bias, i.e. the observer was unaware of the treatment group from which the tissue originated.

Immunohistochemistry

Samples were processed in 4-µm paraffin sections and then subjected to incubation overnight at 4°C according to each protocol developed for each primary antibody. We used the following antibodies: (1:500) monoclonal anti-ED1 (macrophages) (AbD Serotec, Oxford, UK); (1:200) polyclonal anti-Collagen IV (Abcam, Cambridge, UK); (1:400) polyclonal anti-FN1 (fibronectin) (Sigma-Aldrich, Saint Louis, MO, USA); (1:1,000) monoclonal anti-α-smooth-muscle actin (α-SMA) (Millipore, Billerica, MA, USA); and (1:50) monoclonal anti-vimentin (Dako, Glostrup, Denmark). The reaction product was detected with an avidin-biotin-peroxidase complex (Vector Laboratories, Burlingame, CA, USA). The color reaction was developed with 3,3-diaminobenzidine (Sigma Chemical, St. Louis, MO, USA) in the presence of hydrogen peroxide, and the sections were counterstained with Harris' hematoxylin.

For ED1, we analyzed 40–60 renal cortex fields. The result of the immunoreaction was quantified by couting the number of ED1 positive cells per field (0.087 mm^2 each) and averaging the number of cells per field for each section [21]. To evaluate immunoreactivity to collagen IV, fibronectin, α-SMA and vimentin, the volume ratios of positive areas of renal tissue sections, determined by the color limit, were obtained using Image-Pro Plus software (Media Cybernetics, Silver Spring, MD, USA) and the results were expressed as percentages [22].

Statistical Analysis

All quantitative data are mean±standard error of the mean (SEM). Comparisons between groups were made by unpaired t-test. Comparisons among groups were made by one-way analysis of variance followed by the Student–Newman–Keuls test. Values of $p<0.05$ were considered statistically significant.

Results

Body weight and hemodynamics

As described in Table 1, there were no differences in body weight among the studied groups since all animals showed similar food ingestion (~25 g/day) during 90 days. The kidney weight/body weight ratio was calculated and, as expected, IRI and VDD+IRI groups presented an increase of this proportion (Table 1). We did not observe differences among the groups concerning glomerular filtration rate (GFR), renal blood flow (RBF) and renal vascular resistance (RVR). However, we found increased levels (mmHg) of mean arterial pressure (MAP) in VDD (135.2±3.4), IRI (137.3±3.6) and VDD+IRI (134.5±5.2) when compared to Control (119.4±2.3) group ($p<0.05$), Table 1.

Vitamin D and PTH levels

The animals were maintained on a standard or a free-vitamin D diet for 90 days. Over the experimental period, the levels of 25(OH)D from VDD and VDD+IRI groups were undetectable (< 1.5 ng/mL), while Control and IRI groups presented 15.4 and 15.0 ng/mL respectively (Table 2). Concerning PTH data, we found significant higher levels (pg/mL) of the respective hormone in VDD (1,250±155) and VDD+IRI (2,187±336), showing the negative feedback caused by vitamin D deficiency in these groups. Both VDD and VDD+IRI groups presented a significant increase of PTH levels when compared to Control (318±59) and IRI (453±96) groups. Furthermore, VDD+IRI presented significant high levels of PTH when compared to the other groups (Table 2).

Vitamin D deficiency and blood pressure control

In order to further investigate the role of vitamin D on blood pressure control, we evaluated the gene expression (qPCR) of some renin-angiotensin system (RAS) compounds and plasma aldosterone levels as well. The qPCR results showed increased gene expression of renin, angiotensinogen (AGT) and angiotensin converting enzyme (ACE) in VDD, IRI and VDD+IRI when compared to control group (Table 3). In addition, we found higher levels of aldosterone (pg/mL) in VDD (455.8±69.0), IRI

Table 1. Body weight, kidney weight, renal function and hemodynamic measurements after 90 days evaluated in Control rats (C), Vitamin D deficient rats (VDD), rats submitted to Ischemia/Reperfusion Injury (IRI), and Vitamin D deficient rats submitted to Ischemia/Reperfusion Injury (VDD+IRI).

	C	VDD	IRI	VDD+IRI
BW	519.4±11.6	551.4±19.8	515.8±13.6	510.1±14.1
KW/BW	0.36±0.01	0.35±0.01	0.42±0.02 [c,f]	0.44±0.01 [c,e]
GFR	0.62±0.02	0.56±0.04	0.57±0.04	0.57±0.02
MAP	119.4±2.3	135.2±3.4 [c]	137.3±3.6 [c]	134.5±5.2 [c]
RBF	5.61±0.02	5.82±0.06	5.62±0.08	5.83±0.07
RVR	22.02±0.52	24.82±1.09	24.72±0.67	23.4±0.91

BW, body weight (g); KW/BW. kidney weight/body weight ratio; GFR, inulin clearance (mL/min/100 g); MAP, mean arterial pressure (mmHg); RBF, renal blood flow (mL/min); RVR, renal vascular resistance (mmHg/mL/min). Values are mean ± SEM. [c] $p<0.05$ vs. C; [e] $p<0.01$ vs. VDD; [f] $p<0.05$ vs. VDD.

(416.0±89.2) and VDD+IRI (502.5±134.2) when compared to Control (165.7±17.2) group (Table 2). Taken together, our results reinforce the role of vitamin D on blood pressure control.

Proteinuria, calcium, phosphorus and FGF-23 – Klotho axis

As shown in Table 2, we observed a progressive and significant ($p<0.001$) increase of proteinuria (mg/24 h) among the studied groups: Control (5.96±0.53), VDD (17.16±1.56), IRI (23.97±1.43) and VDD+IRI (32.31±0.51). Neither calcium and phosphorus levels nor urinary volume presented differences among the groups (Table 2). Considering the fact that the levels of calcium and phosphorus are closely related to FGF-23 - Klotho axis, we investigated plasmatic levels of FGF-23 and the renal expression of Klotho. We observed decreased levels of FGF-23 (pg/mL) in VDD (41.8±14.6) and VDD+IRI (77.4±18.5) groups when compared to Control (293.1±33.8) and IRI (225.4±24.0) groups (Table 2). Also, we found a decreased expression of Klotho protein (%) in VDD (47.5±6.0), IRI (53.3±7.6) and VDD+IRI (46.7±2.5) when compared to Control (98.8±0.8) group (Figure 1). In addition, similar profile was found concerning gene expression of α-klotho (Table 3).

Histomorphological studies

Light microscopy studies revealed histological alterations such as interstitial fibrosis, tubular atrophy and dilatation, and inflammatory cell infiltrates in the renal cortex of vitamin D deficient and ischemic/reperfusion injury groups (Figure 2). The alterations were subtle, but evident in VDD animals and more prominent in IRI and VDD+IRI groups. In addition, morphometric studies were performed to evaluate the fractional interstitial area (FIA) of the renal cortex. We observed a progressive and increasing involvement of the tubulointerstitial compartment, featuring interstitial expansion and renal fibrosis as follows: Control and VDD groups showed 7.35% and 17.23% of FIA, respectively while IRI and VDD+IRI groups presented 24.41 and 34.87% of FIA, respectively. Based on our results, we could infer that vitamin D deficiency exerts an important role on interstitial expansion and fibrosis formation.

Macrophages infiltration

The number of ED1 positive cells, a marker to macrophages, was evaluated by immunohistochemical studies. We found a significant number of infiltrating ED1 positive cells/per field (0.087 mm^2) in IRI (10.92±1.89) and VDD+IRI (16.93±2.49)

Table 2. Biochemical parameters after 90 days evaluated in Control rats (C), Vitamin D deficient rats (VDD), rats submitted to Ischemia/Reperfusion Injury (IRI), and Vitamin D deficient rats submitted to Ischemia/Reperfusion Injury (VDD+IRI).

	C	VDD	IRI	VDD+IRI
25(OH)D	15.4±1.0	<1.5 (undetectable) [a]	15.0±0.6 [d]	<1.5 (undetectable)[a,g]
PTH	318±59	1,250±155 [c]	453±96 [f]	2,187±336 [a,f,g]
Aldosterone	165.7±17.2	455.8±69.0 [c]	416.0±89.2 [c]	502.5±134.2 [c]
FGF-23	293.1±33.8	41.8±14.6 [a,g]	225.4±24.0	77.4±18.5 [a,g]
P_P	4.8±0.2	5.2±0.2	5.5±0.2	5.3±0.3
P_{Ca}	9.48±0.50	8.81±0.41	9.28±0.15	8.17±0.40
P_{Na}	139.5±1.2	136±0.6	137.4±2.2	137.7±0.6
P_K	4.6±0.1	4.0±0.2	4.5±0.1	4.3±0.2
UV	14.23±0.93	13.40±1.03	14.42±1.71	11.13±1.77
$U_{Prot}V$	5.97±0.53	17.16±1.56 [a]	23.97±1.43 [a,d]	32.31±0.52 [a,d,g]

25(OH)D, 25 hydroxyvitamin D (ng/mL); PTH, parathormone (pg/mL); Aldosterone (pg/mL); FGF-23, fibroblast growth factor 23 (pg/mL); P_P, plasma phosphate concentration (mg/dL); P_{Ca}, plasma calcium concentration (mg/dL); P_{Na}, plasma sodium concentration (mEq/L); P_K, plasma potassium concentration (mEq/L); UV, urinary volume (mL/24 h); $U_{Prot}V$, urinary protein excretion (mg/24 h). Values are means ± SEM. [a] $p<0.001$, [b] $p<0.01$, [c] $p<0.05$ vs. C; [d] $p<0.001$ vs. VDD; [f] $p<0.05$ vs. VDD; [g] $p<0.001$ vs. IRI.

Table 3. Relative gene expression of α-klotho and renin-angiotensin system (RAS) compounds after 90 days evaluated in Control rats (C), Vitamin D deficient rats (VDD), rats submitted to Ischemia/Reperfusion Injury (IRI), and Vitamin D deficient rats submitted to Ischemia/Reperfusion Injury (VDD+IRI).

	C	VDD	IRI	VDD+IRI
renin	0.68±0.49	2.28±0.28 [b]	1.85±0.47 [c]	2.34±0.28 [c]
AGT	0.95±0.45	2.95±0.69 [c]	4.02±0.60 [b]	4.53±0.63 [b]
ACE	1.10±0.63	3.94±0.82 [c]	5.28±0.94 [c]	5.90±1.28 [c]
α-klotho	3.27±1.15	2.07±0.41	2.39±0.38	1.74±0.46

AGT, angiotensinogen; ACE, angiotensin-converting enzyme. Values are mean ± SEM. Relative gene expression values were evaluated with the $2^{-\Delta\Delta Ct}$ method using GAPDH as housekeeping gene. [b] $p<0.01$ and [c] $p<0.05$ vs. C.

when compared to VDD (2.18±0.14) and Control (1.14±0.19) groups. Vitamin D deficiency enhanced this alteration since VDD+IRI presented an increased number of ED1 positive cells than did the other groups (Figure 3).

Extracellular matrix components

As described above, our histological results showed that vitamin D deficiency is an aggravating factor for the expansion of tubulointerstitial compartment and fibrosis formation. This process is complex and involves the production and secretion of many extracellular matrix (ECM) components. So, we performed immunohistochemical studies for type IV collagen and fibronectin, two fibrous components of ECM. Our results showed increased expression of type IV collagen (Figure 4) and fibronectin (Figure 5), demonstrated as percentage of positive area, in the renal cortex of VDD, IRI and VDD+IRI groups when compared to Control group. Vitamin D deficiency enhanced the immunostainings for both ECM markers (Figures 4 and 5).

Phenotypic alteration of renal cells

Besides ECM markers studies, we also aimed to evaluate the presence of phenotypic alteration of renal tubular cells. We used the expression of vimentin to detect tubular injury and α-smooth muscle actin (α-SMA) as a marker for interstitial fibroblast activation. In Control group, the expression of vimentin and α-SMA was identical to that described in normal rats: vimentin was confined to smooth muscle cells and glomerular compartment (mensangial cells and podocytes), and α-SMA to arterial smooth muscle cells [23]. The percentage of positive area for vimentin was increased in IRI when compared to Control and VDD groups. Moreover, VDD+IRI group presented higher vimentin expression than did the other studied groups (Figure 6). A similar profile was found concerning α-SMA expression, even though without statistical difference between IRI and VDD+IRI groups (Figure 7). In addition, vitamin D deficiency may be involved in this cellular phenotypic alteration, since the animals from VDD+IRI groups presented a significant expression of vimentin and a slight increase of α-SMA expression when compared to IRI group (Figures 6 and 7).

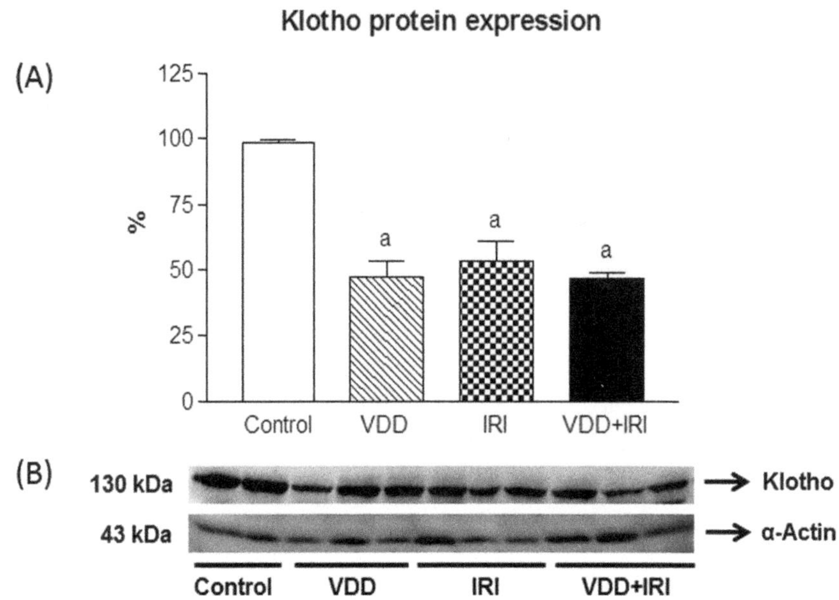

Figure 1. Semiquantitative immunoblotting of kidney fractions. (A) A densitometric analysis of samples from control (n = 4), VDD (n = 6), IRI (n = 6) and VDD+IRI (n = 6) rats is shown. (B) Immunoblots reacted with anti-Klotho revealing a 130-kDa band. Values are mean ± SEM. [a] $p<0.001$ vs. C.

I

II

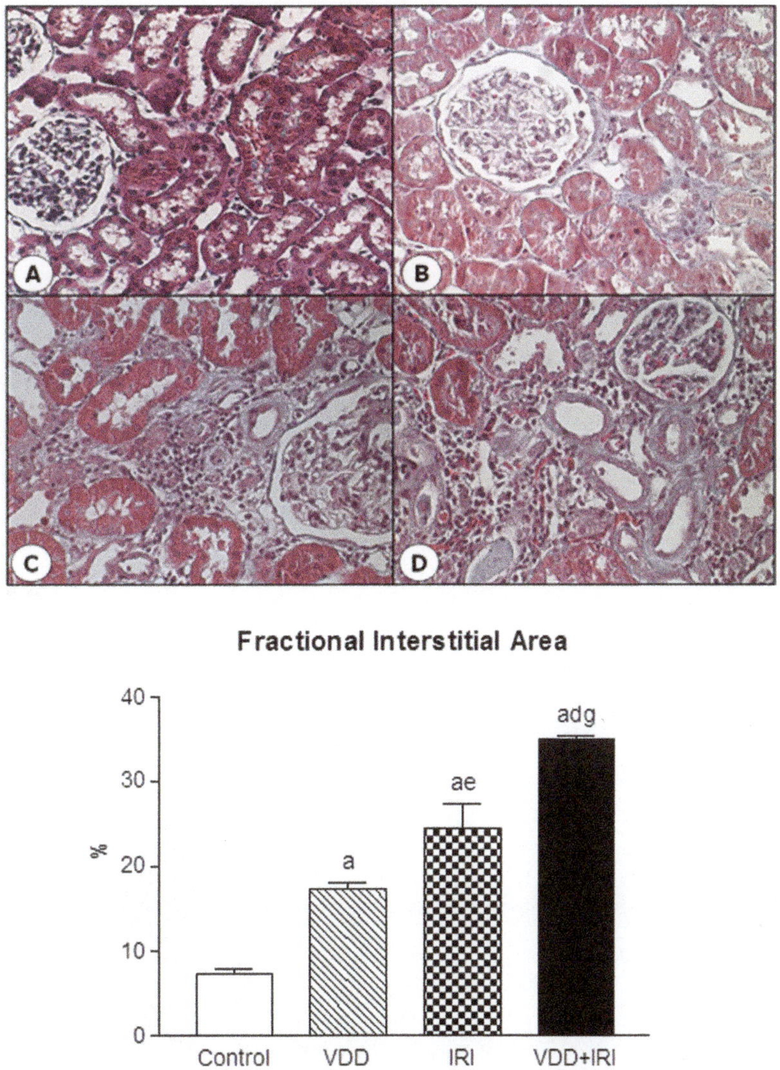

Figure 2. [I] Representative photomicrographs of renal histological changes after 90 days observed in a control rat (A), a vitamin D deficient rat (B), in a rat submitted to ischemia/reperfusion injury (C), and in a vitamin D deficient rat submitted to ischemia/ reperfusion injury (D). [II] Fractional interstitial area evaluated 90 days after in Control (C), Vitamin D Deficiency (VDD), Ischemia-Reperfusion Injury (IRI), and Vitamin D Deficiency and Ischemia/Reperfusion Injury (VDD+IRI) groups. Values are mean ± SEM. [a] $p<0.001$ vs. C; [d] $p<0.001$ vs. VDD; [e] $p<0.01$ vs. VDD; [g] $p<0.001$ vs. IRI.

Vitamin D deficiency, VDR and fibrosis formation

Our results related to histological and immunohistochemical studies revealed a potential involvement of vitamin D with renal fibrosis. To assess the possible link between vitamin D deficiency and fibrosis formation, we decided to study the role TGF-β expression, the most important pro-fibrotic cytokine, and its relationship with the vitamin D receptor (VDR). For that, we analyzed the renal expression of VDR and TGF-β in both IRI and VDD+IRI groups, since these groups presented expressive percentages of interstitial expansion and fibrosis. We observed a significant decrease in VDR expression (%) in VDD+IRI group (44.3±7.6) when compared to IRI group (100.0±22.0) (Figure 8-I). Concerning TGF-β, we found a significant increased expression (%) of this cytokine in the kidneys of VDD+IRI animals (196.3±41.9) when compared to IRI group (100.1±14.9) (Figure 8-II). So, analyzing the results, we observed that vitamin D deficiency caused a decrease in VDR expression and an increase in TGF-β expression in VDD+IRI group, which had the highest ratio of fibrosis.

Discussion

In our experimental ischemia/reperfusion injury model, we found renal hypertrophy, increased levels of blood pressure and proteinuria in both ischemic animal groups. Furthermore, we observed enlargement of the interstitial area, including increased infiltration of ED1 positive cells and presence of fibrosis, and phenotypic modification of renal tubular cells. Vitamin D deficiency contributed to the elevation of plasma PTH and decrease of plasma FGF-23 levels as well as for important chronic tubulointerstitial changes. In addition, we found increased expression of cytokine TGF-β1 and decreased expression of VDR receptor and Klotho protein in vitamin D-deficient animals submitted to ischemia/reperfusion injury.

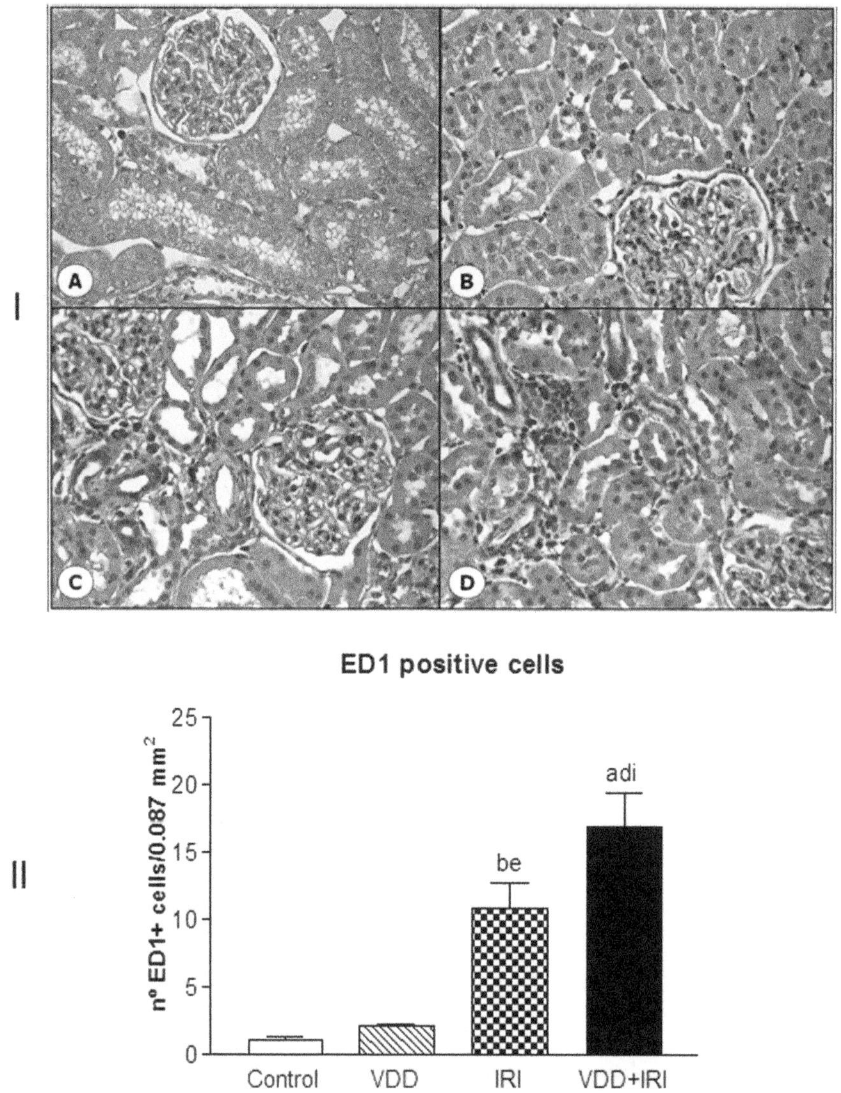

Figure 3. [I] Expression of ED1 positive cells in the renal cortex of a control rat (A), a vitamin D deficient rat (B), in a rat submitted to ischemia/reperfusion injury (C), and in a vitamin D deficient rat submitted to ischemia/reperfusion injury (D). [II] Number of ED1 positive cells per field (0.087 mm^2) evaluated 90 days after in Control (C), Vitamin D Deficiency (VDD), Ischemia-Reperfusion Injury (IRI), and Vitamin D Deficiency and Ischemia/Reperfusion Injury (VDD+IRI) groups. Values are mean ± SEM. ^{a} $p<0.001$ vs. C; ^{b} $p<0.01$ vs. C; ^{d} $p<0.001$ vs. VDD; ^{e} $p<0.01$ vs. VDD; ^{f} $p<0.05$ vs. IRI.

Our results clearly show that animals fed the vitamin D-free diet presented undetectable levels of 25(OH)D. The plasma level of 25(OH)D reflects vitamin D intake from foods and supplements, as well as cutaneous synthesis [24]. In addition to calcium and phosphorus, another important compound related to vitamin D synthesis is PTH level. Our results showed high levels of PTH in VDD, mainly in VDD+IRI group. These alterations were expected since the lack of vitamin D reduces intestinal calcium absorption, leading to a lower level of calcium and higher production of PTH by the parathyroid gland. PTH, in turn, acts on bone tissue in order to attenuate the decrease in serum calcium and the increase in phosphorus excretion [25].

We also investigated the role of vitamin D on blood pressure control. In our study, ischemic and vitamin D deficient rats showed higher levels of blood pressure. This alteration was accompanied by an increased mRNA expression of some RAS compounds, including renin, angiotensinogen and ACE. Furthermore, we found increased levels of plasma aldosterone in VDD, IRI and VDD+IRI groups. So, our data reinforce an important role of vitamin D in blood pressure control. In fact, strong evidences from studies conducted in humans and animals show that vitamin D can be related to a decrease in the renin-angiotensin activity [26,27]. Also, it has been demonstrated that vitamin D deficiency can led to an upregulation of the RAS, changes in the endothelium, and vascular smooth cells as well [27–29]. Li *et al* [30] demonstrated that VDR knockout mice showed increased renin expression and hypertension, and these changes were suppressed by an analogue of vitamin D.

Studies have shown that vitamin D deficiency is associated with increased prevalence of proteinuria in adult population, a marker of CKD progression [31,32]. Our results showed a progressive and significant increase of proteinuria among the studied groups (C, VDD, IRI and VDD+IRI, respectively). In addition, it was noteworthy that vitamin D deficiency enhanced proteinuria in

I

II

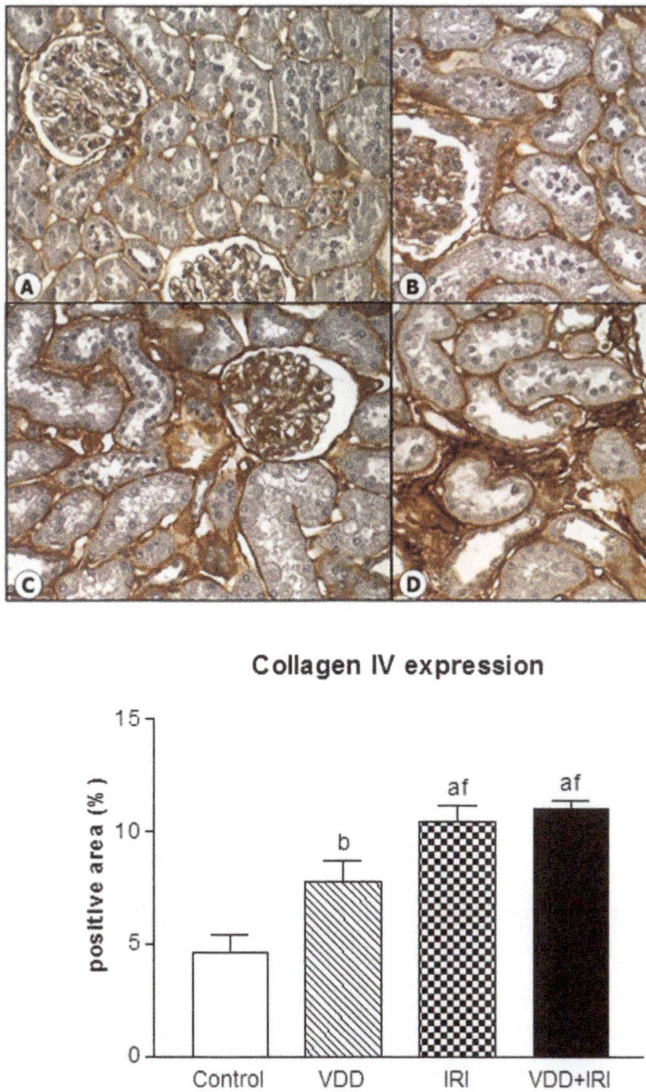

Figure 4. [I] Expression of type IV collagen in the renal cortex of a control rat (A), a vitamin D deficient rat (B), in a rat submitted to ischemia/reperfusion injury (C), and in a vitamin D deficient rat submitted to ischemia/reperfusion injury (D). [II] Evaluation of type IV collagen expression 90 days after in Control (C), Vitamin D Deficiency (VDD), Ischemia-Reperfusion Injury (IRI), and Vitamin D Deficiency and Ischemia/Reperfusion Injury (VDD+IRI) groups. Values are mean ± SEM. [a] $p<0.001$ vs. C; [b] $p<0.01$ vs. C; [f] $p<0.05$ vs. VDD.

VDD and VDD+IRI. However, the mechanisms by which proteinuria leads to reduced levels of vitamin D in the body or vice versa are not fully understood [32]. It is known that vitamin D levels can trigger proteinuria by direct and indirect factors. Through direct cellular effects, low levels of vitamin D induce loss of podocytes and development of glomerulosclerosis, damaging the integrity of the glomerular filtration membrane [33]. Indirectly, vitamin D suppresses renin transcription contributing to a reduction in proteinuria by hemodynamic effects [34].

As previously described, the conversion of vitamin D into biologically active form is tightly regulated by several factors, including FGF-23 [12]. In addition to promote renal phosphate excretion, FGF-23 suppresses the production of vitamin D by inhibition of 1-α-hydroxylase and stimulation of 24-hydroxylase [8,14–16]. Recent findings have been supporting an increasingly and important role of FGF-23 as the initial event in the development of CKD. The first step for that is featured by increased levels of FGF-23 preceding changes in calcium, phosphorus, PTH, or even calcitriol levels [35], that is, its respective regulatory factors [36]. Curiously, in our study we found decreased levels of FGF-23 in both VDD and VDD+IRI groups. According to Rodriguez-Ortiz et al [37], this decreased FGF-23 levels could act as a compensatory response to prevent further reductions in calcitriol levels, which could exacerbate the hypocalcemia already expected by the evolution of CKD. So, a plausible explanation for our results is that we evaluated FGF-23 levels in a very early development of renal disease, without loss of renal function. Moreover, we must consider the diet used in our study for feeding the VDD and VDD+IRI animals. Besides being totally depleted of vitamin D, the diet also presented low levels of calcium and phosphorus, which may have contributed for the low levels of FGF-23 found in VDD and IRI+VDD groups.

An important partnership between FGF-23 and Klotho has been described [17]. Klotho proteins form binary complexes with FGF receptors, increasing Klotho affinity and selectivity for FGF-23 [17]. During kidney disease progression, there is reduced

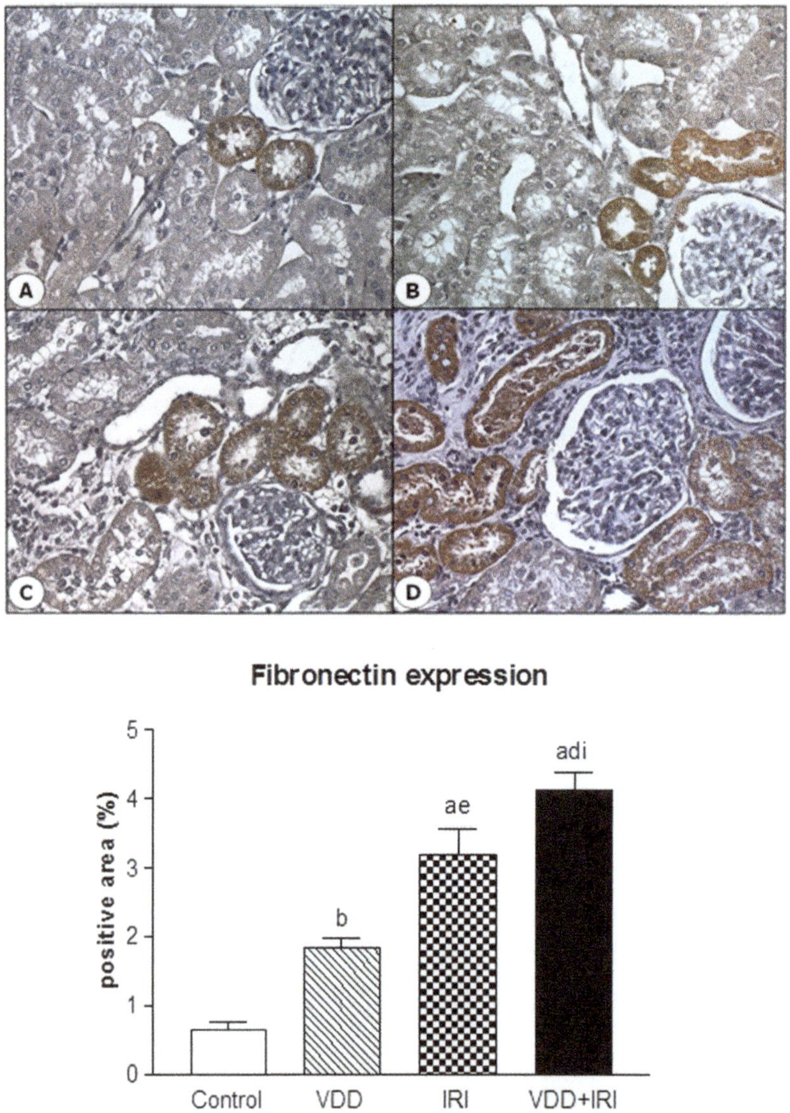

Figure 5. [I] Expression of fibronectin in the renal cortex of a control rat (A), a vitamin D deficient rat (B), in a rat submitted to ischemia/reperfusion injury (C), and in a vitamin D deficient rat submitted to ischemia/reperfusion injury (D). [II] Evaluation of fibronectin expression 90 days after in Control (C), Vitamin D Deficiency (VDD), Ischemia-Reperfusion Injury (IRI), and Vitamin D Deficiency and Ischemia/Reperfusion Injury (VDD+IRI) groups. Values are means ± SEM. [a] $p<0.001$ vs. C; [b] $p<0.01$ vs. C; [d] $p<0.001$ vs. VDD; [e] $p<0.01$ vs. VDD; [i] $p<0.05$ vs. IRI.

expression of Klotho [38], a finding also confirmed in our study. We found a significant reduction in Klotho expression in VDD, IRI and VDD+IRI groups when compared to Control group. In addition, our data showed that vitamin D alone reduced Klotho expression in VDD animals, followed by a similar profile of gene expression for α-klotho. It is described that renal ischemia/reperfusion injury is related to Klotho deficiency. Ming-Chang Hu *et al* [39], using a murine model, showed that ischemic AKI was able to induce an acute and transient state of Klotho deficiency with recovery levels after seven days of injury. Most important, epidemiological studies have shown that increased levels of FGF-23, PTH and low levels of $1,25(OH)_2D_3$ are features that precede hyperphosphatemia during progression to CKD. Moreover, such alterations in FGF-23, PTH and vitamin D levels is usually followed by a progressive decrease in secreted Klotho protein in urine of CKD patients [39].

It is known that the pathological syndrome of CKD frequently does not heal but becomes self-sustaining, stimulating further kidney injury, resulting in progression of CKD [40]. In our study, a very relevant result related to morphological changes was found mainly in the kidney of vitamin D-deficient rats. Although no changes in renal function have been noticed, we observed an enlargement of the tubulointerstitial compartment associated with histological alterations (fibrosis, tubular atrophy and dilatation, and inflammatory cell infiltrates). Further, we analyzed the expression of two fibrous ECM components (fibronectin and type IV collagen) and infiltrating ED1 cells. We observed increased renal expression of both ECM markers and ED1 positive cells in VDD, IRI and VDD+IRI groups. Moreover, vitamin D deficiency enhanced the respective expressions of fibronectin, type IV collagen and ED1 cells.

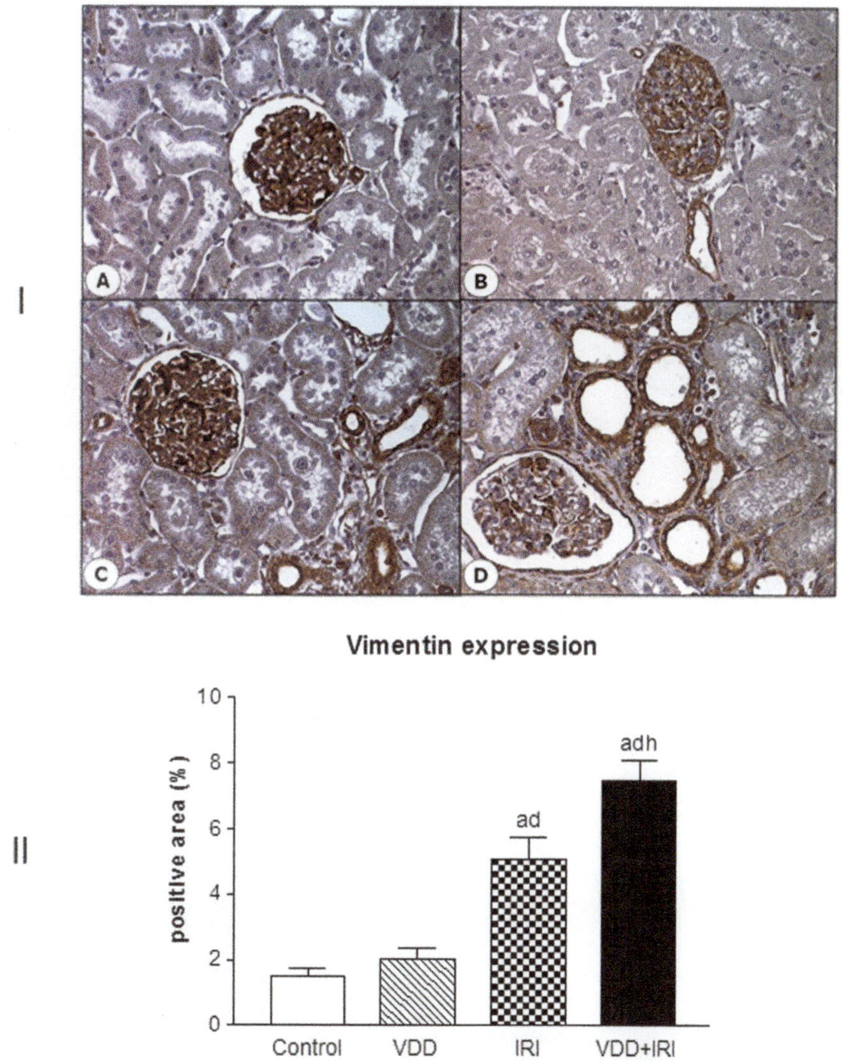

Figure 6. [I] Expression of vimentin in the renal cortex of a control rat (A), a vitamin D deficient rat (B), in a rat submitted to ischemia/reperfusion injury (C), and in a vitamin D deficient rat submitted to ischemia/reperfusion injury (D). [II] Evaluation of vimentin expression 90 days after in Control (C), Vitamin D Deficiency (VDD), Ischemia-Reperfusion Injury (IRI), and Vitamin D Deficiency and Ischemia/Reperfusion Injury (VDD+IRI) groups. Values are mean ± SEM. [a] $p<0.001$ vs. C; [d] $p<0.001$ vs. VDD; [h] $p<0.01$ vs. IRI.

Several studies have shown that the factors of initial injury to renal cell lead to: (a) vascular damage, including platelet aggregation and cytokine release; (b) activation of inflammatory responses with recruitment of neutrophils and monocytes, with subsequent pro-inflammatory cytokines releasing; and (c) fibrotic process, including pro-fibrogenic cytokine releasing such as TGF-β and CTGF (connective tissue growth factor) by macrophages and apoptotic parenchymal cells and activation of collagen-producing cells, among others [41]. These factors of initial injury can be initiated by many insults to the kidney, including toxic, ischemic, endocrine, infectious and immunological diseases [42]. In our case, we must consider two main conditions: endocrine and ischemia/reperfusion insult. As a matter of fact, our results showed morphological alterations associated with increased expression of fibrous ECM components and macrophages, including those observed in VDD group even without ischemic kidney injury. Regardless of the initial insult(s), CKD is characterized by stereotyped kidney injury responses seen pathologically as interstitial fibrosis, tubular atrophy, peritubular capillary rarefaction, inflammation and glomerulosclerosis [43]. Moreover, pathologic deposition of fibrillar collagenous matrix, i.e., fibrosis, results when tissues are damaged and normal wound-healing response persist or become dysregulated, usually in response to sustained or repetitive injury. Therefore, our results allow us to infer that our VDD, IRI and VDD+IRI groups were under hemodynamic and hormonal conditions that contributed to the morphological changes found in the renal tissues.

Attempting to establish a link between fibrosis formation and vitamin D deficiency, we evaluated the expressions of TGF-β and VDR in IRI and VDD+IRI groups, both with more prominent interstitial expansion. We observed that vitamin D deficiency caused a decrease in VDR expression and an increase in TGF-β expression in VDD+IRI group, which had the highest ratio of fibrosis. Thus, our data allowed us to infer that adequate levels of vitamin D could help to slow the renal fibrosis formation. In 2006 Tan × et al [44], using the vitamin D analogue paricalcitol in a model of obstructive nephropathy, showed that paricalcitol treatment was able to suppress the expressions of TGF-β and its

I

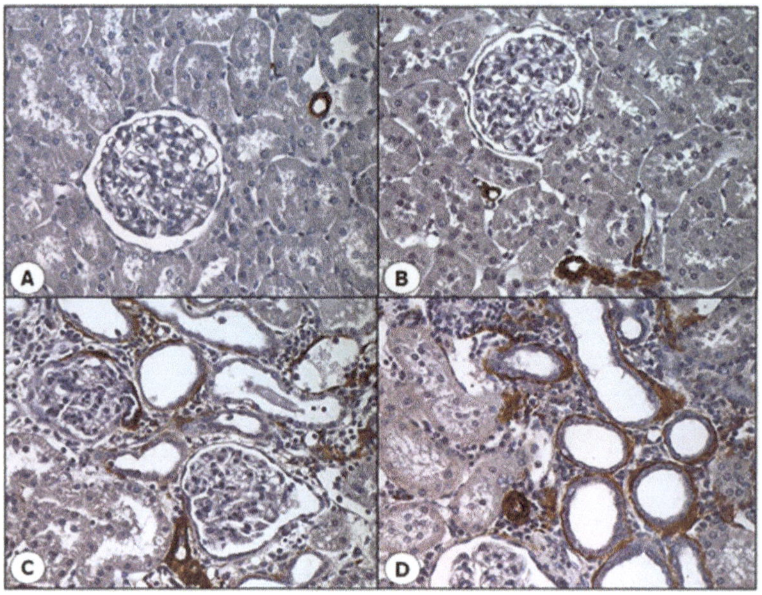

II

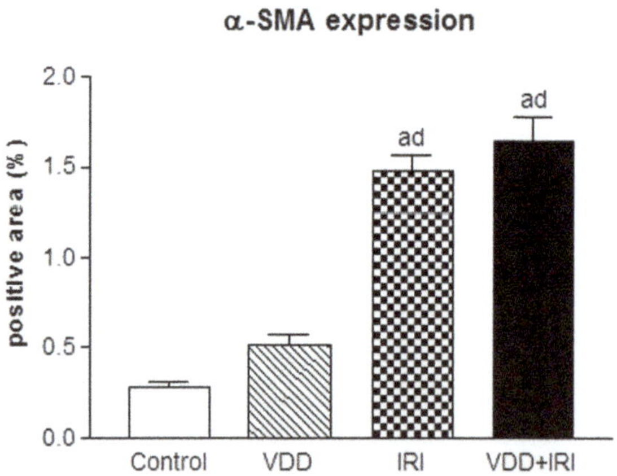

Figure 7. [I] Expression of α-SMA in the renal cortex of a control rat (A), a vitamin D deficient rat (B), in a rat submitted to ischemia/reperfusion injury (C), and in a vitamin D deficient rat submitted to ischemia/reperfusion injury (D). [II] Evaluation of α-SMA expression 90 days after in Control (C), Vitamin D Deficiency (VDD), Ischemia-Reperfusion Injury (IRI), and Vitamin D Deficiency and Ischemia/Reperfusion Injury (VDD+IRI) groups. Values are mean ± SEM. [a] $p<0.001$ vs. C; [d] $p<0.001$ vs. VDD.

respective receptor. In addition, paricalcitol treatment restored the expression of VDR receptor, blocked the epithelial-mesenchymal transition (EMT), and inhibited cell apoptosis and proliferation, showing that vitamin D plays a protective role on cellular integrity against cell injury process [44].

The relation of vitamin D to EMT process and our results concerning index of fibrosis in VDD+IRI group, aroused our interest to study whether renal tubule cells were under phenotypic modification. We observed a significant increase of vimentin expression in IRI and VDD+IRI groups and a similar profile of α-SMA expression, although without statistical difference. Based on that, we considered the involvement of vitamin D deficiency in cellular phenotypic alteration, since the animals from VDD+IRI groups presented more prominent expression of both markers. Xiong et al [45], showed that low expression of VDR in CKD could be a potential mechanism linking inflammation to EMT. It is known that pro-fibrotic effect of inflammation depends partly on EMT process. Such effect was possible by sustained stimulation with inflammatory cytokines (TNF-α or IL-1) on epithelial cells. According to the authors, TNF-α suppressed the expression of VDR in various cell types, and sensitized cells to EMT process induced by TGF-β [45]. In our study, we found reduced expression of VDR and increased expression of TGF-β in VDD+IRI group, supporting the idea that vitamin D deficiency is associated with tubulointerstitial damage and interstitial fibrosis. So, a possible mechanism for that would include an association with inflammatory pathways, suggesting a combination between decreased VDR expression with increased TGF-β1 expression in our animals subjected to ischemia/reperfusion injury.

Based on our data, we can conclude that vitamin D deficiency is an aggravating factor for tubulointerstitial damage and formation of interstitial fibrosis after ischemia/reperfusion injury.

Acknowledgments

The authors thank Dr. Luciene Machado dos Reis from LIM-16 – Nephrology Department for her assistance in preparing the FGF-23 experiments.

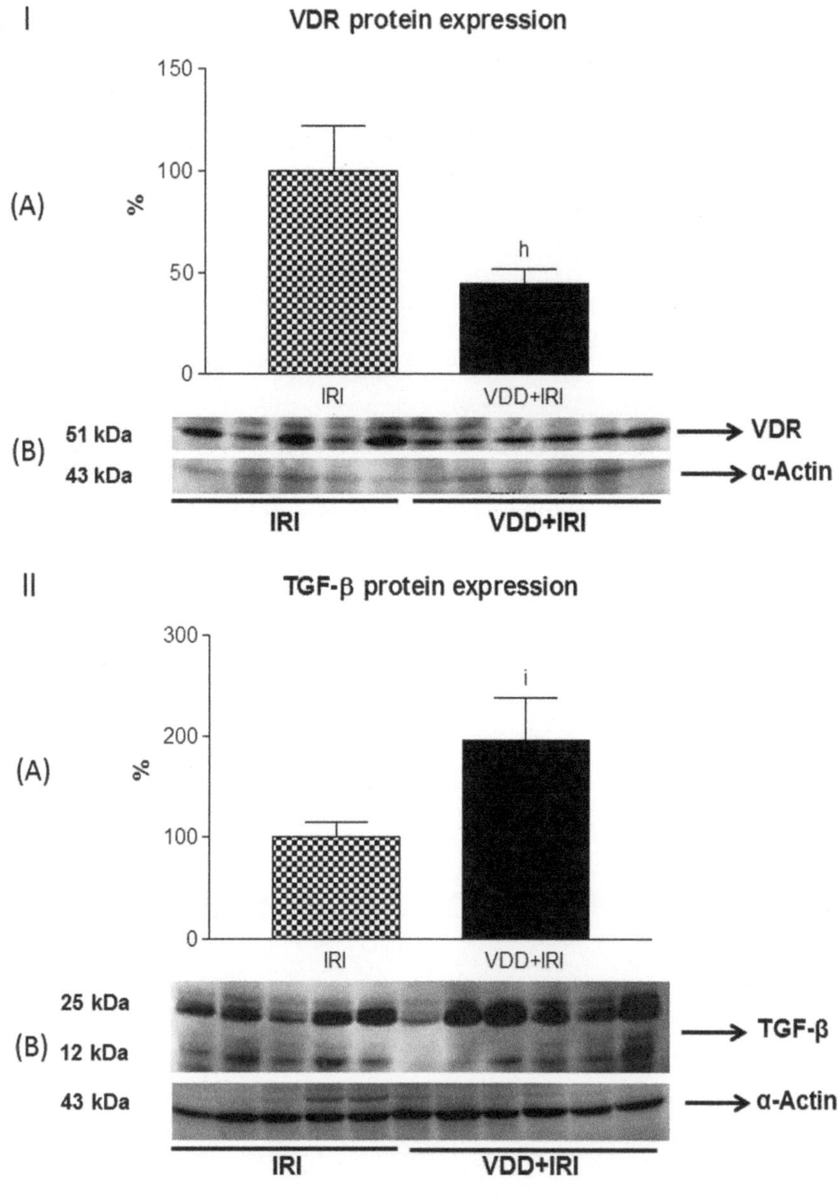

Figure 8. [I] Semiquantitative immunoblotting for VDR in kidney fractions. (A) A densitometric analysis of samples from IRI (n = 5) and VDD+IRI (n = 5) rats is shown. (B) Immunoblots reacted with anti-VDR revealing a 51-kDa band. Values are mean ± SEM. [h] $p<0.01$ vs. IRI. [II] Semiquantitative immunoblotting for TGF-β in kidney fractions. (A) A densitometric analysis of samples from IRI (n = 5) and VDD+IRI (n = 6) rats is shown. (B) Immunoblots reacted with anti-TGF-β revealing a 25 and 12-kDa bands. Values are mean ± SEM. [i] $p<0.05$ vs. IRI.

Author Contributions

Conceived and designed the experiments: RAV JGG ACS. Performed the experiments: JGG ACB DC MHMS TRS LA RAV. Analyzed the data: RAV JGG ACB LA RMAM TRS. Contributed reagents/materials/analysis tools: JGG ACB DC MHMS TRS RMAM LA ACS RAV. Contributed to the writing of the manuscript: RAV.

References

1. Francois H, Jacquet A, Beaudreuil S, Seidowsky A, Hebibi H, et al. (2011) Emerging strategies to preserve renal function. J Nephrol 24: 133–141.
2. Hagiwara S, Kantharidis P, Cooper ME (2012) What are new avenues for renal protection, in addition to RAAS inhibition? Curr Hypertens Rep 14: 100–110.
3. de Araujo M, Andrade L, Coimbra TM, Rodrigues AC, Jr., Seguro AC (2005) Magnesium supplementation combined with N-acetylcysteine protects against postischemic acute renal failure. J Am Soc Nephrol 16: 3339–3349.
4. Bonventre JV (2010) Pathophysiology of AKI: injury and normal and abnormal repair. Contrib Nephrol 165: 9–17.
5. Zhang Y, Kong J, Deb DK, Chang A, Li YC (2010) Vitamin D receptor attenuates renal fibrosis by suppressing the renin-angiotensin system. J Am Soc Nephrol 21: 966–973.
6. Patel TV, Singh AK (2009) Role of vitamin D in chronic kidney disease. Semin Nephrol 29: 113–121.
7. Baeke F, Gysemans C, Korf H, Mathieu C (2010) Vitamin D insufficiency: implications for the immune system. Pediatr Nephrol 25: 1597–1606.
8. Li YC (2011) Podocytes as target of vitamin D. Curr Diabetes Rev 7: 35–40.
9. Cuppari L, Garcia Lopes MG, Kamimura MA (2011) Vitamin D biology: from the discovery to its significance in chronic kidney disease. J Ren Nutr 21: 113–116.
10. Gonzalez EA, Sachdeva A, Oliver DA, Martin KJ (2004) Vitamin D insufficiency and deficiency in chronic kidney disease. A single center observational study. Am J Nephrol 24: 503–510.

11. Ulerich L (2010) Vitamin D in chronic kidney disease-new insights. Nephrol Nurs J 37: 429–431.
12. Holick MF (2007) Vitamin D deficiency. N Engl J Med 357: 266–281.
13. Braun AB, Christopher KB (2013) Vitamin D in acute kidney injury. Inflamm Allergy Drug Targets 12: 262–272.
14. Andress DL (2006) Vitamin D in chronic kidney disease: a systemic role for selective vitamin D receptor activation. Kidney Int 69: 33–43.
15. Perwad F, Azam N, Zhang MY, Yamashita T, Tenenhouse HS, et al. (2005) Dietary and serum phosphorus regulate fibroblast growth factor 23 expression and 1,25-dihydroxyvitamin D metabolism in mice. Endocrinology 146: 5358–5364.
16. Shimada T, Hasegawa H, Yamazaki Y, Muto T, Hino R, et al. (2004) FGF-23 is a potent regulator of vitamin D metabolism and phosphate homeostasis. J Bone Miner Res 19: 429–435.
17. Kuro-o M (2013) Klotho, phosphate and FGF-23 in ageing and disturbed mineral metabolism. Nat Rev Nephrol 9: 650–660.
18. Kuro-o M, Matsumura Y, Aizawa H, Kawaguchi H, Suga T, et al. (1997) Mutation of the mouse klotho gene leads to a syndrome resembling ageing. Nature 390: 45–51.
19. Burnette WN (1981) "Western blotting": electrophoretic transfer of proteins from sodium dodecyl sulfate-polyacrylamide gels to unmodified nitrocellulose and radiographic detection with antibody and radioiodinated protein A. Anal Biochem 112: 195–203.
20. Livak KJ, Schmittgen TD (2001) Analysis of relative gene expression data using real-time quantitative PCR and the 2(-Delta Delta C(T)) Method. Methods 25: 402–408.
21. Volpini RA, Costa RS, da Silva CG, Coimbra TM (2004) Inhibition of nuclear factor-kappaB activation attenuates tubulointerstitial nephritis induced by gentamicin. Nephron Physiol 98: p97–106.
22. Campos R, Shimizu MH, Volpini RA, de Braganca AC, Andrade L, et al. (2012) N-acetylcysteine prevents pulmonary edema and acute kidney injury in rats with sepsis submitted to mechanical ventilation. Am J Physiol Lung Cell Mol Physiol 302: L640–650.
23. Coimbra TM, Janssen U, Grone HJ, Ostendorf T, Kunter U, et al. (2000) Early events leading to renal injury in obese Zucker (fatty) rats with type II diabetes. Kidney Int 57: 167–182.
24. Powers JG, Gilchrest BA (2012) What you and your patients need to know about vitamin D. Semin Cutan Med Surg 31: 2–10.
25. Moe SM (2008) Disorders involving calcium, phosphorus, and magnesium. Prim Care 35: 215–237, v–vi.
26. Li YC (2003) Vitamin D regulation of the renin-angiotensin system. J Cell Biochem 88: 327–331.
27. Tamez H, Kalim S, Thadhani RI (2013) Does vitamin D modulate blood pressure? Curr Opin Nephrol Hypertens 22: 204–209.
28. Lucisano S, Buemi M, Passantino A, Aloisi C, Cernaro V, et al. (2013) New insights on the role of vitamin D in the progression of renal damage. Kidney Blood Press Res 37: 667–678.
29. Vaidya A, Williams JS (2012) The relationship between vitamin D and the renin-angiotensin system in the pathophysiology of hypertension, kidney disease, and diabetes. Metabolism 61: 450–458.
30. Li YC, Kong J, Wei M, Chen ZF, Liu SQ, et al. (2002) 1,25-Dihydroxyvitamin D(3) is a negative endocrine regulator of the renin-angiotensin system. J Clin Invest 110: 229–238.
31. de Boer IH, Ioannou GN, Kestenbaum B, Brunzell JD, Weiss NS (2007) 25-Hydroxyvitamin D levels and albuminuria in the Third National Health and Nutrition Examination Survey (NHANES III). Am J Kidney Dis 50: 69–77.
32. Lee DR, Kong JM, Cho KI, Chan L (2011) Impact of vitamin D on proteinuria, insulin resistance, and cardiovascular parameters in kidney transplant recipients. Transplant Proc 43: 3723–3729.
33. Kuhlmann A, Haas CS, Gross ML, Reulbach U, Holzinger M, et al. (2004) 1,25-Dihydroxyvitamin D3 decreases podocyte loss and podocyte hypertrophy in the subtotally nephrectomized rat. Am J Physiol Renal Physiol 286: F526–533.
34. Freundlich M, Quiroz Y, Zhang Z, Zhang Y, Bravo Y, et al. (2008) Suppression of renin-angiotensin gene expression in the kidney by paricalcitol. Kidney Int 74: 1394–1402.
35. Isakova T, Wolf MS (2010) FGF23 or PTH: which comes first in CKD? Kidney Int 78: 947–949.
36. Silver J, Naveh-Many T (2013) FGF-23 and secondary hyperparathyroidism in chronic kidney disease. Nat Rev Nephrol 9: 641–649.
37. Rodriguez-Ortiz ME, Lopez I, Munoz-Castaneda JR, Martinez-Moreno JM, Ramirez AP, et al. (2012) Calcium deficiency reduces circulating levels of FGF23. J Am Soc Nephrol 23: 1190–1197.
38. John GB, Cheng CY, Kuro-o M (2011) Role of Klotho in aging, phosphate metabolism, and CKD. Am J Kidney Dis 58: 127–134.
39. Hu MC, Shi M, Zhang J, Quinones H, Griffith C, et al. (2011) Klotho deficiency causes vascular calcification in chronic kidney disease. J Am Soc Nephrol 22: 124–136.
40. Campanholle G, Ligresti G, Gharib SA, Duffield JS (2013) Cellular mechanisms of tissue fibrosis. 3. Novel mechanisms of kidney fibrosis. Am J Physiol Cell Physiol 304: C591–603.
41. Kisseleva T, Brenner DA (2008) Mechanisms of fibrogenesis. Exp Biol Med (Maywood) 233: 109–122.
42. Snyder JJ, Foley RN, Collins AJ (2009) Prevalence of CKD in the United States: a sensitivity analysis using the National Health and Nutrition Examination Survey (NHANES) 1999–2004. Am J Kidney Dis 53: 218–228.
43. Grgic I, Duffield JS, Humphreys BD (2012) The origin of interstitial myofibroblasts in chronic kidney disease. Pediatr Nephrol 27: 183–193.
44. Tan X, Li Y, Liu Y (2006) Paricalcitol attenuates renal interstitial fibrosis in obstructive nephropathy. J Am Soc Nephrol 17: 3382–3393.
45. Xiong M, Gong J, Liu Y, Xiang R, Tan X (2012) Loss of vitamin D receptor in chronic kidney disease: a potential mechanism linking inflammation to epithelial-to-mesenchymal transition. Am J Physiol Renal Physiol 303: F1107–1115.

PERMISSIONS

 Every chapter published in this book has been scrutinized by our experts. Their significance has been extensively debated. The topics covered herein carry significant findings which will fuel the growth of the discipline. They may even be implemented as practical applications or may be referred to as a beginning point for another development.

The contributors of this book come from diverse backgrounds, making this book a truly international effort. This book will bring forth new frontiers with its revolutionizing research information and detailed analysis of the nascent developments around the world.

We would like to thank all the contributing authors for lending their expertise to make the book truly unique. They have played a crucial role in the development of this book. Without their invaluable contributions this book wouldn't have been possible. They have made vital efforts to compile up to date information on the varied aspects of this subject to make this book a valuable addition to the collection of many professionals and students.

This book was conceptualized with the vision of imparting up-to-date information and advanced data in this field. To ensure the same, a matchless editorial board was set up. Every individual on the board went through rigorous rounds of assessment to prove their worth. After which they invested a large part of their time researching and compiling the most relevant data for our readers.

The editorial board has been involved in producing this book since its inception. They have spent rigorous hours researching and exploring the diverse topics which have resulted in the successful publishing of this book. They have passed on their knowledge of decades through this book. To expedite this challenging task, the publisher supported the team at every step. A small team of assistant editors was also appointed to further simplify the editing procedure and attain best results for the readers.

Apart from the editorial board, the designing team has also invested a significant amount of their time in understanding the subject and creating the most relevant covers. They scrutinized every image to scout for the most suitable representation of the subject and create an appropriate cover for the book.

The publishing team has been an ardent support to the editorial, designing and production team. Their endless efforts to recruit the best for this project, has resulted in the accomplishment of this book. They are a veteran in the field of academics and their pool of knowledge is as vast as their experience in printing. Their expertise and guidance has proved useful at every step. Their uncompromising quality standards have made this book an exceptional effort. Their encouragement from time to time has been an inspiration for everyone.

The publisher and the editorial board hope that this book will prove to be a valuable piece of knowledge for researchers, students, practitioners and scholars across the globe.

LIST OF CONTRIBUTORS

Jonathan A. Lorch
Department of Medicine, Weill Cornell Medical College and The Rogosin Institute, New York, New York, United States of America

Victor E. Pollak
Department of Medicine, University of Colorado Health Sciences Center, Aurora, Colorado, United States of America
MIQS, Inc., Boulder, Colorado, United States of America

Tsung-Chieh Yao, Kuo-Wei Yeh and Jing-Long Huang
Division of Allergy, Asthma, and Rheumatology, Department of Pediatrics, Chang Gung Memorial Hospital and Chang Gung University College of Medicine, Taoyuan,
Taiwan Community Medicine Research Center, Chang Gung Memorial Hospital at Keelung, Keelung, Taiwan

Yu-Ling Tu
Division of Allergy, Asthma, and Rheumatology, Department of Pediatrics, Chang Gung Memorial Hospital and Chang Gung University College of Medicine, Taoyuan, Taiwan
Community Medicine Research Center, Chang Gung Memorial Hospital at Keelung, Keelung, Taiwan
Graduate Institute of Clinical Medical Sciences, Chang Gung University College of Medicine, Taoyuan, Taiwan

Su-Wei Chang
Clinical Informatics and Medical Statistics Research Center, Chang Gung University College of Medicine, Taoyuan, Taiwan

Hui-Ju Tsai
Division of Biostatistics and Bioinformatics, Institutes of Population Health Sciences, National Health Research Institutes, Miaoli, Taiwan
Department of Pediatrics, Feinberg School of Medicine, Northwestern University, Chicago, Illinois, United States of America
Department of Genome Medicine, Kaohsiung University, Kaohsiung, Taiwan

Po-Wen Gu and Hsian-Chen Ning
Department of Laboratory Medicine, Chang Gung Memorial Hospital, Taoyuan, Taiwan

Man-Chin Hua, Sui-Ling Liao, Ming-Han Tsai and Chih-Yung Chiu
Community Medicine Research Center, Chang Gung Memorial Hospital at Keelung, Keelung, Taiwan
Department of Pediatrics, Chang Gung Memorial Hospital at Keelung, Keelung, Taiwan

Shen-Hao Lai
Division of Pediatric Pulmonology, Department of Pediatrics, Chang Gung Memorial Hospital, Taoyuan, Taiwan

Martin J. Raftery
Department of Renal Medicine, Barts Health NHS Trust, London, United Kingdom

Gavin Dreyer and Muhammad M. Yaqoob
Department of Renal Medicine, Barts Health NHS Trust, London, United Kingdom
Department of Translational Medicine and Therapeutics, Queen Mary University of London, London, United Kingdom

Rupert M. Pearse
Department of Critical Care Medicine, Barts Health NHS Trust, London, United Kingdom

Steven M. Harwood3,
Department of Translational Medicine and Therapeutics, Queen Mary University of London, London, United Kingdom

Arthur T. Tucker
Ernest Cooke Microvascular Unit, Barts Health NHS Trust, London, United Kingdom

Sarah Hanieh
Department of Medicine, Melbourne Academic Centre, University of Melbourne at the Doherty Institute, Parkville, Victoria, Australia

Beverley-Ann Biggs
Department of Medicine, Melbourne Academic Centre, University of Melbourne at the Doherty Institute, Parkville, Victoria, Australia
The Victorian Infectious Diseases Service, Royal Melbourne Hospital, Parkville, Victoria, Australia

Tran T. Ha, Tran T. Thuy and Tran Tuan
Research and Training Centre for Community Development (RTCCD), Hanoi, Vietnam

Thach D. Tran
Research and Training Centre for Community Development (RTCCD), Hanoi, Vietnam
Provincial Centre of Preventive Medicine, Hanam, Hanam Province, Vietnam

Julie A. Simpson
Centre for Epidemiology and Biostatistics, Melbourne School of Population and Global Health, University of Melbourne, Parkville, Victoria, Australia

Nguyen C. Khuong and Dang D. Thoang
Provincial Centre of Preventive Medicine, Hanam, Hanam Province, Vietnam

Jane Fisher
The Jean Hailes Research Unit, School of Public Health and Preventive Medicine, Monash University, Clayton, Victoria, Australia
The Victorian Infectious Diseases Service, Royal Melbourne Hospital, Parkville, Victoria Australia

Marcia A. Luna-Leite
Carlos Chagas Filho Institute of Biophysics, Federal University of Rio de Janeiro, Rio de Janeiro, Brazil

Paulo A. Silva, Gustavo Monnerat-Cahli, Amaury Pereira-Acácio, Ricardo Luzardo, Marcelo Einicker-Lamas, Luzia S. Sampaio, Emiliano Medei and Adalberto Vieyra
Carlos Chagas Filho Institute of Biophysics, Federal University of Rio de Janeiro, Rio de Janeiro, Brazil
National Institute of Science and Technology for Structural Biology and Bioimaging, Rio de Janeiro, Brazil

Lucienne S. Lara, Rogério Panizzutti and Caroline Madeira
National Institute of Science and Technology for Structural Biology and Bioimaging, Rio de Janeiro, Brazil
Institute of Biomedical Sciences, Federal University of Rio de Janeiro, Rio de Janeiro, Brazil

Leucio D. Vieira-Filho, Carmen Castro-Chaves, Valdilene S. Ribeiro and Ana D. O. Paixão
National Institute of Science and Technology for Structural Biology and Bioimaging, Rio de Janeiro, Brazil
Department of Physiology and Pharmacology, Federal University of Pernambuco, Recife, Brazil

Bo L. Chawes, Klaus Bønnelykke, Pia F. Jensen, Ann-Marie M. Schoos and Hans Bisgaard
Copenhagen Prospective Studies on Asthma in Childhood, Health Sciences, University of Copenhagen, Danish Pediatric Asthma Center, Copenhagen University Hospital, Gentofte, Denmark

Lene Heickendorff
Department of Clinical Biochemistry, Aarhus University Hospital, Aarhus, Denmark

Pei Li, Xiaoyong Xu, Ehong Cao, Xin Su and Yi Shi
Department of Respiratory and Critical Care Medicine, Jinling Hospital, Nanjing University School of Medicine, Nanjing Jiangsu Province, People's Republic of China

Bo Yu and Wanchun Li
Department of Pathology, Jinling Hospital, Nanjing University School of Medicine, Nanjing Jiangsu Province, People's Republic of China

Ming Fan and Mei Huang
Department of Clinical Microbiology, Jinling Hospital, Nanjing University School of Medicine, Nanjing Jiangsu Province, People's Republic of China

Lining Shi and Rong Zeng
Department of Clinical Laboratory, Jinling Hospital, Nanjing University School of Medicine, Nanjing Jiangsu Province, People's Republic of China

Benjamin Udoka Nwosu
Division of Endocrinology, Department of Pediatrics, University of Massachusetts Medical School, Worcester, Massachusetts, United States of America

Louise Maranda
Department of Quantitative Health Sciences, University of Massachusetts Medical School, Worcester, Massachusetts, United States of America

Felix Maurer
Dept. Biosciences-Plant Biology, Saarland University, Saarbrücken, Germany

Maria Augusta Naranjo Arcos and Petra Bauer
Dept. Biosciences-Plant Biology, Saarland University, Saarbrücken, Germany
Institute of Botany and Cluster of Excellence on Plant Sciences (CEPLAS), Heinrich Heine University, Düsseldorf, Germany

Maija E. Miettinen and Leena Kinnunen
Diabetes Prevention Unit, National Institute for Health and Welfare, Helsinki, Finland

Jaana Leiviskä
Disease Risk Unit, National Institute for Health and Welfare, Helsinki, Finland

Sirkka Keinänen-Kiukaanniemi
Institute of Health Sciences, University of Oulu, Oulu, Finland, 4 Unit of Primary Health Care, Oulu University Hospital, Oulu, Finland

Eeva Korpi-Hyövälti
Department of Internal Medicine, South Ostrobothnia Central Hospital, Seinäjoki, Finland

Leo Niskanen
Finnish Medicines Agency, Helsinki, Finland
Faculty of Health Sciences, University of Eastern Finland, Kuopio, Finland

Mauno Vanhala
Faculty of Health Sciences, University of Eastern Finland, Kuopio, Finland
Primary Health Care Unit, Central Finland Central Hospital, Jyväskylä, Finland

Heikki Oksa
Tampere University Hospital, Tampere, Finland

Timo Saaristo
Pirkanmaa Hospital District, Tampere, Finland
Finnish Diabetes Association, Tampere, Finland

Jaakko Tuomilehto
Diabetes Prevention Unit, National Institute for Health and Welfare, Helsinki, Finland
Department of Internal Medicine, South Ostrobothnia Central Hospital, Seinäjoki, Finland
Center for Vascular Prevention, Danube-University Krems, Krems, Austria King Abdulaziz University, Jeddah, Saudi Arabia

Matti Uusitupa
Institute of Public Health and Clinical Nutrition, University of Eastern Finland, Kuopio, Finland
Research Unit, Kuopio University Hospital, Kuopio, Finland

Markku Peltonen
Department of Chronic Disease Prevention, National Institute for Health and Welfare, Helsinki, Finland

Nora Adriana Hernández-Cuevas, Christian Weber, Chung-Chau Hon and Nancy Guillen
Institut Pasteur, Unité Biologie Cellulaire du Parasitisme, Paris, France
INSERM U786, Paris, France

Ching-Hui Huang
Division of Cardiology, Department of Internal Medicine, Changhua Christian Hospital, Changhua, Taiwan
Department of Biological Science and Technology, National Chiao Tung University, Hsinchu, Taiwan

Tzai-Wen Chiu and Chih-Sheng Lin
Department of Biological Science and Technology, National Chiao Tung University, Hsinchu, Taiwan

Chia-Chu Chang
Division of Nephrology, Department of Internal Medicine, Changhua Christian Hospital, Changhua, Taiwan
School of Medicine, Chung Shan Medical University, Taichung, Taiwan

Chen-Ling Kuo Ching-Shan Huang
Vascular and Genomic Research Center, Changhua Christian Hospital, Changhua, Taiwan

Chin-San Liu
Vascular and Genomic Research Center, Changhua Christian Hospital, Changhua, Taiwan
Department of Neurology, Changhua Christian Hospital, Changhua, Taiwan Graduate Institute of Integrative Medicine, China Medical University, Taichung, Taiwan

Sara Balesaria, Vernon Skinner and Surjit K. S. Srai
Research Department of Structural and Molecular Biology, Division of Biosciences, University College London, London, United Kingdom

Marija Lesjak
Research Department of Structural and Molecular Biology, Division of Biosciences, University College London, London, United Kingdom
Department of Chemistry, Biochemistry and Environmental Protection, Faculty of Sciences University of Novi Sad, Novi Sad, Serbia

Rukshana Hoque and Paul A. Sharp
Diabetes & Nutritional Sciences Division, King's College London, London, United Kingdom

Edward S. Debnam
Research Department of Neuroscience, Physiology and Pharmacology, Division of Biosciences, University College London, Royal Free Campus, London, United Kingdom

Holger Schmidt, Carmen Günther and Michael Weber
Department of Plant Physiology, University of Bayreuth, Bayreuth, Germany

Stephan Clemens
Department of Plant Physiology, University of Bayreuth, Bayreuth, Germany
Bayreuth Center for Molecular Biosciences, University of Bayreuth, Bayreuth, Germany

Cornelia Spörlein and Sebastian Loscher
Department of Organic Chemistry, University of Bayreuth, Bayreuth, Germany

Christoph Böttcher
Department of Stress and Developmental Biology, Leibniz Institute of Plant Biochemistry, Halle/Saale, Germany

Rainer Schobert
Department of Organic Chemistry, University of Bayreuth, Bayreuth, Germany
Bayreuth Center for Molecular Biosciences, University of Bayreuth, Bayreuth, Germany

Daniele Canale, Ana Carolina de Bragança, Janaína Garcia Gonçalves, Maria Heloisa Massola Shimizu, Talita Rojas Sanches, Lúcia Andrade, Rildo Aparecido Volpini and Antonio Carlos Seguro
Nephrology Department, University of São Paulo School of Medicine, São Paulo, Brazil

Kimberly B. Zumbrennen-Bullough
Program in Anemia Signaling Research, Division of Nephrology, Program in Membrane Biology, Center for Systems Biology, Massachusetts General Hospital, Harvard Medical School, Boston, Massachusetts, United States of America

Lore Becker, Helmut Fuchs and Valerie Gailus-Durner
German Mouse Clinic, Helmholtz-Zentrum München, German Research Center for Environmental Health, Neuherberg, Germany
Institute of Experimental Genetics, Helmholtz-Zentrum München, German Research Center for Environmental Health, Neuherberg, Germany

Lillian Garrett and Sabine M. Hölter
German Mouse Clinic, Helmholtz-Zentrum München, German Research Center for Environmental Health, Neuherberg, Germany
Institute of Development Genetics, Helmholtz-Zentrum München, German Research Center for Environmental Health, Neuherberg, Germany

Julia Calzada-Wack, Ilona Mossbrugger and Leticia Quintanilla-Fend
German Mouse Clinic, Helmholtz-Zentrum München, German Research Center for Environmental Health, Neuherberg, Germany
Institute of Pathology, Helmholtz-Zentrum München, German Research Center for Environmental Health, Neuherberg, Germany

Ildiko Racz
German Mouse Clinic, Helmholtz-Zentrum München, German Research Center for Environmental Health, Neuherberg, Germany
Institute of Molecular Psychiatry, Life & Brain Center, University of Bonn, Bonn, Germany

Birgit Rathkolb
German Mouse Clinic, Helmholtz-Zentrum München, German Research Center for EnvironmentalHealth, Neuherberg, Germany
Institute of Molecular Animal Breeding and Biotechnology, Gene Center, Ludwig-Maximilians-Universitat, Munich, Germany

Andreas Zimmer
Institute of Molecular Psychiatry, Life & Brain Center, University of Bonn, Bonn, Germany

Eckhard Wolf
Institute of Molecular Animal Breeding and Biotechnology, Gene Center, Ludwig-Maximilians-Universitat, Munich, Germany

Thomas Klopstock8,13,14,
Department of Neurology, Friedrich-Baur-Institute, Klinikum der Ludwig-Maximilians-Universitat, Munich, Germany Deutsches
Zentrum für Neurodegenerative Erkrankungen, Munich, Germany
Munich Cluster for Systems Neurology, Munich, Germany

Wolfgang Wurst
Institute of Development Genetics, Helmholtz-Zentrum München, German Research Center for Environmental Health, Neuherberg, Germany
Chair of Developmental Genetics, Technische Universitat München, Freising-Weihenstephan, Germany
Max Planck Institute of Psychiatry, Munich, Germany
Deutsches Zentrum für Neurodegenerative Erkrankungen, Munich, Germany
Munich Cluster for Systems Neurology, Munich, Germany

Martin Hrabĕde Angelis
German Mouse Clinic, Helmholtz-Zentrum München, German Research Center for Environmental Health, Neuherberg, Germany
Institute of Experimental Genetics, Helmholtz-Zentrum München, German Research Center for Environmental Health, Neuherberg, Germany
Chair of Experimental Genetics, Center of Life and Food Sciences Weihenstephan, Technische Universitat München, Freising, Germany
German Center for Diabetes Research, Neuherberg, Germany

Steven J. Romney and Elizabeth A. Leibold
University of Utah, Department of Medicine, Division of Hematology and Hematological Malignancies, Salt Lake City, Utah, United States of America

Sujan Mamidi, Rian K. Lee and Phillip E. McClean
Genomics and Bioinformatics Program, North Dakota State University, Fargo, North Dakota, United States of America
Department of Plant Sciences, North Dakota State University, Fargo, North Dakota, United States of America

Jay R. Goos
Department of Soil Science, North Dakota State University, Fargo, North Dakota, United States of America

Fiona Noronha and Kazem Behbehani
Department of Biostatistics & Epidemiology, Dasman Diabetes Institute, Kuwait City, Kuwait

Naser Elkum
Department of Biostatistics & Epidemiology, Dasman Diabetes Institute, Kuwait City, Kuwait
Clinical Epidemiology, Sidra Medical and Research Centre, Doha, Qatar

Fadi Alkayal, Maisa M. Ali, Motasem Melhem and Osama Alsmadi
Genetics & Genomics Unit, Dasman Diabetes Institute, Kuwait City, Kuwait

Jehad Abubaker
Biochemistry & Molecular Biology Unit, Dasman Diabetes Institute, Kuwait City, Kuwait

Monira Al-Arouj and Abdullah Bennakhi
Clinical Services, Dasman Diabetes Institute, Kuwait City, Kuwait

Sanjana Dayal, Melissa Jensen, Jeff W. Stevens and Steven R. Lentz
Department of Internal Medicine, University of Iowa Carver College of Medicine, Iowa City, Iowa, United States of America

Ilya O. Blokhin
Department of Internal Medicine, University of Iowa Carver College of Medicine, Iowa City, Iowa, United States of America
Interdisciplinary Graduate Program in Molecular and Cellular Biology, University of Iowa Carver College of Medicine, Iowa City, Iowa, United States of America

Rochelle A. Erger
Department of Internal Medicine, University of Iowa Carver College of Medicine, Iowa City, Iowa, United States of America
Veterans Affairs Medical Center, Iowa City, Iowa, United States of America

Frank M. Faraci
Department of Internal Medicine, University of Iowa Carver College of Medicine, Iowa City, Iowa, United States of America
Department of Pharmacology, University of Iowa Carver College of Medicine, Iowa City, Iowa, United States of America
Francois M. Abboud Cardiovascular Center, University of Iowa Carver College of Medicine, Iowa City, Iowa, United States of America

Erland Arning and Teodoro Bottiglieri
Baylor Institute of Metabolic Disease, Dallas, Texas, United States of America

Shaonong Dang, Hong Yan, Lingxia Zeng, Quanli Wang, Qiang Li, Shengbin Xiao and Xiaojing Fan
Department of Epidemiology and Health Statistics, School of Public Health, Xían Jiaotong University Health Science Center, Xían, Shaanxi, People's Republic of China

Janaína Garcia Gonc¸alves, Ana Carolina de Braganc¸a, Daniele Canale, Maria Heloisa Massola Shimizu, Talita Rojas Sanches, Rosa Maria Affonso Moysés, Lúcia Andrade, Antonio Carlos Seguro, Rildo Aparecido Volpini
Nephrology Department, University of São Paulo School of Medicine, São Paulo, Brazil

Index